A HISTORY OF INTELLIGEN[CE]
AND "INTELLECTUAL DISAB[ILITY]"

Starting with the hypothesis that not only human intelligence but also its antithesis "intellectual disability" are nothing more than historical contingencies, C.F. Goodey's paradigm-shifting study traces the rich interplay between labelled human types and the radically changing characteristics attributed to them. From the twelfth-century beginnings of European social administration to the onset of formal human science disciplines in the modern era, *A History of Intelligence and "Intellectual Disability"* reconstructs the socio-political and religious contexts of intellectual ability and disability, and demonstrates how these concepts became part of psychology, medicine and biology. Goodey examines a wide array of classical, late medieval and Renaissance texts, from popular guides on conduct and behavior to medical treatises and from religious and philosophical works to poetry and drama. Focusing especially on the period between the Protestant Reformation and 1700, Goodey challenges the accepted wisdom that would have us believe that "intelligence" and "disability" describe natural, trans-historical realities. Instead, Goodey argues for a model that views intellectual disability and indeed the intellectually disabled person as recent cultural creations. His book is destined to become a standard resource for scholars interested in the history of psychology and medicine, the social origins of human self-representation, and current ethical debates about the genetics of intelligence.

C.F. Goodey has researched and published on the history of "intellectual disability," including the ethical and social implications of the concept, for more than 20 years. His articles have appeared in a number of scholarly journals, including *History of Science*, *Medical History*, *History of the Human Sciences*, *Political Theory* and *Ancient Philosophy*. He formerly held teaching and research posts at Ruskin College, Oxford, the Open University and the University of London Institute of Education, and is currently an independent consultant working for national and local government services on learning disability in the UK.

A History of Intelligence and "Intellectual Disability"
The Shaping of Psychology in Early Modern Europe

C.F. GOODEY

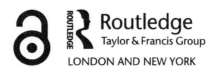

LONDON AND NEW YORK

First published in paperback 2024

First published 2011 by Ashgate Publishing

Published 2016 by Routledge
4 Park Square, Milton Park, Abingdon, Oxon OX14 4RN

and by Routledge
605 Third Avenue, New York, NY 10158

Routledge is an imprint of the Taylor & Francis Group, an informa business

Copyright © C.F. Goodey 2011, 2016, 2024

The right of C.F. Goodey to be identified as author of this work has been asserted in accordance with sections 77 and 78 of the Copyright, Designs and Patents Act 1988.

The Open Access version of this book, available at www.taylorfrancis.com, has been made available under a Creative Commons Attribution-Non Commercial-No Derivatives 4.0 license.

Trademark notice: Product or corporate names may be trademarks or registered trademarks, and are used only for identification and explanation without intent to infringe.

Publisher's Note
The publisher has gone to great lengths to ensure the quality of this reprint but points out that some imperfections in the original copies may be apparent.

British Library Cataloguing in Publication Data
Goodey, C.F.
A conceptual history of intelligence and "intellectual disability": the shaping of psychology in early modern Europe.
   1. Intellect. 2. Intellect – Social aspects. 3. Intellect – Religious aspects. 4. Intellect – Early works to 1800.
5. Mental retardation. 6. Mental retardation – Social aspects. 7. Mental retardation – Religious aspects.
8. Mental retardation – Early works to 1800. 9. Stereotypes (Social psychology) – Europe – History.
10. Psychology – Europe – History.
   I. Title
   153.9'09–dc22

Library of Congress Cataloging-in-Publication Data
Goodey, C.F.
A history of intelligence and "intellectual disability": the shaping of psychology in early modern Europe / C.F. Goodey.
   p. cm.
   Includes bibliographical references and index.
   1. Thought and thinking—Europe—History. 2. Intellect—Europe—History. 3. Psychology—Europe—History. I. Title.
BF441.G656 2011
153.909—dc22

2011001042

ISBN: 978-1-4094-2021-7 (hbk)
ISBN: 978-1-03-292069-6 (pbk)
ISBN: 978-1-315-56483-8 (ebk)

DOI: 10.4324/9781315564838

Contents

Acknowledgements		*vii*
Introduction		1
Part 1	**Problematical Intellects in Ancient Greece**	
1	Ancient Philosophy and the "Worst Disability"	15
2	Aristotle and the Slave's Intellect	25
Part 2	**Intelligence and Disability: Socio-economic Structures**	
3	The Speed of Intelligence: Fast, Slow and Mean	39
4	Quick Wit and the Ingenious Gentleman	49
Part 3	**Intelligence and Disability: Status and Power**	
5	In-group, Out-group: the Place of Intelligence in Anthropology	63
6	Honour, Grace and Intelligence: the Historical Interplay	77
7	"Souls Drowned in a Lump of Flesh": the Excluded	93
Part 4	**Intelligence, Disability and Honour**	
8	Virtue, Blood, Wit: from Lineage to Learning	103
9	"Dead in the Very Midst of Life": the Dishonourable and the Idiotic	125
Part 5	**Intelligence, Disability and Grace**	
10	From Pilgrim's Progress to Developmental Psychology	151
11	The Science of Damnation: from Reprobate to Idiot	179
Part 6	**Fools and Their Medical Histories**	
12	The Long Historical Context of Cognitive Genetics	207
13	The Brain of a Fool	219
14	A First Diagnosis? The Problem with Pioneers	235
Part 7	**Psychology, Biology and the Ethics of Exceptionalism**	
15	Philosophy, the Devil and "Special People"	253
16	The Wrong Child: Changelings and the Bereavement Analogy	261
17	Testing the Rule of Human Nature: Classification and Abnormality	281
Part 8	**John Locke and His Successors**	
18	John Locke and His Successors: the Historical Contingency of Disability	313
Works Cited		*347*
Index		*369*

Acknowledgements

This book would not have been possible without all those people and their families who, by swapping experiences and ideas with me in the course of applied research and practice, have encouraged my belief in the practical applicability of history. Direct support came from Priscilla Alderson, Istvan Hont, Linda Jordan, Patrick McDonagh, the late Roy Porter, Lynn Rose, Roger Smith, Richard Sorabji and Tim Stainton. I would like to thank the many others who have contributed along the way: students, friends, colleagues and those in the medical and psychological professions who have discussed these topics openly and without fear. The Leverhulme Trust financed the first stages of research. Parts of the book exist in more primitive form in articles written for various journals to whose editors and referees I am also indebted (details are in the list of Works Cited).

Historians should know that freaks, if tolerated – and even flattered and fed – can show astonishing influence and longevity. After all, to any rational mind, the greater part of the history of ideas is a history of freaks.

—E.P. Thompson, *The Poverty of Theory*

Introduction

Intelligence stands at the core of modern lives. It marks us out from the rest of nature. It is crucial to our sense of self and an instant yardstick for sizing up others. Psychologists measure it, biologists search for its DNA, women demand it of sperm donors; learned professors from Harvard to Heidelberg foresee our descendants turning into transhuman, bodiless intelligences able to migrate as software to other planets. If these are the dreams of intelligence, the nightmare is its absence. This means being denied family, friends and ordinary relationships; doctors give us treatment without our consent and withhold it when we need it; social workers stop us having sex, sterilize us or take away our children; psychiatrists lock us up without right of appeal; police officers frame us; courts acquit the parents who kill us; and politicians fund geneticists to make sure people like us never turn up again. Both dream and nightmare are so vivid it seems they must be based on some hard scientific reality, but the question "What is intelligence?" has only ever been answered by a shifting social consensus. So perhaps, like the stuff of dreams and nightmares, it too belongs in a realm of mere appearances. But in that case so does intellectual disability. Indeed, our anxieties about it may one day seem as strange as some of our ancestors' anxieties do to us. The pioneers of modern science such as Robert Boyle and Isaac Newton were certain that the devil was real, as real as this chair I am sitting on is to me; and while we now know he was a mere figment of their imaginations, this is no guarantee that some of the objects to which we apply our own, twenty-first-century scientific method are not just as fantastical.

Nevertheless, even if intelligence is only a matter of appearances, appearances matter. Social structures have not only flattered and fed the concept but set it to work to ensure their own survival. It is socially active, helping to bind social structures together, to alienate their human creators from themselves and from each other, and to dull our brains with alternating doses of self-flattery and self-abasement. It also identifies certain people we do not like having around, and only if intellectual disability is also seen as mere appearance can the speciousness of intelligence itself be exposed. The concepts of intelligence and intellectual disability are mutually reinforcing. While this book chiefly explores pre- and early modern concepts of disability, it is also about intelligence. Without each other they are nothing.

We tend to assume that "intellectual disability" is a permanent historical fixture, that all societies would have recognized the same thing in the same human type. But the idea of an intelligence that defines membership of the human species is itself modern. And if we sent people we now call intellectually disabled in a time machine to ancient Greece and asked if they resembled the people in that society with some seemingly equivalent label ("fools," etc.), the answer would be no, even though such an experiment would yield a positive result for physical disability and in part for mental illness. Of course there are always people around who seem unable to grasp certain complex everyday activities. What changes, though, is the content of those activities and their centrality to the life which the rest of us in any one era expect to lead. At any given historical moment, the people thus excluded seem to be a separate and permanent natural kind, but in fact their psychological profile alters radically in the long term along with the social context feeding it.

All this may seem to reflect a current propensity to turn differences previously thought of as natural into identities (ethnic, gendered, sexually oriented, etc.) that have been socially constructed by human beings themselves. And yes, it is certainly true that people may be "intellectually" disabled in one social institution or context but not necessarily disabled in some other, concurrent one. It is true, too, that labelling and separation from ordinary life may be causes of disability rather than outcomes; a person's identity, who they are or might be, is stolen from them in infancy or at diagnosis and is then refashioned by the special institutions in which they are segregated and which turn their personal characteristics into a "psychological object." Nevertheless, to say that intellectual disability is a mere social construction is to ignore problems of everyday life which, even if they are only the creation of a particular society, are for certain people and for the time being real enough, or oblige us to behave as if they were; some of us will need greater support to lead the ordinary lives that others take for granted (even if the various professions and services are institutionally primed to avoid, at all costs, the provision of support for just such a purpose). Disability is always *historically* constructed, however, because the problems change from one era to the next. History is anthropology with time rather than place the variable.

My starting hypothesis, therefore, is that intelligence and intellectual disability, likewise intelligent people and intellectually disabled people, are not natural kinds but historically contingent forms of human self-representation and social reciprocity, of relatively recent historical origin. Following this introduction, Part 1 discusses the relationship between psychological and social inferiority among the ancient Greeks. This is a necessary exercise because early modern writers use Plato, Aristotle and others as a reference point and modern psychology often identifies them as the first primitive stabs at a psychological science, when in fact the gulf between the Greeks and ourselves is profound. Part 2 analyzes the history of intelligence and disability in European socio-economic and administrative structures, and the ever-increasing importance attached to speed of thought. Parts 3 to 5 look at the conduct manuals and the religious and literary texts that present intelligence ("wit") as a self-referential mode of bidding for status, classifiable with concepts such as honour and grace, and juxtaposes these with their corresponding concepts of disability. Part 6 pursues the same themes into the history of medicine, looking at doctors' changing descriptions of problematic intellectual states and of their relationship to the structure and functions of body and brain. Part 7 examines the historical roots of the modern doctrinal fusion between biology, psychology and ethics, and at the early modern invention of abnormality, its place in natural history and accompanying doctrines of cause. Part 8 describes the influence of the sixteenth and early seventeenth centuries on Locke's extensive comments on "idiots" and "changelings," and how his essentially theological doctrine in turn influenced eighteenth-century theories of behaviour and thence modern educational and cultural practices.

Each chapter begins by looking at long-term, cross-historical elements which modern and pre-modern concepts may share in spite of my starting hypothesis, and then briefly at relevant aspects of the recent, short-term history of the formal disciplines (psychology, medicine, etc.): briefly, because there is already a substantial literature on this. There then follows the main business, which is the medium term: the shaping of modern psychological concepts of intelligence and disability, starting in the late Middle Ages but concentrated in the "early modern" period that runs from the Reformation to the Enlightenment. It can be used as a starting point for further investigation into other areas of early modern psychology. I regret not having had the time to extend this investigation beyond intelligence and intellectual disability to other basic psychological concepts of the early modern era: the emotions, for example, or the will (and the first question would be whether in fact such conceptual categories were then or indeed can now be safely distinguished from each other). Others will have to have to take up where I have left off.

Research and debate: opening a new arena

Previous writers have examined the history of the segregated long-stay institutions, hospitals and schools that have legitimized social rejection and distaste, plus something of the lives of people incarcerated there.¹ Yet about the origins of the underlying concepts we know little. Institutional records and official publications are easily located, whereas the conceptual roots are spread across disciplines and periods and so are harder to find. But similar problems have not deterred researchers in the early conceptual history of other disciplines. This research gap reflects social segregation itself: out of sight, out of mind. Moreover, to research the origins of a concept is to admit it had origins in the first place. If a category so basic had a historical starting point, it might imply that there was a time before that when it went unrecognized, and therefore that it could lose its currency again in the future. Unstable categories undermine professional confidence. As a result the history has been trivialized, in two ways. First, the disability as we see it today must have always existed, whether people in the past recognized it or not; historical study is irrelevant or unproblematic ("positivism"). Secondly, if the aim is to make things better, then pulling basic concepts up by the roots for historical investigation won't help; history must be seen instead as a march of progress, towards the triumph of current ideas and the right way of doing things, which just so happens to be our own ("presentism").

What we know about the history of the concept so far has come piecemeal from the extra-curricular interests of a few professionals with varying approaches. The first of these says that since disability is a natural, biological-psychological entity that has always existed in the same type of person, we can unproblematically match current human types to those of the past. Physiologist Paul Cranefield sees certain Renaissance medical writers as the "discoverers" of "mental deficiency" because they seem to describe its symptoms and to use a modern disease model.² Neurologist Richard Neugebauer sees in early accounts of legal competence a proto-modern psychiatric distinction between "mentally retarded" and mentally ill.³ Psychologist Richard Scheerenberger, aiming at an encyclopaedic history of mental retardation and sometimes coming across periods in which no seeming correspondences with the modern concept appear, simply plugs these gaps with primary sources on physical disability or mental illness instead.⁴ A second approach says that the scientific concept becomes actual only with its psychiatric description in modern times. Psychiatrist Leo Kanner, for example, one of the inventors of autism, largely follows the same disease model as the first group but excludes from his history all the unscientific primitives who lacked a modern expertise; consequently, he says, a history of mental retardation is impossible before the nineteenth century.⁵ A third approach is based on a seemingly more sceptical view. Psychologist Inge Mans, for example, begins with the words "Once upon a time there were no mentally retarded people." Like the literary historian Sandra Billington, she puts their early history under a broader heading encompassing professional fools and carnivalesque jesters.⁶ Nevertheless, ignoring the difference among these types means somehow preserving certain assumptions about a cross-historical condition; "retarded" people may well have existed all along, it is just that there

---

[1] James Trent, *Inventing the Feeble Mind*; Philip Ferguson, *Abandoned to their Fate*; Mathew Thomson, *The Problem of Mental Deficiency*; David Wright, *Mental Disability in Victorian England*; Mark Jackson, *The Borderland of Imbecility*; Trent and Steven Noll (eds), *Mental Retardation in America*.

[2] Paul Cranefield, "A seventeenth-century view of mental deficiency," *Bulletin of the History of Medicine*, 35 (1961); Cranefield and Walter Federn, "Paracelsus on goiter and cretinism," ibid., 37 (1963); "The begetting of fools," ibid., 41 (1967); Cranefield, "The discovery of cretinism," ibid., 36 (1962).

[3] Neugebauer, "Medieval and early modern theories of mental illness," *Archive of General Psychiatry*, 36 (1979); "Mental handicap in medieval and early modern England," in David Wright and Anne Digby (eds), *From Idiocy to Mental Deficiency*.

[4] Scheerenberger, *A History of Mental Retardation*.

[5] Kanner, *A History of the Care and Study of the Mentally Retarded*.

[6] Mans, *Zin der Zotheid*; Billington, *A Social History of the Fool*.

was once a Golden Age when they had no separate social identity – for these authors a good thing, for Kanner not.

I have tried to open up a new arena. The reader will find positivism and presentism here too, of course. I want to add to a store of sound historical knowledge on the topic; and I believe that if the past is a foreign country where they do things differently, there is a future country where they do things differently and better. Others in the field, too, have called for an "inclusive anthropology."[7] Now this should arouse suspicions. Although the history of ideas is useless if it does not generate new ideas, it may also fairly be asked whether evidence can be proof against contamination by some political or ethical agenda, and whether the evidential base for the history of psychology is not just as prone to fabrication as for psychology itself. However, suspicions can only be justified or relieved by engaging with the evidence on a scale no one else has done till now. Moreover, I do not draw on the usual models of radical policy-making in this area ("rights," "citizenship," "justice," etc.), borrowed from liberation movements of black people, gays or women, as not only are the people we are talking about deprived of such things, they are not entitled to them in the first place because they do not qualify for the founding premise of all such models: namely, that human beings are equal and autonomous by virtue of being rational. Nor on the other hand does my agenda owe much to that seductive form of conflict avoidance which says that, as "bearers of discourse," we cannot stand outside even the thinnest and airiest of concepts, among which the concepts under discussion in this book undoubtedly belong. Finally, to all those who still think that science can speak to our topic, I have to confess that the scientific and ethical questions (How do we know what intellectual disability really is? How do we value the people it describes?) are as inextricable from each other for the historian as they are, minus any acknowledgement of the fact, for the psychologist or cognitive geneticist.

We can begin tackling these questions of definition at the most superficial level, that of names. Here our psychological object seems more problematic than most. On the one hand, the disabled are defined more dogmatically than any other human group. They are still seen as a natural category, the last justifiable bastion of essentialism in an era when gender, race and sexuality (for example) are no longer natural or essential. This definition allows things to be done to them that are no longer justifiable for those other groups; denigration, segregation, elimination and prevention belong to their recent and continuing history. On the other hand, do we really know who they are? I ask because it seems we don't know what to call them. Even within the last century the multiplicity of names for their condition has been extraordinary: backwardness, cognitive impairment, complex needs, cretinism, developmental delay, developmental disability, dullness, educational subnormality, fatuity, feeble-mindedness, idiotism, imbecility, intellectual disability, intellectual handicap, intellectual impairment, learning difficulties, learning disability, mental defectiveness, mental deficiency, mental disability, mental handicap, mental impairment, mental retardation, moronism, neurodisability, neurodiversity, oligophreny, slowness, special needs, etc. One could double the number. This instability of names surely points to a deeper conceptual problem and, as Murray Simpson has demonstrated for the nineteenth century, to the absence of any stable nature linking the people thus described.[8] Histories of the topic, supposing that names denote the same natural kind across the ages, have tended to proceed in parallel with traditional histories of physical disability, treating it as a history of freaks when actually it is the history of a freak idea.

In defining intellectual disability, psychology comes up with a list of particular deficits in what it sees as intellectual ability and (which amounts to the same thing) as characteristically human.

---

[7] Herman P. Meininger, "Authenticity in community: theory and practice of an inclusive anthropology," *Journal of Religion, Disability and Health*, 5 (2001).

[8] Simpson, *Modernity and the Appearance of Idiocy: Intellectual Disability as a Regime of Truth*.

In other words, definitions are circular. Now it is professionally acceptable, even commonplace, to say that sanity consists of the absence of mental illness. But it would no doubt be professionally crass to say the same thing about intelligence, which is not just an absence of disability but self-evidently positive, the crowning feature of our species. If intelligence has any historically continuous characteristic at all, this circularity of definition is it. The content of the definition itself changes from one era to the next, making it not only circular but contingent at each point on historical circumstance. Today definitions come, ostensibly, from a theoretical base in the academy, proceeding from there to applied psychology or the genetics laboratory for their evidence base, and thence to the social institutions such as health, education, human and social services, employment, etc.; their final destination is the everyday mind-set, which closes the cycle by feeding back into the academy and providing a covert rationale for the latter's hypotheses. The student, having stumbled across psychology by being "interested in people," makes this journey in reverse. He or more often she, prompted by the mind-set, must at some point face the fact that her chosen profession is not interested in people in any way she may have so far thought of them, but only as parts and props of a vulnerable institutional order which she herself will help to police and of which intelligence is the supreme membership criterion. At this point psychology's enchanted forest will either swallow her up, or she will come to ask about its idea of people, in W.H. Auden's words, "Was it to meet such grinning evidence / We left our richly odoured ignorance?"

At the centre of the forest – somewhere – is the holy grail of scientific status. Meanwhile the ideological core of intelligence can be glimpsed from the very claim that its social critics are the ideologues. Take cognitive ability tests (IQ), and the fact that they have regularly been modified in response to criticism of their inherent cultural bias. Many psychologists have seen this criticism as an ideological intrusion, motivated by an unscientific egalitarianism which the science disproves. However, the psychometrician's very act of responding to criticism, by moving away from culturally relative tasks towards apparently more abstract ones seemingly possessed of universality, is itself a necessary ideological collusion; the fact that modification takes place at all belies any claim to exact-science status that might be made for intelligence as such, exposing the emptiness of psychology's "Newtonian fantasies" about parity with physics or chemistry, about objectivity and calculability.[9] Its extremely short-term historical shifts undermine not just the claim that one can measure intelligence but also that intelligence in itself has the long- or even medium-term stability of content that an exact science might expect from its object of study. Of course there is already a whole discipline, the philosophy of science, devoted to doubting whether the subject matter even of physics is real; but doubts about intelligence are of a different and deeper order entirely.

Intelligence is a social construction: enough said?

Disenchantment leads to scepticism. Any champion of the idea that intelligence has a real essence, scientifically classifiable in nature, is countered by others for whom it is relative and changeable and who regard the attempt to produce "culture-fair or -free" estimations of it as a nonsense.[10] But this sceptical position usually turns out to be mere bravado. Beneath superficial disputes about whether intelligence is measurable or absolute, in the deeper recesses of the mind-set we still need to make shorthand judgements of our fellows and to establish our own intelligence: otherwise,

---

[9] Thomas Leahy, *A History of Modern Psychology*, 6.
[10] See J. Berry, "Radical cultural relativism and the concept of intelligence," in Berry and P. Dasen (eds), *Culture and Cognition*.

to borrow a classic argument, how could our scepticism be a more intelligent stance than the positivist's? For the sceptic, intelligence is relative or absolute according to where advantage lies; there are moments in one's life when the concept cannot be lightly dismissed. At the same time, it seems readily deconstructable in the popular mind: "Rabbit's clever," says the famously slow Winnie-the-Pooh, "and he has Brain. I suppose that's why he never understands anything." And as far as academic critiques are concerned, many have come from within the discipline of psychology itself. But anyone who claims to have dispensed fully with the essential reality of intellectual ability must have dispensed fully with that of intellectual disability too. The moment one takes (say) "severe mental retardation" as a positive concept describing a natural kind, one automatically reactivates the positive concept of intelligence itself. Even among historians who write about "social constructions" and "inventions," the content of the analysis rarely matches the aim: for example, Paul Michael Privateer's *Inventing Intelligence* presupposes the natural reality of its opposite, "mental disability," while James Trent's *Inventing the Feeble Mind*, despite its title, does not challenge the transhistorical psychological identity of the population it describes.

Disengagement from the whole farrago is not easy, then. Most sceptics, academic or lay, living in a segregated society, are unlikely to have had much to do with people whose disability they cannot deconstruct unless they can first know some people thus constructed. A professional will at least know the person at first hand, even if social and conceptual segregation has distorted the relationship between them. And as one of those professionals, without a positive belief in intelligence and disability I could not exist. My job is to pass expert judgement on people in a way that distributes and perpetuates these appearances formally, as a series of crediting operations that endow this natural object, intelligence, with social power. It is in this realm, in social institutions rather than the ivory tower, that disputes occur, personal destinies are fought over and injustices become visible. In some institutions, such as education and examination systems, they affect the majority of the population, but how this happens is often hard to pin down. One stark reality alone is universally obvious: the absence of intelligence in the disabled, a separate population whose deficiency is to be regretted, quarantined and prevented. "Intellectual disability" is the reserve tank into which anyone who needs a justification for other, supposedly more arguable discriminations, can dip momentarily, an insurance policy guaranteeing that some of the normal population are more intelligent than others: that is, both individually (I more than you, my child more than yours) and in groups (men more than women, whites more than blacks, self-improvers more than the underclass). A society that congratulates itself on celebrating diversity must understand that signing up to an intelligence hierarchy among individuals necessarily entails, in the small print, signing up to and keeping on the back-burner an intelligence hierarchy among ethnic, gendered and class-based groups.

Intelligence as the psychologist conceives it owes its existence to metaphor. The early psychometrician Karl Pearson saw it as being like gas particles or planets, at that time the commonest objects for statistical treatment in the exact sciences. Intelligence could be handled *as if* it were, like them, a material object. They were all things that could be mass-measured; this similarity of method overrode any category difference among them (mind and matter, for example). But stretch our imaginations as far as we like, intelligence is not the same sort of thing as a gas particle or a planet. So we have to ask: if the similarity of intelligence to material objects is merely metaphorical or methodological and no more, then to what class of things *does* it belong, and what other kinds of thing belong with it?

Calling it a social construction and leaving it at that leads only to the same question begged by the positivist. Countless books and articles of the last generation have had the word construction in the title, as Ian Hacking has pointed out: for example "Constructing the self", "Constructing oral history," "Constructing quarks," "Constructing youth homelessness," even "Constructing the social" – not to mention, in the history of psychology, Kurt Danziger's *Constructing the Subject*.

What do all those nouns have in common? Obviously nothing. The scope of "constructing" is so broad as to be useless; it comes to mean simply "the concept of," which can be attached to absolutely anything.[11] If I say something is socially constructed, I add nothing to my understanding of it because I have not indicated how it differs from anything else so constructed, let alone how the more general categories to which they might belong differ. Talk of the construction of intelligence or its disabilities sidesteps the same question we asked of the positivist: the construction of *what* exactly? As a member of which class of things? This book tries to answer such questions. Unanswered, the definition and use of the term will always go to the highest and most powerful bidder.

Positivism and social constructionism share a common problem, as we can see from the fact that they often drift across each other's flight paths. Just as the constructionist has to be a bit positive about intelligence in order to think that constructionism is the more intelligent stance, so the positivist suffering from physics envy will admit when convenient that there is no such thing as intelligence. Replying to someone who denied that it exists, the experimental psychologist and militant psychometrician Hans Eysenck claimed he had never said it did: "Its existence is neither here nor there; intelligence is a concept" or, as we might say, a construction. Admittedly he goes on to spoil his unlikely constructionist credentials when he adds "a concept like gravity" (not for nothing do gravity and general intelligence share the same symbol, g).[12] Nevertheless he was following a tradition in psychometrics of being defiant and dismissive about defining one's object of study. As well as Eysenck, Alfred Binet ("inventor" of intelligence testing), Truman Kelley and Cyril Burt (pioneers of educational psychology in the USA and Britain respectively) can all be found at some point saying openly that a scientific definition of intelligence is impossible, *and that this does not matter*. It is whatever one likes.[13] The reason it does not matter is that it can be measured, and measurement alone is what matters, since it makes the psychometrician a fully fledged experimental scientist at par with the measurers of gas particles or gravity.

The question as to what class of things intelligence belongs with and what other historical concepts it resembles is dealt with in detail in the course of this book. For the moment, we can say that till now that question has had answers that are either misleadingly metaphorical (intelligence is an honorary member of the class of measurable material objects) or uselessly trivial (it is a member of the class of concepts). Of course, philosophers of science have given far subtler accounts of the general debate between constructionists and positivists than the crude opposition I present here. But where the particular topic is intelligence, any reader who probes the subtleties of this debate further (and I do not do so in this book) may well find that they are all ultimately reducible to one position or the other.

Psychologists, for example, frequently modify their position by saying they cannot aspire to absolute truth, only to the closest approximation the evidence will allow. This is false modesty, however – a covert self-identification with physicists and other exact scientists who routinely apply this falsifiability rule to their own objects of study. Then there are Howard Gardner's "multiple intelligences," some of which do not correspond to psychology's usual application of the term; or the (James) "Flynn Effect," which shows how the average person of a century ago would score as "mentally retarded" in a modern IQ test.[14] Yet both authors feel obliged to retain a core concept of intelligence as some specifically human essence that is fixed in nature, when all the while their very

---

[11] Ian Hacking, *The Social Construction of What?* 1 ff.
[12] Hans Eysenck, "The concept of intelligence," *Intelligence*, 12 (1988).
[13] Binet, "Méthodes nouvelles," *L'année psychologique*, 11 (1905), 191; Kelley, *Scientific Method*, 77; Burt, *Mental and Scholastic Tests*, 9.
[14] Howard Gardner, *Frames of Mind*; James Flynn, *What is Intelligence?*

own theories make it redundant. It makes no difference whether intelligence is unitary or modular. Which particular abilities come under the heading of intelligence and which not? Who decides? Such questions are not just constructionist fooling, since without answers not only the content of intelligence but its actual existence remains open to challenge. Perhaps it is those who do not attempt answers but carry on as before who are fooling.

Critical approaches, too, have sometimes had a greater depth than I have room to indicate here. There is the idea of social intelligence, for example, which distinguishes between intelligence as the ideological product of a social niche whose particular interests it serves and intelligence as the general intellectual labour that goes into social production. This critique has had major successes in tackling the racial, sexual and class biases of psychometrics and their roots in concepts of individualized intelligence.[15] Its counter claim is that there is a genuinely existing, universal "social" intelligence, in which sense, for example, "there has probably been a concept of intelligence, and a word for it, since people first started to compare themselves with other animals and with one another."[16] Does the author mean there have been many different words for roughly the same concept? Or does he mean there have been many different words for many different concepts, which have all turned out to be culturally relative, but that in "social intelligence" we at last find a non-relative concept, and it just happens to be his? Either way there is an assumption of historical permanence, and of progress. A new and more genuinely positive intelligence will rise from the ashes; so it is still, at least potentially, a real object of science, and one that has been mapped with increasing accuracy over the centuries.

A self-defeating consequence of this universalist, cross-historical notion is that all one's contemporaries are as entitled as oneself to insert their own project into the universality slot ("this is what intelligence *really* is"), and that this includes one's opponents. Everyone is entitled to take part in the game: promoters of individualized intelligence, psychometrians using it for the purposes of institutional segregation, eugenicists, cognitive geneticists looking for an intelligence gene, not to mention cosmologists for whom human intelligence is preordained from the evolution of the first cell and inherent in the Big Bang.[17] All these idiocies are nourished by powerful socio-economic forces with deep historical roots. "Social intelligence" therefore does not compete on a level playing field. It says what the social character of intelligence is as a form of *being* (in intellectual labour, for example) without telling us why or how, as a way of *perceiving* other human beings and thus as a component of social action, we can make it prevail over individualized intelligence. And it takes for granted a division between intellectual and manual labour when, even in the marxist theory from which it stems, that division is itself merely a passing illusion given off by alienated production relations at a particular stage of economic development.

Constructionists have tended to ignore the historical roots of our topic. Georges Canguilhem asked what if the madman were rational – but not what if the idiot were. Madness may be the sign of an exceptional intelligence that then rubs off on the historian; often quoted in this context is John Dryden's line "Great wits are sure to madness near allied," its satirical intent passing unnoticed. The idiot is a less glamorous character. Radical assumptions about the *relativity* of reason, as demonstrated in the madman's supposed lack of sanity, remain entangled in conservative assumptions about the *absoluteness of its absence* in the idiot's presupposed lack of intelligence. Disability as absence is not a matter of interpreting the world this way as against that way, but of whether someone interprets the world at all, in any way. Constructionist historians such as Danziger may have shown how psychological objects such as "mind," "perception," "memory,"

---

[15] Steven Rose, *Not in our Genes*, 83 ff.
[16] Ken Richardson, *The Making of Intelligence*, 3.
[17] Simon Conway Morris, *Life's Solution*, 66.

"emotion," etc. are not natural kinds at all but values, since they can be shown to have undergone fundamental historical change; but while implying that intelligence belongs on this list, Danziger probes not so much the underlying concept as the limited psychometric version of it.[18]

Furthermore, one can use constructionist language to support a positive account of the disabled intellect. Take, for example, the claim that disabled people have abnormal difficulty coping with bereavement, and thus that they are a discrete group, "a population for whom the very meaning of life is unclear."[19] The authors' conceptual framework here is Danziger's "dark construction" and the idea of multivocality. However, inasmuch as intellectually disabled people are distinct from a majority for whom the meaning of life is clear, their reaction to bereavement is not part of some multivocal relativity: rather, they are not comparable to the rest of us in the first place, but an anomaly. Using constructionism to support the absolute exception of this one group reinforces univocality rather than refuting it. Such adaptations of scepticism to positive ends lie in a respectable tradition. As we shall see later in detail, John Locke asks us to be sceptical about whether there can be any "real" definition of the species "man," but only so that he can establish the deeper reality of his own seminal redefinition of it as an aggregate of logically reasoning individuals, founded upon the exception of intellectually disabled "changelings." In a similar way, Danziger's scepticism can be cited in support of a positive account of abnormality, even though his premise was that intelligence and (we may infer) its disabilities are mere values. At the end of this process is the entry of the constructionist language into professional practice, where it lays down how something such as intellectual disability should be conceptualized or "constructed" (just as "discourse" is now a routine usage in psychology and has thus become itself, in Foucault's critically intended sense, a discourse).

The idea that intelligence is relative and socially constructed is a truth which, if left at that, conceals other truths. Certainly Western societies have at one moment favoured one definition of it, at another moment another. But how did we come in the first place to class certain human activities as intelligent and others not? It is not just testing that requires critique. It is the entrenched medium-term historical inheritance informing our broader, everyday notions of intelligence that inhibits critical analysis. We single out a certain assembly of human characteristics – let's assume for the sake of argument that each characteristic, taken singly, does indeed have a real, empirically verifiable existence in nature – then we leap to the conclusion that the assembly itself ("intelligence" or "intellectual ability") is real in the same sense as the single characteristics are, and that it too exists in nature. This assembly now appears to differ from other supposed assemblies of characteristics ("emotion," for example, or "will") as distinctly as any of the single characteristics do from each other, as chalk from cheese. This is more than some technical example of a merely nominal category being made to seem real. It is downright obfuscation, the concrete historical details of which will emerge later in this book, as part of a game of social advantage.

Critique of psychology's value-based cognitive claims can always be deflected or absorbed unless one can establish the *spuriousness*, and not just the relativity, of the overall concepts of intelligence and intellectual disability upon which they depend, and the social realities they support. To say that intelligence is pure appearance might imply that its strength is the strength we continue to give it, and no more. We mistake it for reality: remove that misapprehension and the thing itself would vanish. Would it? There is no getting away from appearances. They have a big stake in our lives because they have their own structured reality. Intelligence matters because, as appearance, it gives rise to major injustices overlooked daily within a society that invokes it to underpin certain

---

[18] Danziger, *Constructing the Subject*, 161.
[19] Jennifer Clegg and R. Lansdall-Welfare, "Death, disability and dogma," *Philosophy, Psychiatry, and Psychology*, 10/1 (2003).

accepted rationales of consent, rational choice and personal autonomy. These nurturers of our intelligent self-image continue to determine our futures because the image is socially active – and it can only be understood as such from a historical perspective.

Unscientific method and necessary precautions

Psychology claims to be ahistorical. The assumption that intelligence and its disabilities are more or less stable concepts with some core that survives importation across the borders of historical enquiry helps psychology to claim universality and therefore scientific status. Historical stability underwrites scientific stability. The idea of intellectual disability on this view is by no means a freak. Quite the opposite: it is what the evolutionary psychologists would call a "meme," an idea that has gradually evolved and proved its viability by the scientific law of natural selection, as if the idea itself were a living biological creature. As a non-scientist myself, I do not feel confident enough to make such a leap. I need to undergo certain laborious preliminaries, such as keeping the descriptive characteristics, x, separate from human type, y.[20] I take human types of the past ("idiot," "natural fool," etc.) and research the historical source-materials to see what descriptive characteristics were then attached to them; and I take modern descriptive characteristics (inability to abstract, reason logically, process information, maintain attention, etc.) and research the historical source-materials to see to what human types these modern psychological characteristics were then attached. It is no good bypassing this precaution, which for a historian should be as rudimentary as is sterilizing one's pipettes for a biotechnician, and just assuming that modern descriptor x describes historical type y. On the evidence, it does not.

The Virgin and Child depicted on the front cover of this book, the *Madonna del Bordone* of 1261 by Coppo di Marcovaldo, is an illustration of what can happen if this procedure is ignored.[21] A few paintings in this genre are regarded as tokens of an early recognition of our own "intellectual disability," indicated by certain significant physiognomic features.[22] In one from the school of Andrea Mantegna, both the Madonna and the infant Jesus appear to have a goitre, which – subsequent to the fifteenth-century date of the painting – became associated with cretinism, whose characteristics then fed into nineteenth-century accounts of "idiocy" and the creation of Down's syndrome. Another, by Mantegna himself, appears to depict Jesus with hypotonia or weak muscle tone and with fleshy folds round the neck (both characteristic of Down's). A further painting, of the Dutch school, gives a pair of young adults similar features.[23] Yet a swathe of modern assumptions will have informed the conclusion that these are pre-modern takes on a cross-historical phenomenon. Mantegna in particular is noted for his precision in respect of the science of physiognomics popular in his time. If these painters saw a distinctive physical feature in their sitters, including inherited ones, why not represent it? We seem to be under several urges at once, evidence for which in the mind-sets of these painters is lacking. In two of these paintings, the baby has a big gap between the big toe and the next one, as well as marked epicanthic folds on his eyelids: are these not among

---

[20] German Berrios, "Mental retardation," in Berrios and Roy Porter (eds), *A History of Clinical Psychiatry*, 225.

[21] Church of Santa Maria dei Servi, Siena, Italy. Foto LENSINI Siena.

[22] For example Brian Stratford, "Down's syndrome at the court of Mantua," *Maternal and Child Health*, 7 (1982); Andrew S. Levitas and Cheryl S. Reid, "An angel with Down syndrome: a sixteenth-century Flemish nativity painting." *American Journal of Medical Genetics*, 116 (2003).

[23] Follower of Andrea Mantegna, Virgin and Child, Museum of Fine Arts, Boston; Mantegna, Virgin and Child, Accademia Carrara, Bergamo; Follower of Jan Joest, The Adoration of the Christ Child, Metropolitan Museum of Art, New York.

the first things a paediatrician looks for when diagnosing Down's syndrome in a baby? Were the painters deliberately representing disability in an iconic religious format, thus attributing a positive value to a condition which in modern times we view negatively? That would be to assume that they interpreted whatever it was they observed in an exceptional light – good or bad – rather than as an ordinary part of life that did not need remarking on other than by its simple physical representation.

By contrast, no one has ever made any suggestion of the above kind about Coppo's *Madonna del Bordone*. It is the earliest in a clutch of Madonnas that mark the beginnings of Renaissance art and of a humanist narrative style that moves away from static adoration or mere idolatry towards engaging its viewers in active thought and rational understanding. Not only does the Madonna, remarkably for her time, look at the viewer eliciting a response, the infant Jesus seems to be doing the same to her, exhibiting his divine intellect. Yes, but look at his toes, which his mother is fondling: there is the gap. And close up, there too are the epicanthic folds. Stop for a moment as you hurry through those early rooms in whatever large gallery you are in, with their endless and seemingly identical Virgins-and-Childs. You will find that many of the baby Jesuses have that gap between the toes, and nearly all of them the folds on the eyelids and/or a fleshy neck: this seems to be a painterly technique, a way of enhancing ordinary physical features. The hypotonia of the other sitters mentioned above can be explained by the fact that these are typical features of the "phlegmatic" type – slow and lethargic to be sure, but ordinary too, since the then-dominant medical theory of the four humours (of which phlegm was one) meant that people of this disposition might have made up a quarter of the human race. Now it is true that we read into the images our own values, whether negative or positive. It is entirely appropriate, for example, that the phrase "an angel with Down syndrome" should be coined in the journal of a discipline routinely devoted to the elimination of angels. But that is not the prior problem. Before embarking on the question of values, we have made assumptions about what is actually there – those "intellectual" characteristics – in the first place.

What all these paintings – the Mantegna as much as the *Madonna del Bordone* – are in fact depicting, beyond the limits of their era and beyond religion and dogma of any kind, is a social relationship that is unconditional. "Intelligence" and "intellectual disability" are thus *conditions* set, in the last resort arbitrarily, upon human relationships in a certain historical period. Any historian concerned with the social world at all, let alone with questions of social justice, has a responsibility to negotiate a way round these swamps of deconstruction, to cope with the doubts about our topic and to account for them. My preliminary step in this direction has been to divide the history into three overlapping periods. One is long term, which Mary Douglas describes in *Purity and Danger* as having its roots in the history of dirt, that basic pattern-making habit whereby we classify and separate what belongs from what is rejected or scapegoated, of which "intellectual disability" is a current and temporary manifestation; related to this is our urge to seek certainty about each other and about who belongs where, which manifests itself in determinism of various historically interchangeable kinds (divine, genetic, etc.). Another period is medium term, and extends from the beginnings of modern social administration around 1200 to the present. The roots of the cultural concept we are dealing with lie in this initial expansion of social administration and West European capitalism: a long period certainly, but a historically specific one. If any such concept can be perceived at the start of the period, it is at most a ripple among countless others and was virtually undetected by people of the time. The third period is short term and starts with the beginnings of the modern discipline of psychology and its doctrines of human intelligence and disability (under various names), from the mid-nineteenth century to the present. This book spends most of its time tracing the medium term: the growth, amidst social change, of ripple into wave.

Certain problems of terminology should be noted. "Intelligence" is a term that has to be defined precisely by its context, the more so the further the history goes back. Its various usages and its contexts, as well as those of different but cognate terms such as "wit" and "reason," are explained as I go along; if sometimes I use "intelligence" anachronistically, it is to avoid overburdening the reader and myself. Likewise I sometimes use the word "psychology" for theories that predate the first appearances of that word at the end of the sixteenth century. Like most human science disciplines, psychology is descended from medieval scholasticism and has so far not enjoyed the transformational scientific moment that (say) physics had with the law of gravity; that is why I occasionally feel justified in using the word to describe the entire descent, from Thomas Aquinas to Steven Pinker.

Usually I call the pre- or early modern doctrine "faculty psychology" and the later one "modern psychology." Two caveats are needed here. The first is that psychology, once the word was invented, still had to wait another three centuries to become a formal academic discipline, while faculty psychology survived beyond the early period and well into the nineteenth century. The second is that I use "modern psychology" to cover everything since 1700. This too begs questions. In fact, it is usually shorthand here for something more limited, namely the psychology of human intelligence as it appears in its subdisciplines – clinical, cognitive, behavioural, educational, developmental, genetic – and at their point of interface with social practice. Furthermore, one cannot really speak of the history of a single discipline with Locke as founding father, or indeed of a discipline at all as distinct from a fluctuating constellation of social anxieties. However, this book ends with Locke, and that is because even if the history of modern psychology is highly complex, as a significant social practice it is recognizably Lockean. Whenever psychologists are paid to assess someone or to deny social participation – on the grounds, for example, that this or that person lacks the ability to think abstractly, reason logically, process information, maintain attention, etc. – they are using criteria which Locke, in his seminal refashioning of theological doctrine, also used, and from which he created for such people a separate space in society and therefore in nature.

I have tried to make the telling of this story accessible to anyone with an interest in the history or indeed the future of ideas in the human and social sciences. The range of reference will mean that parts of the road ahead are steeper than others, depending on readers' familiarity with this or that stretch of it. Sometimes they may feel I am throwing evidence or mere assertions at them which, without previous knowledge, they are in no position to question. But that is because we are looking at a greenfield site. The problem will only be solved by others taking up these historical themes. Scholars with a deep historical knowledge of early modern culture, if not of our particular topic, will know exactly where I have strayed or taken short cuts. However, the road is steep in more than one sense. Accessibility is not just a matter of understanding the historical material, but of being morally prepared for what one has access to. While there are hard facts to be established, there are also hard truths to be faced. Of these, truths about our self-esteem – which is where, ultimately, I locate the subject matter of this book – are among the hardest.

PART 1
Problematical Intellects in Ancient Greece

Chapter 1
Ancient Philosophy and the "Worst Disability"

When we assume that in the distant past intelligence and its disabilities, under any label, existed in a sense we might understand them today, we turn a history that is rich and strange into a recital of our own prejudices. "Intellectual (dis)ability" presupposes an entire modern conceptual apparatus whose basic components would have been altogether obscure to the Greeks or indeed to Europeans of more than a couple of centuries ago. When Charles Dickens and William Henry Wills, in the 1853 edition of *Household Words*, claimed under the entry "Idiot" that this "hopeless, irreclaimable, unimprovable being" is a "main idea," meaning a universal truth independent of time or place, they belonged to the specific generation which was just at that moment inventing such a being, as a complement to the middle-class identity their journal sought to establish: 1853 was also the foundation year of the Royal Earlswood Hospital, the world's first mass, long-stay segregated institution.

    The conceptual apparatus of modern psychology, a product as well as a producer of mass segregation, forms a huge barrier to historical enquiry, resting as it does on the following presuppositions, each of which will be challenged in more detail at various points in this book. (1) Intelligence follows certain laws of human nature, just as atoms and molecules follow the laws of the physical universe. (2) These psychological laws determine our place in natural history, as strictly as biological laws do; intelligence marks what is fully or typically human, rendering doubtful the species membership of those who lack it. (3) Such laws are exhibited in a common set of detailed intellectual operations that all members of the species bar a few reveal under observation, to varying degrees: logical reasoning, abstraction, information-processing, attention, etc., all of which boil down to cognitive competence. (4) The mind can be separated from the body, at least for purposes of method, as a distinct object in natural history: hence "intellectual" disability, running in parallel with physical disability. (5) Personal identity (which includes intellectual ability) is a temporal unity, defined by the permanent state of an individual mind taken as a whole over the period between birth and death or senile dementia. (6) Intelligence is a possession of the individual, like height or eye-colour. (7) There are many more or less normal people, and otherwise a small minority of abnormal ones who deviate from the norm in their cognitive abilities and are situated at the furthest extremes: highest in the genius, lowest in the idiot. (8) The causes of intelligence and disability belong either to nature or to nurture, or to both, or to some interaction between the two. (9) Cognitive psychology (educational, developmental, etc.) is an exact science, based on empirical data drawn from the human subject's performance under observation; hence performance is evidence of ability, or simply *is* ability. (10) Rights are separable from competence; the first is a legal concept, the second a scientific one, based on expert assessments of an intelligence that has its own objective existence and is prior to the sphere of law as such. (11) Intellect is quite separate from morals; how we know about people's intelligence is one thing, a matter for science, but how we value them quite another.

    If today all this goes without saying as part of the modern mind-set, among ancient and early modern authors it simply was not said. We can find occasional traces of some of it, but not all at the same time or as part of an overall mind-set. That is not because those authors were primitives, struggling for a scientific explanation of human nature which transcends history and which we have finally come to understand. It is because people did not then ask the same questions about each other as we do now, nor will in the future.

When, as it so often does, a history of ideas starts with the Greeks, it maps out the remaining journey as an ascent towards the summit that is the modern discipline. In the case of psychology, this helps create the impression that categories describing the mind are stable, permanent historical objects. It follows then that they are sound: primitive Greek speculation about them has matured into an exact modern science. But if the claim is that Plato and Aristotle are psychology's founding fathers, we ought in the era of DNA forensics to administer a paternity test. We then find that this role does not suit them at all. In the history of modern psychological concepts, Plato and Aristotle are not ancestors but outsiders, barbarians even. The role of ancestor better suits their intellectual opponents of the time, the sophists, who shared certain values with modern psychologists, among them the information-processing model of intelligence and the importance of speed. This was what Athenians liked to hear about themselves, and the sophists pandered to it. They coached people in the skills needed for social advancement, sold their expertise in a market economy as complex in its way as ours is and held a place in the society's formal structures. Hence they earned the enmity of philosophers such as Plato and Aristotle, members of a leisured but politically marginalized landowning class. Unlike the sophists, the philosophers did not charge fees and were detached from power and the entire public arena; they preferred under the democratic circumstances to remain *idiotai*, that is, in a private capacity.[1]

It is easy to misappropriate Plato or Aristotle to underwrite modern doctrine. They certainly valued some human activities more than others, some of which can be compared with things we ourselves call intellectual. But which of these exactly did they regard as better, and what was the out-group thus created (since it was not some golden age without scapegoating or stereotyping)? We cannot just assume that the philosophers had concepts such as "ability" or "intellect" to match our own, or that it was even possible to yoke two such concepts together in the first place. The texts are foreign territory. All we can do is reconnoitre the relevant vocabulary and try to reconstruct its meanings.

Ease of learning, "learning difficulty" and sophistry

It is easy to read into Plato the "scale of nature," that central Western image of a natural hierarchy in which what is lowest in human beings is closest to the animals. But while he does indeed have a problem with animals, that is mainly because of their hedonism rather than absence of reason *per se*. We can detect in Plato the ascending series existence-life-intelligence, intrinsic to modern human sciences, but only very roughly – not as an obsessive need to maintain the sharpest possible separation between species. Instead, human abilities and disabilities are closely related to the more fundamental problem of ignorance, in which psychological, epistemological and ethical questions are inseparable from each other.

Plato presents Socrates in a constant state of puzzlement – part feigned, part real – when people confront him with an argument that seems too pat. His claim to be ignorant, as he worms their pre-packaged thoughts out of them, is a way of claiming intellectual ability for himself. One thing Socrates knows for sure: that other people's knowledge claims are grounded in ignorance, plausible only because they happen to be popular or ideologically dominant. The intentions behind this ironic method often spiral beyond our understanding. Nevertheless Plato is not being playful

---

[1] Lene Rubinstein, "The Athenian political perception of the *idiotes*," in Paul Cartledge et al. (eds), *Kosmos*.

for the sake of it; a stable world-view lies beneath. Although it is hard to pin him down to a system of thought holding good over his entire output, the late dialogues have a consistent terminology and scale of values related to intelligence and disability.

Sifting through these terms, we find only one that is specific to humans alone: "making calculations" (*logarizesthai*). Thomas Hobbes, a shrewd interpreter of classical source-texts, noted how minor an item this was in ancient thought; he viewed calculation, central to his own mechanistic psychology, as the down-to-earth reality behind his contemporaries' preposterous claims to higher intellectual abilities. He rightly thought they were misappropriating the Greek terms. *Episteme* ("understanding") is not specific to humans, nor does it pretend to distinguish subjective operations of knowing from the knowledge at which they aim. Likewise *nous* ("intuited intellect") is attributed not only to humans but also to divine beings, planets and occasionally to other animals. Other terms such as *dianoia* and *noiesis*, meanwhile, are too narrow, since the Greeks saw "intellect" in this sense as a succession of thinking states rather than as a prior capacity ("it consists of thoughts; these are one in terms of their succession, like numbers, not like sizes or spaces," said Aristotle).[2] *Phronesis* (prudence or civic intellect) was less than specifically human, being restricted to citizens. Finally, there is *logos* ("rational account"), which is central to Greek philosophy. Plato nowhere says that this is exclusive to humans. Of all such terms it is the most susceptible to context. It can be good or bad, support false opinion as well as true and does not seem to cover subjective "ability." Moreover it is the failed rational accounts that are described as "monsters," not the struggling humans who submit them to Socrates's withering cross-examination. Plato's *Theaetetus*, which deals with the difficulties of giving a rational account, is peppered with such metaphors.

Then there are secondary operations, such as "ease of learning" (*eumathia*) and its opposite "learning difficulty" (*dusmathia*). These terms came from the sophists: enough reason to doubt whether Plato takes them seriously. Ease of learning is a "demotic" quality, he says – not something with which his Academy would want to be associated.[3] In any case, according to the prevailing doctrine of the mean, there are desirable limits to intellectual activity.[4] Moreover, ease of learning does not necessarily mean having a good memory; it is a necessary condition for the philosopher-ruler's "understanding," but not a sufficient one. The scope of learning difficulty is likewise limited; it is not pathological, and can go with having a good memory. Although Plato says in his *Timaeus* that it is a component of "ultimate ignorance" (*amathia*, the worst kind), they remain conceptually separate.

The difference between ease of learning and genuine understanding becomes clearer over the course of Plato's work. In *The Republic*, from the middle period, he says that ease of learning cannot be of use to the philosopher-ruler unless it is accompanied, paradoxically, by the kind of plodding steadiness more often observed in people who find learning difficult.[5] He does not, however, suggest the converse: that "learning difficulty" may be a positive value. In his late dialogue *The Laws*, where he describes the ideal state of Magnesia, he makes good this silence. He suggests unprecedentedly (for him) that even if people are illiterate, slow-witted and lack any specialized ability of the kind associated with the highest, reasoning part of the psyche, they can be rulers, simply on condition that the modicum of rational judgment they do possess is in harmony with the part of their psyche that deals with pleasure and pain.[6] Whereas the rulers of *The Republic* rule

---

[2] Aristotle, *On the Soul*, 407a. References are to the paragraph numbers given in the margins of most English or original-language editions of classical texts; the bibliography lists the most frequently used dual-language editions. Translations here and throughout the book are my own unless otherwise indicated.
[3] Plato, *The Republic*, 494b.
[4] Plato, *Timaeus*, 88a.
[5] *The Republic*, 486a ff.
[6] Plato, *The Laws*, 689d.

in the name of the Absolute Good, the rulers of Magnesia seek the good for ordinary people. The unlearned can rule and possess civic intellect because what they are judging is everyday affairs, and this they are capable of.

Plato's "ease of learning" and "learning difficulty" therefore cannot be identified with modern notions of a specifically human intelligence or disability. And people who learn slowly and with difficulty are not those whom he wants excluded from public life. They are not the real defectives or the real threat to society. Elimination is warranted for some people simply because of the particular way in which their humanity is expressed. But who exactly is on Plato's hit list? If disabled people of our present type were *the* enemy for Plato, they would surely appear in a form recognizable to us. Many historians have called him a eugenicist because in *The Republic* he seems (the text is ambiguous) to hint approvingly at an alleged Spartan practice of exposing defective new-borns at the foot of Mount Taygetos.[7] However, it is not clear how the Spartan example could refer to anything except visible physical weakness: diagnosing anything else in early infancy would have been impossible at the time. Nor is there a clear historical distinction between purposeful infanticide and simply abandoning babies in public places. We project a modern, eugenicist impulse on to Plato; he recommended it, so it is all right for us. Whereas *The Laws* describes a state that is "ideal" in terms of everyday, second-order reality, *The Republic* is a poetic account of the first-order reality of ideal forms, particular that of justice. We should be wary of seeing everything in it as a policy recommendation.

Alternatively, one might try to locate the sources of modern "intellectual" disability in the psychological make-up of slaves, which would then justify their enslavement (as it would later for European colonialists). But the Greek texts on slavery are not a reliable source for modern psychological differentiations of any kind. There is no such thing as a slave psychology, says Plato. The nature of slaves cannot be reduced to such simple elements – they are capable of civic intellect, of which some free citizens are incapable – nor is it any use for a citizen to be capable of a rational account but incapable of communicating it.[8]

When Plato decides who is to fail the humanity test, the intellectual criteria are not, as we would construe them, dissociated from moral ones; the acid test for deciding who is human has to do with the supremacy of the Good, though that does not make it any the less an intelligence test. In his late dialogues he singles out three types of deficiency, outlining a precise classification that was missing from his earlier texts. It has a systematic vocabulary, prefigured in a key passage at the end of *Timaeus*.[9] Here he lists the reincarnations merited by certain types of intellect and behaviour. In the highest rank, men are reborn as men, and in the next highest as women. Below are three further ranks (discussed below). Of these, the highest are those who in their previous life suffered from "simple-mindedness" (*euetheia*). They are wise enough to study astronomy but stupid enough to think that it comes from using one's eyes rather from theory: in other words, they are seduced by appearances and sense-perception. Such people are "harmless" and are reincarnated as birds. Lower down come those suffering from "civic ignorance" (*aphrosune*), who are reincarnated as land animals. This is the only rank that contains subgrades within it (four-legged, multi-legged, legless); these internally differentiated levels of reincarnation reflect the hierarchical differentiation of civic functions. The lowest rank are reincarnated to live in water, thus breathing the foulest air and inhabiting the lowest region, furthest from the divine heavens: those who have lived in "ultimate ignorance" (*amathia*) and "unreason" (*anoia*), and the only ones whose reincarnation is described as a punishment. These three ranks are associated with

---

[7] *The Republic*, 460c.
[8] *The Laws*, 776b; 817e.
[9] *Timaeus*, 91d.

heaven, earth and water, and with the three hierarchical divisions of the psyche portrayed earlier in *Timaeus*. We shall see now how all three feature in the late dialogues.

Simple-mindedness

In *The Republic*, someone who judges things by appearances and sense perception rather than by apprehending their ideal forms is said to be suffering from simple-mindedness (the conventional meaning of the Greek term was naivety, or taking things at face value). Plato continues to use this term in all the post-*Republic* dialogues; but whereas in that earlier work it had just meant an inability to see beyond surface appearance, in the later dialogues it has a broader range. It is deployed ironically, opposing sincere, "simple-minded" ignorance to that of the sophists.[10] Simple-mindedness occurs in Plato's account of the first stage of human development after the flood. It is characteristic of a peasant society with no experience of civilization, that is, "of the skills and machinations that people in cities use against each other in their desire to get the upper hand." Peasant society had no distinctions of power or wealth; consequently, "when people heard things labelled good and bad, being simple-minded they thought the absolute truth was being spoken, and they believed it." The machinating city-dwellers stand for the power-holders in Plato's Athens; the labellers of good and bad are the sophists and rhetoricians. Simple-mindedness belongs to the unlamented past but is more desirable than the Athenian present. Plato even puts simple-mindedness up there alongside courage and temperance in his list of the "virtues" of primitive society.[11] Since it also means taking things at face value, this comes close to an acceptance of the world of appearances Plato had rejected in *The Republic*. Ironic it may be, but he is only half in jest. In these late texts Plato has learned to live with the appearances.

Civic ignorance

Second, more severe than simple-mindedness is lack of the intellect one needs to function as a citizen: civic ignorance. Coming as it does in varying degrees, it concerns not the Absolute Good but the exact skills required for this life: good conduct towards the state, one's family and oneself. One needs it both to rule and be ruled. Some people never acquire it, or do so in negligible amounts – though whatever its differential distribution, its actual quality remains unchanged from lowest to highest. Civic ignorance (*aphrosune*) is, correspondingly, an inability to see the need for social curbs on the unlimited possibilities of life (in this sense it can also cover madness, *paraphrosune*). The word's everyday sense means something like thoughtlessness – not thinking when you are capable of doing so – and this sense is clearly present in Plato too. He says, for example, that pleasure and pain are "thoughtless" educational advisers; obedience to them prevents one from "setting limits." The context is one of education for citizenship, of learning to set and accept political and legal constraints. If one lacks civic intellect, one will lack justice, temperance and bravery since it is the first cause of these other three virtues. Inability to exercise this primordially intellectual virtue, the key to an ethical social life in the treacherous second-order world of appearances, is more serious than the simple-minded inability to see beneath them.[12]

---

[10] *The Laws*, 679a ff.; Plato, *The Statesman*, 276e; 309e; *The Sophist*, 267e.
[11] *The Laws*, 677b; 679c.
[12] *The Laws*, 689a; 733a ff.; 630c; 927a; 769d; 644c; 927a; 649d.

Ultimate ignorance

Even civic ignorance is not public enemy number one. What is the greatest threat to the city state or *polis*? It is what in *Timaeus* Plato calls "ultimate ignorance": *amathia*. He also calls it "the greatest disease," "ignorance of humankind's greatest concerns" and an "alien" state of mind. It answers the question, "Why do states fail?" and is vital to the scheme of *The Laws*. Still being worked out through the late dialogues, its complex significance is only reached here in the last of them, where he introduces it with a flourish that rounds off a long purple sentence.

In the developed form it acquires over the late dialogues, ultimate ignorance is multi-faceted. Its starting-point is the ignorance that Socrates congratulated himself on not having, to compensate for not having wisdom either: that is, the belief that because you have knowledge about some things you have knowledge about everything, and consequently that you know everything when in fact you don't. Initially Plato labels this alone as ultimate ignorance. However, in the late dialogues he assigns a separate name to it: "self-deceptive wisdom" (*doxosophia*). He states also that he will not be using *amathia* in its everyday Greek sense, as the ignorance of the artisan who knows only one skill.[13] He is now free to use the term for something more complex.

One new feature is that to be ultimately ignorant, one must have power over others. To explain this, we need to bring in the much-discussed question of whether Plato thinks one can do wrong willingly or be punished for crimes committed in ignorance. The usual conclusion is that he is ambiguous. But the ambiguity is in our own minds. Even in earlier works he was already employing two separate terms. One type was simple ignorance or lack of knowledge (*agnoia*), which is *prior* to the other, morally corrupt type. The latter (*amathia*) was also called "double ignorance": an abuse of personal power over others, which deserves punishment. This distinction becomes more explicit in *The Laws*, where Plato juxtaposes the two terms in a single passage. One cannot be overcome by simple lack of knowledge; one *can*, however, be overcome by ultimate ignorance, because it arises out of the pursuit of selfish pleasure (a point not established in the earlier works).[14] This identification of ultimate ignorance with abuse of power has a sweeping range: mismanagement of the state, "disorderly" sexual behaviour, mistreatment of partners, abuse of slaves. At its root is the ultimately ignorant person's reliance on rhetoric and sophistry, on self-seeking relativities that threaten the cosmic and social order as portrayed in *Timaeus* and the laws of Magnesia.[15]

In addition, then, to self-deceptive wisdom and abuse of power, the ultimately ignorant are intoxicated with the pleasures obtainable through that power. Intoxication indicates a disjunction between the pleasure principle and rational justification of one's opinions (the highest intellectual ability that can be expected of mere humans). Plato's example is the Persian rulers, whose loss of power he ascribes to their selfish and irrational belief that what was honourable and good for the state was unimportant compared with gold and silver; their notion of the good was momentary, with no thought of what might constitute the absolute good.[16] Plato's concern here is the balanced integration of a second-best, because human, realm: the ultimately ignorant are a bar to this integrated society, its real aliens. And because ultimate ignorance causes the destruction of the state, people suffering from it are to be excluded from power. They only need to be excluded from power because they are in a position to wield it; put another way, they have to be excluded

---

[13] *The Laws*, 689a ff.; *Timaeus*, 88b; Plato, *The Seventh Letter*, in *Epistles*, 344c; *The Laws*, 679d; *The Sophist*, 231b; Plato, *Philebus*, 49a.

[14] *The Laws*, 863a ff.; Plato, *Protagoras*, 357a ff.; 312c ff.

[15] *The Laws*, 784c; 777d; 886b ff.

[16] *The Laws*, 698a.

from power in utopian Magnesia because they wield it in the actual society in which Plato lived. Its constitution requires a supervisory body of examiners, and examiners of examiners, to weed out rulers who, in spite of Magnesia having given them a decent Platonic education, do not live up to expectations. No one graduates with a certificate guaranteeing a permanent right to rule. The examiners are a check on backsliding rulers, whom Plato wishes could be put to death twice. His final, elaborated concept of ultimate ignorance defines the backsliding: it is the disease of advanced society.[17]

Plato reinserts "ease of learning" into this ultimate ignorance. His doubts about it have now increased. He takes the crucial step of crediting ultimately ignorant people with outstanding learning abilities, of the kind that belong to the highest, divine part of the psyche: arithmetical reasoning, forethought, making judgements, etc. These abilities are "fully rational"; perhaps the phrase is ironic (the word "fully" evokes Socratic misgivings about any kind of claim to complete knowledge), but it does not work as irony unless we read it in a positive sense first. According to Plato, the desires of the lowest part of the psyche (say, for gold) may harness even the most expert and divine "calculative faculty" (*logistikon*) for their own ends: the first and only time Plato ever uses the latter term in a pejorative sense. Whereas in *The Republic* the very idea of such a fall from grace was out of the question, in the more practical context of *The Laws* it has become a real threat, the greatest danger to the state, and the reason why there can be no innate and thus incorruptible virtue among rulers. Virtue can be learned, but it can be unlearned too; ultimate ignorance in a specifically educational setting is given its own term (*apaideusia*) – not the simple lack of an education but the unravelling of a good one.[18]

In ultimate ignorance, then, we have found the real enemy. What has it got to do with "intellectual disability" in any sense that we might understand it today? If Plato's "ultimate ignorance" seems not to tally with some kind of intellectual disability in our own sense, it is not some dichotomously conceived moral incompetence either. Though "the cause of great and brutal sins," it is not some psychopathic exception.[19] It embraces all sorts of people, not only ancient Persian rulers and backsliding Magnesian ones but people of influence in Plato's own society: materialist philosophers whose teachings persuade the masses away from piety and hence from social deference; the political careerists heading the democracy; sophists who think education should be relevant and pragmatic, and that the divine cosmological disciplines (arithmetic, astronomy, etc.) are mere frills; and King Dionysios of Sicily, whom Plato himself had tutored but who nevertheless suffered from the self-deceptive wisdom and abused his power. The *Seventh Letter* attributed to Plato tells this latter story. It was his one known foray into political activity, as tutor to a future ruler – and it failed. Ultimate ignorance is here in all but name when he describes the pointlessness of Dionysios having been a quick and easy learner when he was "by nature" (i.e., ingrained habit) bad. Ease of learning, if Dionysios is anything to go by, is an "alien disposition."[20]

Plato does at times discuss something closer to modern notions of psychopathy and moral incapacity: a "disease of the psyche" akin to madness, in which the calculative faculty is absent because these "wicked" and "unjust" people have always sought pleasure immediately. The ultimately ignorant, on the other hand, are reasoners able to calculate the relative merits of pleasure and pain and to make a convincing pretence of civic intellect; they can postpone the gratification of desire, and use their reasoning skills to plan for it.[21] Now whereas we can readily

---

[17] *The Laws*, 945a ff.; 677b.
[18] *The Laws*, 689c; 641c.
[19] *The Laws*, 863c.
[20] *Epistles*, 344a.
[21] *The Sophist*, 227d; *The Laws*, 644c; 886b.

envisage knowledge being abused for immoral ends, Plato regards unvirtuous knowledge as a nonsensical notion. Ultimate ignorance is not just moral ignorance; the moral is inseparable from the intellectual. Whereas we are used to the notion that intelligent people may have moral flaws, Plato asks a harder question: why is amoral intelligence unintelligent? Why does it lead not only to the destruction of the state and the misery of the powerless, but eventually to the downfall of the intelligent person? That it does so is taken for granted. And if the ultimately ignorant are said to have great intellectual abilities, including some that are by definition divine, how can this simultaneously involve intellectual failure?

While *amathes* in its everyday sense meant ignorant of a particular skill, it could also mean being unteachable, as animals are. Plato knows this resonance will be heard within his own complex philosophical usage. He says that the sophists call certain people ignorant just because they find learning difficult, and suggests the label should apply to *them*, his know-all peers.[22] He classifies ultimate ignorance under the genus "unreason" (*anoia*), a broad category of cosmic disorder.[23] By contrast with ignorance as simple lack of knowledge (*agnoia*, referred to above), which though "ugly" is merely an absence, unreason as it occurs in the human realm is positively evil. In *The Laws* it covers a wide range of conditions: being mad, immature, senile, female, drunk or a poet. It is a sign, in the individual, of an absence of intuited intellect (*nous*) and thereby of his due portion of cosmic order and purpose. It is "the absolute unreason of motion that is never uniform or regular."[24] There is an organic link between the cosmological dimensions of intellectual activity and the human ones: between, say, the planets revolving on their circular orbits and Magnesia's school curriculum, designed to wean children away from the absolute unreason of their disorderly motions driven by sense-perception and towards the perfect order of the circle, through the teaching of mathematics.

In human beings, intuited intellect is specifically associated with the highest, divine part of the psyche. How then can the opposite condition (*anoia*), which encompasses the "disease" of ultimate ignorance, sit alongside an outstanding calculative faculty in certain individuals? The answer is that the reasoning of the ultimately ignorant person contributes to his downfall.[25] It is certainly present initially; you cannot think you know, let alone actually know some expert thing without being a good reasoner to start with. Now while the reasoning faculty seems to be present at the outset in the ultimately ignorant person, it is also by definition *absent* in his state of unreason. Unhinged by desire, which originates in the lowest part of the psyche but has used reasoning abilities to lay long-term plans for gratification, those abilities eventually self-destruct. Ultimate ignorance is unvirtuous knowledge, or rather the upshot of trying to attain this unattainable prize. It is a dynamic process that, in coming to fruition, renders useless the reasoning faculty with which its possessor undoubtedly set out. You cannot wield power without reason, and initially it is compatible with your state of ultimate ignorance. But to the extent that it also gets embroiled in excess and attachment to money or to power over others for its own sake, it leads to the loss and destruction of power, and of the state. You will end up alone in old age, deserted by companions and even your own children.[26] Through this process, power becomes not-power. The contradiction of suffering from unreason while possessing an expert reasoning faculty unfolds over time, in the social and political realm.

---

[22] Plato, *Theaetetus*, 195a.
[23] *Timaeus*, 86b; *The Laws*, 689b.
[24] *The Laws*, 898a.
[25] *The Laws*, 689c.
[26] *The Laws*, 730c.

Plato's supreme disability is embodied in the person who (a) has power and (b) is ignorant of its dialectic: that is, someone who in both respects is the exact opposite of himself. If we want to look for cross-historical links from Plato to ourselves, it is in this solipsistic way of thinking that we shall find them, rather than in any supposedly positive definition of human intelligence or disability. Such definitions are always self-referential, thus bound to time and place. The time and place of early modern writers are quite other.

Chapter 2
Aristotle and the Slave's Intellect

Broadly, Aristotle agrees with Plato that the intellectual alien is someone with uncontainable desires. The ideal is the mean: a balanced life, centred on the theoretical and civic intellect. Aristotle's modern commentators, however, have had their eyes not only on the man of excess but on certain social distinctions, and we shall examine here what Aristotle has to say about these. Just as man has a finer sense of touch than the other animals – a sign that he "is the most intelligent (*phronimos*) of all creatures" – so, in relation to each other, humans can be ranked morally and intellectually by whether they have hard or soft skin.[1] For hard skin, read manual labour.[2] These stray references aside, his social distinctions centre on slavery. In Book 1 of *Politics*, he writes about a separate population of "natural slaves," as distinct from slaves by "convention" or "law" such as prisoners of war. Were the former the intellectually disabled people of his time?

Aristotle against the sophists, ancient and modern

It is commonly thought that this distinction, between slaves press-ganged by brute force and "natural" ones whose enslavement is due to some innate slavelike characteristic, was Aristotle's own. However, the nature/convention polarity does not appear anywhere else in his works. On the other hand we do know, because he himself tells us, that it was popular with the sophists. They asserted that all slavery, even that which others called natural, was in fact conventional: that is, that the usual polarity does not apply in this case. Aristotle, like Plato, was dismissive of polarity; as an analytic tool it was inadequate.[3] He starts his discussion of slavery with the nature/convention polarity not because he endorses it but because this is his customary method: he begins with a received formula, then seeks to undermine it. He will look for elements of convention in nature, and of nature in convention.

What does it mean to label some people slaves "by nature"? Most of us, weaned on liberal theories of rational consent and autonomy, might think he is saying that certain people are born with an inferior or disabled intellect, a natural psychological condition that is prior to their socio-political status, and that one is therefore justified in denying them citizenship. If "man is a rational animal" (to use a phrase misattributed to Aristotle), then natural slaves are just like modern disabled people: the exception that tests the rule of human species membership. Many commentators have supposed that Aristotle was also being racist, attributing this disabled or inferior intellect to non-Greek "barbarians." From the later Middle Ages the *Politics* was often cited to justify contemporary forms of discrimination. Juan Ginés de Sepúlveda used it to justify the enslavement of first-nation South Americans, who he said were "slaves by nature."[4] North American

---

[1] Aristotle, *On the Soul*, 421a.
[2] Lynn Rose, "The courage of subordination: women and mental retardation in ancient Greece," unpublished ms.
[3] Plato, *Gorgias*, 482e; *Protagoras*, 337d; *The Republic*, 381a.
[4] Juan Ginés de Sepúlveda, *Tratado sobre las justas causas de la guerra contra los Indios*, 153; see also Anthony Pagden, *The Fall of Natural Man*.

anti-abolitionist intellectuals used it to justify slavery in the Confederate states.[5] In Victorian Britain, Benjamin Jowett – the Master of Balliol who in Thomas Hardy's fictional caricature sent Jude back to his obscure labouring ghetto and who in real life was responsible for placing the eugenics of Plato's *Republic* at the centre of the classics curriculum – cited the naturally slavish mentality of the English working classes in order to justify barring them from the "common ideas" of philosophy, which should remain the inherited preserve of "the higher classes." (Jowett's own father, as is often the way, kept a haberdasher's shop.)[6]

In the shadows of Nazism, commentators suggested that Aristotle believed slaves to be subhuman, interstitial creatures "of neither species [man or beast] but *sui generis*," and that he "trivialize[s] the distinction" between slaves and animals. Often they have tried to extricate Aristotle from his apparent culpability over race precisely by reaching for a disability model instead. His doctrine of natural slavery was "neither inconsistent" nor "morally repulsive" since apparently it was designed to demonstrate an injustice: that most so-called natural slaves were wrongly categorized because actually they had been enslaved by convention, i.e., as prisoners of war.[7] By true natural slavery, then, he must have meant a small "feeble-minded" group, people with "the psychology of the childlike adult." These commentators' transhistorical view of disability is a necessary antidote to the idea that he thought some racial groups to be of naturally inferior intelligence. He was not, it is said, justifying the enslavement of foreigners, but simply talking about "a few people" who really are "naturally deficient," the "backward individual[s] in any society" – and this, of course, poses no ethical problems.[8] We may note here that rather than eradicating the racist interpretation, such comments merely displace it. In implying that one *is* entitled in these exceptional cases to order people about for their own benefit, intellectual disability remains intact as a positive principle, lurking there to be applied once again to other groups (such as ethnic ones) when the political wind changes. Rather than an antidote to racism, then, the modern "intellectual disability" interpretation of natural slavery can be a reserve pool for discrimination of all kinds.

In fact, Aristotle needs to be rescued from those who would force him either into a liberal gentleman's club blazer or into an SS uniform. Nowhere does he say that natural slaves have less ability at their job than conventional ones.[9] They are all "partners in the masters' lives."[10] His concept of slavery was largely economic. He does not discuss the slave mind or indeed superior and inferior intellects at all (other than brief references to the hard-skinned and the senile) in *On the Soul*, his account of the human psyche. In *Politics*, the topic is mainly confined to a single section on household management. Fifteen hundred years later, the early scholastic commentators on *Politics* still treated slavery as an economic concept.[11] Only later – in fact, when their own contemporaries began enslaving

---

[5] Harvey Wish, "Aristotle, Plato, and the Mason-Dixon Line," *Journal of the History of Ideas*, 10 (1949).

[6] E.V. Quinn and J.M. Prest, *Dear Miss Nightingale*, Introduction, xxiv.

[7] R. Schlaifer, "Greek theories of slavery," *Harvard Studies in Classical Philology*, 47 (1936); O. Gigon, "Die Sklaverei bei Aristoteles," in Fondation Hardt (ed.), *La 'Politique' d'Aristote*; A. Baruzzi, "Der Freie und der Sklave," *Philosophisches Jahrbuch*, 77 (1970); W. Fortenbaugh, "Aristotle on slaves and women," in Jonathan Barnes et al (eds), *Articles on Aristotle*, 2.

[8] Malcolm Schofield, "Ideology and philosophy in Aristotle's theory of slavery," in G. Patzig (ed.), *Aristoteles 'Politik.'*

[9] Abraham Shulsky, "The 'infrastructure' of Aristotle's *Politics*," in C. Lord and D.K. O'Connor (eds), *Essays on the Foundations of Aristotelian Political Science*.

[10] Aristotle, *Politics*, 1259b.

[11] Albertus Magnus, *Commentari in Octo Libros Politicorum Aristotelis*, in A. Borgnet (ed.), *Opera*, viii, 77; Jean Buridan, *Quaestio in Octo Libros Politicorum Aristotelis*, 24.

people – did they start to assume that Aristotle was making natural intellectual capacity and incapacity the basis of people's political status. Many modern political philosophers do now acknowledge that he is more interested here in the nature of power than in the nature of slaves as such. But there remains an assumption that he saw some people in terms of modern doctrines of competence, as being "so framed by nature that they were incapable of full human development."[12] In this view, the *nature* of slavery is already covertly present in its *political* character: there is/was "by nature a position to be filled and there were people who by nature occupied it."[13] In the modern relationship between a psychology of intelligence and a politics of consent, this is true: rationality is a precondition for autonomy. But looked at historically, the concept of a universal human type lacking rationality is a relatively recent invention, by people who have found ways of asserting that autonomy.

The slave mind: social, natural or necessary?

If Aristotle did not say what we think he said, what actually did he say? Certain themes are intertwined: the slave population's inferior position in the nature of the community; the individual slave's natural lack of certain intellectual operations; and the metaphorical expression of both these as a relationship between psyche and body.

We must begin by being pedantic about translation. Aristotle's exact phrase is not "natural slave" (adjective plus noun) but "slave in respect of nature" (*doulos phusei*). Grammatically, "slave *by* nature" is another possible reading, but although this rolls temptingly off the modern tongue it evokes the idea of natural or biological causes and, as we shall see, Aristotle does not argue for any such thing. What does "nature" mean here? He tells us at the start that a search for nature involves digging beneath the foundations of a given formula, trying to obtain a better account than the current one. He warns against taking for granted what "nature" means when we apply it to slaves, or to politics in general, and particularly against two sophistic assumptions: (1) that there is an abstract set of techniques for ruling that encompasses all the specific forms of power; and (2) that because one rules over slaves by force, it is therefore a matter not of nature but of convention alone.

Assumption (1) is inadequate, he says, because it does not start in the right place. We need to know the nature of man, and particularly his social nature, before we can say anything about techniques by which he rules. Man is a creature belonging in a community of some kind. The supreme human community is the *polis* or city-state; this, then, is the supreme authority. Aristotle's train of thought from here on is dialectical, in the Greek sense of the word. Starting from a single term, "rule" or authority, he asks how it subdivides. Where is "nature" in all its various branches and subtypes? It is false to suppose that there is one abstract technique of ruling that can be applied across all of them. There are kings, statesmen, heads of large estates, heads of small households; these forms of authority are not equivalent or interchangeable. The differences among them are qualitative, since each of them has its own distinct goal (*telos*) and therefore differs from the others "with respect to nature." The same is true of those who are ruled. For example, although women are naturally subordinate, their subordination is not the same as that of slaves, as if by some abstract common denominator. The distinct nature of the slave is functionally specific to the management of the household, a "community in accordance with nature" whose own specific goal is to satisfy everyday needs.[14] The slave exists in opposition to the "master" (*despotes*) of the

---

[12] P. Brunt, *Studies in Greek History and Thought*, 343; R. Müller, "La logique de la liberté," in Aubenque (ed.), *Aristote politique*.

[13] Bernard Williams, *Shame and Necessity*, 110 ff.

[14] *Politics*, 1252b.

household. Simple opposition applies only to this lowliest level of authority. (In larger units such as the landed estate or the city-state, relationships among social classes are more complicated.)

In response to assumption (1), then, Aristotle says that the nature of authority consists in specific differences. However, all these relationships are subordinate to the supreme goal of the city-state, which "circumscribes all the other [forms of] community."[15] The specific nature of the slave is expressed in terms of wider *goals*, in which (as always in Aristotle) *causes* are already inscribed. The causes of slavery lie in the realm of necessity. What determines the slave's natural difference is not biological but technological, a "necessary utility." If shuttles wove by themselves (robot shuttles were not in prospect), masters would not need slaves. Necessity of this type describes two particular dialectical pairings that come under the general metaphysical principle "Rule and be ruled."[16] One pairing is between slave and master, the other between slave (tool of action) and inanimate object (tool of production). So when Aristotle says that some people are marked out "from birth" to rule and others to be ruled, the cause is not some congenital deficiency but the managerial requirements of the household economy.

If the causes of slavery spring from economic necessity, it hardly seems to matter whether it is natural or conventional. Why, then, is Aristotle interested in this question? Typically, he is playing along with a formula his contemporaries have confronted him with. Like our social constructionists, the sophists were good at seeing mere social convention beneath what their contemporaries saw as natural. But Aristotle typically wants to deal with the unnoticed converse of this: that elements of nature may lurk beneath a social convention. This brings him to assumption (2), the sophistic claim that *all* slavery is mere convention. The sophists do not object morally to this; they are not abolitionists. Slavery may be "not just," but we do it anyway. It is one of those things that have to be. Aristotle agrees, for reasons of economic necessity.[17] But unlike the sophists, he feels a need to try and square slavery with justice. He could have agreed that all slavery is conventional and simply added that it was unjust, as the Stoics did.[18] But they only objected to it speculatively: no Greek could have imagined a slaveless social system. Aristotle, on the other hand, wants to square slavery with justice because he wants to square it with nature. He objects to the sophists' picture of a dog-eat-dog world where anyone who is powerful enough can enslave anyone else for no good reason. There *is* such a thing as society: man is a "political" (*polis*-inhabiting) animal. It is the community itself that is human nature, with its own clear goal; it is not just a set of changeable conventions. If so, and if slavery is a part of it, then one is obliged to find something natural in the slave. In addition, it is not clear how a "feeble-minded" population group – even if the Greeks had been able to conceive such a thing – could have contributed positively to the natural goal of community as Aristotle's slaves do.

Not every natural slave, then, is actually a conventional one. But also, as Aristotle accepted, not every conventional slave is a natural one. All Athenians would have understood the political background to this. Plato had described barbarians, non-Greeks, as natural enemies, indeed "enemies in respect of nature" (*polemioi phusei*), by contrast with natural friends such as the Hellenic peoples; true, they fought each other, but this was seen as institutionalized factionalism rather than war.[19] Natural justice said that foreign enemies could be treated like slaves, but that among Greeks certain conventions applied, or ought to: enslavement of Greek by Greek was against nature, natural justice and natural friendship. After their victory at Syracuse in 413 BC, however,

---

[15] *Politics*, 1252a7.
[16] *Politics*, 1254a.
[17] *Politics*, 1253b.
[18] Dio Chrysostom, *Discourses*, 15.
[19] *The Republic*, 470c.

the Spartans had sent their Athenian captives, fellow-Greeks, into slavery. The folk memory of this was still raw in Aristotle's time. Thucydides, to whom we owe the story, went out of his way to say how unnatural the humiliation was. A core Athenian narrative, it may explain why Aristotle was so keen to find "natural" characteristics in some slaves. While slavery in general was determined by the necessities of the household economy, what made you this or that kind of slave was the concrete circumstances of your enslavement. Perhaps then, all slaves were naturally so apart from the Athenians seized at Syracuse.

One of the most embarrassing moments for the modern reader comes when Aristotle says it is the "nature and ability" of a slave to be someone else's possession. Translators try to excuse him by rendering the second of these terms as "office," or "quality," rather than ability. To say, not just that slaves are other people's possessions, but that it is their ability or capacity to be so, seems cruel, even perverse (though if they were our modern "intellectual disabled" people rather than racial others the denial of their autonomy might seem less embarrassing). However, we can see Aristotle's intentions better by considering a passage from *Nicomachean Ethics*, the companion piece to *Politics*. Here he writes about natural as opposed to conventional justice. Natural justice is "that which has the same potentiality everywhere" and (unlike the conventional type) "is not a matter of what seems good or not": that is, it is not relative or a might-is-right issue, as the sophists would have it.[20] Natural slavery is a part of natural justice. We know this because the subjective "ability" he writes about in *Politics* is the objective "potentiality" he writes about in *Ethics*; the same word (*dunamis*) is used for both. In other words, slavery was a ubiquitous aspect of social organization whose horizon no one at the time, not even Aristotle, could see beyond.

Slave mind and slave body

In a couple of passages Aristotle is said to create a crude picture of the master as pure psyche and the slave as a mere body whose humanity is therefore in question. But we need to examine these passages closely.

In the first passage, the absolute and fundamental division "rule or be ruled" operates in the domain of "nature as a whole."[21] He divides this nature into animate and inanimate. "Animate" is then subdivided into psyche and body, male and female, intuitive intellect and appetite, humans and non-humans. From this list he selects humans ("all humans") for further subdivision. Who would the ruled portion of "all humans" be? The answer is self-evident: we can see them all around us. It is those who are ruled now: slaves, or (in this context) so-called "natural" slaves. In short, Aristotle does not model the relationship between master and slave on that between psyche and body.[22] Both pairings merely happen to turn up in the same context, as quite separate examples of how the "rule and be ruled" principle operates in "animate nature."

It is true that he draws a couple of passing analogies between the two pairings, and that in pre-modern philosophy analogies are never *mere* analogies but have some extra, explanatory force. However, we need to establish exactly where that force lies in each case. In the first analogy, all he says is that using their bodies is what slaves are best at.[23] In the other, he says that psyche rules like a head of household whereas intuited intellect (*nous*) rules like a king. Here he merely

---

[20] Aristotle, *Nicomachean Ethics*, 1134b; 1094b.
[21] *Politics*, 1254a.
[22] N. Smith, "Aristotle's theory of natural slavery," in D. Keyt and F. Miller (eds), *A Companion to Aristotle's Politics*, 142.
[23] *Politics*, 1254b.

wants to show that "being ruled" is not a unitary or abstract condition, but (as we have seen) varies according to the specific social institution; it is as harmful, he says, to lose sight of such specificities as it is to ignore the difference between ruler and ruled overall. In each case, if the analogy *as a whole* held an explanatory force, one would have to conclude, absurdly, that natural slaves are automata, or psyche-less bodies. Instead, he goes out of his way to avoid any simplistic polarity that denies slaves their humanity. The explanatory element consists only in showing that slavery is a natural function of the community. Moreover, being ruled gives them protection. We have of course heard the same argument used about social inferiors in our own era: about women for example, or about black people under apartheid, and we hear the same argument being used today against the social inclusion of people labelled with intellectual disabilities. A conservative would suggest that we owe them protection as a benevolent duty, towards quasi-human creatures whose prior lack of rationality raises doubts about dealing with them as species members. For Aristotle, however, protection was something more positive; it was an aspect of the slave's positive socio-economic function.

In a second passage he says that slaves are like domestic animals, at least in terms of their bodily usefulness. Nature accordingly "seeks to make different bodies for free men and slaves," but sometimes misses its aim.[24] This idea of a gap between intention and achievement, so different from the quasi-logical classifications of modern biology, is characteristic of Aristotelian nature. A slave may sometimes have the bodily features of a free man, and a free man (we are to infer) the body of a slave. Aristotle, always determined to cover every angle, does not however appear to have thought the unthinkable: that the slave might have the psyche of a free man. In any case it is difficult, he says, to deduce intellectual features from physical ones. Experts on the mind have long since claimed to possess the answer, from bumps on the skull to DNA strings, but Aristotle was far more cautious. He does say that women's social inferiority is mirrored in the constitution of their bodies; but generally speaking, the weakness of boundary lines in his concept of nature means that the confusion between free and slave-like bodily types is not even a puzzle, it is just a fact of life, an everyday reality. "If free men were born as different in body as the statues of the gods, everyone would say that inferior people would be worthy of being their slaves," and it would certainly be "more just." But free men are not born that way. If a slave can resemble a free man physically, no clear proof is possible that beneath this bodily appearance lies an inferior psyche. Aristotle's frame of reference is far from that of twentieth-century alarms about racial mixing or the reproductive menace of the feeble-minded, let alone today's liberal eugenics.

A possible objection arises. Doesn't Aristotle contrast the "master in respect of nature ... *able* to look ahead by his thinking" with the slave who is "*able* to do such-and-such by his body"?[25] This is not a deficit model, however. Both abilities are positive functions of the household and polis. Where Aristotle does discuss a deficit in ability, the creature who pops up is the citiless individual who is "*un*able to belong to a community," "not part of a polis" and who must therefore be "a wild beast."[26] Even here there is no suggestion that the deficit is in the intellect as such. He may be thinking of fellow philosophers such as Diogenes the Cynic, who adopted the life of a homeless beggar. Where Aristotle describes the natural slave in negative terms, the context is essentially socio-economic: "He who in nature is not in possession of himself but of another, precisely this man is a natural slave."[27] It is in this context that we must take Aristotle's assertion that the slave's "ability" is to be someone else's possession.

---

[24] *Politics*, 1254b.
[25] *Politics*, 1252a.
[26] *Politics*, 1253a.
[27] *Politics*, 1254a.

Natural slaves in a natural community

Aristotle's gestures towards the humanity of natural slaves can, to be sure, seem precarious. He says, for example, that slaves "participate in reason (*logos*) so far as to apprehend it but not to possess it, for the animals other than man are subservient not to reason, by apprehending it, but to feelings." I have quoted a standard translation.[28] The word translated here as "participate" (*koinoneo*) echoes the book's initial reference to the city-state as the supreme community (*koinonia*). A better translation might therefore be that slaves "belong to the community of reason," rather than simply participating in it. Moreover, to "apprehend but not possess" reason sounds suspiciously self-contradictory, and needs closer inspection. Apprehensions or perceptions, says Aristotle in his *Metaphysics*, are things one either "possesses" or not; a halfway state is out of the question, just as a soldier can only be either armed or unarmed.[29] It is the most clearcut type of opposition. And in the practical context of *Politics*, "possessing an apprehension of good and bad, just and unjust" is a quality that is "prior to the household" and therefore holds true of all humans, regardless of their subsequent division into masters and slaves.[30] This communal awareness of justice "makes the household and the city-state." So "possessing an apprehension of justice" is already contained within the overall idea of "apprehending reason," whatever the social status of the possessor. When, therefore, Aristotle goes on to say that despite slaves apprehending reason they do not possess it, is he "hopelessly confused"?[31] Perhaps he is being extra clear. The particular Greek word he chooses for "possess" (*ekhein*) is one that emphasizes use over acquisition. Slaves do not fully use their reason because the structure of the community is such that it is not required of them. This does not stop them from "having" it in a broader sense. The notion of some modern commentators that Aristotle's so-called natural slaves were an interstitial type between humans and other animals, defined by differential intellect, therefore seems unsustainable. Little remains of the frequently noted conflict between the slave's apprehension of reason and Aristotle's later claim, at the end of Book 1, that people "get it wrong" when they say slaves are destitute of reason (*logos*).

It is true that of all the terms that might translate as reason, *logos* is the most mundane and susceptible to social context and relativism. It also has juridical overtones; slaves would have been incompetent to give a reasoned account in court – but only because they had no legal personhood, not on some separate psychological grounds. Another possible objection comes when Aristotle says that the slave lacks civic intellect (*phronesis*) and that his psyche lacks a "deliberating" component.[32] Surely these are natural intellectual deficits, by any stretch? Once again we need some context. If slaves belong to the community of reason, they also have its properly human virtues: bravery, justice, temperance. The fourth in the standard quartet of virtues, civic intellect, is self-evidently absent because the slave is not a citizen. The other three virtues, like the absence of the fourth, are specific to his social function. Accordingly, they operate differently from those same virtues in the master. Aristotle illustrates this with a further psyche/body analogy. The rational part of the psyche rules and its irrational part is ruled, "like the body."[33] He does not say that masters possess only its rational part and slaves only its irrational part. Although the idea of a bipartite, rational/irrational psyche turns up several times in Aristotle's ethical writings, the two

---

[28] *Politics*, 1254b: see Works Cited.
[29] Aristotle, *Metaphysics*, 1017b.
[30] *Politics*, 1253a.
[31] Schlaifer, "Greek theories of slavery."
[32] *Politics*, 1259b.
[33] *Politics*, 1260a.

parts never correspond to two congenitally different types of human being.[34] Here as elsewhere, he is using them to explain different social functions.

Although science, in the sense of a natural science of the mind, plays no part in Aristotle's discussion of slavery, psyche itself nevertheless has a scientific significance of sorts. It is the overarching principle of movement in living things and thus constitutes a metaphysical boundary, like gravity in Newtonian physics. In humans, it is divided into various parts, of which one is the "deliberating" part, responsible for ethical choice and the planned life. In the ruler, this part is "fully formed." Women have something of it but "without authority," children have it but "not complete." As for the slave, Aristotle says nothing beyond the bald fact that his psyche lacks this part. Slaves "cannot" plan their own lives, and a group of slaves on their own would not be a *polis* because they would not "share in the planned life."[35] Could he mean that their lack of a deliberative psyche is congenital? This would indicate a strictly biological cause quite foreign to all his other remarks about slaves (though other Greeks such as the Stoics posed the idea of hereditary slavery).[36] Could he mean that the deliberating part is triggered only at a certain stage in the human lifespan, and that in the slave it simply fails to do so? This looks more plausible to us, if only because we have grown up with modern developmentalist notions of a "plateau" in disabled people, who are "retarded" inasmuch as they fail to develop beyond a certain stage. However, the notion of a trigger would be inconsistent with Aristotle's clear implication that the free child already has the deliberative part, albeit incomplete, at birth.

We can align the psychological characteristic of deliberation and forward planning with a certain social status. The Greek word for this part is *bouleutikon*. This was originally the name for a theatre seat reserved for members of the *boule* or ruling council; as a metaphor for high status in public life, it subsequently entered discussions of the psyche. As Lynn Rose, citing the philosophical conundrum as to whether a tree falling in a forest makes a noise if no one is there to hear, asks: "If a person is, by modern standards, intellectually disabled, but the concept of intellectual disability has not yet been invented, is that person really intellectually disabled? To take it another step, if a person is by his own culture's standards mentally deficient [such as slaves or women], but mental deficiency is the expected and appropriate quality, can we still say that he is disabled in any way?"[37] Aristotle's answer to the question of what causes the deliberative part of the psyche to be absent in the slave is implicit in his ideas about the nature of politics and community; it can no more refer behind these, to some "science" of the mind, than Newtonian physics looks to any deeper-lying discipline for an answer to the question "What force causes gravity?" The opposite, in fact: Aristotle explicitly warns us against trying. Study of politics and the psyche should not exceed "the extent proportionate to the things investigated."[38] Nothing beyond psyche *causes* it, or any aspect of it. There is no mention of natural slaves in his *On the Soul*, the text that describes the general workings of the psyche, though later commentators have more than made up for this omission.

This is not simply to substitute political science for psychological science. Aristotle never argues outright for slavery as a structural necessity in Greek society. He has no reason to, because for him, it is simply a given. The parts of the psyche explain various everyday aspects of civic virtue. The ruler's intellectual virtue is the supreme social function, of which deliberation is a necessary part. A slave's virtue is relative to his master's.[39] It is positive, and belongs precisely to the function of

---

[34] *Politics*, 1249b.
[35] *Politics*, 1260a; 1280a.
[36] Dio Chrysostom, *Discourses*, 15.
[37] Rose, "The courage."
[38] *Nicomachean Ethics*, 1102a.
[39] *Politics*, 1260a.

being ruled; it is not that he is less virtuous than his master when measured on some single scale. True, the slave's virtue is "small" – seeming to imply difference of degree. Is this a deficit model, though? That is another matter. His virtue is small because the natural community needs it to be small for the purposes of his particular social function, which renders his virtue different in kind rather than degree. Unlike free children, slaves should not be taught virtue because they already have as much of it as they need for the community to function properly. There would be no point teaching them beyond their station. The virtues they do possess for that station are already inherent in it. This may be harsh; the rule of life for slaves was not the Delphic command to the free man, "Know your self," but Jowett's to Jude, "Know your place." However, Aristotle does not say slaves *cannot* be taught. Indeed, this discussion about the lack of a deliberative part of the soul is precisely the point in the text at which he goes out of his way to say that we get it wrong if we deny reason to them. It is also the place where he points out that there is considerable overlap between the natural slave and the free artisan. In a natural community the artisan's occupational niche differs from the slave's but, says Aristotle, both require exactly the same virtues.

So much for the slave's nature. If, then, slavery does not have a psychological basis in any sense that we would understand it today, what then remains of the distinction between natural and conventional? Why is all slavery not just a socio-political phenomenon? The problem is the nature/convention antithesis itself, which does not neatly correspond to our current obsessions: nature versus nurture, genes versus environment and so forth. Our own concept of nature as necessity, a deterministic influence on the perceived intellectual disabilities of individuals that are prior to decisions about their social and political status, would have been foreign to Aristotle. That is because for him necessity and nature were not identical, and indeed hardly overlapped at all. And this renders equally questionable the other half of the antithesis, convention. If the slave's intellectual shortcomings were merely some socially constructed stereotype about barbarians, Aristotle would have had to agree with the sophists: there is nothing to slavery except how things have actually worked out in society, and therefore no real distinction between conventional and natural slaves – they would all be conventional. Yet he still clearly regards the distinction as useful.

The reason for this is that, at least sometimes, he talks about nature as something deeper than a mere set of descriptive categories, and attributes goals and intentions to it. Moreover, it is this strand that predominates in *Politics*. Nature here is an ideal. He personifies it: as well as trying (not always successfully) to differentiate between the bodies of free men and slaves, nature tries to create good offspring from good parents.[40] Nevertheless, such differentiations among human beings are not simply read off from an external, scientific account of nature assumed to say the same thing to everyone. Rather, Aristotle theorizes his so-called natural slave from *within* social participation and shared ethics. He sees the acquisition of intellectual virtue as natural in the sense that it is based on natural causes, or more precisely on natural goals inherent in those causes. This is hardly scientific in any sense that we might understand it, since the causes are dispositional rather than determined; they hinge indiscriminately on biology or just plain luck – and social status. Any teleological components in the slave's nature refer to the larger nature of the community rather than to that of the individual. Aristotle was no scientific racist, either; if the barbarian character is inferior, it is not in terms of some deterministic schema. He says plenty about natural origins and natural causes elsewhere in his philosophy, so there was certainly an opening for him to talk about "natural barbarians" if he had wanted to. No such creature appears in his writings. If he had seen slaves as a separate species in nature on grounds of their inferior intellect, whether in terms of race or disability, it would be inconsistent with the way he talks about humans in all other contexts.

---

[40] *Politics*, 1255b.

"Man is a rational animal": Did Aristotle say it? Could he have said it?

Broadly speaking, then, Aristotle's work provides us with no metaphysical or scientific basis for sharply defined intellectual subcategories of human being. Yet he was reputedly author of the phrase "Man is a rational animal," cited ubiquitously across the Middle Ages and the early modern period. This phrase seems like the very foundation of the discipline of psychology; the truth it contains seems so obviously a classificatory fact of the natural world that it is hardly surprising the Greeks had a word for it. Even classicists with an eye for the historical distance of Greek thought from the modern world somehow fail to realize that in this instance we are reading modern psychology back into Aristotle. They assume he was saying something like "rationality is the essence of man" when in fact he said nothing of the sort, nor – given the way his biological works divide up the natural world – could he have done.[41] And if the phrase "Man is a rational animal" were a principle of Aristotelian psychology, it would obviously place a question mark over the species membership of individuals lacking rationality, especially those lacking it throughout their lives. But no such creature ever appears in his works. What Aristotle had actually written was: "It is the essential property of man to be a creature receptive of understanding."[42] But this too is much less than it seems.

First, the "essential property" of something in Aristotle is not the same as its "essence." (Two were elided by later Stoic philosophers.)[43] An *essence* is the most consistently important aspect of something: in other words, it has a scientific status. Nowhere does he say that understanding, intuited reason, civic intellect, *logos*, or any other relevant Greek concept is, scientifically, the essence of the human species. The modern mind-set tempts commentators to gloss him as saying so. An otherwise reliable expert, commenting on the vast gulf between Aristotle's biological classification system and ours, writes that his definition of an animal "is described by selecting the appropriate disjunctives," which in the case of man is "biped not quadruped, many-toed not hoofed, reasoning not unreasoning."[44] Search as we may, however, we will not find this last pairing in the text (though biped and many-toed are there), nor anywhere else in his output. And we cannot just assume that Aristotle did not feel like stating the obvious. It is obvious only to us. An *essential property*, by contrast, is not a scientific category at all. It is simply that which establishes the relationship of a thing to other things in its external environment. Moreover, when Aristotle writes about the essential property of man being related to the "understanding" (*episteme*), it is merely, he says, a "well-established doctrine" (*endoxon*): generally accepted and thus solid enough to start a debate, but no more. Its truth content is not at issue.

Secondly "receptive," though this is indeed a literal translation of the Greek, was not some psychological metaphor but a technical term in logic. Aristotle was echoing his immediate predecessors' "well-established" attempt to develop a more sophisticated approach to logic. The old logic, such as it was, had distinguished between classes of things only in the crudest way. Things were either the same or different; they were grouped by identity or by polar opposition – and that was that. Aristotle's older contemporaries, seeking a subtler conceptual apparatus for logic, drew it from music and arithmetic. Overtones in music, they said, suggest that sameness and difference are not the only possibilities; a single note contains several other different pitches,

---

[41] Jonathan Lear, *Aristotle*, 211.
[42] Aristotle, *Topics*, 132b and *passim*.
[43] Sextus Empiricus, *Against the Mathematicians*, 11.8; Cicero, *Topics*, 7.31; Diogenes Laertius, *The Lives of the Philosophers*, 7.60.
[44] David Balme, "Aristotle's biology was not essentialist," in A. Gotthelf and J. Lennox (eds), *Philosophical Issues in Aristotle's Biology*.

each of which can also have its own separate existence with its own overtones. Numbers have a similar characteristic. And so in logic: some classes, though different, are just contiguous rather than mutually repellent, while others, though alike, overlap only partly and are not just identical with each other. Plato refers to this as the "mixing" of classes, and he too uses "receptive" to describe the relationship of some classes to others.[45]

The word usually translated as "receptive" (*dektikon*), then, signifies logical contiguity in the above sense. It is not that human beings "receive" some intellectual content in their subjective understandings. Rather, they belong objectively to that class of living beings which has some possible point of contact with the class of things to which "the understanding" belongs. Man and the understanding, in terms of logic, are not mutually repellent or exclusive categories. Nor do they overlap. Overlap, he says for the sake of contrast, occurs in the essential property of certain other living beings, i.e., divine or eternal ones. An eternal being "partakes of" (*metekhon*) the understanding (this was again a term in logic that Plato had briefly used); no part of the class "eternal beings" lies outside the boundaries of the "understanding." Aristotle draws a sharp contrast between "partaking of" (overlap) and "receptive of" (contiguity). In short, the relationship between "man" and "understanding" is an illustration (one among many) of how classes of things relate to each other in logic; it is not a grand statement of man's subjective receptivity to reason. "Receptive of understanding" cannot be "capable of understanding," though this is often how it is translated. In Aristotle's *Metaphysics* any kind of "potentiality" (*dunamis*) is something that can change, come and go, may or may not develop. Its subjective, human aspect of "capability" although it can be part of the "nature" of something, is therefore insufficiently stable to be an essential property, or indeed to bear any conceptual relation to it, other than at the remotest level of both being aspects of "the good."[46]

The "well-established doctrine" therefore does not come under the heading of psychology at all, ancient or modern. And there are further reasons for disconnecting Aristotle from the Western tradition as we know it. One involves his account of "nature" (*phusis*). Nature as such does not contain essential properties. If something is an essential property, it has to be true of every man *qua* man; it cannot differentiate among individual men. Moreover, an essential property renders the class "man" unambiguously recognizable; in this sense it is more fundamental than a "temporary property" or even than a "permanent property." Although there is in man a calculative or reasoning faculty (*logistikon*) absent from other animals, it is sometimes in control of the psyche but sometimes not; therefore it can only be a temporary property, and so is not essential. "Permanence," meanwhile, suggests a need to keep checking whether the features of the property are still there. An essential property must be more than all this, and "must *necessarily* belong" (emphasis added).[47] There was nothing necessary, on the other hand, about nature. Greek "nature" did not distinguish between biological species by watertight Linnaean rules akin to those of logic. According to Aristotle, the correct description of the nature of something is insufficient for a correct description of its essential property, but the correct description of the essential property of something *is* sufficient for a correct description of its nature. The "nature" of a thing does not have the same classificatory rigour as its "essential property."

He gives the example of a one-legged man. In this case, the supposed property "biped" seems not to apply "by nature," since "it is possible for that which belongs by nature not actually to belong to that to which it belongs by nature." Unscrambled, this means: natural classification is flexible as to particulars. An individual may exhibit a contradiction in nature without this depriving

---

[45] Goodey, "On Aristotle's 'animal capable of reason'," *Ancient Philosophy*, 16 (1996).
[46] *Metaphysics*, 1019a.
[47] *Topics*, 130b; 129a.

him of the essential property "man." Blindness, says Aristotle, is a similar case. He includes within the boundaries of the natural any apparent exceptions or deficiencies that might test its relatively weak classificatory boundaries. He is not trying to say, as we might, that people with physical and sensory disabilities are of the same intellectual or moral worth as anyone else, since he has a similarly inclusive attitude towards mad people and even to intractable "wild" men.[48] This last case is especially significant, because as we saw earlier, the wild man living beyond the *polis* contradicts the very principle that is closest in Aristotle to a species definition of man, as creatures living in a "natural community." All exceptions imaginable are thereby covered. Neither two-footedness and eyesight, nor even sanity and civilization, are in the last resort essential properties, precisely because nature will always throw up certain exceptional individuals whom we would still want to call human.

In short, there is a radical discontinuity between the "well-established doctrines" of Greek philosophy and the Western convention of "Man is a rational animal." Moreover there is a world of difference, within Aristotle's own output, between those doctrines and his own supposedly "psychological" text *On the Soul*, which is mainly restricted to general principles. He does briefly mention a "recipient" of understanding there, but only as one example illustrating the principle that the psyche is the form of the body's matter ("one can no more separate body from psyche than the wax from its shape"). One might be tempted to infer here that the human species is defined by its reception of the understanding, in a modern sense – raising the possibility of exceptions who do not receive it. But in fact this passage only refers to particular individuals who already have that understanding; the ability is not that of every individual human *qua* human, merely of someone who in a specific context may be said to know something.[49]

There are certain inklings of a more exclusive approach in the Stoics. Where Aristotle had said that to lack understanding is not like being limbless – understanding and ignorance can turn into each other and back through imperceptible degrees, while the limbless do not grow back their limbs – the Stoics said that the understanding *is* tied thus to the human subject: it is a matter of possession and privation. Privation, then, means that some individuals are excluded from the category of universal man. However, this turns out to mean most of us except Stoic philosophers. The ethics of exceptionalism and its interplay with biology and psychology are largely (as we shall see in Part 7) a European and modern phenomenon.

---

[48] *Topics*, 134b; 143b; Aristotle, *Categories*, 10a.
[49] *On the Soul*, 414a; 417a.

PART 2
Intelligence and Disability: Socio-economic Structures

Chapter 3
The Speed of Intelligence: Fast, Slow and Mean

We now turn to the socio-economic framework of intelligence and its disabilities. Within this framework, psychology sets a special value on *speed*. The present section deals briefly with this modern phenomenon, its premises and its immediate history since the birth of the formal discipline of psychology, as a prelude to examining in detail the complex relationships between intelligence and speed in earlier times.

A choice of models

Modern social life presents certain people, from birth, as problematical at best, and at worst positively harmful. "Intellectual disability" is a product of certain historical idiosyncrasies: the complexity specific to modern social organization, the atomization of modern living arrangements, the demand from the market and a marketized bureaucracy that each of us answer to it individually (rational choice), and a shift in the typical Western proletarian activity from manual labour to services – the latter usually involving intellectual components, however minimal. The person whose disability is thus generated is also disabled by its characteristic speed. We are dealing here with long-term social forces. Concepts of socio-economic development and of personal and child development arose in one and the same historical context. The microcosm-macrocosm picture of man's place in the universe, a central feature of medieval cosmology, has been transformed in the modern era into a picture where the horizontal axis of time replaces the vertical one of space, and a future godlike human intelligence replaces God himself as its point of aspiration. In this developmental world-view, the fit between intelligence as a status concept and the hard realities of socio-economic structure is so tight as to be barely visible. In both respects the norms and goals of development appear as targets, the value of which lies in being achieved sooner rather than later. It is true that psychometrics has seen some rivalry between speed and accuracy; in the 1920s, for example, some psychologists were observing that because first-nation Americans valued accuracy over speed, they needed fewer attempts to get something right.[1] By and large, however, "quick thinking" has become so ingrained in the administrative structures of West European capitalism that it feels like the only kind.

What, more precisely, are the abilities in which speed is a positive value? Psychology marks out a limited number of abilities as intelligent. One of them is logic, first given a subjective location in the human mind in the late medieval period; Jean Piaget's "mental logic" has become now a formal descriptor of intelligence. Another is abstraction, the ability to generalize from particulars or from one context to another, which dates from the same period. A further ability, albeit mentioned as far back as the Greek sophists, is information processing or the storage and retrieval of information. The practicing psychologist regards these abilities as permanent features of human nature; and the historian of psychology often regards the belief that this is the case as itself a permanent feature of Western thought, in addition to the abilities themselves. Both, however, are at most a medium-term phenomenon.

---

[1] Otto Klineberg, "An experimental study of speed," *Archives of Psychology*, 93 (1928).

Those abilities, it is suggested, occur in time: for example, that the measured speed of immaterial mental processes matches the measured speed of certain corresponding material entities. Take "the cortical glucose metabolic rate correlates of abstract reasoning."[2] The presupposition is Cartesian: that if machine-like bodies can be measured, so too can minds. Nevertheless, it raises problems. Measuring metabolic rates in the brain is in principle an uncomplicated business, at least on the biochemist's own terms. But "What is abstract reasoning?" is a much knottier question than "What is cortical glucose?" The speed of an intangible cannot be measured so straightforwardly. The very possibility of correlation is therefore in question. Even some psychometricians have asked whether intelligence is measurable at all if one cannot establish its independence from time.[3] In fact the very notion of speed in intelligence is historically contingent. The assumption that mental processes exist in time and are therefore measurable became embedded only in the nineteenth century, when "mental physiologists," as they then called themselves, got interested in measuring reaction times, and subsequently in measuring the intellectual abilities listed above. Underlying the relationship between intelligence and speed is a deeper, tripartite framework that appears to run across cultures. It seems to be always the case that human intelligence is fast and efficient, or slow and deliberative, or a mean between the two. Each of these three models comes with inseparable cultural baggage: each is *better* than the others. Each dominates a particular period or culture, though closer inspection reveals that at any period of history all three are at work, and that the dominance of one or another is a matter of political and cultural bias.

In the first model, speed is the absolute value. The question "Can the speed of intelligence be measured?" has, buried within it, a positive answer to the quite separate question, "Does quicker mean better?" As victims of the currently dominant model, we instinctively view the other two from its perspective. Where intelligence is by definition fast, the disabled mind must be slow. A mind said to be fast, or even just of average speed, has one prospect, that of intensified productivity; a mind said to be slow, to the point of disability, is marginalized on just these grounds.

The second model is a mean between fast and slow. In classical texts this was axiomatic, the ethical principle being "Nothing to excess." In the Hippocratic medical corpus, intellectual/moral soundness (*phronesis*) consists in a correct blend between fire and water, these being the basic material elements of the universe whose balanced combination makes up the human psyche. Excess fire makes thinking too quick, excess water too slow; in some cases the psyche "rushes forward to too many objects," while in others "the senses meet their objects only spasmodically."[4] In the writings of the Roman medical authority Galen, the mean dominates, with the exception of a single passage that focuses on speed (discussed in detail in the next section). Galenist medical writers of the Renaissance described mental states by the workings of invisible but supposedly material "elements," "humours" and "soul spirits" (more usually called "animal spirits," the living embodiment of *anima* or soul). Mental health consisted in a mean state between excesses and deficiencies such as phrenitis (fast) and lethargy (slow), or mania (fast) and melancholy (slow) or some such. (Renaissance melancholy could in fact express "delirium" as well as "stupidity.") The mean did not exist in a cultural vacuum. Melancholy often meant laziness, a social disorder, or despair, a religious one. Seventeenth-century religious norms in England posed a mean between sectarian Protestant enthusiasm (fast, mad) and Romanist idolatry (slow, idiotic). The big difference in modern psychology is that the mean is no longer a balance between opposing elemental qualities but quantitative, the average value of a single parameter; the ethical desirability of the mean in the ancient model has vanished, though it survives in mutterings about people who are "too clever by half."

---

[2] R. Haier, "Cortical glucose metabolic rate," *Intelligence*, 12 (1988).
[3] Joel Michell, *Measurement in Psychology*, 42.
[4] Hippocrates, *On Regimen*, in *Hippocrates IV*, 281.

The third model is the retrograde of the first. Here slowness is an absolute value. It can be found in parts of the world beyond the reach of the dominant modern European model.[5] Although there has been a tradition of "learned ignorance" in the West too, it is not so much a positive trait as oppositional and ironic; the most widely cited examples, Nicholas of Cusa's *On the Doctrine of Ignorance* and Erasmus's *In Praise of Folly*, celebrate the piety of unlearned people (*idiotae*) in order to criticize the venality of ecclesiastics. When intended seriously, the slow model advocates slowing down one's rational operations to the point of non-existence: knowledge is reached by emptying them from one's mind. Slow and fast model thus meet at their respective extremes, in a state of immediacy: they are alternative ways of being with God.[6] The fool, who is void of rational thought and therefore wide open to divine truths, is somehow similar to the prophet, who intuits them without having to work through a laborious syllogistic process, since in both cases knowledge is achieved in zero time.

The appearance of the fast model in modern psychology

The fast model opposes disability to genius, a word that originally had connotations of frenzy. In the late seventeenth century it began to shake these off, though it remained a form of external inspiration with overtones of instantaneousness and divinity. In this sense genius could seize anyone across the whole social spectrum, from "happy" to "poor," as Issac Watts put it. If it increasingly singled out the exceptional individual, he scarcely yet constituted a type: he was rather a man *of* genius.[7] In science Newton was the exemplar, and following him the late eighteenth-century mathematician Carl Friedrich Gauss, whose genius consisted in the exceptional speed of his arithmetical computations. Meanwhile the Romantics reassigned genius from computation to the imagination. It remained external to the self, however. William Wordsworth's boyhood self is possessed by this genius in *The Prelude* (so too is Newton, whom he mentions there), while the alter ego of that self, *The Idiot Boy*, is possessed by exactly the same force of immediacy.[8]

Science itself subsequently demoted calculation from being the mind's greatest gift to something mechanical.[9] A major example is Charles Babbage, inventor of the calculating machine and an early advocate of time-tested exams. He reassigned the computing tasks to social inferiors, and the mundane information processing to a machine. The genius of the human subject, by contrast, lay in the "maximum efficiency of [the] mental power" that enabled one to rule over computers both mechanical and human, by writing and directing the requisite algebraic calculus of abstraction. According to Babbage, this kind of genius (i.e., his own) models the supreme intelligence of the Almighty.[10] His concern with speed as mental labour saving came partly from his religious upbringing. It can be traced back to the popular seventeenth-century Christian literature of men like Richard Baxter, whose doctrine of social utility ("saving time") was partly an attack on the idleness of "idiots and illiterates" and the threat they posed to social order: a reaction against the corrupt Catholic practice of paying ecclesiastics to buy out time spent in purgatory ("killing time").[11]

---

[5] M. Wober, "Towards an understanding of the Kiganda concept of intelligence," in Berry and Dasen, *Culture and Cognition*.

[6] Michael Dols, *Majnun: the Madman in Medieval Islamic Society*, 370.

[7] See Clive Kilmister, "Genius in mathematics," in P. Murray (ed.), *Genius: the History of an Idea*.

[8] See Patrick McDonagh, *Idiocy: a Cultural History*, 24 ff.

[9] Lorraine Daston, "Enlightenment calculations," *Critical Inquiry*, 21 (1994).

[10] William Ashworth, "Memory, efficiency, and symbolic analysis," *Isis*, 87 (1996).

[11] Richard Fenn, *The Persistence of Purgatory*, 73 ff.

Time had to be redeemed on this earth. It was in any case becoming increasingly important to measure it for the purposes of social administration and production. To this Protestant ethic of time Babbage added the value of speed. It was his "machine intelligence" that Marx had in mind when he described factory production as endowing material forces with intellectual life, and as disabling or "stultifying" (rendering stupid) the human intellect itself by turning it into an adjunct of material force.[12]

The status of calculation within "genius" was subsequently refurbished by Francis Galton, who offered himself as its archetype. One was no longer *possessed by* this genius, one simply *possessed* it. The statistical law of normal distribution, the famous bell-curve, was used at the time only in public administration (risk) and the trajectory of physical objects (weapons design, astronomy). Inspired by Belgian Astronomer Royal Adolphe Quételet's extension of it to human beings – their height – Galton extended it further, to the psychological subject. But do measurers of height, let alone actuaries, arms manufacturers or astronomers, start from the same place as observers of human personality? Study of the latter lies not in an empirically verifiable realm but in the partisan observations made by one group (this group) about what other groups (those people over there) are like. All psychology of intelligence and the emotions is a temporarily formalized manifestation of what the long anthropological and historical view reveals to be just gossip. Galton, like the modern psychology he helped create, did not start from something that was real in any empirical sense. What he did was *first* posit the hypothesis of a quantitative mean and *then* say that, because a mean had been posited, the quantity he was observing must be of something real (Chapter 5 unpicks how this subterfuge works in detail, in Binet's case). A purely abstract mathematical concept was thus prestidigitated into a psychological fact. To amplify an argument of Hacking's, the mean *became* the fact of normal intelligence, while the smallness of the numbers at the extremes of dispersion *became* the facts of outstanding genius and egregious disability.[13]

Intelligence measurement came about as a more or less direct replacement for measurement of reaction times. The seeds for this latter had been sown in 1796 when another Astronomer Royal, the British one, sacked his assistant for making observations of stellar transit that lagged behind his own.[14] He complained not about the assistant being slow, simply about his "confused method"; his observations were simply wrong. (They might equally have resulted from taking the reading too quickly.) The astronomical problem was solved in 1850 with the invention of a reliable chronograph, but it had meanwhile alerted the mental physiologists. For them 1850 was a beginning. In that year Hermann von Helmholtz made his claim that nervous impulses are of finite and therefore relative velocity, and thereby measurable. The idea that "nervous action" was not instantaneous had already been tentatively proposed by astronomers to explain the disparity between the two Greenwich observers. It was resisted by Helmholtz's teacher, the great nineteenth-century physiologist Johannes Müller, who dismissed the astronomers' observational discrepancies as being due simply to the brain's inability to deal with more than one sense-impression at a time.[15] He couched this in terms of faculty psychology, the descriptive system which had dominated discussions of psychology from the Middle Ages and which located the source of human abilities in certain static "faculties" of the brain (imagination, judgment, memory). The quality of these was paramount, and their active operations secondary to it. However, a crucial assumption was already shared on both sides of this dispute, namely that speed is a main constituent of mental activity. It merely had to be decided where these all-important variations of speed should be sought: in the intellectual "faculties" as traditionally conceived, or in experimental study of the nervous system.

---

[12] Simon Schaffer, "Babbage's intelligence," *Critical Inquiry*, 21 (1994).
[13] Hacking, *The Taming of Chance*, 107.
[14] Edwin Boring, *A History of Experimental Psychology*, 133.
[15] Müller, *Elements of Physiology*, 678 ff.

The emergence of modern psychology as a discipline owes much to this victory of mental physiology over faculty psychology. If the speed of the mind was already an issue, its measurability was now in prospect. Gustav Fechner coined the term "psychophysics" for it in 1860. Three years later Wilhelm Wundt succeeded, on the basis of Helmholtz's observations, in showing that perception times vary. The first phase of practical *psycho*metry consisted in a technique known as mental *chrono*metry: time and the mind were one. Mental chronometry, though "a paragon of exactness," was not at first applied to tasks measuring supposedly intellectual abilities of any seriousness.[16] A big leap was still needed. In the 1860s the Dutch physiologist Frans Donders researched reaction times in terms of thought reactions. He asked his subjects to discriminate and choose, rather than simply react to a single stimulus or to stimuli involving only one sense.[17] However, the thoughts involved were little more than perceptions; they merely involved differential rates of reaction between sight and hearing, which hardly seems like the "abstract thinking" that was later to be demanded in cognitive ability tests. Donders himself denied that any but the simplest mental processes could be measured. Wundt tried to complexify them but all he did was bring in the other senses; he added to the experimental conditions (for example, by fuelling the subject with brandy), but not to the intellectuality of the task. At some point, however, speed was to become *constitutive of* intelligence; this took three successive forms.

(1) From Galton's own writings we can detect how the interest in measuring speed in terms of reaction gradually shifted to measuring it in terms of ability. There is a glimpse of it in his comments on the work of Wundt's former assistant James Cattell. Most of the items which Cattell observed under the heading of "mental time" involve reaction to and perception of simple external stimuli; a couple of them seem to involve more complex abilities ("the time of mental association" and "the time it takes to remember and to come to a decision"), but they do not necessarily involve abstraction, logical reasoning or information-processing. Galton's criticism, appended to Cattell's publication of the results, ran:

> One of the most important objects of measurement is hardly if at all alluded to here and should be emphasized. It is to obtain a general knowledge of the capacities of a man by sinking shafts, as it were at a few critical points. In order to ascertain the best points for the purpose, the sets of [reaction-time] measures should be compared with an independent estimate of the man's powers.[18]

In other words, Galton thought there might be a correlation between stimulus-response times and a separately estimated set of "powers" or abilities. The wobbly syllogism must have run, subconsciously: "Fast = good, able = good, therefore able = fast." Now there would have been a problem about measuring some of the actual powers Galton specifies here: being "eager, energetic; well-shaped; successful at games requiring good hand and eye; sensitive; good at music and drawing." This is hardly the stuff of IQ. It resembles rather Gardner's multiple intelligences, or better still the Elizabethan educationist Richard Mulcaster, for whom the sum of human abilities was "to read, to write, to draw, to sing, to play, to have language, to have learning, to have health and activity."[19] It hardly mattered, though, that the powers suggested by Galton were so diffuse as to resist measurement. By 1890 the Wundt-Cattell project of mass measurement of reaction times,

---

[16] See Ruth Benschop and Douwe Draaisma, "In pursuit of precision," *Annals of Science*, 57 (2000).
[17] Josef Brozek and Maarten Sibinga, *Origins of Psychometry*, 12.
[18] James Cattell, "Mental tests and measurement," *Mind*, 15 (1890).
[19] Richard Mulcaster, *Positions wherin those Primitive Circumstances be Examined, which are Necessarie for the Training up of Children*, 208. I have modernized the spelling and (where necessary) the punctuation for quotations, but have maintained the original spelling for book titles.

their master-plan for mapping the whole of "the generalized mind," was itself about to collapse under the weight of its own unmanageable arithmetical detail, and with it therefore (temporarily) any possible hypothesis about correlation between reaction times and general "powers."

Wundt's failure probably helped to divert psychologists' motivations towards measuring the as yet vaguely outlined "powers" and "capacities" instead. Measurement as such, the pursuit of mass data in a society of mass institutions, was the driving principle, and took precedence over whatever object of study it happened to light upon. It was Galton's disciple Karl Pearson who refined the idea of a mass-measured "intelligence." Meanwhile another disciple, Cyril Burt, and another of Wundt's pupils, Charles Spearman, singled out what they chose to nominate as the strictly intellectual component among Galton's "powers." They proposed a unitary or "general" intelligence, g, giving Lewis Terman the conceptual tools with which to refine Binet's mental age scores into IQ. Their reification of intellectual ability (Binet himself had not regarded the individual's score as an immutable fact) made its measurement more feasible. It promised to justify psychology's exact-science status, more so than reaction times. Several decades therefore lapsed before there was a serious effort to reinvestigate the correlation between speed of reaction and the measured set of abilities we now call intelligence. Binet hypothesized a relationship between reaction times and attention span, and there was occasional discussion in the 1920s and 1930s, but these attempts led nowhere (though they did revive the question of speed versus accuracy).[20] Indeed, there was a tradition derived from Herbert Spencer claiming that the correlation was an inverse one, since inferior races had faster reaction times and this was compensation for their inability to abstract or "generalize" as Europeans did.[21]

One factor influencing the revival of interest in speed was information theory, introduced into the study of intelligence in the early 1950s. The human subject no longer received and reproduced information from the environment but "processed" it, in "bits." This inspired two new moves. One was in educational psychology where a member of Eysenck's school, drawing on this doctrine, posited a "complex structure of time" within tests, and concluded that time should be factored independently. A slow accurate performance and a fast inaccurate performance could yield the same score, the score itself being the overriding scientific fact.[22] The other move, closer to Galton's original hypothesis, was Arthur Jensen's. His claim was that fast reaction times do strongly correlate with intelligence and are indeed its best indicator. It involves a fudge, since his definition of information processing covers *both* reaction to stimulus *and* complex reasoning itself. Be that as it may, his claim differs from the way in which predecessors envisaged the relationship between intelligence and reaction time. Reaction time was not then an independent variable (Galton's hints to the contrary being an exception) but just one among several items within the battery of tests itself. For Jensen, on the other hand, intelligence – chiefly "racial intelligence" – is the point, and reaction time not only separate but secondary.[23]

(2) With the shift of interest from reaction times to ability, speed has become a constitutive and practical component of the latter. Tasks have time limits, over which the test administrator has discretion. The pseudo-clinical environment requires precision, a formal termination of the task so that the participant can move on to the next one. The tester has a stopwatch, or at best will ask the subject beforehand to say "I don't know," as a way of identifying the appropriate moment to move on. Limiting the time is more than a banal administrative convenience. It deserves a name of its

---

[20] Edward Thorndike, *The Measurement of Intelligence*, and the series of responses that make up *Archives of Psychology*, 93 (1928); see also Raymond Fancher, *The Intelligence Men*, 59.

[21] Graham Richards, *"Race", Racism and Psychology*, 21, 32.

[22] W.D. Furneaux, "Intellectual abilities," in Eysenck (ed.), *Handbook of Abnormal Psychology*, 167.

[23] Arthur Jensen, "Reaction time and psychometric g," in Eysenck (ed.), *A Model for Intelligence*.

own: *ability time*. The social processes at work here had already been operating on the Astronomer Royal. On his observations depended not just the calibration of the Greenwich clock but thereby all observations of place and time in industry and social administration. Meanwhile speed and its measurement became fundamental to educational psychology at the same time as it became fundamental to factory labour and Frederick Taylor's industrial psychology. Commodification of time was the basis both for psychology and for the wider demands of the economy. (This is also the historical context in which the British colonial service became the first European working environment to assess abilities by time-tested exams.)[24] The Book of Ecclesiastes can be ignored: the race is to the swift. In the test situation you may puzzle at length over the very concept of a correct or incorrect response to some task; in fact this will be quite probable if you have a philosophy of science doctorate or an extra 21-chromosome. But as in the world of manual and intellectual labour, the clock dictates. You are moved on to the next task, having scored zero.

(3) More recently a third phenomenon has emerged: the *constant intensification of ability time*. This is reflected in the information-processing components of cognitive ability tests. In the abstraction tasks of the Wechsler psychometric scales which now dominate the field, a correct answer given quickly scores higher than a correct answer given more slowly. Its historical context is the increased concentration of intellectual labour in the economy, and the intensification of the flows by which communications networks dominate social space. Meanwhile the "efficiency theory" of brain function now claims that the brain achieving a higher IQ score and working more quickly uses proportionately less energy. This doctrine is based on studies of people with disabilities labelled intellectual in whom inefficiency is presupposed to be a neurological slowness of intellect – a method not only circular but demonstrating just how co-dependent the concepts of intelligence and intellectual disability are. Moreover, this biochemical efficiency (fast intellect as energy-saving) seems to have its roots in fiscal efficiency: fast intellects are time-redeeming, the eugenic elimination of slow intellects a saving on public costs.[25] In the vanguard of this movement towards constant intensification are the transhumanists, who warn that human beings must aim at developing their intellects sufficiently to compete with the exponentially increasing information-processing speeds of computers. Their inspiration is artificial intelligence, itself modelled on the neuronal networks of the human brain, which envisages (as in the recent title of Gregory Stock) a "Metaman: the merging of humans and machines into a global superorganism," and an incorporation of machine speeds in human thought processes to pursue Babbage's mission.[26]

The fast model and the distortion of the mean

Psychometrics, in the form of IQ, now presupposes the fast model. The sophisticated reader may already consider IQ a dead duck, and there have indeed been enough lethal critiques of it to stuff a museumful of ducks, the most effective coming from within the discipline itself.[27] But IQ remains active theoretically because all the abilities deemed to define what is specifically human (information-processing, logical reasoning, abstraction, etc.) seem to consist in something

---

[24] Gillian Sutherland, *Ability, Merit and Measurement*, 97, 115.

[25] F. Song et al, "Screening for fragile X syndrome," *Health Technology Assessment Publications*, 7 (2003).

[26] See also Nick Bostrom, "How long before superintelligence?" *International Journal of Futures Studies*, 2 (1998).

[27] Michell, *Measurement in Psychology*; Richards, "Getting the intelligence controversy knotted," *Bulletin of the British Psychological Society*, 37 (1984).

measurable, even if one might want to ask whether they are not specifically human *because* they are measurable. And it remains active institutionally because psychology is now, as Burt more or less acknowledged it to be, a sub-branch of social administration, providing a rationale for rulebooks that differentiate and segregate "intellectually disabled" people from the rest of us.[28] IQ has also been given a fresh lease on life by biotechnology; in association with twin studies, it constitutes the very *raison d'être* of the new cognitive geneticists, whose anxieties tend to hone in on the same group of people. We do not yet know the total number of shots that must be fired into IQ's corpse for a pronouncement of death to be forensically sound; the answer lies not with psychologists or historians but in social processes in which the importance of speed is currently increasing, not diminishing. IQ's rise has been well documented and I do not propose to go over it again.[29] Its history is relevant here only to illustrate how it has incorporated notions of speed. Speed was perhaps the first object of psychological investigation that looked as if it might exist in the same realm as physics. But even if one accepts that mental processes exist in time and therefore their speed is measurable, this in itself does not itself supply the exact-science status which psychology seeks, because the reality of any "intelligence" whose speed might be measurable is – unlike a stopwatch – dependent on a shifting human consensus across history and social groups.

Since the emergence of psychology as a formal discipline, the case for the fast model has seemed to need no justification. It is simply a part of a socio-economic machine that demands maximum yield from commodified ability-time: a machine in which psychology is a cog. In a sense, the fast model has not obliterated the others even now. The idea of the mean persists in today's doctrines. However, it would have been unrecognizable as such to pre-moderns. The classical mean meant "moderation in all things." The statistical mean presents us with a bell-shaped curve in which at one end speed is desirable and superior, while at the other end the slow intellect is to be avoided as self-evidently pathological. One would not describe as *too* fast a brilliant mathematician whose ability score lies at the opposite deviation from people labelled with severe disability, even if he or she is looked on as a freak. Greek philosophers would have been bemused by a mean where a greater value is placed on one of two extremes; that is why early statisticians decided to change the terminology so that genius ceased to be described as "error" (the original term in statistical physics) and became, less pejoratively, an upward "deviation from the mean."[30]

If the ethical aspect of the mean does still register with modern psychology, the ways of dealing with it are necessarily tortuous. The Nazis, for example, noted that non-whites were slow and unintelligent, but also that the Jews were pre-eminent in intellectual life. They lacked racial strength and character, however, since according to Ernst Rüdin, the founding father of psychiatric genetics and author of Hitler's Law for the Prevention of Hereditarily Diseased Offspring, their "quickness of understanding" made them *too* clever.[31] A more recent example is the cognitive diagnosis known as hyperlexia, a "developmental disability" whose symptoms are "reading too soon … a precocious ability to read words far above what would be expected at [the child's] chronological age." Hyperlexia fills the vacant deviation opposite dyslexia, balancing out reading norms with a bell curve of their own. But it can only do so by accommodating the contradictory terms "ability" and "disability" in the same diagnosis, as above. On the websites, parental excitement at the advanced development of their children is reflected paradoxically in their adoption of a "Why me?" profile otherwise ascribed to parents of children with severe

---

[28] Burt, *Mental and Scholastic Tests*, Preface to second edition.
[29] See Daniel Kevles, *In the Name of Eugenics*; Richard Lewontin et al., *Not in Our Genes*.
[30] Donald Mackenzie, *Statistics in Britain*, 56.
[31] Cited in Joseph, *The Gene Illusion*, 25.

disability; conversely, the parental literature on dyslexia is at pains to emphasize the child's intellectual normality and to remove the moral taint of disability.[32]

If the mean survives in this strange form, the slow model is marginal as never before. People marked out by modern intellectual disability face a dilemma. Do they resist the dominant fast model and pursue a radically slow existence, admired for the traits that make them different and making a virtue out of their supposed developmental plateau? In this sense they are a residue of Rousseau's natural man, setting a moral example by their uninhibitedness and other childlike characteristics. Or do they try their limited best to catch up with the norm, getting their small achievements recognized just as the coat tails of the last non-disabled person vanish into the distance ahead of them? Both of these prospects for slow people marginalize them. Either: disabled people are a type that constitutes a complete difference in kind, celebrating diversity in defiance of conformism and prevailing norms; marginalization then ensues because these norms are in fact proof against defiance, and the psychological difference thus celebrated can only reinforce the social segregation which the norms themselves have created. Or: the modicum of abilities they do possess, constituting a difference in degree only, is pursued as far as possible, thus showing that they are more or less the same as anyone else; marginalization then ensues because in fact it always turns out to be "less": norms are engineered to ensure that they never catch up. Slow people have the prospect of a futile running backwards and forwards from one to the other model. Any further alternative would presuppose a deep change in the structures of social organization.

---

[32] See P.G. Aaron, *Dyslexia and Hyperlexia*.

Chapter 4
Quick Wit and the Ingenious Gentleman

We saw above that there is a world of difference between the ancient philosophers and the Western tradition which has claimed them as the fountainhead of its own ideas, at least in respect to the topics we are discussing – if not quite so much difference between the Western tradition and those sophists, ideologues and educators who were bound to the political and social institutions of Greece and Rome. Nevertheless, the classical philosophical texts were the starting point, however interpreted and read, for most writers on faculty psychology and human behaviour from the late Middle Ages onwards. What sources did they use in placing an increasing value on the fast model?

The classical source-texts

We can begin with Plato's *Theaetetus*, in which the relationship between mind and external reality appears as a receipt, processing and storage of information. This passage is much cited by early modern writers.[1] Modern historians have claimed it to be a primitive, "incomplete and tortuously argued" account of modern cognitive psychology.[2] *Theaetetus* is not in fact a psychology text but a philosophical one, about the difference between knowing and believing, and concludes that while we cannot know anything for sure, we can at least say whether or not our opinions are rationally justified. At one point Socrates slyly coaxes his promising young interlocutor Theaetetus into saying that of course we can achieve certain knowledge. Socrates disingenuously agrees with him. The psyche is – or is like – a wax tablet, he says. We perceive objects in the external world through our senses, and these objects reach the human soul as "signs" on the wax. (Stoic philosophers used the word "impressions" for the same thing, thereby launching a still prevalent way of speaking about the mind.)[3] The signs should be of optimum clarity, depth and duration. Ideally, the person who "learns easily" (he is *eumathes*) remembers what he has learned and does not confuse one sign with another. The result is certain knowledge. However, the soul's wax may be too soft, or too hard. Where it is soft and can receive signs, the person may be a good learner; but wax tends to melt and so his memory is bad, because the signs become difficult to distinguish from each other. The result in this case is false opinion. Where the wax is hard, he "learns with difficulty" (he is *dusmathes*). What he does learn he remembers well, but the signs are once more unclear, this time because they are only faintly impressed. The result again is false opinion: "When such people see or hear or think, they cannot assign each [external object] to its corresponding [sign] quickly; they are slow, and because they assign them to the wrong places they largely see, hear and think incorrectly."

Plato is at the very least ambiguous about speed here. Quick impressions seem at first sight to be a good thing. But if being quick means having a bad memory, speed cannot lead to rationally justifiable opinion. Perhaps one can simply be *too* quick, making a mean speed preferable? But Plato's criticism runs deeper. At the start of the dialogue, he has Socrates praise Theaetetus for possessing *both* a good memory *and* "quick thinking" (*agkhinoia*). Praise from Socrates usually means that the interlocutor is going to be taken down a peg, and indeed it turns out he has encouraged

---

[1] Plato, *Theaetetus*, 194c.
[2] Daniel Robinson, *An Intellectual History of Psychology*, 52.
[3] A.A. Long and D.N. Sedley, *The Hellenistic Philosophers*, 236 ff.

the speedy young tyro to approve the wax tablet model with the precise purpose of informing him forthwith that it is nonsense.

All this suggests that Plato positively distrusts speed. We have already seen that in his Utopian state of *The Laws* people who are slow, illiterate or find learning difficult are qualified for political office as long as they use the abilities they do possess to moderate their pleasures. His distrust of immoderate people with fast-moving psyches is reflected in the wax tablet model. This model seems to be someone else's, which he is lampooning because it reduces the search for knowledge to something mechanical. He refers here to the "all-wise Homer's" admiration for "rough, dirty" psyches, and any time Plato mentions poets we know his intentions are ironic. His target is the sophists. They are the ones with the dirty minds. From everything we know about Plato, he would surely have thought it trivial to describe the act of knowing in quasi-material terms drawn from the first thing that happens to be lying around, namely the wax tablet on which the student was taking his lecture notes (about the wax tablet); he would have mocked, on the same grounds, a model of human cognitive ability based on the information-processing properties of the psychology student's laptop. His attack on the sophistic ideology of knowledge as merely instrumental – a matter of self-advancement – involves attacking their predilection for speed.

Aristotle touches on the wax tablet model in his own account of the psyche.[4] Some have taken this as a gloss on Plato's text.[5] More probably both men were referring to an already prevalent idea, independently of each other (it also turns up in the Greek drama).[6] Aristotle's most influential text on speed was not these passing remarks, however, but certain others in *Posterior Analytics*, a work that deals with logic. His logic is a set of objective structures; inasmuch as some corresponding subjective element is involved, it consists in the individual's laborious elaboration of demonstrative proofs, from intuited first principles. In a brief aside, Aristotle asks us to distinguish this logic-related understanding (*to epistasthai*) from three other things: opinion, sense perceptions and "quick thinking" (*agkhinoia*).[7] The first two obviously bear no resemblance to a logic-related understanding. Quick thinking, however, reaches conclusions similar to the latter. It too discovers the middle term of a syllogism, the connection between two intuited givens. It differs, however, in that it occurs "without pause for thought." It is not just that a fully elaborated logic-related understanding takes longer; the length of time is a mark of its value, whereas quick thinking is mundane, takes short cuts and thus does not really follow logic at all. It arises only in chaotic situations that for practical reasons *resist* the careful building up of syllogistic proof. Aristotle uses as an example the decisions made by military commanders or midwives: empirical ones, by contrast with logic-related understanding, which involves philosophical and mathematical first principles. Nevertheless it was "quick thinking" that Renaissance medical writers would find interesting in Aristotle. And more importantly, in claiming adherence to Aristotle, they were to confuse quick thinking with a full-blown subjective capacity for logic, and to pass it off as the latter.

The Renaissance writers' chief reference point on speed was in fact neither Plato nor Aristotle but Galen. Where today we speak about mental processes and abilities, Galen in *The Art of Medicine* was concerned with the health of a bodily organ, the brain, of which mental processes were just one organic facet. Unusual brain states were not ultimately fixed or determinate in any individual; pre-modern medicine held no place for geniuses or idiots. As for speed, a key passage (much commented on by Renaissance Galenists) ran:

---

[4] Aristotle, *On the Soul*, 430a; *On Memory*, 450b.
[5] Draaisma, *Metaphors of Memory*, 24.
[6] Aeschylus, *Prometheus Bound*, l.789.
[7] Aristotle, *Posterior Analytics*, 89b.

Quick apprehension indicates a fine brain substance, slowness a thick one. Ease of learning indicates a good receipt of impressions, and [good] memory indicates a stable one. Correspondingly, difficulty in learning indicates a difficulty in receiving impressions, and forgetfulness a fluidity in this respect.[8]

Galen seems less critical of speed here than Plato or Aristotle, but in the ensuing passage he recommends a balance between too much and too little "stability of opinion." Galen's treatment of mental states usually has some moral twist, so perhaps by juxtaposing quick thinking with excessively shifting opinion he wants to contrast them: the first is a desirable type of speed, the second an undesirable one. Be that as it may, even if Galen does take fast to mean good, he means good in a narrow sense: speed indicates that the substance of the brain is physically healthy.

We see from the classical texts how all three models can be at work simultaneously. Plato and Aristotle are so suspicious of quick thinking that their insistence on the mean actually seems to approve the slow. The fast model dominated public life. The Odyssean quick-wittedness on which Athenians prided themselves was appropriate to a febrile merchant economy in which the sophists forged their mercenary vocations; quick thinking was supposedly Pericles's outstanding characteristic, and he spun this image of itself to the democracy. It was an image foreign to the land-owning class to which the philosophers mostly belonged. Their disdain for it is evident in Socrates's ironic references to himself being slow on the uptake. Gentlemen of leisure did not have to hurry; Plato's and Aristotle's student Theophrastus, in his seminal study of character types, allocates speed of movement to the labouring classes. Galen's more ambiguous attitude to speed may have been due to his closer personal links to Roman state power, its sophists, rhetoricians and educators.

The arrival of quick wit on the medical curriculum

The seeds of an intelligence specific to humans were sown during the twelfth-century beginnings of modern capitalism, with the expansion of trade and urban populations and consequently of ecclesiastical and state administration. The universities arose partly as training schools for these purposes. In this context, intelligence was both a theological concept that would gradually lose its divine connotations and descend to earth, and a quotidian concept ("wit") that would eventually rise to a higher, quasi-divine level.

We can trace the importance of speed to this process from standard medical textbooks. Most important were the many Renaissance commentaries on *The Art of Medicine*, which of all Galen's works had the most influence on European medicine. In one or the other of its two Latin translations this work had a permanent place, together with Avicenna's *Canon*, in the many versions of the basic compendium supplied to all medical students from the mid-twelfth century onwards. Known as the *Articella*, this compendium also had a cultured readership well beyond the medical realm. Galen's brief remark on the relationship between speed and mental states thereby entered the mind-set of the learned doctor and of other professionals with the arrival of university-based medical teaching. There it stayed, variously reinterpreted, until the eighteenth century. In addition to the two Latin translations, at least eight commentaries on *The Art of Medicine* had appeared before 1500; a century later this number had doubled.[9] Two books in particular, from the Italian heart of European medicine, were added to the standard curriculum: Pietro Torrigiano's commentary on Galen, written in Bologna around 1300 and first printed in 1489 with the two translations, and

---

[8] Galen, *Ars Medica*, in C. Kühn, *Opera*, i, 319.
[9] Per Gunnar Ottosson, *Scholastic Medicine*; Timo Joutsivuo, *Scholastic Tradition*.

Niccolò Leoniceno's revision of these latter, first published in 1508. These are the authorities most often cited by Renaissance doctors.

In paraphrasing the classical source-texts Torrigiano, possibly inspired by his teacher Taddeo Alderotti, made certain crucial elisions. First, he created a short circuit between logic as a set of objective structures and a logical reasoning that goes on in the human subject. Whereas for Aristotle syllogisms had their own objective structures from which the subject's "logic-related understanding" was well separated, for Torrigiano logical structures arise directly from human reasoning; "composing and separating phantasmata," the human ability for abstraction, somehow just "end up in" a syllogism, i.e., in the phantasmata correctly abstracted.[10] Secondly, he identified Aristotle's logic-related understanding, a patient elaboration of syllogisms, with the "quick thinking" that Aristotle had dismissed as having nothing to do with logic. Torrigiano took them to be the same thing. And of the two, it was the "quickness" term (*agkhinoia*, Latin *solertia*) that he used to describe this new amalgam. Quick thinking now just *is* logical understanding, rather than a spurious, rushed imitation of it. Thirdly, he solemnized the marriage of Galen to Aristotle. He assumes that when they wrote about quick thinking they were sharing a mutually comprehensible concept, though there is nothing in either author to suggest that Galen had been referring to his predecessor.

Leoniceno's revised Latin translation of *The Art of Medicine* reinforced these elisions, in such a way that speed started to invade the domain of ability. In one of the two standard translations, "quick thinking" (*agkhinoia*) had been rendered as *solertia* (an exact Latin equivalent) or *praesentia*, "presence of mind"; in the other it was rendered as "ease of learning," probably as a result of this latter appearing in an adjacent passage of Galen's original. Leoniceno retranslated *agkhinoia* as *ingenium*, and this then became standard.[11] It was usually rendered as "wit" in English, though I shall retain the Latin term to avoid confusion with other contemporary resonances of wit (superficial cleverness, the external senses or "five wits," etc.). Leoniceno claimed here to be getting closer to the original Greek. But in fact *ingenium* was ambiguous. In late medieval philosophy it had been something quite unlike quick thinking: it was the technical term for the meticulous discovery of the linking terms in syllogisms, the "logic-related understanding" described by Aristotle; it was used thus by Albert the Great, doyen of the early scholastic philosophers.[12] Leoniceno, by contrast, was a pioneering humanist who made a point of distancing himself from medieval convention. When he used *ingenium* for "quickness of apprehension" he had in mind not the scholastics' term but the everyday Roman sense of the word, which did indeed signify an everyday cleverness. Moreover, it had speed as its foremost quality; the humanists' authority Cicero commends *ingenium* for precisely this reason.[13] With his "improved" translation Leoniceno was therefore making a point. Humanist writers, in their dedicatory prefaces to books on medicine, law and other professional disciplines, praise each other interminably for their "ingenious" qualities. That was how they liked to see themselves: clever and up to speed.

Two quite distinct primary meanings of *ingenium* were therefore available: one descriptive (of an operation of the intellect), the other normative (a judgement on its performance, in terms of speed). In medieval and early modern psychology, operations and performances were sharply distinct categories, even if for today's psychologist operations just *are* performances. Renaissance writers would still have been aware of the distinction; in Shakespeare's *Love's Labour's Lost*, for

---

[10] Pietro Torrigiano, *Plusquam Commentum in Parvam Galeni Artem*, 39v–54r.
[11] Niccolò Leoniceno, *Galeni Ars Medicinalis*, 295.
[12] Albert, *Summa de Creaturis*, in Borgnet (ed.), xxxiv, 516.
[13] Cicero, *On Oratory*, 80; see also E. Hidalgo-Serna, "The philosophy of 'ingenium'," *Philosophy and Rhetoric*, 13 (1980).

example, the comic parody of scholastic debate between Moth and Don Armado hinges precisely on whether or not "ingenious" means quick. Nevertheless, the boundary between the two usages would gradually erode.

The fast model in Renaissance Europe

Before tracing this erosion in detail, we need first to know something about the conceptual framework in which they lay, the Renaissance's overall doctrines of soul, mind and intellect. One important aspect of this was the tension between doctors' pagan-derived medical theories and the demands of Christian theology.[14] Galen was known to have been sceptical about the soul or psyche being immaterial, since he seemed to say that it was just a variety of combinations of bodily temperament, which then explained the individual "differences in character that make people spirited or otherwise, thoughtful or otherwise."[15] Aristotle seemed to be more ambiguous; he regarded the psyche as the set of abilities that animates and maintains the body, rather than something simply inextricable from it. And in an isolated and much-touted remark in *On the Soul*, he said that intuited intellect (*nous*) comes to human beings "from outside"; theologians cited this as evidence that he thought of the soul as immaterial, perhaps even immortal. If Aristotle could be reconciled thus with religion, and Galen and Aristotle with each other, then it might be possible to make Galen a quasi-Christian, despite his evident materialism. Medical writers tried to match theological truths with their own expert ones, which had uncomfortably pagan origins in these classical writers. They asked themselves: in pursuing medicine, how do we defend the immateriality and immortality of the soul against arguments to the contrary – heretic and atheist arguments which may (heaven forbid) even suggest themselves to us, since our textual authorities are pagan? Defence of the soul's immortality was central to Christian Galenist theory about the human intellect and (as we shall see later) to early modern psychology. It was driven by the same degree of obsession as defence of the white ruling class's superior minds later drove Galton.

Another important element in the conceptual framework was the theory of faculty psychology. Closest to God, or in some versions overlapping with him, is man's "rational soul" (sometimes called the "intellective" soul). Closest to corrupt, mortal flesh and its passions are the five "external senses." In between are the "internal senses," consisting of certain intellectual faculties organically linked to the body: imagination, "reason" in the sense of human reasoning (also "judgement," or some such term) and memory. Imagination is anatomically located in the front ventricle of the brain. This receives images from the external world via the external senses and brings them together in a "common sense," which then assigns these particulars to certain universal ideas. Reasoning or judgement, in the middle ventricle, contemplates the ideas, joining premises to conclusions (though this part of the picture is especially prone to variation). The ideas are then stored in memory, in the rear ventricle. Some version of this model remained intact for centuries.[16] It survived the arrival of new theories of brain anatomy that rejected ventricular localization; and it proved adaptable to the wholesale changes in medical theory of the mid-seventeenth century, influencing medical education well into the eighteenth. It also entered the wider culture. Locke

---

[14] See Pietro D'Abano, *Conciliator Controversiarum*, 114.
[15] Galen, *Quod Animi Mores*, in Kühn (ed.), *Opera*, iv, 786.
[16] See Ruth Harvey, *The Inward Wits*; George Bruyn, "The seat of the soul," in F. Rose and W. Bynum (eds), *Historical Aspects of the Neurosciences*; Katharine Park, "The organic soul," in C. Schmitt and Q. Skinner (eds), *The Cambridge History of Renaissance Philosophy*; Eckhard Kessler, "The intellective soul," in ibid.

preserves the basic faculty psychology framework for his discussion of intellectual operations in the *Essay concerning Human Understanding*, and John Milton uses it in Book 5 of *Paradise Lost* to describe God's creation of Adam: two works which no educated British person of the eighteenth century could fail to know.

This crude outline of faculty psychology will do for the moment, but a caveat is needed. Whereas in the classical texts the soul (*psyche, anima*) has plenty of work to do, in medieval philosophy this sense of activity has been taken over by the understanding (*intellectus*), now the more "animate" entity of the two. Early modern medical and philosophical sources tend to remain unclear whether by "soul" they mean the Christian idea of some divine, semi-detached haze that just hovers around us, or our working faculties (in which sense it is often indistinguishable from *mens*, "mind"). In the mainstream of scholasticism, the character of the faculties involved in *intellectus* to a certain extent drifted towards the realm occupied by *anima*. Aquinas, for example, is interested in the faculties mainly because their existence deductively proves the nature of the soul, and he is therefore less interested in their active operations. In the fourteenth century there was a minority view, prefiguring Juan Luis Vives, Michel de Montaigne and Locke among others, which sought a detailed account of those operations, proceeding empirically after a fashion.[17] However, this belonged to a rarified, metaphysical school of thought; in the broad scheme of things, the concretization and reification of the detailed operational activities of the mind is a historical development of the early modern period.

Resuming now our discussion of the rise of wit or *ingenium*, we shall see that (1) the operations increasingly took precedence over the faculties to which they belonged and to which they had once been secondary; (2) the distinction between performance and operation began to be elided, with the result that speed becomes normative; and (3) regardless of whether the description of faculty psychology becomes simplified or more complicated, the operation of *ingenium* tends to assume leadership. Strictly speaking, *ingenium* was one operation of one faculty, the imagination. Indeed, that is what it remained in many texts through to Galenism's last eighteenth-century gasp. But there was also constant renaming and reclassifying of certain operations from one faculty to the other, in which *ingenium* was often reassigned to the superior reasoning faculty.[18] Once Leoniceno's humanist contemporary Pietro Pomponazzi had disrupted European intellectual life by asserting that the existence of the rational soul was a matter for faith alone, not scientific demonstration, the desire for a demonstrable knowledge of man's place in nature refocused on the detail of intellectual activity. As one of his disciples put it: "the soul of man is a substance by which man is man, that is one in its essence and many in its virtues and faculties: to which … many instruments are available," and it was the latter with their operations that needed investigation, rather than the faculty as such.[19]

In addition, an already existing minority theory which said that the faculties were localized in various sections of the brain, always controversial, became increasingly so. It had materialist implications. If an injury occurred to imagination or memory, did it only affect that faculty, or might it not affect the reasoning faculty too? And if so, why not the immaterial soul as well? To the usual examples of brain injury or sleep, the sixteenth century's philosophy curriculum now added that of "the stupid" (*stulti ac fatui*), though as usual whom the author means by this is an open question.[20] It highlighted the more fundamental question: if there is an immaterial rational soul,

---

[17] J. Zupko, "What is the science of the soul? A case study in the evolution of late medieval natural philosophy," *Synthese*, 110 (1997).

[18] For example Nicolas Coeffeteau, *A Table of Humane Passions*, Preface.

[19] Simone Porzio, *De Humana Mente*, 36.

[20] Gregor Reisch, *Margarita Philosophica*, 457.

how does it link to intellectual faculties that belong to a material bodily organ, the brain? Are these organic intellectual faculties partly separate from the higher rational soul, or merely (as Albert had described them) "accidents" or secondary "qualities" of it?[21] Under such sceptical questioning, the initial instinct was to add categories or subdivide existing ones. But some writers clearly felt that this increased complexity only made things worse. Instead, they simplified. Many went so far as to treat the numerous conflicting names for various faculties and operations as a homogeneous lump, a unitary "mind."[22] From the 1630s, René Descartes's mind/body dualism was there to encourage them, but medical men interested in the psychological faculties had not waited for him to tell them.

Over time, then, the word *ingenium* often came to describe not just the operation (one among several) of one faculty, but a whole faculty or ability in itself. Speed became entangled with the notion of a single overarching *ingenium*, especially among medical writers. This Ciceronian usage of the term dominates commentaries on *The Art of Medicine*. Oddo degli Oddi writes not about *ingenium* alone but about *ingenium et ars* (skill), as if they were equivalent, whereas in scholastic philosophy they had represented a contrast between the theoretical and the mundane.[23] Oddi also fuses *ingenium* with previously suspect "ease of learning": both "belong to the [immaterial] rational soul itself." *Ingenium* "not only discourses, composes and divides easily, but previously apprehends singulars easily," thereby straddling both the imaginative and reasoning faculties. Salvo Sclano employs *ingenium* and *tarditas* (slowness) as a contrasting pair, while Giovanni Argenterio criticizes a fellow commentator for using "speed" (*celeritas*) as a synonym for *ingenium* on the grounds that the latter is not *only* speed, it is synonymous with the intellect as a whole.[24] Jérémie de Dryvere uses this latter argument about *ingenium* being an overarching principle to refute the localization of faculties in the brain and its materialist implications, which seduced the vulgar, "common herd of physicians"; partly, then, this move towards homogenization under the aegis of wit was a move towards sounder theological principle.[25]

The humanistic *ingenium*, with its connotations of speed, gained prominence through this reduction of complexities. Scholastic philosophers had allocated speed no special value in any of the various operations of the reasoning faculty such as *discursus* (the relating of premises to conclusions), *contemplatio* ("study" or meditation on these) or even *discretio* (their subsequent application), let alone the *ingenium* as they conceived it. On the rare occasion when operations are described in terms of speed, they are *so* quick as to take place in zero time, and then only in angels, "prophets" or exceptional humans who have "an extemporary knowledge, and upon the first motion of their reason do what we cannot do without study or deliberation."[26] But in the Renaissance this territory was invaded by the more everyday quick-wittedness of *ingenium*, as the humanists conceived it. The basic stuff of the soul – its "substance" – came to be homogenized with its various faculties; the faculty was homogenized with one of its operations, *ingenium* or wit; and the whole came to be homogenized with the performance criteria – speed included – of that operation, blurring the previously fundamental category distinction between potentiality and actuality.

The distinction between everyday intellectual activity and the immaterial intellect formerly located "beyond the wit of man" also began to disappear. "Wit" is already ambiguous in the fourteenth-century *Piers Plowman* of William Langland, who at one point personifies it as

---

[21] Albert, *Summa de Creaturis*, 335.
[22] Katharine Park, "Albert's influence on late medieval psychology," in J.A. Weisheipl (ed.), *Albertus Magnus and the Sciences*.
[23] Oddo degli Oddi, *Expositio ... Artis Medicinalis*, 132.
[24] Salvo Sclano, *Commentaria ... Artis Medicinalis*, 319; Giovanni Argenterio, *In Artem Medicinalem*, 218.
[25] Jérémie de Dryvere, *In Τεχνην Galeni*, 120.
[26] Thomas Browne, *Religio Medici*, 37.

the lazy, henpecked swine of a husband before whom Dame Study (*contemplatio*) casts her pearls of wisdom, while at others Langland already clearly sees wit as close to wisdom itself.[27] The social sources of this elevation in the status of wit lay in a growing bureaucracy of clerks and *literati*, who administered the burgeoning fields of canon and civil law for their rulers and developed authentification systems for establishing the status of their superiors, both social and religious, through canonization. R.I. Moore has described this shift, starting in the eleventh century, as the triumph of aspirational clerks over the illiterate. Sucking up also meant spitting down: "Common interests, common values and common loyalties were expressed in bottomless contempt for those who did not share their skills: ... the illiterates, *idiota*, *rusticus* – all words used regularly to describe those accused of heresy, and expressing perhaps the broadest and most universal of the stereotypes ..., like those of heresy, leprosy [and] Jewry."[28] Around 1200 lepers were banned from inheriting property, as idiots were later to be, and were segregated by law; leprosy was a "disease of the soul." Fear was expressed in the language of contamination, contributing both to the solidarity of the group operating the administrative systems and eventually to the status elevation of wit in general; melancholia and then idiocy replaced leprosy as better approximations to the opposite of whatever it was the administrative caste prided itself on. This was a lengthy process, as gentry and episcopate – i.e., those with an ability to present themselves as the channels of social and religious status – continued trying to beat off fellow-*literati* further down the ladder. If only very loosely, we can associate speed with more radical individuals among the latter group, encouraged by the onset of humanism.

Resistances to the fast model

With exactly the same theological intent as those who were reducing faculty psychology to an all-important *ingenium*, some commentators took the opposite line and resisted the erosion of category boundaries. Francisco Vallés, physician to Philip II of Spain, warned against confusing *ingenium*, which as a mere operation can vary according to individual performance, with the unalloyed immaterial intellect "which is in all of us *per se* by its own perfection."[29] Battista Fiera's commentary of 1515 attributed speed to *ingenium* alone, a discrete and subordinate "operation" which "moves very quickly to track down the middle term and cause." He warns against identifying it with the whole faculty or ability (*potentia*) and in particular with the immaterial rational soul, attacking the dunces "who believe that Galen thought of the faculty and the operation as the same thing."[30] Whereas Torrigiano had earlier *assumed* the existence of an immaterial soul, Fiera is now having to *defend* it, though of course that was what the homogenizers were trying to do, too. He interweaves biblical authority with earthly, often pre-Christian ones: a rhetorical intrusion of theology into faculty psychology and medical theory about the brain that was to become routine a century later, among those who coined the term "psychology."

A different form of resistance to this trend towards homogenizing *ingenium* with speed can be seen in Giambattista da Monte, an unlikely conservative since he had studied with Leoniceno and was himself, in many respects, the most radical innovator of Italian Renaissance medicine. For him it was not just the blurring of boundaries between faculty and operation, ability and performance, that was the mistake, but the actual value placed on speed. He criticized "the new men" not just

---

[27] Langland, *The Vision of Piers Plowman* (B-Text), 10.5; 5.587.
[28] *The Formation of a Persecuting Society*, 139.
[29] *Galeni Ars Medicinalis*, 31.
[30] *Commentaria ... in Artem Medicinalem*, ii, unpaginated.

for over-simplifying the elaborate apparatus of scholastic tradition but on the more particular grounds that they judged performance by speed when it should really be judged in terms of depth and penetration. Albert had thought of *ingenium* as "subtlety," says Da Monte. "It conceives the minutest thing ... so that it contains all the differentiations of that thing, completely and perfectly, and nothing is lacking from those differences ... all the way to the bottom."[31] Endorsing Plato, Da Monte insists that *ingenium* and "ease of learning" are quite distinct: "those who learn easily or rather apprehend easily, are not *ingeniosi*. People like this, while they very easily learn, just as easily forget." And whereas *ingenium* consists in "weighing carefully," easy learners use their powers "precipitately" and "suddenly." It may in fact be better to be slow. For Da Monte, speed is simply excess: rashness and nothing else. As in Plato, it precludes accuracy, and for Da Monte it also precludes comprehensiveness. Where Plato had made his point ironically, Da Monte makes his by straining the vocabulary of speed and forcing its terms (*agkhinoia, solertia*) to mean "depth" and "penetration" instead.

The concept of depth was not in fact so conservative, since it suggested a greater *complexity* of the mind, which may thereby be empirically observable, even if it does not reveal its secrets at all quickly. Montaigne's disciple Pierre Charron held "the mind of man" to be "a dark and deep abyss, an intricate labyrinth, full of corners and creeks, and secret lurking places: such is the disposition and state of this exalted part of the soul, distinguished by the term of *intellectual*, which consists of vastly many ... faculties, and operations, and different movements, each of which have their proper names and each of them infinite doubts and difficulties peculiar to them."[32] The soul should be studied, he says, not via the faculties but via these operations. Vives, in his description of *ingenium* as one of the human or "natural graces" and "a universal virtue of our minds," was "less interested in what the soul is, but rather *how* it is and which are its *effects*."[33]

The Cartesian mind, on the other hand, might seem the ultimate reduction of faculty psychology. But Descartes himself looks backwards as well as forwards. The text that lays the groundwork for the famous "method" of "the ingenious Descartes," as he was called, bore the title "Rules for the Direction of the *Ingenium*." He uses this term for the general activating principle of all the faculties. He prefers the one disembodied half of a dualistic model to the complexly arranged faculties noted above; but in so doing he also in some sense preserves them. In the sense that it is an activating principle, his *ingenium* has the characteristics of an operation, which is what the scholastics had said it was; but precisely because it activates faculties (imagination, reasoning, memory) which the scholastics had seen as prior but somehow inert, it somehow becomes a faculty itself. It is above all *ingenium*, not the static faculties nor even mind, reason, intellect or soul (*animus*), that separates man from beast-machine: "Nothing quite like this power [of *ingenium*] is found in corporeal things .... According to [the] different functions the same power is also called either pure intellect, or imagination, or memory, or sense-perception; but it is *ingenium* in the proper sense when it is forming new ideas."[34] What about its relationship to speed? Descartes says that the *ingenium* appears to grasp propositions and the connections between them immediately, but that this "simultaneous" understanding is deceptive. It is achieved only by training the faculty of memory. Once the thinker has laboriously worked out a chain of reasoning, the temporal aspect of the chaining can be discarded, so that he seems to be "intuiting the whole thing at once" even though it has actually been memorized: "so in this way the slowness of the wit (*tarditas ingenii*) is improved upon and the ability enlarged." Descartes is using here Galen's phrase from

---

[31] *In Artem Parvam Galeni*, 310.
[32] Pierre Charron, *Of Wisdom*, i, 130.
[33] Juan Luis Vives, *De Anima*, 77; Américo Castro, *Spanien, Vision und Wirklichkeit*, 556.
[34] René Descartes, *Regulae ad Directionem Ingenii*, 136; 139.

The Art of Medicine, quoted above. However, whereas earlier commentators saw Galen's "slowness" as a condition that was defective and organic to the body, Descartes sees it as normal (at least for the first outing of any new propositional synthesis), and *ingenium* as operating independently of the body.

Reductionism continued, fed by the Cartesianism it had formerly prefigured. By the time of Luca Tozzi's late seventeenth-century Galen commentary, *ingenium* has become a whole empire. It is (1) "the power of discovering very quickly the middle terms leading to the knowledge of causes," (2) generalized across the brain and (3) coterminous with the "immaterial rational soul."[35] Cognitive speed is no longer a quality of invisible matter such as the humours or soul spirits, but of an invisible immateriality, the Cartesian mind. *Ingenium* is now important enough to be a species marker in natural history, the main distinction between man and beast. Nor does this overarching concept retain any element of overlap with medieval philosophy's "divine intelligences" at the other end of the scale; it is "proper to humans alone."

However, alongside the reductionist trend in faculty psychology and the resistances to it, there was also stasis. Accounts of *ingenium* as just one particular operation of the imagination, as it had been for Albert in the thirteenth century, can be found in works written or consulted in the middle of the eighteenth century. The *Art of Medicine* commentaries, even later ones, do not pursue the relationship between speed and ability systematically. Moreover, in most other medical contexts, the health of brain and intellect still consisted in a mean between fast and slow. The continuing strength of the mean in the wider culture is pithily expressed in the example Blaise Pascal chose to give for its definition, which happens to have a bearing on our topic: "*Mean*. When we read too quickly or too slowly, we do not understand anything."[36] This casts doubt on whether the speeding-up process was purposive or even conscious. The Galen commentators, whose approach to any topic would always start with pasting together a variety of seemingly relevant classical texts, can be found approving Galen on the desirability of speed in one and the same paragraph as approving Hippocrates on that of a mean.[37] (It was more important to present the Hippocratics, only recently revived, as being at one with Galen than to deal with the contradiction.) Speed, though sometimes preferable, was never *necessary* to intellectual ability, as it is in modern educational psychology. On the other hand, the idea of an overarching, specifically human intellectual ability whose performance is estimated in terms of (among other things) its speed was undoubtedly becoming dominant in the society beyond the learned doctor's study.

Quick wit as cultural capital: the ingenious gentleman

"Fast equals good" was for a long time a minority habit, in the routine discussion of one or two passages in an ancestral medical curriculum. Meanwhile, in the everyday world, the clock had become not only a model for the workings of the universe but had altered urban and commercial perceptions of time. Replacing the craftsman's balance as the core technological metaphor, it supplied a new way of measuring intellectual activity and facilitated notions of productivity. (We could also note here the rise in the 1650s of the first coffeehouses, where the early Royal Society held its meetings; speedy caffeine was more suited to calculative skills than beer, its melancholic predecessor.) If speed of wit was an esoteric corner of theoretical medicine, in the real world its profile was increasing, and feeding, if slowly and unevenly, into the professional mind-

---

[35] Luca Tozzi, *In Artem Medicinalem Galeni*, ii, 42.
[36] Pascal, *Pensées*, 244.
[37] Santorio Santorio, *Commentaria in Artem Medicinalem Galeni*, 200.

set and finally the academic one. Professional intellectuals, among them the medical humanists whose texts we have been analyzing, had the precarious job of both advising power and toeing its line, and the tension between speed and the traditional convention of the mean reflected this. In Elizabethan England, for example, Roger Ascham revived Plato's seeming ambiguities about the wax tablet in a widely consulted handbook on education. The pupil with a "hard and rough wit" (evoking the hard, rough hands of his labouring family) will grow up to be a mere steward or an apprentice, even though he may be "wiser" than the pupil whose wit is "quick and light" and who will therefore get on in the world. Nevertheless, asks Ascham, who is to say that these "natural graces," quickness and lightness, are not also signs of divine grace?[38] It would have been tactless for a courtier (Ascham was Elizabeth's secretary) to say outright that a quick-witted climbing of the greasy pole was incompatible with divinity when most of the Tudor court were upstart commoners who had done just that.

At the end of the seventeenth century Locke, though he defined wit as "the assemblage of ideas, and putting those together with quickness," was more concerned about the mean, and the pathology of "wrong judgement" that lay on both sides of it.[39] There is "heat and passion" on one side and "sloth" on the other; if the latter is a mark of the "idiot" and his "want of quickness ... in the intellectual faculties," the former are marks of a politically dangerous sectarian religious enthusiasm. Speed remains largely insignificant in Locke's psychology. The same is true of his eighteenth-century readers. The nonconformist educator Isaac Watts warns, "Presume not too much upon a bright genius, a ready wit, and good parts; for this, without labour and study, will never make a man of knowledge and wisdom ... When they ha[ve] lost their vivacity ..., they bec[o]me stupid and sottish."[40] More scientifically oriented writers such as David Hartley wrote about the internal movement and association of ideas in terms of physics, likening them to the "vibrations" of Newton's *Optics*; on this basis he differentiated individual intellects from each other by their strength, vividness, intensity and (in the case of "idiots") their educability – but not their speed.[41] James Mill noted the time it takes for ideas and thoughts to animate the muscles; he saw speed as an operation of the faculty of will, but did not discuss differences in speed among individual wills or intellects.[42] At this theoretical level, then, the relationship between intellect and speed plateaus in the eighteenth and early nineteenth centuries, precisely on the threshold of the momentous leap in machine speeds and in the complexity and speed of social life.

However, the history of eighteenth-century theories of the mind needs complementing with the developments at a more mundane level, as described in Graham Richards's *Mental Machinery*. Speed was as much an indicator of social status as of psychological status. While the arrival of an overarching *ingenium* in the later medical texts coincides with its attribution to ever wider social strata, its elite character is nevertheless preserved in the "ingenious gentleman," a stock character in tales of intellectual exploration from the mid-seventeenth century onwards. In the immediacy of his abilities he is a descendant of medieval philosophy's "prophet." The Royal Society itself was modest on this score: the title page of the early issues of its *Philosophical Transactions* announced that they were drawn from "the labours of the ingenious." But there was also a consistent tendency to believe that elite brains could perform intellectual activity without having to labour at their studies whereas from other people, however healthy their brains, the same activity required time. Traditionally angels, and at inspired moments philosophers themselves, had been exempt from

---

[38] Roger Ascham, *The Scholemaster*, 25.
[39] John Locke, *An Essay concerning Human Understanding*, 156; 160.
[40] Isaac Watts, *The Improvement of the Mind*, 6.
[41] David Hartley, *Observations on Man*, i, 30.
[42] James Mill, *Analysis of the Phenomena of the Human Mind*, ii, 345.

the labour of constructing syllogisms, their understandings being not just quick but instantaneous.[43] Like them, the ingenious gentleman had an instant understanding that exempted him from the opprobrium of apprenticeship. The fact that the ingenious gentleman did not need training, unlike the artisans with whom he now had to associate and who assisted with his experiments, helped to shore up his (often dubious) social status, and to offset any depreciation resulting from the fact that the road to knowledge in increasingly important areas of life now required base mechanical skills.

Instant performance had its objective counterpart in "natural magic," which was distinct from ordinary nature not by being *super*natural but by the extraordinarily reduced time it took to operate. Latent within nature, magic was a legitimate source of scientific inquiry (Robert Boyle's quest to tap into it led to some of the first principles of modern chemistry). The founding narrative of genius in this sense was the story of the Pentecostal descent of the holy spirit. A typical example from everyday life in the medieval period was speaking in tongues, like the old peasant woman who suddenly spoke fluent Latin when seized by melancholy, only to lapse into monolingualism upon recovery.[44] The ingenious gentleman, and thence the Galtonian genius, are her natural successors.

---

[43] See Noel Brann, *The Debate over the Origin of Genius in the Italian Renaissance*.
[44] D'Abano, *Conciliator Controversiarum*, Differentia 37.

PART 3
Intelligence and Disability: Status and Power

Chapter 5
In-group, Out-group: the Place of Intelligence in Anthropology

One's intelligence is not determined by the hard realities of time and labour alone but also, and equally concretely, by the realm of appearances. In this and the following two parts, we shall look at the social manifestation of these appearances alongside certain other concepts with structural similarities to intelligence, and then at the historical interplay among them.

Forms of self-representation

It is by appearances that we judge others, they judge us and mutual recognition or misrecognition occurs. Intelligence is one such form of mutual (mis)recognition. Disputes about it are disputes over status. Status is usually seen as a two-tiered structure: at the upper level, an abstraction of social goals; at the lower, any concrete evidence or collateral one might have for claiming it. Lower-level evidence varies with the values of a given historical or cultural context. For instance, it may be that I own a diamond mine, or my great aunt's second cousin was a Duke or I am completely chaste. Hypothetically at least, the reality of each of these can be externally confirmed; they are more than just concepts. In our own meritocratic mind-set, intelligence too belongs on this level; it is something to be called upon as concrete collateral when claiming status, and is assumed to compete for recognition on the same taxonomic level with (for example) wealth.

But this two-level structure is inadequate. Looking at the sheer variety of candidates for status across history and cultures, we find another level mediating between abstract status and its collateral. This level consists of what are indeed only concepts (though as such they play an active social role). Nor are they externally verifiable – indeed, that is often their whole point. Concepts such as honour, for example, or grace, have been described by anthropologists in such terms. Honour and grace are not themselves concrete collateral: they bring no offering to the great god Status except the promise offered by the word itself. That is because they are wholly internal to the game of bidding for status; they are, so to speak, its "modes."[1] *Modes of bidding* belong in the realm of appearances and mutual recognition alone. To people claiming status on grounds of their honour or state of grace, a request for hard evidence is insulting because it would expose that very flimsiness. This point has often been made. Aristotle rejected honour's claim to constitute the good life, because "it seems rather to exist in those doing the honouring than in him who is honoured."[2] The seventeenth-century theologian Pierre Nicole recognized its modal role. If honour has any reality, he says, it lies not even "in our inclination to love it, nor in the belief that such an inclination is natural" but in the mere "inclination to attach it more to one thing than to another."[3] As a nobleman in a much-quoted phrase from Lope de Vega's *The Commanders of Cordoba* admits, "Honour is something one does not possess .... It is that which exists in the other," a homage paid to power. Evidence is therefore always contingent and arbitrary. Honour is that which the person in

---

[1] Don Herzog, *Happy Slaves*, 92.
[2] Aristotle, *Nicomachean Ethics*, 1.5.4.
[3] Nicole, *Honneur*, 365.

power says it is. Ultimately, said Hobbes, my honour is just my assertion of my social rank against others, the display or "manifestation" of "the value we set on one another."[4] Likewise with my being in grace: God has predestined my soul for salvation, and this gift of grace obviates the need for any evidence base such as absence of sin. If I know I am in grace, that is enough. True, only God can know what is "essential and constitutive of [the] being of grace"; but it is also a human and social phenomenon, since we discern it in each other "mediately and secondarily, by the effects and operations ... manifestative of such a being."[5]

Honour and grace, then, are examples of bidding modes: they connect status at its higher level, as an abstraction of values and goals, to its lower level, as concrete collateral to be used in support of a bid. That is why such modes are not susceptible to objectivist definition, why there is endless controversy about what constitutes them and why people claiming status will talk about their honour or state of grace as if it were self-evident when actually the terms are purely self-referential.

Back, then, to intelligence. In what class of things does it belong? We tend to answer this in two ways. One is scientific: it belongs in the same class as gas particles or planets. The other is sociological: it belongs in the same class as (for example) money, against which it competes. Usually we think of it in both ways at the same time. But intelligence no more resembles a pound coin than a planet. In the universal poker game of self-representation, its only collateral is its own name and the deference this commands. Intelligence is thus the same kind of thing as honour and grace: it belongs to the class of *claims to status that are purely self-referential*. Like honour and grace, it is a mode of bidding for status and nothing else. Like them, it belongs in the realm of appearances, even if it never lets us forget the reality of these appearances in any social interaction where someone is pulling rank. Like them, it is located midway between status as a sum of general goals and status as the array of concrete items upon which one calls when making a bid. Like them, it fills the round hole of individual human uniqueness with the square peg of abstract hierarchy. And like them, it creates not just an in-group but an out-group that is definitively disqualified from entering the bidding in the first place.

The idea of an intelligence that is (a) specifically human, distinct from any other creature animal or divine, and (b) an individual possession, is not something universal and transhistorical but arises out of early modern games of social bidding. In this period, honour, grace and intelligence ("wit") at times occupied or fought over the same conceptual space. In its age of innocence, contemporaries sometimes saw intelligence in this way themselves. When Descartes remarked, "No one desires a larger measure of good sense than he already possesses," he could equally have been talking about the other two modes.[6] Conversely, when the Jesuit authority on human behaviour Balthasar Gracián wrote "With the world full of fools, there is none who thinks himself one or even suspects it," his readers would have understood "fool" in terms of disablement from any or all three.[7]

Intelligence and the structure of status

Honour, grace and intelligence are not the only possible "modes" of this type, but in the early modern period there is a dynamic, historically formative interplay between them. We can start by establishing their common structural components. I draw here on the anthropology of Julian Pitt-Rivers, who first noted the structural similarities between honour and grace and who (along

---

[4] *Leviathan*, 62.
[5] John Flavell, *The Method of Grace*, 405.
[6] Descartes, *Discours de la méthode*, 7.
[7] *Oráculo manual y arte de prudenza*, Aphorism 201.

with Pierre Bourdieu) also touched, if very half-heartedly, on their resemblance to intelligence. I will flesh out that passing intuition.[8]

First of all, honour, grace and intelligence all entail *personal destiny* and *collective perfectibility*, a permanent place in the cosmos that transcends the temporality of individual lives. Death with honour, the traditional motto of the defeated, signifies that one may forfeit life itself so that honour can live on; with honour, wrote Edmund Spenser, we are "eternized ... in th'immortal book of fame."[9] The constitutive element of selfhood lies in the group identity of "the honour society" (the *societas*, as contemporaries called it), where honour lifts one so far above the nonentity of the mass that withdrawal of status is the difference between life and death. Similarly, with grace come salvation and a life everlasting among the company of the elect, thereby marking one off from the reprobate and doomed. Likewise intelligence is the individual possession of the intelligence society – that is, the 98 per cent or so of the population who participate collectively in a future intellectual perfection, marked by developmental goals and the practices of genetic enhancement and eugenics. Perfection can be retrospective too: the honourable man's glorious ancestors (Spenser's "eternal brood of glory excellent"), whose precedent seems impossible to reproduce; Adam's state of grace, corrupted by the Fall; the gene pool that has degenerated from its original state, as in Galton's fears about racial degeneration and regression to the mean.

All three modes *sanctify the person*. Each confirms the legitimacy of an individual's behaviour by referring it to external authority. In a form appropriate to the mode (the king disburses honourable titles, God dispenses grace, the psychologist allocates IQ scores), selected individuals are invested with some of the superior's sacred authority. Although this authority is in fact arbitrary, in receiving its blessings we abnegate our right to question it, thereby binding ourselves to accept practices which a different generation, in different historical circumstances, might regard as utterly wrong.

With sanctification of the person comes purity of the group, raising anxiety about *inauthenticity* and *pollution*. The *arriviste* buys the coat of arms which only a person's bloodline entitles them to; by pretending to be honourable, he pollutes the group. The hypocrite fakes the outward behaviours signalling confirmation of grace at holy communion; he thereby defiles it, since the devil himself is able to "counterfeit all the saving operations and graces of the spirit of God."[10] People called intellectually disabled are stereotypically good mimics but also *mere* mimics, of intelligent behaviour; educational psychologists are at their most alert when someone already labelled as severely autistic appears to give eye contact, thus mimicking human interaction, or when someone with a supposedly deficient intelligence appears to be reading but is merely, like a dog, "barking at print." The disabled person is not *really* interacting, reading, thinking, self-aware, ambitious, in love or expressing opinions, like everyone else, but merely copying surface behaviours he sees around him. In all these examples, the physical presence of the polluter threatens to destabilize the group and its internal bonds. Bastards adulterate noble and honourable blood; reprobate communicants pollute the truly Christian receiver; the disabled contaminate the gene pool and defile the community of the intelligent. (If this were not the case, one would not need segregated social activities and institutions.)

We find too an anxiety about *self-authentification*, directed inwards at one's self-esteem and personal autonomy. A gentleman's ancestry is the permanent guarantee of his honour, yet depends also on an unattainable certainty as to who his real father was; if his pure bloodline falls in doubt,

---

[8] "Postscript: the place of grace in anthropology," in J. Peristiany and Pitt-Rivers (eds), *Honour and Grace in Anthropology*; *The Fate of Schechem*; "Honor," in E. Sills (ed.), *International Encyclopedia of the Social Sciences*.

[9] *The Faerie Queene*, 1.10.59; 1.5.1.

[10] Jonathan Edwards, *A Treatise concerning Religious Affectations*, 40.

so does his autonomy and freedom from having to bow to the will of others, and perhaps he must join the servile out-group which by definition has no such autonomy. People otherwise certain of their own salvation worry about their status with God whenever they suffer a personal setback, however clearly the Bible says that grace is conferred once and for all. And one's intelligence, that which endows modern personhood with its sense of permanence, may be denied by the formal entrance requirements of educational and social institutions. The genealogy that certifies the nobleman's continuous honourable bloodline; the gift of grace by which the godly man is born again forever; the autobiographical "self" whose intelligence has a birth-to-death consistency and permanence: all are ways of whistling in the dark of transience, as we veer between self-flattery and self-abasement.

There is also in each mode a *tension between self-authentification and authentification by others*: between the felt, internal aspects of each mode and the verifiable, external ones; between what I advance as a claim and others' recognition of it; between private and public behaviour; between potentiality and assessable performance. Honour, grace and intelligence each form a nexus between the ideals of a society and the reproduction of those ideals in individuals who are able to extort from others a validation of the image they cherish of themselves. Authentification is in each case a source of socio-cultural conflict or coherence; it underpins the rituals specific to a mode (interpersonal violence, prayer, command of grammar), its rites of passage (dubbing, confirmation, developmental assessment) and forms of verification (jousting, trial by ordeal, academic exams).

All three are forms of *apparently equal exchange* amongst creatures who are *actually unequal*. The man of honour exchanges forms of honourable address with the socially inferior stranger, out of "politeness." The quality of being polite or "polished" (clean) oneself obliges one to attribute this quality, if only whimsically, to the unclean. The cost of this ambiguity is the eventual collapse of the mode itself. First the merchant or yeoman farmer and then even the road sweeper has to be addressed as Mr or Esquire. In religion, where inequality is at its starkest, grace is often known as "the friendship of God," while in secular terms grace is a form of social reciprocity illustrated (as Marcel Mauss observed) by words such as *gracias*, *grazie* and so forth, which show that the reciprocity is actually an obligation from one party to another and therefore intrinsically unequal. The case of intelligence remains obscure to most of us, because it is the form of exchange in which we remain enmeshed today. The relationship between the intelligent and the intellectually disabled is nevertheless one of exchange, inasmuch as the credit of the one could not exist without the debit of the other; it takes place without the awareness of either, or perhaps only with the awareness of the latter. (A milder version is the advanced meritocratic principle of rule by exam-passers.) To deal with ambiguities about equality, all three modes place seals of official public recognition on reputations that would otherwise stand in doubt, giving them the illusion of permanence. The effect is to suppress the immediacy of human reciprocity, objectifying and depersonalizing it in the form of contracts and sanctions. Intelligence itself is a contractualized form, internalized within each individual, of this felt need for social reciprocity and exchange.

Each mode is a *legitimation* of certain kinds of behaviour, relating the world as it is to the world as the in-group would like to see it. Honour is a disculpating factor, rendering admissible the motive for any behaviour so long as one is a member of the honour group. Grace brings "justification," God's suspension of sentence for the elect few; in the extreme version of this doctrine known as Antinomianism, no action can be sinful if the actor knows he is in grace. Intelligence, too, can legitimize otherwise reprehensible behaviour, such as the genius's neglect of spouse and children. Grace, honour and intelligence are the halo that surrounds power. They turn its brute facts into moral arguments, and have all been used to moralize the language of politics. Though they appear to be evaluated by some objective knowledge system, they are in fact evaluated from within in-groups of honourable, graced and intelligent people. The fact that with intelligence the in-group boundaries extend more or less to the boundaries of the human species should not blind us to the fact that in the past both honour and grace entailed exactly the same claim; they cast the out-group (commoners, hypocrites) as "monsters of nature," even if at that time such monsters formed the majority of the population. If this claim with regard to honour and grace seems ludicrous to us and with regard to intelligence does not, it is because intelligence is our own preferred way of bidding for status; the out-group may be very small, but that does not alter its structural similarity to those other out-groups. All these legitimations belong to the extensive medium-term period of centralization of power that runs from the surge in administrative outreach in the thirteenth century to the globalized information societies of the twenty-first. Bidding modes are characteristically pushed forward by ambitious groups not quite at the centre of power; consequently they become a preoccupation of state power itself, as it responds to the threat. Henry VIII's governmental revolution, for example, centralized the honour codes that had till then been policed by semi-autonomous groups of nobles. Jean Calvin's godly government of Geneva transformed grace, which the Reformation held to be a matter of the individual's relationship with God, into a monopoly of the state. The totalitarian tendency of modern liberal societies is obscured by its offer to individual citizens of a spurious access to social power against a previously entrenched elite, through their certifiable intelligence ("meritocracy"). In adopting the principle of each mode, state power renders illusory any promise of personal autonomy which that mode may have begun by offering, and uses it to bind individuals more tightly to the social order.

Important to legitimation is *precedence*. Each mode is competitive within itself: struggles take place wherever precedence is intrinsic but the outcome in doubt. Each in-group has its own technical gradations of excellence (honourable title, canonization, Mensa membership) that are also presented as moral gradations. In addition, if communities of honour, grace and intelligence are circumscribed by the vulgar, the ungodly and the disabled respectively, there are also groups whose bid is ambiguous. Alongside honourable gentlemen are gentle women, whose honour is something quite different from men's; alongside the godly are those whose state of grace mere mortals cannot know; alongside the intelligent are those whose status is ambiguous because postponed, such as children (hence that thoroughly modern notion, "cognitive development").

Friction also arises from the contradiction within each bidding mode between the *porousness of borders* (a steady trickle of people being admitted to the in-group or expelled) and the fact that membership is super-determined by a necessity that is beyond time or place. Thus there is tension between status *ascribed* and status *achieved*. Is my innate honour subject to fate, or can I act to rescue it? Am I saved by God's predestined grace, or can I work at my salvation? Is my intelligence determined by my DNA, or is it improvable by nurture? These debates are the contentious political face of the modes. Lives, and potential lives, hang on the outcome. The tensions are only ever resolved temporarily, by quota systems which impose a conceptual discontinuity and social frontier between the back row of the elite and the front row of the excluded, and which reserve a place for the offspring of the in-group in each mode.[11]

There is also a struggle to maintain the inherently abstract and general character of a mode, without which it would break down because hard evidence would be needed instead – a need that contradicts the very principle of the modes themselves. The struggle is against *concretely verifiable and therefore degraded accounts* of the mode. Honour cannot be substituted with ersatz alternatives such as mere honesty, which can be properly monitored and is therefore bourgeois. "Special" or "saving" grace, which inexplicably guarantees salvation regardless of mere earthly merit, must be sharply distinguished from "natural" graces, the empirically verifiable gifts or abilities that entitle

---

[11] Pierre Bourdieu, "Epreuve scolaire et consécration sociale," in *Actes de la recherche en sciences sociales*, 39 (1981).

one to command others in the secular realm. And intelligence as generalized intellectual ability exists over and above the specificity of particular abilities, with their susceptibility to mundane forms of verification.

To avoid calls for evidence, all three bids are forced instead to blur the distinction between individual, *subjective ability* and *objective abilities or powers* (property differentials, contractual freedoms, verifiable scientific knowledge and so forth), creating the illusion that certain objective powers are the personal, internal quality of individuals. It then turns out that personal ability consists in facing down people who might otherwise feel they were your equal. Just as in property disputes nine-tenths of the law is possession, so nine-tenths of intelligence is the silencing of anyone who would dispute your claim to it. A psychometric test may sometimes be called upon, though usually all that is needed is the minutest of signs given off. Since each mode can in fact be used to signify more or less anything one likes, or its opposite, according to the power of the parties involved, such randomness has to be disguised by an apparently stable theoretical basis in the form of a script that is read off from some external, objective source and means the same thing to everyone. In this way personal abilities acquire the same ontological certainty as the corresponding objective powers.

Randomness also involves what Mauss calls a *general theory of magic*: each mode can vanish and pop up again anywhere with fresh principles, differing from one time or place to another. Its principles are refreshed by appealing to the new "facts" of the mode that establish one's right to give instructions or to talk first, and down. These principles usually involve only tacit consensus, since the mere hint of spelling them out may cause offence or threaten the principle itself. Only when the threat becomes real does it become necessary, despite everything, to codify the consensus explicitly, producing (as we shall see) grace and honour quotients, GQ and HQ, as well as IQ. These codes are the official signs of one's rank in a universal order, identically social and natural, where it might otherwise stand in doubt. Bidding modes for status start out by being sensed emotionally, as reciprocal but unverifiable "states of the heart"; but at certain historical points, the pressures of socio-economic change call for desperate measures, not to say desperate measurements.[12] Detached, objectified, abstract, impersonal accounts are drawn up as a last resort against the impending meltdown of a mode, and this new pseudo-legal, pseudo-scientific hierarchy is then inserted in the minds of individual subjects who internalize it informally as a new state of the heart and a new source of social cohesion – and of friction. The friction occurs within spaces so homogeneous, at least to an outside observer, that difference is created out of nothing. A newly arrived Martian, for example, asked to consider variations in intelligence among earthlings, would surely be baffled by the question.[13]

There follows, in all three modes, a *confusion of sign with substance*. In a technique characteristic of power, the insignia of a mode precede its facts. The sign of a lion rampant on a coat of arms may not make the owner brave, but it helps to enhance his power: "reputation of power, is power."[14] Calvin and Oliver Cromwell took their earthly triumphs as the sign they were in grace and therefore fit to rule. This confusion of sign with substance renders the "nature" of the mode deterministic and elevates it into something unchangeable. Accreditation operates in reverse order: the sign, with its exactitude, arrives first and the thing it codifies comes after, in a clearly identifiable historical sequence. The same happens with IQ and cognitive ability scores, as we shall see shortly. Social tensions are relieved by this constant turning of the sign or outer manifestation into inner truth, display into identity (honourable, elect, intelligent). However, the relief is never enough because there can be no guarantee that one has really reached the heart of the onion. Always controversial, signs indicate differential degrees of a mode as they are constantly readjusted to the objective

---

[12] Pitt-Rivers, "Postscript," 215.
[13] Bourdieu, *The Logic of Practice*, 136.
[14] Hobbes, *Leviathan*, 62.

structures legitimizing it. The natural distinction they identify correlates with one's distance from the swamps of vulgarity, reprobation or intellectual disability, and legitimizes social segregation.

Finally, the necessity of each mode is confirmed by that most clearly verifiable aspect of human beings, their physical make-up. Grace, honour and intelligence are all *associated with the body*: blood in the gentry, "soul spirits" in God's elect, genes in the intelligent. The head especially, as the point of control, ritually signals the authenticity of a bidding mode: the crowning of a monarch, the sign of the cross over the head, or the touch on it with a book in academic degree ceremonies. The body's importance also means that all three modes are the business of physicians. The body can be decisive in proving group membership, and in ousting certain individuals from full membership of the natural human kind.

The structural, historically continuous feature of these self-referential status bids is precisely their modal function, their ability to block our view of the facts of power. "After all," to quote the historian Marc Bloch, "what is a social hierarchy other than a system of collective representations that are by their very nature mobile?" The name of any bid smells as sweet as any other, even if in concrete historical contexts they compete with each other because each is implicated in its own respective political ideology. Despite their similarities, the modes are structurally different in one respect. While they all command charismatic recognition, intelligence seems to stand out from the other two because of the numbers involved. The possessors of honour and grace were few and proud of it. But if the proud possessors of intelligence are a group consisting entirely of charismatic individuals, there are by now an awful lot of us, about 98 per cent of the population. The only people in awe of us, one hopes, are the "intellectually disabled." Intelligence is a *generalized* charisma, its historical roots lying in the Protestant dispersal of sacredness to the laity. Bourdieu, in describing charismatic honour and grace as forms of symbolic capital, dips a toe in this water when he puts educational qualifications in the same category as the other two modes. However, he does not put intelligence as such there; he assumes it has a genuine, untouchable substance that is somehow separate from the sign. One can only think that this is because he is seduced by one of the "realist typologies" he himself criticizes elsewhere. Intelligence, though absent from his analysis, ought to be a supreme illustration of his own definition of symbolic capital as "the self-consciousness of a dominant class." As our political leaders keep telling us, "We are all middle class now." And inasmuch as intelligence characterizes the middle classes above all, the dream Marx ascribed to them of "a bourgeoisie without a proletariat" is also the dream of an "intelligence society" eugenically cleansed of the unintelligent.

"Merit" and modern intelligence: the immediate historical background

By the late nineteenth century, the shift in ideological balance from honour and grace to intelligence – from "arms" to "letters," seminary to seminar – and the split between religious and secular-scientific learning were more or less complete. Revisiting the concept of the genius in this context, we find that as scientific knowledge began to be thought of as the genius's *possession*, the branch of it known as psychology gave rise to scientific knowledge *about* the genius (and, of course, its opposite). A status concept was thereby transformed into an objective scientific entity, subsuming the characteristics of grace and honour under those of a supreme intuited intellect (*nous*, for which "intelligence" was the preferred translation).

Hints of this were already around in the eighteenth century, when a descendant of the (Robert) Boyle family received the following piece of flattery from an expert on human behaviour: "Every one must see, in what an abundant measure you inherit the same genius, and with what an increase of honour ... you are likely to transmit the revered name to future generations."[15] Honourable line and intellectual line are one here. (Boyle himself had, in fact, died childless.) To take another example, what could have postulated an invisible and universal force – gravity – if not an invisible and universal force – intelligence – with Newton at its summit? Newton was the last historical exemplar of the medieval prophet, that is, someone whose route to knowledge was an unmediated, intuited intellect; but by the same token he was a prototype of the modern genius, the era's most honoured mind and, in terms of grace, God's elect instrument. "God said, let Newton be, and all was light." The public deference he obtained confirmed the honourable and elect status of all those who bestowed it, endowing them with a third, intellectual claim to status that reflected Newton's own intellectual glory. However, by contrast with the honourable person's disdain for labour and God's preference for faith over works, intellectual status of this sort seemed to demand quite hard works, at least for ordinary mortals. Mathematical puzzles became acceptable pursuits in *The Gentleman's Magazine or Monthly Intelligencer* and (because they did not threaten female honour either) *The Ladies' Diary*, and were a prototype for the first written, time-tested exams.[16] The year 1682 saw the launch of the *Weekly Memorials for the Ingenious*, a digest of the latest intellectual pursuits. The elite still aspired to the emblems of honour and the signs of grace; now they also sought the accreditation of their intelligence. And if "elite" is, as sociologists have observed, a nebulous concept, then so much the better: it is entirely appropriate to the bidding modes and their unwavering superficiality.

Two names stand out in the history of forms of accreditation: Galton and Binet. The roots of modern intelligence in honour and grace were nurtured by Galton, even if he rarely used the word itself. The stimulus for his first book *Hereditary Genius* was his own youthful record, disapproved by his family, of intellectual failure. Cousin Charles (Darwin) was a genius, their mutual grandfather Erasmus Darwin had been a genius, so Galton naturally aspired to genius too. He needed a field in which it could be expressed, and he found it in his theory that genius runs in families.[17] Although he excluded people whose reputations were due solely to hereditary title from his underlying principle that "high reputation is a pretty accurate test of high ability," Galton's description of the genius remains steeped in the vocabulary of honour. Genius and esteem were close, not necessarily because esteem was the *outcome* of having high ability but because they were conceptually alike. True, the anthropometrical laboratory he went on to construct measured people from all walks of life. But he had been right the first time: the families of "men of reputation" are precisely where to find genius, provided one can keep slipping in one's own definition of the abilities that comprise it. To complain that such families are not a proper population sample is to presuppose that intelligence can be an object of scientific investigation with an observable essence across social classes, rather than simply another bidding claim cognate with honour.

Historians have written much about Galton's role as innovator, but little on what got him there. The nonconformist culture of Galton's family background had long ago turned optimistic about the general availability of grace; elect status was not some blind Calvinist conundrum solved only in one's afterlife destination, it was manifest here on earth in the inner light of (nearly) every individual's nature.[18] It nevertheless had the deterministic overtones of earlier predestinarianism. These overtones entered psychology partly through the work of the eighteenth-century dissenting clergyman Joseph Priestley, whose studies both of exact science and of human nature found room for what he now termed "necessitarianism." Galton took this term and squeezed what had been

---

[15] Thomas Salkeld, *The Compleat Gentleman*, Dedicatory note.
[16] Andrew Warwick, *Masters of Theory*, 130; C. John Somerville, *The Secularization of Early Modern England*, 185.
[17] Adrian Wooldridge, *Measuring the Mind*, 75.
[18] See Geoffrey Cantor, *Quakers, Jews and Science*.

a trinitarian mind-set (divine necessity, malleable nature, human nurture) into a new, dualistic one of nature versus nurture.[19] No doubt in using the term he was just pitching his tent on the clergy's lawn, but he was also refurbishing the causal basis on which geneticists might account for intelligence. As for nurture, when Galton wrote about improving the human stock, he used metaphors of "husbandry" and "grafting." If these look quasi-biological and therefore modern, we must remember that priests had been routinely using them a couple of centuries earlier in their advice on how to rear the children of the elect. Galton's "powers" and abilities therefore had a subliminally divine element. They were to take precedence over mere high breeding of an earthly kind. He reconstituted grace and election on a scientific basis that justified the claims of an intellectually elite family like his own to the same status as the older aristocracy, which had so far ranked above it in terms of bloodline and honour.[20] The same is true further down the social scale. When Burt justified IQ tests by their raising of a few innately intelligent working-class children to their proper station through entry into grammar schools, he was of this same tradition. If one were to say that social selection by intelligence testing leads to the company of the elect, it would be more than mere metaphor; there is an organic historical link. The contemporary prominence of Plato's *Republic* is again relevant, with its "noble lie" about the golden child who, having been born into a bronze family, is reallocated to a golden one.[21]

We have already seen that the procedure for establishing intelligence as a scientific concept consists *first* in conjuring up the notion of a mean purely as such. Subsequently, and only subsequently, this mean becomes something concrete; as "intelligence," it in fact consists in whatever is lying around in the conjuror's mind-set at that point. The sign becomes the thing itself. It is therefore nothing more than what those with the power say it is, as were honour and grace: a dummy category, a magic hold-all into which they can pack whatever they like according to purpose. Binet is a classic case. In 1904 a radically anti-clerical government commissioned him to deal with the consequences of its closure of thousands of church schools, the central plank in its separation of church and state. The left-wing parties were full of men of science and physician-legislators, the prime minister Emile Combes being himself a doctor who had specialized in psychology; the Third Republic's prominent medical interest in hereditary degeneration was linked to its sense of political and social malaise.[22] The closure seems to have decanted into the recently established state educational system certain children whom it did not want. As a network of separate special schools was just then being established, Binet was required to design a stricter system that could identify those children to be quarantined, or "helped," as historians have put it. Where did the idea come from in the first place, that some children might need to be ejected? The existence of some notional out-group is *a priori* for those fearing pollution. *Someone* must be ejected, but who? At this stage the slate was blank. No criteria existed for what exactly defined a problem child in the new system. Binet's underlying criteria were as arbitrary as the means of assessing them needed to be precise.

He began by noting that certain things are absent in certain children. What things, exactly? He fell back, as one does, on his own previous and somewhat desultory professional history, which was a mix of theoretical remnants of faculty psychology and disparate empirical studies that had largely led up blind alleys. He notes that what is absent in problem children – that is, those already shortlisted for segregation, on a pure hunch – is the faculties of attention span, judgement, adaptation, critical spirit, abstraction and generalization. He then takes the unilateral decision to let precisely these things comprise a standard, which he calls "mental age." Finally he goes back and

---

[19] Francis Galton, *Inquiries into Human Faculty and its Development*, 234.
[20] Wooldridge, *Measuring the Mind*, 75.
[21] *The Republic*, 547a.
[22] See Daniel Pick, *Faces of Degeneration*; Jack D. Ellis, *The Physician-Legislators of France*.

applies this standard to each individual "mentally defective" child on the shortlist; he compares the child's performance with the norm by establishing the (inevitably lower) age of the average child at whose level the defective one is operating. The child might look at this process slightly differently: he or she is being measured precisely according to those criteria which it is suspected in advance he or she will fail to meet. Binet, by contrast, is looking at success: a chance government summons has led him to the holy grail that will redeem the psychology of intelligence, and perhaps all psychology, by curing it of its inexactness.

Binet, unlike Galton, was a worrier, whose work underwent anxious recensions: there is probably no unitary intelligence, it is not actually a concrete characteristic like height, people will over-systematize my ideas, we must prevent teachers from trying to eject normal children who are merely disaffected or uninterested and so forth. Yet his only major effort to deal with his anxieties was to say that it does not matter what the tests are of so long as there are plenty of them.[23] In the 1920s, following the failure of the new applied disciplines to agree on a common definition of intelligence, Kelley's blunt closure to the debate ran: "Mental tests measure something, we may or may not care what …. The measuring device as a measure of something that is desirable comes first, and what it is a measure of comes second."[24] The whole claim to exact-science legitimacy was loaded off from the substance of this elusive target, intelligence, and on to measurement alone, the codification of status. For the psychometrician the arbitrariness of content is not a failing but an endorsement, since the closer one is to measurement the closer one is to *experimental* psychology and thus to the aura of an exact science. Here is the point at which a subjective bid for status convinces itself that it is objective scientific knowledge. Our own everyday presuppositions about intelligence are the product of this psychometric turn. Pychometrics was the vehicle through which the reification of social relations was transferred from the domain of honour/degeneracy and grace/reprobation to that of intellectual ability/disability.

Intellectual disability and meritocracy

If intelligence is purely self-referential, then those first psychometricians were right to conclude that it cannot and need not be defined. Nevertheless, it does have one core constituent that covers all contexts and might point to its rightful place in a dictionary of synonyms: intelligent means better. The word can only function as a disguised comparative. So, it is true, do all descriptive terms in the human sciences. None is neutral. But "intelligent" is not only value laden, it is content free. Its comparativeness is synonymous with biological hierarchy *as such*. That is because (as we shall see in Chapter 17) intelligence not only describes but in some sense also *is*, first, the place of humans in relation to other animals, and second, the place of some humans in relation to other humans. It is the scale of nature itself.

The ideological thrust of intelligence can be meritocratic, or conservative, or both at the same time. Currently meritocracy predominates. When Michael Young coined this term in *The Rise of the Meritocracy*, he was being ironic; he was describing how modern social systems and their forms of accreditation block access to people without educational qualifications. Our present political class has detoxified and repackaged it as apple pie, alongside freedom, democracy and choice. In fact it has been stood on its head, to become rule by exam-passers. There is a long tradition of such ambiguity over the usefulness of the concept of merit to political power. In the early

---

[23] Alfred Binet, *A Method of Measuring the Development of the Intelligence of Young Children*, 67; *Les idées modernes sur les enfants*, 103.

[24] Kelley, *Scientific Method*, 77.

seventeenth century there was a prevalent ideological tension between honour and merit, sparked by the monarch's sale of honourable titles to state-employed commoners and rich merchants. In religion, the tension was between grace and merit; the latter one could earn by accumulating good works, while grace came from God (it was external, "gratuitous"). Could one achieve grace by one's own merit? Whereas Aquinas had seen the relationship between grace and merit as "a synthesis of divine condescension and human effort," Luther and the Reformation saw them as mutually exclusive, as did many Counter Reformation Catholics. The absolutist political doctrine of rule by divine grace was partly an attempt to control these tensions.[25] And as John Carson's *The Measure of Merit* has shown, the residue of such anxieties would help shape the formal disciplines of psychology in countries whose political cultures have had strong meritocratic pretensions such as France and the USA.

In a meritocracy, to rise by merit means to rise by ability, not by inherited title or a hotline to God. Does this include the abilities of road sweepers? Does each ability command equal status regardless of what the ability is? One has to ask because *status* by its very definition consists of ranks; and if that is the case, then *abilities* too must come in ranks, otherwise there would be no way of pegging one to the other. Hence some abilities have a higher value than others. But by what criteria? What constitutes the merit of one sort of ability against another? Although the vague impression often given is that abilities are equal but different, meritocracy (some abilities are more equal than others) is at one with conservatism (hierarchy is natural). One's level of intelligence both determines one's vocation or calling and *is* that calling, one's place in a natural social hierarchy – a principle already announced in a seminal text of the 1590s familiar to all historians of psychology, Juan Huarte's *The Examination of Men's Wits*. In fact keeping the streets clean may require such abilities as coherence, comprehensiveness and empirical adequacy (if not in so many words), but these abilities are ranked below the same abilities as applied to trading hedge funds, running a government department or writing books on conceptual history. Meritocracy cannot favour "ability" over bloodline or wealth without passing hierarchical judgements that involve matters intellectual and their concomitant social and political interests. This Whig-Tory hybrid existed embryonically as early as 1659. At the point when restoration of the English House of Lords was under consideration, some suggested that henceforth it should be based on appointed life peerages alone, so that "no asses with golden trappings, may be admitted to sit and bray upon our tribunals and seats of judicature" – while taking care that the elected House of Commons keep out those who have "no better education ... than their shops or exchange."[26]

Even in a meritocracy, then, the merits of intellectual ability cannot exist in the abstract. It seems more like *professional* ability. The latter covertly assimilates the former. Young himself compounds this, by thinking (like Bourdieu) only of educational levels. The failure of both writers to go for intelligence as such neuters their critical intent. It is a form of intellectualocentrism, to use Bourdieu's own term. The assumption remains that behind the insignia of qualifications is some abstract substance. And certainly, from the standpoint of the successful meritocrat, professional knowledge just *is* intelligence. Why else would medical and psychological professionals come to choose a label such as "intellectually disabled" for their clients? It is an officialization strategy (to use a term of Bourdieu's), which raises their own specific expertise to the level of a generalized intellect. The professional identity that constitutes their interest in the social hierarchy is elevated into a disinterested science governing the sphere of public reason; this is achieved by disconnecting certain other people from that sphere and reducing them to a purely private condition (the stereotypically private thinker at the moment is, of course, the "autist"). Status is a zero sum: it can

---

[25] B. Gerrish, *Grace and Reason*, 133.
[26] Anon., *A Modest Plea for an Equal Commonwealth, against Monarchy*, 120.

only be acquired by one person by being taken from another. "Intellectual ability" – divine reason, now become human – maintains the due distance between professionals in psychology and their disabled clients. It makes them high or lowly, and orders their estate.

Reducing "intellectual" ability to professional merit is a way of defending one's status against the threat from external structural necessities. It provides the grounds on which people in a higher calling (of which psychology is merely one, though it supplies the rest with a rationale) can establish or hold their ground, against the threat from potentially equalizing counter tendencies that might want to corner some intelligence for themselves. In this way, it is also a form of mutual awareness and political bonding between fellow-members of a status group. A constant maintenance and renewal of the self-referential bid for status is crucial to systems of social administration and order as they respond to external threat. It enables them to obtain the consent of the minds they structure. In labelling someone intellectually disabled, I am defining myself as intellectual. This word, intellectual, claims a universal value and precedence for certain expertises required by the dominant political ideology and institutions, and which my group possesses as bearers of intellect on behalf of the rest of society – reducing the whole of "intellect" to the sum of our expertises and thereby closing down any subversive potential or inherent freedoms the word may suggest. This group, because its self-definition constitutes a vested interest in the argument, can invent and reinvent intelligence at will: that is, until extreme circumstances demand the invention of a whole new bidding mode.

Underlying all concepts of intelligence is the conservative assumption that one cannot have order without hierarchy, either in society or nature. And undoubtedly it seems a bedrock truth that some people are more able than others at some particular thing. This general acknowledgement of hierarchy explains why the psychometricians, just when you thought you had seen the back of them with some irrefutable critique, keep popping up again to say that men are more intelligent than women or whites than blacks. The game is never up with such assertions. The psychometrician may say he wishes the figures didn't turn out this way but they do; to object, he says, is to be deluded by an egalitarian ideology which, however worthy, is not borne out by the regrettable scientific facts – and in any case he is only talking about averages, not individuals.[27] But the egalitarianism he claims to be opposing is a straw man. Belief in equality before the law or before God may by now be a commonplace, but is there anyone who believes in equality of ability? Even a diehard constructionist would be hard pressed to deny that some people are better than others at some things (at deconstructing, for example). Unequal ability, it appears, has some incontestable essence to it. Nevertheless, what is certainly arbitrary and constructed is the classification of some of those things as intellectual and some not. Assessing whether one person is more able than another at some particular thing is one kind of thought, and may in some cases be empirically verifiable. Naming a general category – intelligence, for example – and putting some abilities into it while excluding others is at root another kind of thought, to which the idea of empirical verification is irrelevant. They do not belong together. The first is a judgement, the second a sorting of terms. The confusion between those two entirely different types of thought process is key. To clear it up would be not to relativize intelligence but to annihilate it. Yet abandoning a concept so socially powerful requires a revolution.

Concealed within this arbitrary sorting of human beings is an absolute judgement on the performance of things deemed to be intellectual. Today's professionals exercise a monopoly of power over that judgement, while in a fit of displaced egalitarianism they relativize other kinds of judgement whose claims to be absolute are perhaps not so tenuous (moral or aesthetic ones,

---

[27] Paul Irwing and Richard Lynn, "Is there a sex difference in IQ scores?" *Nature*, 442 (2006); Lynn, "Skin color and intelligence in African Americans," *Population and Environment*, 23/4 (2002).

for example). In this confusion, the purely nominal classification of certain abilities as intelligent or intellectual is passed off as real. I may be especially able at maths, for example, or ironic humour, or orienteering, or recognizing another person's concealed emotions. The only thing they have in common is that I can be judged as being better or worse at them. That judgement may in some cases be real enough. But to be useless at maths or orienteering is a chosen characteristic of intellectual disability, to be useless at ironic humour or perceiving hidden feelings is not; and in fact some people labelled with severe intellectual disability are better at ironic humour and perceptiveness than some people classed as highly or just normally intelligent. No distinction between intellectually better and worse can exist unless some temporary, subjective and purely human consensus has been reached as to which particular abilities "intellectual" or "intelligent" covers and which not. Talking about emotional intelligence, which might seem to cover humour and perceptiveness, does not solve the problem, since exactly the same point can be made here too. Indeed it is on these flimsy grounds (the consensual sorting of intellectual from emotional) that some "high-functioning" people with the Asperger label, despite supposedly being humourless, bad mind readers, are not intellectually disabled at all and may indeed be geniuses.

Finally, like Leo Kanner, one might agree with all the above and assume that the critique of intellectual hierarchy just outlined is entirely valid, but – it goes without saying – cuts out at some point near the bottom of the scale, where the selection of certain abilities as intellectual becomes no longer merely consensual but is indeed objective, separating off a discrete set of *really* intellectually disabled people who are therefore exempt from an otherwise historically constructed group.[28] Surely there must be *some* such creatures. But the exemption would only work if one were already assuming that they exist separately in nature as some biological subspecies, which is indeed the historically contingent premise on which the modern notion of intellectual disability has been built. They are exempt from egalitarian principle only because that principle, in order to exist at all, has already exempted them.

---

[28] Gil Eyal et al., *The Autism Matrix*, 87.

Chapter 6
Honour, Grace and Intelligence: the Historical Interplay

Having dealt with structural similarity of the three modes of status bidding (honour, grace and wit), we are now in a position to look at how they interact in the early modern period, at their historical similarities and mutual displacements. All three belong to the same early modern socio-cultural matrix, occupying at times a single conceptual space. Sometimes all three, or any two, are competing with each other. Sometimes they coalesce. Or they morph into and out of each other. Any one of them may be used to moderate tensions between the other two, between their invisible, internal aspects and their visible, external ones. A change of mode may temporarily disguise the redistribution of privilege, or its defence, in the face of excessive social mobility.

The nature of ability

The three modes are a rough frame of public reference by which judgement is passed on other people. The honourable, the elect and the intelligent are cognate groups, as at the other end are the masses, the reprobate and the intellectually disabled. No doubt a Venn diagram would yield only a small number of primary sources where contemporaries saw intelligence as overlapping with the other two modes. But sometimes it is the only way a text can be understood.

A prime example will suffice for the moment. Richard Mulcaster, Elizabeth's education policy adviser, was also head teacher of Merchant Taylors' School. In this role he had to deal with the porousness of in-group boundaries, as many of his pupils were tradesmen's sons. It was a long-standing problem that had surfaced during the Peasants' Revolt two centuries earlier, when Parliament unsuccessfully petitioned Richard II to prevent serfs' children from going to school, so as to "save the honour of all freemen of the realm."[1] When Mulcaster discusses his own school's admissions policy, he seems uncharacteristically muddled. Discussing "the difference of wits" in children, he writes about the "natural ability" of the gentry and the "natural towardness" of the non-gentle. Both groups should be "set to learning ... as the whole common weal standeth upon these two kinds. If all rich be excluded, ability will snuff, if all poor be restrained, then will towardness repine." This distinction between ability and towardness seems to us redundant, since he identifies the same cognitive components in both: wit, memory, numeracy and so on.[2] Is he is just trying to please two different audiences at once, to give the nod to intelligent commoners without alarming his gentle readership? At any rate he is ambiguous at best, impenetrable at worst, until we realize that by this word ability he means, indiscriminately, both wit *and* the inheritability of a landed title. There is no essential category distinction between the power of noble blood with its concomitant external (political, legal) qualities, and internal reasoning powers. "Towardness," meanwhile, was generally identified with "the multitude" who stood at two removes from the genuine virtues of "honour."[3]

---

[1] Cited in Nicholas Orme, *Medieval Schools*, 220.
[2] Mulcaster, *Positions*, 138 ff.
[3] Robert Ashley, *Of Honour*, 69.

On the one hand, genteel landed property is the source of an ability that could not exist without it; as an earlier Tudor authority had put it, "such men having substance in goods by certain and stable possessions ... may (if nature repugn not) cause them to be so instructed and furnished toward the administration of a public weal, that a poor man's son, only by his natural wit ... seldom may attain."[4] On the other hand, there *is* a difference, a fundamental one, between honourable and dishonourable property ownership: between the rich who "bear the cognizance of virtue, whereto honour is companion" and those "counterfeit gentlemen ... too filthy to be honoured upon earth with either arms by herald, or honour by any," or between land as synonymous with honour and land as what it was increasingly becoming, a commodity. The moment one realizes where the category boundaries are and are not drawn, the difficulties of interpretation disappear. Towardness can only be observed once children are in school; ability precedes it, since it is *given* in the gentle and not in the commoner. It is not so much that one expects ability in the former but not always in the latter; rather, ability as innate intelligence and ability as social power are inseparable. Ability is "answerable to their parents' estate and quality."[5] It lies in the gentleman's "freedom of his cunning, and not to strain her for need": in other words, distinguishing intellectual ability from wealth might look suspiciously like having something to prove. Of course, the wealthy commoner may "be in the same case for ability, though far behind for gentility"; but in that case his cleverness has "the worst effects." That is why, as is exactly the case with honour too, "it is not wit, that carrieth the praise, but the matter, whereon, and the manner how it is, or hath been ill or well employed."

Mulcaster goes on to discuss the bottom end of the intellectual scale: "infirmities in nobility by descent." The modern reader has to make similar adjustments here. Such disabilities exist "either naturally by simpleness, or casually [sc. accidentally], by fortune." Natural simpleness in the gentry, though "to be moaned in respect of their [social] place" (it was the assumed natural condition of most non-gentles), "yet is to be excused in respect of the [individual] person." To "rail upon nobility as too much degenerate" and morally responsible for their own infirmities was to usurp the divine role in allocating or withholding grace. (Degeneracy was also a "fall from grace.") In any case, at the opposite pole to the ability of the genteel and noble stood not simpleness but "idleness" or neglect of "the honour of their houses," and thus of the abilities inscribed in their own social rank – going into business, for example, or marrying a tradesman's daughter. All three modes are in play at once here, as they often were for Mulcaster's contemporaries.

Honour and grace in crisis

In order to appreciate the part played by "wit" and human reasoning in settling the tensions between honour and grace, we need first to understand the relationship between these latter two. "When Adam delved and Eve span / Who was then the gentleman?" was a rhetorical question, the answer obvious to any religious egalitarian: Adam's spade symbolized the tiller of the soil, who was the equal of any gentleman in his ability or inability to receive God's grace. But its shape also resembled a heraldic shield, and in this sense it symbolized the honour society with Adam as its founder: an elite that singled out certain people from within the generality of the commonwealth. In the Middle Ages honour had referred to military valour, and this tended to exclude grace; the man of honour could offload responsibility for his state of grace to monastic types who would intercede for him, or he could defer it to old age, when he could be "unmanned" (grace had feminine connotations) without shedding honour. However, by the early seventeenth century grace had muscled its way to

---

[4] Elyot, *The Governour*, 15r.
[5] Mulcaster, *Positions*, 51; 193 ff.

the centre of the political and ideological stage. On the one hand, even in the republican England of the 1650s people were still being beaten at the magistrate's orders for not raising their hat to their landlord ("hat honour"); on the other, criticism of traditional honour norms, based on the idea of the creaturely equality of souls before God, had been mounting for decades.

One type of criticism was sceptical. Montaigne, for example, described honour as foolishness and the typical earthly illusion, an "empty image ... with neither body nor form." Honourable birth and religious virtue positively precluded each other. Not only a gentleman's honour but his very substance was "a quality dependent on others"; real virtues were inner, religious ones, even in his public role as a governor. Honour was located in the *imaginatio* – a random and dangerous place; "men place [honour] where they want," by contrast with the ultimate reality of grace.[6] This link between honour and the imaginative faculty was widely made, often satirically (the symptom of Don Quixote's diseased imagination, for example, is his obsession with chivalry).

Other critics of honour tried instead to co-opt its terms. Calvinist theologian William Perkins, a stickler for the strict division between elect and reprobate, makes honour a mark of our creaturely equality. Access to grace and election may be restricted, but all of us – "Jew and Greek, slave and free," as St Paul had put it – share honour, by virtue of God's love. To be *dis*honourable was therefore, paradoxically, to have power (particularly intellectual power) here on earth, like the Pharisees, whose hubristic sense of their own honour lay precisely in their assumption of a superior wit and learning. It was a mark of original sin: "Such a one is every man by nature, he lifteth up himself, saying, *I am the man*, and treadeth his brother under his feet." The hubris comes from thinking "of all other men beside ourselves: *such and such a man is far inferior unto me, a base and contemptible fellow in regard of me*" (emphasis in original).[7] Catholics too co-opted the violence of traditional honour codes for divine purposes in their notion of the "church militant." Paintings of the Archangel Michael display him in full armour, spear in hand, leading the nine orders of angelic intelligences in the heraldic attire of their rank; and eventually any old bishop could have his official portrait taken against the background of an altar cloth emblazoned with his own personal coat of arms. Conversely the traditional honour clans of the nobility co-opted religious terms when resisting the incursions of an increasingly centralized state. Their last-ditch rebellion against the Tudors named itself the Pilgrimage of Grace. A century later, Bunyan's famous hymn would reverse the emphasis, insisting that "true" valour is Christian perseverance.

These tendencies to fuse honour and grace can be seen at the symbolic level of coats of arms. Abuse of heraldry, that "sacrament of knightly dignity," was also a pollution of the sacraments of religion:[8]

> None can by order of arms ... put to vile use any Christian's banner ... [nor] pollute any sign or token of arms. Therefore gentlemen should not suffer .... Much the Miller's son, to be arrayed in coats of arms, as I have seen some wear at Whitsuntide ... in maypole mirth, which have been pulled down and given to them by the churchwardens.

Plebeians pollute heraldry as reprobates pollute the eucharist; these churchwardens' negligence was a threat to the social order in both respects. A cosmological abyss separated "the vessels of honour, the elect, the children of promise" from "the vessels of dishonour and wrath, the reprobate."[9] St Paul, discussing the gift and refusal of grace, asks the Romans: "Hath not the potter power over

---

[6] Montaigne, *Essais*, i, 41; Nicole, *Essais de morale*, 39.
[7] William Perkins, *Workes*, ii, 467.
[8] Gerard Leigh, *The Accedence of Armorie*, 239.
[9] Cited in John Bray, *Theodore Beza's Doctrine of Predestination*, 86.

the clay, of the same lump to make one vessel unto honour, and another unto dishonour?" Satan's angels were dishonoured by their apostasy; Cain's progeny became servants. Philip Sidney, who as a devout Calvinist slain in battle represented the late Elizabethan ideal of a combined grace and honour – possibly the original of the phrase "a paragon of virtue" – himself represented reprobation and dishonour as identical in his *Arcadia*; Spenser's *The Faerie Queene* personifies them both in the venal knight Sans Foy ("Faithless" or "Disloyal").

The honour society's ideologues depicted the substance of a gentleman in terms of his soul. Gentility was "spiritual," a "quality of the soul," "a secret disposition of the soul to honourable things."[10] Certain tensions were inherent in this picture. A "new man" is someone reborn in Christ, but the same phrase also indicates an upstart who has arrived in society via his appointment by a new, state-controlled honours system; a "man of means" is someone capable of living independently on the interest from his estate, but the same phrase is used for being in possession of the means to salvation. The anxiety provoked by these contradictions (Do I really belong socially? Can I really get through the eye of the needle?) focused the gentleman's attention inwards, on how he stood with God as well as with his peers, and hence on the consistency of his personality over time. This was to prove fertile soil for later notions of human intelligence as a natural constituent of personhood, an individual possession.

These nervous accommodations between honour and grace occurred in shifting political contexts and national cultures. In England, when Puritan gentry make appeals to creaturely equality and claim that only God could know whether someone is in grace or not, it is sometimes as a power play against the bishops, who did indeed claim to know. A Puritan leader might assert that power should lie with "those of best rank according to God's account," but did so as a way of attacking the government's depredations on his estates, so that he could defend "the luster of this house" and his family name, which "is and ever shall be precious to me." His appeal to creaturely equality was thus an appeal to a not-so-new earthly hierarchy: fellow Puritans were to infer that his family ranked rather better with God than theirs.[11] At the same time, there was a blurring of the lines between "common" or "natural" grace, that is to say the gifts required here on earth to maintain social order, and "special" or "effective" grace, which is divine and is not necessarily a reward for earthly merit but simply elects some and ensures their salvation. His Gracious Majesty the King of England was dispenser of all the earthly honours that went with natural graces, but he was also the chief distribution channel for divine grace. Secular power, both over people's estates and their access to the sacraments, could properly exist only in someone who was himself in grace. Although the monarch was "but a servant to execute the law of God and not to rule after his own imagination," in practice honour did not so much concede ground to grace as join with it, as the arbitrary possession of the ruler. Henry VIII could therefore say both "I rule therefore I am in grace" and "My state of grace entitles me to rule."[12] Special and natural grace unite here, as instruments of divine necessity and social control.

This erosion of earthly and divine boundaries can be traced in Baldesar Castiglione's *The Book of the Courtier* of 1528, translated and read throughout Western Europe. Castiglione's notion of "imitative grace" (*sprezzatura*) confounded honour with grace in similar ways. As one of his disciples put it, the distinctive mark of a gentleman is "a certain *natural* grace, which shines like a *divine* light in all his exercises and even his least important activities" (emphasis added): in other words, a kind of acting ability. It was paramount to avoid giving offence, even if you knew that the requisite virtue

---

[10] Gilles de la Roque, *Traité de la noblesse*, 17.

[11] J.H. Hexter, "The English aristocracy," *Journal of British Studies*, 8/1 (1968).

[12] William Tyndale, *The Obedience of a Christen Man*, 229; see also G.R. Evans, *John Wyclif, Myth and Reality*.

was absent in the person you were honouring and that he was merely acting; one avoided doing so "for courtesy's sake ..., because it belongs to the conversation of human society" and to the social order.[13] The real boundary was therefore not so much between genuine and false claims to social rank as between those who had got themselves into the position of being entitled to put on an act in the first place, and those who had not. Francis Bacon provides us with a similar example. Though he locates honour mainly in religious virtue, this virtue is nevertheless the property of an already closed group. Your social peers will honour you for the virtues you really do possess, but the honour that comes to you "from the common people ... is commonly false and naught," so "shows, and *species virtutibus similes* [appearances that resemble virtues], serve best with them." Unlike Castiglione, Bacon thought the gentry should reserve their acting skills for social inferiors.[14]

In England, as across Europe, religion not only refurbished the ruler's earthly honour by designating him the "godly prince" but internalized this image within each of his subjects. There had to be something within human beings that would respond to God's external, supernatural gift and to royal decree alike. Political and military decisions now required not just the priest's blessing but an inner religious motivation. Troops on the eve of battle were told, "No man can be honourable without divine inspiration and inward motion."[15] Some people probably adopted religious language from cynical motives, but generally talk of grace indicated a genuine obedience to secular authority. The crucial text in this respect was John Foxe's 1563 *Book of Martyrs*, read by nearly every literate English person for the next half century: to the idea of monarchy as a divine calling, Foxe added a providential pattern of history that explained the past and pointed the elect nation of the English towards its future destiny, with which the obedient Protestant could identify. Purely secular honour was a sinful worship of the individual will; conversely, the faith bestowed by God's grace gave men courage in battle. The violence of the honour mode was thereby transferred to that of grace, rather than merely suppressed. Puritans, borrowing their language of violence from the honour mode, fantasized about an Anti-Christ who was making war against the elect and whom a godly ruler (Cromwell, as it turned out) must defeat.

In Spain too, justifications of earthly honour were increasingly made in the Counter Reformation language of grace. In the dramas of Lope de Vega and Calderón, the king makes regular appearances in the final scene to confer grace in a way that takes no account of the recipient's earthly status. Rather than merely parodying sacramental powers, the royal act is sanctified by its divine connotations. The suggestion of the equality of souls before God is sometimes used to raise the profile, while obscuring the continuing subservience, of the peasantry, who at times might even be considered an entire elect caste. (Foxe too exemplified the elect in the lower and middling orders.) This idea was invoked to counterbalance the social importance of the rising professional castes, who were in merit-based competition with the old nobility for honours and titles. The latter perceived the professions to be dominated by descendants of forcibly baptized Jews and Moors, a counterfeit nobility with contaminated and polluting blood. Via this radicalized route, the idea of the elect nation – where uniform faith and national honour are the same thing – came very early in Spain, lasting at least until Franco. The Inquisition fought heresy "in the service of God and his majesty, and for the honour of the Spanish nation." The discriminations involved become natural ones; as one of Lope's characters says to a Moor, "Without my faith there is no nobility ... whoever has God is noble, whoever doesn't is a dog."[16]

---

[13] Nicole Faret, cited in Mark Motley, *Becoming a French Aristocrat*, 13; Baldesar Castiglione, *The Book of the Courtier*.

[14] Francis Bacon, "Of praise," *Essays*, 133.

[15] John Norden, *The Mirror of Honour*, 15.

[16] Cited in Américo Castro, *Le drame de l'honneur*, 23 ff.

In Geneva, Calvinist playwrights (among them Calvin's political successor, Théodore Beza) wrote popular didactic dramas that used contemporary social anxieties around land inheritance, primogeniture and bloodline as metaphors in the teaching of grace and predestination.[17] The landed inheritance was the Promised Land, which was reserved for the Calvinist elect, the bloodline of Abraham; Catholics, stripped of their coats of arms, were a disinherited line. Reprobation and disinheritance were one and the same. The key biblical characters in this genre were the twins Esau and Jacob. Esau was born first, but God decreed that he serve the younger, through whom the bloodline of Abraham would continue. The story shows how personal salvation is predestined, a product of grace. Neither legal primogeniture nor moral merit – Jacob gets his father's blessing by trickery – can alter God's predeterminate decision. Honour and grace then pass through a single, elect bloodline from Jacob through to the community of Geneva itself, having prevented the dispersal of the Promised Land among a multitude of heirs and protected its latter-day saints against disinheritance. Echoes of Esau and Jacob remain in Alexandre Dumas's *The Man in the Iron Mask*, where Louis XIV turns out to have a dastardly twin who claims his inheritance, and indeed in the obsession modern cognitive genetics has with twin studies (even if the emphasis here is on sameness rather than difference).

In France, the political tensions between honour and grace arose out of the nobility's anxieties about social status and religious belief, which reinforced each other. Many nobles thought they partook of the purity of Christ's blood not only at communion but by direct descent in their own noble veins – an idea that eventually found its way into the racism of Gobineau. But at the same time, they had to endure public investigation into false claims to nobility. These were conducted by non-noble functionaries who went under the unfortunate professional title of *les élus*, at the same time as Protestant nobles were using this term to describe their own religious status.[18] Humiliated by such inquisitions, and alarmed at the state's mass sale of honourable titles to commoners, they insisted that "nobility should remain the endowment of a minority, of the elect" and promoted a eugenics of virtue.[19] Election was, in a more than merely homonymous sense, an earthly as well as a heavenly status; religious writers had in any case long noted the irony in having both a "company of the elect" of God and a Pope "elected" by mortal cardinals. Accordingly, ordinary guides to earthly social rank were presented in hyperbolic terms of religious purity and defilement. One such writer introduces the topic thus: "Since it was proposed to me to discourse on true Nobility, it seemed to me that I should do as those do who seek religiously and in good conscience to enter a Temple, and who must first be purified and prepared for divine thoughts and holy meditations, leaving at the door all those affections which might prevent them from raising their spirits above temporal things."[20]

During the European fiscal crises and spectacular advancement of merchant capital of the 1590s, the increasing grants of titles to commoners for cash or services began to demand theorization. Some behavioural authors took an openly bourgeois line, attacking the idea that purity of blood was a product of ancestry. Virtue, especially that which consisted in wisdom and learning, could accumulate over a couple of generations and in that way become hereditary; a law of acquired characteristics arose, with metaphors drawn from animal husbandry. Other writers strayed even further from the criterion of bloodline. The most essential aspect of man was the soul, whose gradations were subject not to laws of nature but to divine necessity. There were indeed "rights of

---

[17] Daniel Smail, "Predestination and the ethos of disinheritance," *Sixteenth Century Journal*, 23 (1992).

[18] James Wood, *The Nobility*, 3.

[19] Christophle Bonours, *Eugeniaretologie*, cited in Devyver, *Le sang*, 68.

[20] Claude Marois, *Le gentil-homme parfaict*, 1.

blood"; it was just that they were not the product of ancestry or nature but donated by the King, who stood in for God and filled the role of necessity here on earth by handing out titles.[21] These writers projected the same principle back into history. The origins of honour, they said (correctly), lay in the feudal ruler's allocation of fiefdoms to his personal warrior servants, rather than anything more ancient: "hence ... our ancient and immemorial nobility of which the commencement is unknown, does not come by right of nature, as liberty does, but from the ancient right and disposition of the state." The ruler could likewise remove at a stroke any taints in nature – pollution by marriage to a merchant's daughter, for example – with a "restitution of native rights." While it was true that only God could "make someone a bloodline noble who is not one by nature," he delegated this job to earthly rulers. Necessity, at once divine and political, could override nature.

A huge theoretical apparatus was wheeled in to justify this position. Aristotle's theory of the final cause, in which natural causes are explicable only in terms of their goals, was used to justify divine right: honour and titles belonged to the science of nature because their true goals lay in their source, which was the monarch.[22] By Louis XIV's time, strict social practices had been generated to deal with tensions over honourable precedence and the rivalry among those immediately below him. A formalized prestige fetish came into existence: a set of rituals upon which courtiers, all signed up into an Order of the Knights of the Holy Spirit, depended both for their spiritual salvation and for their degree of social distance from the out-group and from each other, and consequently for their whole personal identity.[23] To be demoted or ejected was at once social death and death of the soul. The minutest discriminations of the external honour insignia conferred by the king were also those of the inner, divine grace he transmitted; these involved elements of public performance at court. Verification by insignia was also naturalization; the visible hierarchical signs presented at court were drawn from nature, following earlier authorities who had ranked coats of arms by the emblematic creatures which were displayed on them and each of which had their place in a biological hierarchy. The arrival of new forms of biological classification in the eighteenth century among naturalists such as Buffon may owe something to the wider mind-set created in the interim by the strict courtly ranking of the emblems of honour and grace.

Wit to the rescue

Such were the tensions, combinations and recombinations between honour and grace. How did specifically human intelligence ("wit") come to resolve them? Was this somehow a progressive change? Intelligence is a change of nomenclature for the way the abstract goals of status are accommodated to the brute facts of life; it is the bourgeoisification of honour and the secularization of grace. But if honour and grace really were principles of a value-rational society and intelligence of a succeeding goal-rational one (as Weber might have put it), the first two should have been withering away during the gestation of the third – and the opposite is the case. The language of honour and grace became increasingly central to early modern politics, and only as its accompanying codifications became increasingly rigid were they absorbed within that of wit. The absorption process was facilitated by another of the structural similarities noted above. Each mode has three elements: an in-group in whom the mode is embodied (the gentle and noble, the godly and elect, people within the band of normal intelligence and above) and a set of external signs (coat of arms, catechism, cognitive ability score). A team of experts (heralds, pastors, psychologists)

---

[21] Charles Loyseau, *Traité des ordres*, 29 ff.
[22] Guillaume de Oncieu, *La précédence de la noblesse*, 13; 38.
[23] See Norbert Elias, *The Court Society*, 147.

operates border controls, distinguishing genuine from counterfeit, maintaining in-group quotas and verifying the external insignia that confirm these borders as natural ones. Command of the public sphere takes place in the name of the appropriate mode, banishing autonomous honour, personal grace and private intelligence (autism, for example) to the margins or worse.

Although the dominance of intelligence today might lead us to think of it as a progressive victory of wit over the other two modes, popular texts of the time dealing with everyday matters of child-rearing, education and personal virtue, often mixed up with accounts of genealogy and heraldic science, reveal a more complex relationship. The competition and complementarity among the three modes rearranged the terms in which political power was justified, and forged new relationships between state power and the "virtues" or types of excellence it required.

Tensions in the relationship between externality and internality, outward show and inward reflectiveness, reality and appearance (central to the Dutch portraiture of the period, for example) are clearly perceptible. The public coat of arms required "the privy coat of a good conscience," but this sense of complementarity is equally matched by that of tension.[24] Grace was in some sense external, since it could not be generated from within oneself; but more often it bore internal connotations of faith and a one-to-one relationship with God. The proponents of grace contrasted it with the pure externality of honour. Hence Cromwell's demand for Sir Peter Lely to paint him, unlike Charles I, with his warts intact (perhaps in mitigation for his acceptance of the Lord Protectorship and retention of the vanquished Antichrist's own official portraitist). Predestinarians of all colours – Protestants first, then the Jansenist school of Catholicism – claimed that honour's externality was surely the positive sign of a corrupt interior. Honour was external also in that to exist at all it had to be recognized by other people. Its official performative rite was heraldic display; the Jansenists' critique of honour would resurface among the Jacobins, who regarded heraldry as "barbarous and arid emblems which speak only to the eyes."[25]

Since this exposed honour to the charge that it was *only* external and therefore superficial, its defenders had to cite in support its internal constituents of blood and lineage, or at least of virtue acquired over generations. Honour was in this sense a "true substance ..., that needeth the mixture of no other colours than its own beauty," by contrast with the "mere popinjays, who glory more in the painting or varnish of honour" – what mattered was one's "natural or original disposition."[26] Yet "natural" here does not indicate biological necessity. And we should note what a recent preoccupation bloodline and the "true substance" of time-honoured ancestry were. The very principle of succession of titles was made law only in the fifteenth century. It then took another two centuries for an English court to deem honourable titles inalienable. It did so on the grounds that they were a natural and "invisible hereditament in the blood." "Hereditament" was a legal term for inherited land. In its new usage here, gentry and honour are the internalization of an external good: the subjectification of an objective ability or power (landed property).

The contrast between honour as external and grace as internal was thus not straightforward. And in fact these attempts to enhance the internality of honour led to a change of mode. Of all its internal virtues, the most honourable had to be an "inward mind" that matched "outward glittering": a gentleman "should surmount the rest in store of wisdom" and, moreover, "*quickness* of invention" (emphasis added).[27] And the *constancy* that had been an external, public value of the honour society – loyalty and promise keeping ("a gentleman's word is his bond") – was increasingly supplanted

---

[24] Francis Bacon, Letter to Lord Henry Howard, 3 December 1599, in J. Spedding, *Life and Letters of Francis Bacon*, ii, 161.

[25] Jacques-Antoine Dulaure, *Histoire critique de la noblesse*, 280; 284.

[26] Francis Markham, *The Booke of Honour*, 4; Richard Brathwait, *The English Gentleman*, 59.

[27] Lawrence Humfrey, *The Nobles, and of Nobility*, A7a.

by the internal value of *consistency* over one's lifetime, a religious quality and, increasingly, an intellectual one in which intelligence was a personal possession. The honour clan's mutual solidarity became individual solidity, a permanence of those qualities, while the external display so important to the old honourable behaviours turned into the mere superficiality of everyday manners. Likewise internality as the sense of personal autonomy and freedom from external compulsion, central to a gentleman's honour, was transmuted into a modern rational autonomy.

Wit, in addition to usurping honour's own internal qualities, began to usurp those of grace, as we shall see. Tensions between all three modes were a source of political disorder and led to attempts at synthesis. Castiglione, for example, by associating gentry with humanist learning rather than the martial valour of the traditional honour code, was addressing the crisis in social identity that followed a long period of civil and religious wars on the Italian peninsula. It was already hard to sustain any pretence that the identity concerned was not bourgeois. Traditional chivalry was codified into a "technically rigorous cultural model, more theoretically trained, more rigidly selected," a virtuous pursuit of professionalism.[28] The trick was to handle the shifting personnel, functions and vocabulary of the honour society while representing it as the immutable hierarchy of a natural order. Men of wit (*ingenium*) and quick soul spirits but no genealogy could obtain honours for services rendered. As recipients of the prince's grace, they then represented themselves as a company of earthly elect (*electi*), by contrast with the out-group of the *plebs*. This instant election not only qualified them as gentlemen (*cavalieri*), it instilled in them a systematic knowledge of their own gentility, at which point any labour they may have expended on acquiring this knowledge suddenly became invisible and unmentionable.

Castiglione's characters politely maintain the fiction that it is hard to be the perfect courtier without being of noble birth; but, and more seriously, those claiming noble birth must have the ability appropriate to their public duties. Wit, as professional merit, therefore achieved pre-eminence because of its place in a system of social exchange: status for skills. This went with the intensified codification characteristic of any bidding mode, an increasing requirement for status to be performed that extended to the most mundane behaviours, such as table manners. The key to a courtier's professional knowledge (*scienza*) was knowing how to imitate natural grace. He had the ability to *perform as* a member of the honour society, and only as a result to *be* one. This ability was an inner quality and even had its own corresponding bodily complexion (the "sanguine"). Grace as imitated to perfection, even if natural and not spiritual, could "correct natural defects," in a parody of Christian rebirth.[29]

The interplay between modes was presented in terms of faculty psychology. One French writer in the Castiglione tradition presents the faculties of the human Soul (capital S) as a descending series: understanding, spirit and soul (small s). Understanding is that which "some call ... a portion of divinity" and comprises the power of cognition and of ordering things wisely. Spirit is "the mediator between terrestrial and heavenly things," and can float upwards to the understanding or be dragged downwards. To soul belong the passions, senses and corresponding bodily temperaments. "Can we find anywhere in nature images that correspond better to the prince, the nobles and the people, than this triple distinction of our Soul?" The prince's equivalence with the ruling faculty is more than metaphorical. He just *is* the "rational Soul" or "understanding," and as such he holds together the macrocosm of external world and the microcosm of the individual psychology. This not only allows him to disburse honours, it *consists in* his disbursing honours, which then become

---

[28] Giancarlo Mazzacurati, *Il Renascimento dei moderni*, 234.
[29] Harry Berger, *The Absence of Grace*, 16.

imprinted physically and materially on his subjects' soul spirits. Hence "honour is the greatest earthly good, and no other; goods are only such to the extent that they participate in honour."[30]

The tensions were particularly great in England. From the late sixteenth century there was a deepening ideological fissure between self-assertive honour and the pursuit of godly behaviour, at a time when the weakness of existing forms of coercion was forcing government to pursue the internalization of social controls. This fissure made room for wit's status to advance within the mix of cultural norms. One of the highest political achievements was to calibrate successfully the fulcrum of the three status modes. Impending social breakdown is always evidenced by a perceived lack of discipline in the upcoming generation, and a famous moral panic of Elizabeth's reign was the strike by Eton pupils against corporal punishment. It led her secretary and former tutor, the alarmed Roger Ascham, to come up with a new handbook on pedagogy, whose opening statement of intent ran: "In writing this, I have had earnest respect to three special points: truth of religion, honesty in living, right order in learning."[31] With these three great goals of public life in mind, educators like Ascham and Mulcaster sought to mould what they called a "monarchical learner." By this they meant someone who, in ruling himself, would therefore accept the rule of another. The honour society had originally been a pluralist system of solidarity among semi-autonomous nobles, with the monarch as first among equals; this pluralism had produced the century of civil strife that was resolved only by the Tudors, along with their monopolization of the honour system. There was now a single seat of authority. Henry VIII tamed semi-autonomous nobles by making the principle of honour obedience to himself, rather than obedience to a separate, self-standing code to which he too might have been bound. Honour, following Cicero's Roman model, now came from service to the state, as a reward for the professional wit of an expanding clerical caste with its administrative and legal abilities.

The most widely consulted advice on behaviour during Henry VIII's governmental innovations was Thomas Elyot's *The Governour*, which advocated replacing military prowess with learning as the core skill of the gentry. Honourable lineage was important as a surface decoration that might help preserve due deference from the lower ranks. But it had to be complemented by inner religious virtues, shorn of any implicit egalitarianism. It was in any case becoming less clear where the virtue of a religious "understanding" or *intellectus* stopped and professional wit started. The governing elite, a lay intellectual caste that had traditionally been inculcated with the public virtues of Aristotle's *Ethics*, had now to be imbued with an internal honour that was achievable through grace. This moralization of politics was reflected in a moralization of administration, though the abrupt end to Thomas More's career shows that the moralizers sometimes pushed their luck. Cultivation of a higher religious learning was now a requirement of public life, intrinsic to the self-image of the man of honour. Perversely, it would in the end fuel opposition to the absolute state.

While Elyot's ostensible theme is honour, which many of his readers might have identified with military valour, his opening chapter is nevertheless entitled "The Understanding." A token nod to intellectual distinctions between the angelic orders, as evidence for the varying degrees of their divinity, yields within a few lines to a discussion of the earthly social differentiations that imitate them. Just as the individual's understanding is the most important part of his soul, "most nigh unto the similitude of God ... so should the estate of his person be advanced in degree, or place, where understanding may profit."[32] God does not distribute natural graces equally. Some men are "set in a more high place" because they "excel other in this influence of understanding ... by the beams of their excellent wit." Unlike Calvin, who kept the spiritual gift of divine grace separate from the natural gift of a corruptible human reason that should therefore not encroach upon religion,

---

[30] David de Rivault, *Les estats ... du Prince, du Noble, & du tiers Estat*, 247.
[31] Ascham, *The Scholemaster*, Preface.
[32] Elyot, *The Governour*, 4r–6r.

Elyot fuses the understanding (*intellectus*), divine origin and all, with natural, everyday human wit (*ingenium*). Wit is an "instrument" of the understanding, a mobile, practical force engaged in "finding out" rather than merely contemplating.

The most usually cited authorities on honour, Ramón Lull and Bartolus of Saxoferrato, had already regretted any lack of learning in a gentleman. However, they saw learning merely as complementary to lineage and valour, whereas Elyot now has a positive agenda for instilling it. He invokes the divinity of the understanding only and precisely in order to sanctify the secular authority of wit. Human understanding thus reconceived hangs on to its divine doppelganger by the thinnest of threads. In replacing one mode with another, Elyot is acknowledging the structural importance of self-referential status modes in general:

> It can none otherwise stand with reason, but that the estate of the person in pre-eminence of living, should be esteemed with his understanding ... whereunto must be added an augmentation of honour and substance: which not only impresseth a reverence, whereof proceedeth due obedience among subjects: but also inflameth men naturally inclined to idleness, or sensual appetite ... to dispose them to study.

In short, honour is kicked upstairs to become a vague aspiration in the moment that it becomes modally subordinate to the understanding. Its role now is to conceal any lingering Calvinistic contradiction between the understanding's divine, spiritual role and its natural, earthly one. And that is how it would feature in Locke's *Essay*, whose very first sentence appeals to this principle: "Since it is the understanding that sets man above the rest of sensible beings, and gives him all the advantage and dominion, which he has over them; it is certainly a subject, even for its nobleness, worth our labour to enquire into."[33] It would become, in the words of his close acquaintance Joseph Glanvill, a matter of defending "the honour of our faculties" against the unreason of sectarian fanaticism.

The erection of wit

Some late Elizabethan writers went further than Elyot and came up with the concept of an "erected wit": a natural grace that, though human, might escape the taint of corruption. Echoing growing millenarian tendencies, they imagined that Adam's total understanding of nature before the Fall might be restored to his descendants. It is true, says one, that Aristotle's "desire to understand" is part of man's (sinful) nature and so can corrupt, as Calvin warned – but only "if special grace, or an excellent education (which cannot be without grace) do not fashion and frame the mind to the right use of it."[34] The second use of the word grace here is syntactically ambiguous: does it refer to the special (i.e., divine) grace of the opening phrase, or to the merely human, natural grace implied by "education"? This ambiguity is the cautious expression of an increasingly optimistic perspective on our ability to develop quasi-divine understandings here on earth. There was, as Mervyn James has described, a "composite Tudor court culture which aspired to be honourable, religious and wise," and the erection of wit coincides exactly with failure to paper over the cracks between the first two.[35]

A major example of this self-conscious search for three-way synthesis is Sidney's *A Defence of Poesy*. Like Elyot's, this was a much-read text aimed at "governors" that sought to improve the

---

[33] Locke, *An Essay*, 44; Glanvill, "Anti-fanatical religion," 20, in *Essays*.
[34] Lodowick Bryskett, *A Discourse of Civill Life*, 15.
[35] M.E. James, "English politics and the concept of honour, 1485–1642," *Past and Present*, supp. iii (1978).

existing classical curriculum with new inputs from religion. Sidney advocated self-examination as a training for good conduct. He had translated and absorbed the French Protestant Philippe de Mornay's *De la vérité de la religion chrétienne*, approving the role of human effort and natural virtue as supplements to faith, as well as the role of rational consent in face of political tyranny. A necessary ingredient of self-examination was the "strengthening" and "purifying [of] man's wit" in order to purge its intrinsic corruption. He presents it in faculty psychology terms: purification is "the enriching of memory, enabling of judgement, and enlarging of conceit" or imagination. The man of honour matures, from his quest for glory in private violence, into the "wisdom" that is true honour and consists in obedience and service to a just public order ("the king his majesty, his councillors, officers, and administrators").[36] More than just everyday cleverness, the "final end" of wit is "to lead ... us to as high a perfection as our degenerate souls, made worse by their clayey lodgings, can be capable of" – to the point where it becomes "erected wit ... not at all corrupted." That the devoutly Calvinist Sidney could express such an un-Calvinist notion, even if tentatively (the text goes on to display some second thoughts), illustrates the depth of the crisis. Only an erected wit could negotiate the abyss between honour and grace.

Wit now seems to be an independent entity, at the same level as the other two modes rather than merely complementing one or the other. Elyot had already put civic intellect (*prudentia*) in the first and most honourable place in the cultural identity of the gentleman. But Sidney's "erected wit," albeit restricted to the gentry, went beyond that old Aristotelian mantra. The idea that honour and nobility might have an intellectual component of sorts was not entirely new, nor was his proposal that wit could yield in part a "knowledge of a man's self" through his conscience. What was startling was his notion that it might shake off original sin and lead to a "*perfect* ... knowledge of a man's self" (emphasis added). Human understanding – that is, *purely* human and thus synonymous with wit – was a political project that could only mediate between honour and grace if it could be hived off from the cosmological and divine associations of the scholastic *intellectus*. Elyot had still seen man's reasoning abilities as a second-hand version of divine ones; they were the road to knowledge but would always be blocked at the last step by the need for some additional, spiritual element beyond the operations of mere wit. Sidney, in contrast, writes about the human understanding as a natural grace with a superadded perfection of its own. His insistence on self-examination is key to this. For Elyot, man's understanding is honourable as long as he contemplates the divine; Sidney's project for man is "to lift up the mind ... to the enjoying [of] *his own* divine essence" (emphasis added). His erection of wit is already aimed at something like the modern psychological project: at intelligence's own (circular) rationale and self-justification.

The political context of Sidney's three-way synthesis was matched in an ecclesiastical one by his contemporary Richard Hooker, Elizabethan England's leading authority on church government. Both men recognized the hubristic implications of promoting a specifically human understanding, but while these made Sidney hesitant, Hooker cocoons them in ambiguity. Sometimes, when writing about human "reason," he claims that the elect have one type of reason that is divine, aided by "special" grace, and another type that is not divine but merely natural. At other times, however, he writes about a reason that is naturally human and exists *irrespective of* whether one is elect or not, and describes *this* as "divine." In other words, human reason can be divinely enhanced even while retaining its role as a merely natural grace. Whereas Calvin restricted the application of reason as a natural grace to earthly matters and warned that any intrusion of it into religion would

---

[36] Philip Sidney, *A Defense of Poesy*, 82; 86; see also Brian Cummings, *The Literary Culture of the Reformation*.

lead to depravity, Hooker uses it to hint that humans may not be totally depraved, that they may have a divinely tinged "ableness" (his term) of their own.[37]

Many behaviour guides (and, later on, Locke) draw on these writings of the Sidney circle and of Hooker. According to one, "those which think themselves gentlemen, only because their fathers ... did descend of noble houses" are exactly the same as those "void of grace which wisheth no order of obedience in commonwealth to be observed."[38] The solution to both is learning; ignorance is the contrary of all three. Learning is "next to the omnipotent God"; its particular disciplines of grammar, logic and rhetoric persuade "by grace, and divine assistance" and hence have supernatural efficiency. But the greatest persuader, Sidney noted, is poetry, reason's supreme expression and an "instrument" of divine grace, with a "utility, power, and virtue" whose movement doctors can trace in the body. It has been said that "the nexus of grammar and grace is found ... at the surface of discourse" in these texts, and must not be "reduced to a doctrinal statement."[39] But this begs the question of how what is at the surface of discourse becomes doctrinal subsequently, and hence enmeshed in material interests. These latter are implicit in the Sidney-inspired practical guides to everyday behaviour just as they are in today's psychology textbook. The Protestant emphasis on reading for oneself, on the principle that "grammar is next to godliness," created a new out-group of the unlearned and illiterate, thus drawing closer to the role of verbal reasoning sections in cognitive ability tests, which help to exclude a group labelled as intellectually disabled. The very existence of such out-groups amounts to a doctrinal statement.

In the early Stuart culture some 20 years after Sidney's death, a fusion of honour, religion and humanist learning was briefly achieved, but as a tool of absolutism. Its court literature represents kingly authority in terms of a supreme honour which, in combination with the other two modes, infiltrates his subjects and enables them to overcome the passions, and more importantly the self, in favour of political obedience. In order to achieve this, honour as old-fashioned vainglory (one of Bacon's idols of the tribe) is effaced, in favour of what Ben Jonson in his court masque *The New Inne* calls the "honour that springs from reason." With this the elite took on a particular psychological identity. "Contemplation," formerly typical of the learned monk, now typified the gentleman. It set him on the path of what Bacon called "the great restoration" of man's prelapsarian understanding, and rendered him sufficiently reasonable in the meantime to avoid turning into a "factious or litigious sectist" who might challenge the absolute state.[40] The civil war period was to prove the futility of this line. Parliament's support was supposed to have come from men "of a lower state ... that love freedom and to be something themselves," whereas the king's was said to come from "the nobility and gentry ... men of implicit faith, whose conscience is much regulated by their superiors," i.e., their earthly ones, and "whose honour is predominant over their reason and religion."[41]

The civil wars also saw the rise of the "invisible college" (precursor to the Royal Society), a new attempt at fusion in which wit was even more clearly in the lead – though as Steven Shapin has demonstrated, the other two modes are constantly in play; both Boyle and Newton liked to hint that their extraordinary intellectual abilities proved their descent by blood and faith from King Solomon. Gentlemen of the college built mutual trust by a deliberate, pacific abstention from all discussion of current political conflicts as well as from their loosely associated disputes over honour and grace; the gap was filled by promoting the modal status of the human subject's "ingenuity," embodied in an objective, scientific method which they knew to be secure because

---

[37] Cited in Nigel Voak, *Richard Hooker and Reformed Theology*, 278.
[38] Humfrey Braham, *The Institucion of a Gentleman*, unpaginated.
[39] Cummings, *The Literary Culture of the Reformation*, 281.
[40] Brathwait, *The English Gentleman*, 47.
[41] Cited in Hill, *From Reformation to Revolution*, 132.

"a man of honour would not write a lie." In this milieu at last, it was conceivable that there is "no truth ... so far elevated out of our reach, but man's wit may raise engines to scale and conquer it."[42] And that would include truths *about* man's wit.

Literary treatments of wit and foolishness

The three status modes and the relationships among them leap from the pages of the canonical literary texts of the time. Book 1 of Spenser's *The Faerie Queene*, contemporary with Sidney, portrays a man who arrives at court and is at first denied honourable status because of what the poet in his prefatory letter calls a "clownish" (rustic and stupid) appearance. Sent on a trial mission, the anonymous knight ends up being providentially bathed in a "living well" of saving grace that enables him to restore a family's noble lineage from pollution by a dragon. Evidently capable of noble deeds, he is, as it turns out, one of those creatures whom "men do changelings call, so changed by faeries' theft": in other words, the ploughman who raised him is not his real father. He discovers this when he arrives at the New Jerusalem built by God "for those to dwell in, that are chosen," where faith and reason are one. An old man named Contemplation (this being the supreme function of the reasoning faculty) offers himself as a guide. The knight, on being shown the company of the elect and told that he will be joining them, wonders: "Unworthy wretch ... of so great grace / How dare I think such glory to attain?" Whereupon the old man tells him his true name and genealogy, which are his entitlement to membership: he is Georgos, sprung "from ancient race / Of Saxon kings."

Spenser's readers well knew both that *georgos* was Greek for "peasant" and that St George was patron saint of knightly gentlemen. This ambiguity reflects the poet himself. A journeyman's son claiming aristocratic family connections, Spenser had been educated at Merchant Taylors', where no doubt headteacher Mulcaster had typecast him with plebeian "towardness" rather than innate or landed "ability." This circumstance certainly rounds out for us Spenser's description of the purpose behind *The Faerie Queene* (to Sir Walter Raleigh) as being to "fashion a gentleman or noble person in virtuous and gentle discipline." Here, in the Tudor elite's state of denial about the emptiness of their own claims to ancient lineage (a good proportion of Henry VII's ancestors had been servants), is the source for that canon of obsequious disbelief and disgust at the ordinariness of one's own social origins that pervades English literature through to Dickens and Harry Potter.

The "changeling" explanation offered by Spenser for the knight's (and possibly his own) status re-emerges in a reversed format in Locke's changeling, which was one of the most important textual models for modern concepts of severe intellectual disability. Instead of a country clown who turns out to have been born noble and elect, we have here a creature whose appearance is not clownish, whose physical and bodily matter suggests the "form" of a rational soul, who is born of parents belonging to the human species, but who exhibits no signs of rationality throughout his life and therefore turns out to lack a soul and to be possibly not even human. Translating this back into Tudor terms, we might say that he is intellectually a ploughman even though born to an honourable and elect line: the opposite of Spenser's knight.

Old man Contemplation is only one of Spenser's allegorical descriptions of human reasoning as it interfaces with social and religious status. We also find "workman's wit," which builds the House of Pride. It falls down: so far, so conventionally Calvinist. Then there is "mortal wit," which sways with the winds of Providence; "sudden wit," which is over-quick to counsel despair; "the weaker wit of man," lacking the necessary complement of faith; and "practic wit," i.e., the devil's.

---

[42] Steven Shapin, *A Social History of Truth*; Kenelm Digby, *Observations upon* Religio Medici.

Yet contrasted with all these is something positive, namely "poet's wit."[43] Like Sidney, Spenser promotes poetry not only as the highest form of reason but as a policy tool: the appearance of poet's wit in Book 2 coincides exactly with the appearance of the Queen herself. Elizabeth is represented as Medina (the mean), dispensing honours and transmitting divine grace in order to reimpose a peace that has been shaken by Acrasia (intemperance). To match this public allegory there is also a private, inner one. A knight-errant on a quest for temperance is conducted by Lady Alma ("Soul"), herself dressed in heraldic garments, on a journey through her palace. Each room is named after one of the three psychological faculties.[44] The House of Alma is organic to the knight's inner self: his journey through the palace makes him who he is. After passing through the rooms of imagination and judgement, he arrives at memory, and this is where Spenser chooses to itemize Elizabeth's genealogy; his lengthy recital of her honourable line gives memory a lopsided importance by comparison with the other faculties, just as theological texts tend to devote more space to memory than to the other faculties because of its importance to confession and the conscience. Ending the ancestral list with the present incumbent, he assembles all three modes together to sum Elizabeth up: "Nobler liveth none this hour, / Ne like in grace, ne like in learned skill."

Shakespeare invokes the triad frequently. Hamlet laments that his reflective understanding "quartered hath but one part wisdom, / And ever three parts coward." A heraldic device consisted of four "quarterings." The coward occupying the other three and negating Hamlet's honour is his conscience, which in Puritan doctrine is the one residue of divine reason still lodged within human beings after the Fall: "Thus conscience doth make cowards of us all." *Love's Labour's Lost* opens with the King of Navarre telling his courtiers that the tension between worldly glory (the struggle for a fame "registered upon our brazen tombs") and religion (the struggle against "the huge army of the world's desires") can be resolved, because both offer a window on immortality. Abandoning the usual court life and turning it into "a little academe, / Still and contemplative" will enable them to see this. However, this dramatic intervention by the intellect is subordinate to the main dichotomy between honour and grace, which Navarre is unable to repair; reasoned contemplation can only flourish in withdrawal from the real political world where the dichotomy is being played out.

The best-known texts to evoke the triad of status modes involve Falstaff. His famous soliloquy on honour in *I Henry IV* is often cited to illustrate the decline of the honour-rational society. It is, however, more than that. We can set his dismissal of honour alongside his other famous soliloquy, from *II Henry IV*, which is a celebration of wit. Honour as military valour is the contrary of wit and therefore foolish, a disabled rival in the bidding game of worldly advancement. Falstaff's wit is not just a trivial ability to amuse his companions or the audience. It is the human understanding itself, represented here by the "discretion" (*discretio* or discrimination, a key operation of the reasoning faculty) which Falstaff calls "the better part of valour." If Falstaff is "not only witty in myself but the cause that wit is in other men," he is a cause in the Aristotelian sense: wit is that to which all men, as a species, naturally tend. Hotspur in the opposing political camp calls people who disregard their own honour "foolish"; the fat knight is a fool because his shameful behaviour contradicts his ascribed membership of the honour society. It might be supposed that when each identifies the other as a fool, he is invoking some external referent, specifically the person whom today's psychologist would call intellectually disabled. But no such person yet existed. Lack of a sense of one's own honour is, for Hotspur, foolishness defined, not foolishness by metaphor. He who does not pay attention to his own honour is a fool at root; that is what a fool *is*.

Falstaff's honour soliloquy, parodying conventional eve-of-battle meditations on God and death, is set out in question-and-answer format like a catechism: "What is honour? A word ... Who

---

[43] *The Faerie Queene*, 1.4.5; 1.6.6; 1.9.41; 1.10.19; 2.1.3; 1.4.32.
[44] Ibid., Book 2, cantos 9 and 10.

hath it? He that died a' Wednesday," etc. His sign-off line – "Honour is a mere scutcheon, and so ends my catechism" – juxtaposes two politically hostile ways of claiming status, but can only be understood by its covert reference to a third. A scutcheon was the emblem on a shield that verified its owner's honourable status (in Puritan terms a meaningless outward show), while the catechism verifies the communicant's receptivity to grace. But for Falstaff, neither is an adequate means of authentification. His self-seeking wit is subversive of the other two modes, rather than just a purely hypothetical solution to the tensions between them as it was in *Love's Labour's Lost*. Wit, with Prince Hal's embodiment of it eventually usurping Falstaff's, competes successfully with grace for the role of inner man, as the main opposition to the externality and superficiality of honour.

A similar nexus appears in lines as central to Spanish drama as Falstaff's are to English. Calderón's *The Mayor of Zalamea* features Pedro Crespo, a peasant whose daughter has been raped by a nobleman. He claims, absurdly for a peasant, that his honour has been insulted and therefore he may kill in revenge: absurdly because, as any nobleman knows, honour is lacking in peasants. To justify himself Crespo universalizes the concept of honour, in defiance of existing social norms: "Honour is the patrimony of my soul, and my soul is God's alone." This is not mere metaphor, nor is honour here just some external adornment to the soul. The word "patrimony" suggests property, both in a legalistic sense (God is the soul's ultimate owner) and in a faculty-psychology sense (honour is a property of the soul). The lines are in fact a paraphrase of Aquinas, who had written that the understanding (*intellectus*) was the patrimony of the soul, and the intellective soul from God alone – not from the parental act of conception, and thus not from honourable ancestry.[45] When the Thomist ex-seminarian Calderón substitutes honour for the human intellect here, he is pointing out their kinship; both belong to the same class of things, along with the gift of divine grace that is freely offered to every soul, even a peasant's.

Crespo's social levelling of honour helps bring the *intellectus* down with it into the real social and political world. Honour, intellect and grace are transposable with each other both as status terms and as naturalized "psychological" ones. His claim is both religious (all souls are equally honourable because they come from God) and secular (honour is a quasi-material inheritance, like land – a protectable personal possession). The prospect offered – that horizontal honour might consist not only of equal access to grace but of earthly equality – is nevertheless a ruse of power. The granting to a peasant of his own quasi-autonomous sphere was also a strengthening of the bonds tying him to the state; the King appears in the final scene to endorse Crespo's claim but also thereby his own supremacy, as sole distributor of earthly honours. Like meritocratic intelligence today, horizontal honour helped to naturalize the structures of political authority. Any form of self-assertion, even that of a peasant, was permissible – natural, even – just as long as it did not challenge those structures.

A final, summary example is George Herbert's couplet "The pliant mind, whose gentle measure / Complies and suits with all estates," which encapsulates the three-way relationship in a single poetic breath. Here any tension between the creaturely equality of grace and earthly hierarchy is resolved by the flexibility of the reasoning mind, which is perhaps why this poem had trouble getting past the ecclesiastical censors. "Gentle" refers both to social rank and to the resolution of conflict, while "measure" contains the sense of "pace," a mean speed, as well as being the poem's reference to its own stanzaic structure. The mind's pliancy allows it to negotiate political tensions among "estates" both social (high/low) and religious (elect/reprobate). The poem's title, "Content," implying as it does social and not only personal peace, provides the cloak under which all three modes are interchangeable but have the reasoning mind as their subject and therefore as first among equals.

---

[45] Vera Bickert, *Calderons El alcalde de Zalamea als soziales Drama*, 68; Aquinas, *Summa Theologica*, 1.118.2.

Chapter 7
"Souls Drowned in a Lump of Flesh": the Excluded

On the eve of psychology's birth as a formal discipline, Wordsworth hints at something like the status modes described above. He writes to a friend about the part played in public life by certain "modes of sentiment." Honour and grace are there, in what he calls the "civil" and "religious" modes of sentiment. Intelligence is there too but only in its negative form, in a comment he makes about the "sentiment" of "loathing and disgust which many people have at the sight of an idiot."[1] Readers had criticized "The Idiot Boy" because they claimed it was not a subject fit for poetry. Their disgust is not natural, says Wordsworth, but inspired by class disdain. Ordinary people, who actually live with idiots (the rich board them out), do not have this sense of disgust because for them idiots like the poem's Johnny Foy are just part of normal life; Wordsworth's inclusiveness is a refusal to succumb to the fear of pollution which out-groups inspire and by which their conceptualization is inspired. It is to these various types of out-group and their early modern sources that we now turn. Here we shall be looking in outline at how all three modes work together; a separate and more detailed analysis of each mode comes in Parts 4 and 5.

Children

Certain people are disqualified, by nature, from even entering the bidding for in-group membership. For some, this state is temporary. Modern notions of childhood are inseparable from those of adulthood as a state of fully developed intelligence and the concomitant ability to give rational consent. Take Locke's account of religious toleration and political heterodoxy in the *Two Treatises of Civil Government*, written in response to the publication in 1680, at a politically provocative moment, of an absolutist samizdat from the civil war period, Robert Filmer's *Patriarcha, or the Natural Power of Kings*. Locke's premise is that each human being possesses the light of reason, individually, given that "each man's mind has some peculiarity as well as his face that distinguishes him from all others."[2] The point of this heterodox reason is that it will eventually guide all persons to a single revealed truth if they are allowed to pursue it freely by themselves. In the first treatise, Locke gives us his view of the historical Adam. For Filmer, Adam was first in a chain of rulers over other men; for Locke, he was all human beings, a universal man who had bequeathed to them their right to rule over the animals. In other words, he represents a human equality from which difference emerged only subsequently. The original state of equality was one of original sin. The esoteric biblical exegesis of the first treatise then leads directly into the modern political philosophy of the rest: from the equality of sinful humankind in Adam to the rational property differentials among his descendants. The fence around property is also the fence around the self. It encloses not only differential amounts of material property but differential amounts of interior space, inhabited by the individual's reason.

---

[1] Letter to John Wilson, June 1802, in Ernest de Selincourt (ed.), *The Early Letters*, 292.
[2] Locke, *Some Thoughts concerning Education*, 235; see also Joshua Mitchell, *Not by Reason Alone*, 73 ff.

Our modern notions of intellectual competence, derived partly as they are from Locke, are thus ramifications of the myth of Eden. The individual's reason, says Locke, is constituted in the historical act of freeing itself from the dominion of others: in society from paternalistic political rule, and in families from the father. This sets up a distinction between (a) minors, who are now (more sharply than before) temporary idiots over whom paternal rule is morally justified on grounds of psychological immaturity, and (b) people come of age – "free and intelligent agent[s]" – over whom paternal rule suppresses God's gift of reason because it treats them not as freely developing adults but as unfree children of the monarch ("idiots" in the old sense). Locke separated adult psychological status from that of children *and therefore from childlike adults*. He reinvents "idiots" in order to oppose absolutist politics. If opposition to Filmer's paternalism requires that children will develop into adults and that adults ought not to be treated like children, a narrower but sharper conceptual space is thereby created for the person come of age who ought still to be so treated: a character who had till now lay in obscure corners of jurisprudence and whose diagnostic traits were in any case different. The residual paternalism in Locke's concept of idiotic adults drives his anti-paternalist argument about autonomy for the rest of us.

And just as the child develops into an adult, so immature societies develop into adult ones. In Locke's mind, God is at this very moment intervening in history with a new revelation of which Locke and his contemporaries are the bearers, and which *sanctifies* the reasoning adulthood of the society just then developing around them; this adulthood extends beyond the honour society and the company of the elect to wider sectors of the population who are no longer the children they had been. And so the secularization of psychology, said to start with Locke, is not so much a progressivist replacement of selective, divine "special" grace by a universalized natural grace but rather a universalization of the former. Intelligent adulthood is the new election, brought down to earth and historically located midway between Adam and our redemption at the day of glory, in preparing for which an earthly "application of mind" is now required.[3] The politics of rational consent, to which Locke's Whig political doctrine was the handbook, remains in some sense the road to the kingdom of the saints, with the intellectually disabled – Locke's idiots and changelings – in the out-group role formerly occupied by reprobates.

The lower orders

When the Leveller John Lilburne said, "Christ doth not choose many rich, nor many wise, but the fools, idiots, base and contemptible poor men and women in the esteem of the world," all these groups were parts of a single concept.[4] And when Locke's Quaker friend William Penn prefaced his own account of toleration with the remark that absolutist and paternalist ideologies "cannot convince the understanding of [even] the poorest idiot," did he mean here a wage labourer, or someone who is disabled in their understanding?[5] We cannot tell, nor did he. Locke's own idiots in the *Essay* (as distinct from his purely mindless "changelings") occupy a similarly ambiguous niche between sociological and psychological definition. Where psychology and social class interface, deficiencies of intelligence are never far away. Sometimes the political target is at the top of the social scale, as in the above examples, but more often it is those underneath. The psalmist's much-quoted line, "Man that is in honour, and understandeth not, is like the beasts that perish,"

---

[3] John Dunn, "From applied theology to social analysis," in I. Hont and M. Ignatieff (eds), *Wealth and Virtue*, 119.
[4] Cited in Jacques Barzun, *From Dawn to Decadence*, 270.
[5] William Penn, *The Great Case of Liberty of Conscience*, 3.

was taken to indicate those who do not understand how man's access to divine reason makes him different from the animals. People who do not *understand* their own honour are of a piece with those who do not *have* honour (which in the psalm is a recuperated term for grace). This is what medieval writers meant by *pagani* (literally "country-dwellers"): labouring, illiterate, unbelieving – and therefore semi-bestial. The same line from the psalms was used in the early modern period to attack the Anabaptists. Mainly artisans or traders, they abused the notion of creaturely equality before God by trying to put it into practice on this earth. They did not understand that only some of them – and perhaps in view of their non-gentle status none of them – were elect.

The out-group of social class is "natural" partly in terms of its *degeneracy*. This initially involved all three modes at once. The bloodline virtues of the honour society were something which "nature in her own operation, doth seldom digress [sc. degenerate] from." That word "seldom" is crucial, because it pitches nature somewhere between deterministic necessity and the vagaries of nurture. It leaves room for the existence of certain ascribed members of the honour society who "neither by celestial grace nor by learning, nor endeavour ... aspire unto the habit of virtue," and since this makes them "thereby unfit for all public action," they are to be reclassified with commoners, as merely private individuals. Nicole Faret cited the widely discussed case of a French nobleman who had served as a magistrate, though barely able to sign his name: "How then could he judge matters of honour and human life?"[6]

Faret, expert on honour and a cobbler's son, noted that natural graces cut across class divisions. Some non-gentles may have a "good seed." Even the gentleman's seed has to be "carefully manured." Nature and nurture here overlap, in antithesis to "the sower," who is a personification of divine necessity and its "secret" predestined goals; grace may be read both under the first heading, as natural grace, and under the second, as "a beam of divinity" or superaddition for those who lack the natural eminence of honourable birth. Meanwhile at the bottom end of the scale, there are creatures "so unfortunate, as a man may say they are cast into the world by force, or that they are not made but to serve for objects of sport and scorn to other men." In other words they are fully determined: both by religious necessity, like reprobates, and by social necessity, like household jesters. In such people there is no spiritual grace and no natural grace, but also no nurture that can come to the rescue of the latter. They are an unimprovable, absolute exclusion. This creates space for an intellectually "middling sort ... a mean of those which have not received such extraordinary favours of nature, neither have they any remarkable imperfections." Such people are educable in the natural (professional) graces and, by hard work, come to "deserve the esteem" of the honour society. This middling sort is modern and meritocratic: it is not a point of balance like the classical mean, but an aspiration towards one extreme and away from the other.

Mid-seventeenth century England is especially rich in such ambiguities around class and degeneracy, which are reflected in the very title of Baxter's 1681 *Compassionate Counsel to All Young Men. Especially, 1. London apprentices. 2. Students of divinity, physic, and law. 3. the sons of magistrates and rich men*. Is 1-2-3 a descending or an ascending scale? He would rather, he says, be ministering to 3 or 2 than, as he is, to 1. (The Restoration bishops had just dumped an inner-city parish on the provincial Baxter as punishment for his heterodox views.) Nevertheless, he points out that category 3 contains "the ill examples of too many persons of your rank. You are apt to think that their wealth and pomp and power makes them ... more honourable. And if they wallow in drunkenness or filthy lust, or talk profanely, you may think that such sins are the less disgraceful. But you can dream." The title, self-consciously reversing the honour rankings, hints at the creaturely equality of souls. The Baxter who in the 1650s had seen man's reason as just one preparation among many for an imminent rule of the saints now saw preparation more soberly

---

[6] William Segar, *The Book of Honor and Armes*, 51; Nicole Faret, *The Honest Man*, 18 ff.

as "a good succession of the several generations," demanding a curriculum with a correspondingly greater reasoning element. "A Christian's child," he says, "is born with no more knowledge than a heathen's, and must have as much labour and study to make him wise .... O what a blessed world were it, if the blessings of men famous for wisdom and godliness, were entailed on all that should spring from them! And if this were the common case! But the doleful miseries of the world have come from the degenerating of good men's posterity," from regression to the mean.[7]

Sidelined by political events, Baxter redeploys the surface language of the elite in pursuit of a deeper strategy: the abandonment of a theory of imminent grace in the elect and its transformation into a theory of intellectual development for all. The road to salvation now lies in hard intellectual graft. And the absence of intellect that once denoted degeneracy within the honour society alone, having been taken for granted in the masses and feared only at moments of social disorder, now induces a permanent and generalized fear of any individual displaying such absence, from across the entire range of humanity.

Another concept highlighting pseudo-egalitarian tendencies, religious and secular, was that of the "capable subject." This referred either to those capable of receiving God's grace or to those with earthly capabilities such as landed property, or (more usually) both in the same person. In contrast stood "the uncapable multitude," which was the phrase Charles II reached for when he banned preaching on predestination out of fear that it would stir them up.[8] Uncapable – disabled – in what sense here? Talk about "uncapable" subjects helped smooth over elite disputes about grace by uniting them in defence against the out-group. An out-group is only ever a temporary manifestation, in whatever mode, of a prior category, that of the *representative* otherness which each era seems to manifest in different ways. The modern concept of intellectual disability was just then being inserted in this role. When in the 1670s Joseph Glanvill, a Royal Society member and acquaintance of Baxter and Locke, criticized the doctrine that the elect are few, he appealed to a concept of "general grace." This, he said, had been offered "unto all men, in the light of reason, the [natural] laws written upon our hearts, and common aids of the spirit ... in its universal diffusion through the world without let, or impediment ... communicating itself to all *subjects* that were *capable*" (emphasis in original).[9] However, this subject, in whom divine grace is naturalized by being embedded in human reason and natural law, is still not an everyman. It hovers between the creaturely equality of souls and social hierarchy. In generalizing (divine) grace, Glanvill is not exactly discarding election. "General" grace differs from the divine grace of the elect few not so much by being universal as by being mouldable to fit whatever social boundaries one might want it to fit (like "general" intelligence, in fact).

Locke simply ignores the language of grace, describing capability in terms of its detailed psychological operations. However, that is not because he was a sensible fellow, modern before his time, but because talk of grace was surplus to his requirements. In fact, in founding a seemingly universal and classless psychology, he was not abandoning the mode of divine grace at all, nor indeed that of honour. Rather, he absorbed both within a primarily intellectual vocabulary. The uncapable multitude, the "hydra-headed monster" recently let loose by civil war, very gradually thereafter would become a minority. Two centuries later public education, dominated by Nonconformism and its remaining subliminal beliefs about election, had transformed "a mad, bad and dangerous people" into citizenry of the middling sort, respectable rather than honourable, leaving behind only

---

[7] *Compassionate Counsel*, 386.
[8] Isabel Rivers, *Reason, Grace and Sentiment*, 54.
[9] Joseph Glanvill, "Anti-fanatical religion, and free philosophy," 34, in *Essays*.

a small, pathological intellectually disabled population (alongside and merging into the unskilled working class) to be as feared as the "multitude" once was.[10]

The importance of social class to the interplay between bidding modes and their respective out-groups is apparent also from the detail of church politics. When Hooker outlines the principles or "laws of ecclesiastical polity," he makes human reasoning a back-up to the holy spirit, its job being to persuade us that revelation is authentic. Whereas Calvin would have regarded this as blasphemous because our reasoning corrupts religion, Hooker thought corruption occurs mainly outside the honour society. He notes that the "common people" are "credulous and over capable of … pleasing errors." They have only the holy spirit to go by, and this means they can easily convince themselves that something is from the holy spirit when in fact it is from the devil.[11] His example is religious sectarians who claim powers of "prophecy," or instantaneously achieved reason. "Understanding of the scriptures," he warns, is "dependent not principally of the *sharpness* of men's wits or of their learning" (emphasis added). The common sort take their quick, unreasoning apprehension of the holy spirit to mean that they are elect, whereas in fact no one can know he is elect unless the holy spirit works laboriously through his intellect to convince him of the fact. Questions of election and social class overlap almost completely here. Only "almost," because when Hooker writes about speedy and unreasoning "common people" as above, he is not playing it straight; he is actually referring in coded terms to the Presbyterian gentry, who in Hooker's time formed an opposition tendency within church and state. One dealt with one's opponents' claims to grace and therefore to possession of the right political policy by representing them in the persona of idiots, of the common sort.

A similar interplay can be seen at local level, in authority's management of the hard facts of everyday behaviour. The parish was a unit of social administration; the church was its town hall, and reports on anti-social behaviour among the common people were posted on the door. Honour rankings were marked within the physical space of the church itself, pews arranged by degree of comfort and the amount of rates paid; local social status overrode creaturely equality (though this also meant that fights broke out over who could sit where). During services, the lower sort were barred from the chancel because it was assumed their behaviour would be indecorous, a likely token of reprobation. By the 1650s some churches were lifting the bar, but not completely, as we shall see later. All were agreed that "idiots" should be excluded from communion. But who were now these idiots? If no longer the generality of the common people, did they still include the illiterate, or servants? The latter were not always expected to attend church at all. It was said that gentry who brought their servants "were as good send their horse," that epitome of the reasonless brutes over whom man was born to rule.[12]

Women

As with class, so with gender. At the trial of the charismatic preacher Anne Hutchinson, Massachusetts's blessed magistracy proclaimed that for women – who after all were natural idiots – to get together and think in abstractions, as her all-female caucus did, was to remove honour from men and to strip reason of its inherent maleness.[13] Hutchinson, by claiming that she knew

---

[10] Boyd Hilton, *A Mad, Bad, and Dangerous People? England 1783–1846*.
[11] Voak, *Richard Hooker*, 230.
[12] Cited in Martin Ingram, "From Reformation to toleration," in T. Harris (ed.), *Popular Culture in England*.
[13] Michael Winship, *Making Heretics*, 42.

who belonged to the company of the elect and that the magistrates did not, was impugning their honour. The only honour appropriate to women was that which they derived from their husbands' or fathers' possession of them. The opposition between grace and male honour (at least of the old self-assertive kind) implied an identification between grace and female honour. As Pitt-Rivers notes, to renounce one's honour is also to cry for mercy, like a woman: without self-assertiveness, there is only submission.

The softer side of feminine values could be of considerable use to male power. While woman's rightful place was in the private sphere of home, private *men* were a potential threat. Private male reasoning might lead to heresy or opposition. The Tudor elite had therefore been cautioned to rear its infants in an exclusively female environment, to avoid exposing them to the rough manners of male clan members.[14] The nobility till then had reared its children and those of its feudal vassals in the old martial honour codes, often within the private household. Henry VIII's increasingly centralized state apparatus, with increased control of the honour codes, found this practice suspect. Testostrionic men were to be kept away from the nursery because their private minds and self-assertive behaviours might set a bad example to the young, fostering oppositional defiant disorder or an unreasoning disdain for reasons of state. The young had to be socialized into obedience to its head, though he himself was less radical feminist than serial femicide. The Puritans who grew in political strength over the next generation would have been the first to learn to police themselves in this way. Their rejection of the honour clans' way of bidding for status, in favour of an internal religious grace and regeneration or "new man," was their rejection of machismo for a more feminine quality that would eventually enable Puritan elites, male of course, to manage more softly and delicately the levers of power. "Have a new master: get a new man," was Caliban's advice to his fellow menials in *The Tempest*. (In Shakespeare's ironic inversion, this new man was a libertine, a drunken servant.)

A comparison may be drawn here with modern intellectual disability doctrine, notably around autism, and its involvement in the recuperation of radical feminist values. The autistic brain with its excessively private reasoning, says Simon Baron-Cohen in *The Essential Difference*, is an extreme version of the male one. Therefore we are to think of the female brain as normative. As Cordelia Fine has comprehensively shown, Baron-Cohen is unaware of the socially constructed character of notions of gender.[15] But it should further be noted that when the new man, like his Puritan counterpart, aspires to these feminized behavioural norms – "empathy", for example, as that which the "autist" cannot perform – he finds in them the constituents of a new managerial technique for maintaining, in the long run, a social control that remains patriarchal, and his.

The seminal insult

One final element is to be noted in the three-way relationship and its out-groups: the role of satire and insult. When a satirist of the time, with Socratic irony, calls himself an "idiot," rather than pretending to be intellectually disabled as we would understand it, he is more often representing himself as a member of the out-group in all three modes at once, with the aim of recalibrating the relationship between them. Take, for example, the reaction to Castiglione's elision of the distinctions between divine and natural grace and between honourable lineage and professional merit, with reason subsumed under both and ability reduced to performance and imitation. By way of contrast, his younger contemporary Giovanni Della Casa creates the persona of "an old idiot"

---

[14] Elyot, *The Governour*, 17r.
[15] See *Delusions of Gender: the Real Science behind Sex Differences*.

(*un vecchio idiota*), whose defining psychological characteristic is an inability to enact the performances required of him as a member of the social elite. In an Italian context of great social mobility, where reason is explicitly reinterpreted as imitative grace and honour consists in sham genealogies whose invention is openly admitted to be a mere ritual of office holding, one's only resource is to renounce membership of all three in-groups at once. What Della Casa wants us to infer from that ironic assumption of the title "idiot" is that imitative grace is an actual absence of true grace, and that in a true gentleman, honour does not have to be performed; it simply is. True grace and true honour are, instead, inborn nature *plus reason*. Only if the "nobility" (however dubious) adopts this novel approach, where a natural, specifically human wit reinforces the other two and is at least equal to them in value, can its bid for status remain competitive against the sophistries of the *arrivisti*.[16]

Today's insults ("idiot," "retard," etc.), especially when applied to one's peers, assume a referent. They say: you are like that pathological group over there. In the early modern period, the very existence of any such group or referent is questionable. Where there is textual evidence for such insults, it is in the class sense of the idiot as labourer or layman. When an opponent's argument is said to be "popish, that is very plebeianly and idiotically spoken," we still – this is the later seventeenth century – have no clear sense of the category boundaries between these three descriptive terms.[17] Satire and insult in the primary sources can therefore be read as applying in any bidding mode, and a vast range of reference is often incorporated in the "disabled" identity. This is clear from the many books about character types published in the seventeenth century in the genre inspired by Theophrastus. The satirist Samuel Butler, for example, writes of the man who

> Believes the honour that was left him as well as the estate is sufficient to support his quality without troubling himself to purchase any more of his own; and he meddles as little with the management of the one as the other, but trusts both to the government of his servants, by whom he is equally cheated in both. He is like a fanatic, that contents himself with the mere title of a saint and makes that his privilege to act all manner of wickedness.[18]

To Theophrastus's standard example, involving social class, Butler has added the religious element of an empty Antinomian claim to be among the elect. Or take the following entry, "Dunce," added (allegedly by John Donne) to Thomas Overbury's famous work in the same genre:

> He hath a soul drowned in a lump of flesh ... the most dangerous creature for confirming an atheist, who would swear his soul were nothing but the bare temperature of his body. He sleeps as he goes, and his thoughts seldom reach an inch further than his eyes. The most part of the faculties of his soul lie fallow .... One of the most unprofitable of God's creatures, being, as he is, a thing put clean besides his right use, made fit for the cart and the flail, and by mischance entangled amongst books and papers. A man cannot tell possible what he is now good for, save to move up and down and fill room, or to serve as *animatum instrumentum*, for others to work withal in base employments, or to be foil for better wits, or to serve (as they say monsters do) to set out the variety of nature .... He is mere nothing of himself, neither eats, nor drinks, nor goes, nor spits, but by imitation, for all which he hath set forms and fashions .... He speaks just what his books or last company said unto him, without varying one whit, and very seldom understands himself .... Rip him quite asunder, and examine every shred of him, you shall find him to be just nothing but the subject of nothing:

---

[16] Berger, *The Absence of Grace*, 196.
[17] Glanvill, *Saducismus*, 47.
[18] Samuel Butler, *Characters*, 67.

the object of contempt. Yet such as he is you must take him, for there is no hope he should ever become better.[19]

This is a rich mix: it refers to intellectual opposition ("dunce" is from the philosopher John Duns Scotus), original sin (the drowned soul), atheism, materialism (the soul as merely the "temperature" of the mortal body), lethargy, reliance on the external senses, emptiness or absence, horse-like beastliness, lack of autonomy, unstable opinion, manual labour, natural slavery, monstrosity, imitation, incurability – though little, it seems, that might be recognizable as disability to a modern psychologist. There is no sense that the author might be distinguishing between the people insulted and some separate population that provides a reference point for the insult. Passages like this are not metaphors by which one sneeringly or jokingly compares one's peers with some positive, pre-existing intellectually disabled population, so much as an early co-*creator* of a referent that is itself modern.

---

[19] Thomas Overbury, *Characters*.

PART 4
Intelligence, Disability and Honour

Chapter 8
Virtue, Blood, Wit: from Lineage to Learning

It is not often that we can see all three modes of bidding for status – honour, grace and wit – in full focus at the same time. We have abundant evidence, however, for the separate ways in which each of the two older modes and their corresponding concepts of disability feed into the modern one. In this and the next chapter we shall look at this process in terms of social status (honour), and in the following two, in terms of religious status (grace).

Changes in the types of collateral offered against recognition of status can be gleaned from the widespread early modern genre of conduct manuals and courtesy books: "behaviour guides" as I shall call them. These popular psychology texts form a continuous tradition, taking in key works such as Castiglione's *The Book of the Courtier* (1528), Henry Peacham's *The Compleat Gentleman* (1622) and Francis Nivelon's *The Rudiments of Genteel Behaviour* (1737, much consulted by contemporary portrait painters), through to those of the intelligence society: Edward de Bono's *How to Have a Beautiful Mind* (2004), for example. These guides, whether from the sixteenth century or the twenty-first, reveal the nexus between the ideals of the society and the facsimile of those ideals in the individual who aspires to personify them, and who has the ability to extort from others a validation of the image he cherishes of himself. In modern societies this validation is extorted by the creation of the disability we call intellectual, which can be traced back to the types of disqualification made on the grounds of honour. Before looking at the question of disqualification, however, we need first to examine the positive concept of honour to which it relates, and about which James and Shapin have already written.

We shall start by looking at the relationship of honour to social structure and mobility in the early modern period, and at ways in which honour was scientifically assessed. The discussion will then centre on the modal shift from honour to wit and learning, often via the mediation of "virtue." We need to remind ourselves yet again here how intrinsically slippery such concepts are. Honour may simply mean reputation and glory, or it may mean a supposedly more substantial, class-based "nobility." Nobility itself is sometimes synonymous with gentility, sometimes (and increasingly) a distinctly higher form of the latter. The inflection of these terms in any case varies according to author and/or national context. More than this by way of a general analysis of terms and we shall find ourselves drowning. We will engage with the texts first, and then see.

Social structure and social mobility

For the "real life" landscape of early modern social structure, we must seek elsewhere. We might find, for example, how when the chips were down, gentry would bond with the merchants and yeomen to defend common interests. We are looking here instead at the history of surfaces, of human self-representation. Even if *societas*, "the honour society," was something fairly nebulous, its members knew exactly who each of the others were. This mutual recognition is itself one aspect of social structure, and therefore we need at least a brief account of the latter.

At first sight, intelligence seems to play a quite different role in social structures from the role played by ancestral lineage. The difference lies in the distinction anthropologists make between "achieved" and "ascribed" status. Intelligence seems to be a quality within each individual, on the basis of which people achieve status by replacing each other in the structure: "social mobility." Lineage, by contrast, seems to be ascribed to families and groups by external social codes that pose absolute barriers to mobility, at the same time as creating anxiety about the porousness of those barriers. At first sight the intelligence society has no barriers that can be porous or otherwise, since intelligence is supposedly intrinsic to the species as a whole (allowing for certain differences of degree in individual capabilities and the amount of effort one puts in). But in fact intelligence, too, is an ascribed status: the intelligence society is a caste into which one is born socially, with social restrictions imposed on membership, just as was the case with honour. We have only our notional intellectually disabled people to explain to us that this is the case, and their categorization as intellectually disabled pre-empts all possible critique by disqualifying them from membership of the group that has the ability to explain anything.

The honour society's ideology of limited membership was one thing, actual social mobility quite another. Meritocracy's historical fable runs: once upon a time, you got on because of who you were (i.e., who you were descended from); now you get on because of what you can do, which is chiefly ranked by your intellectual ability. This kind of achievement-based system is supposed to have been suppressed in earlier times by an elite marked out by bloodline and inherited juridical powers. The onset of gentry and nobility is pushed as far back in time as possible, almost to a state of nature, thereby creating the historical myth of semi-permanent rule by an honour group, which in fact mirrors that group's own idea of itself as reaching back to the dawn of the species. The truth is something else. The difference between aristocracy and meritocracy is not between less and more social mobility, but between two different ways of closing off privilege and passing it on to one's offspring. And it is not just that meritocracy is the new aristocracy. Aristocracy, as historians have long known, was the old meritocracy, "governing solely by virtue of birth (not usually that ancient), royal caprice, or flat cash payment."[1] Detailed family records were not kept before the thirteenth century; nor, once they were, could descent be traced back more than a few decades. Partly this was because of structural changes in kinship; strict patrilinealism, which made tracing the family line important, was a relatively new system. And partly it was because even as the system was taking root, the ruling elite was undergoing constant change and infiltration. Let us compare the kinds of advantage people have sought to pass on to their offspring then and now: the gentility qualifications of parents around 1500 (juridical ones attached to landed estates) and the merit-based qualifications of parents today ("intellectual" or educational ones). In modern societies upward mobility is structurally restricted above all by parents' lack of educational qualifications, but this bias evens out over three generations or so. In the earlier period, changes of social rank through land acquisition probably evened out over a similar period. We cannot take it for granted that there was less social mobility in the thirteenth or seventeenth century than in the twenty-first. To do so is just to repeat the meritocratic fable that the undeserving have been replaced by the deserving, who by objectively justified criteria such as intelligence just happen to be us.

The very origin of gentility was meritocratic. In the property revolution of the late medieval period, lands were handed out in return for military service regardless of social background; "honour" could be used synonymously to mean a grant of land. Hereditary titles, and with them early modern notions of inherited honour, only came about once the king, then merely the strongest among equals, needed a system for keeping track of his peers' ambitious sons. Conversely, titles were a guarantee to chosen individuals that the king's favour could not be revoked. Economic capital was a means to the upkeep of these gentle appearances, which were the more real and valued entity. Titles, having begun as a form of ID card, only became systemized during that phase of early

---

[1] Hexter, "The English aristocracy," 72.

modern capitalism which was already beginning to spawn an intelligence-based meritocracy too; it seems to have been possible even then to describe oneself to the Court of Chivalry as "a gentleman by birth and a linen draper by trade" while keeping a straight face.[2]

As the French revolutionaries would (correctly) point out, titled nobility started out as gangs.[3] The system did not settle into one of primogeniture and hereditary surnames until the thirteenth century; in England, hereditary entitlement to a seat in the House of Lords came as late as the end of the fifteenth century, it having been an appointed chamber until then. The system of heraldic assessment and the genre of behaviour guides began immediately after this. The gap between the most pukka gentleman and the *arriviste* "shot up with last night's mushroom" (a frequent trope) was slight. The real question was, exactly *how recently* arrived? Not just in James I's two-a-penny honours sales or in the contemporary mass ennoblement of professionals in France but all along, urban trade or peasant avarice sufficed to buy a title, at some decent interval following purchase of the land. Expansion of the gentry had always occurred from the bottom up because heralds had a direct financial interest in granting coats of arms. In the 1540s the English state monopolized the business of collecting fees for the granting of arms. The nobility's crisis of prestige then came only when monarchs accelerated the granting of new titles, to reinforce the elite with good administrators and merchants who could supply the treasury with ready cash. The value of titles declined with their increase in number; like grade inflation in educational qualifications, these over-rapid shifts in precedence threatened the stability of existing occupants of the social niche. Honour after 1600 increasingly became not just an attribute of caste but concretized in the person, an individual possession emanating from within, even as it was reinterpreted in terms of obedience to the state. Religious authorities attempted, with some success, to replace bloodline with the soul and the mind as the locus of honour, which helped justify a limited extension of status down the social scale. It also sowed the seeds of honour's decline, since it meant the individual might be author of his own code; this semi-classless honour was eventually reduced to bourgeois "honesty" (financial and contractual), thus provoking conflict with the anti-mercenary bias of the old honour codes.

The purity of the in-group had in any case revealed certain inherent structural problems. In 1200 the nobility was tiny, and knighthood a lower, specialist stratum; when they merged, the former's system of primogeniture and hereditary names met up with the latter's codification system of heraldic coats of arms.[4] The problem was that the more tightly codified the patrilineal family, the more easily it died out. Plague exacerbated this. Gaps in the gentry had to be filled by servants from the great houses or men from the religious establishments beyond the honour society, without whom the elite could not have regularly renewed itself. Villeins studied at Paris and Oxford, taking up posts in the expanding ecclesiastical and state administrations and forming a literate secretariat for household economies increasingly reliant on documentation. A leading English recruiter from the ranks was William of Wykeham, himself unashamedly a tradesman's son, Lord Chancellor, and founder of the first Oxford college. Gentry and merchants in England, like nobility and bourgeoisie in France, shared a common cultural space despite the flamboyant noises about honour continually heard from the higher stratum. One of the most popular genres in the first wave of new, printed books among their bourgeois consumers were albums of medallion engravings illustrating the coats of arms to which they aspired; in republican Italy, whose ruling families tended to have very recent merchant origins, the coat of arms at first modestly embossed on the covers of book-keeping ledgers eventually found a prominent place in the portraits these family members commissioned of themselves in ancient dress, proclaiming their direct biological line of honourable descent from the ancient Romans.

---

[2] Cited in George Squibb, *The High Court of Chivalry*, 172.
[3] Dulaure, *Histoire*, 47.
[4] See Georges Duby, *The Chivalrous Society*, 9 ff.; 85 ff.

Some, then, are born honourable and great, some achieve greatness and some have greatness thrust upon them: in the second case through merit, and in the third by one's lord (or in Malvolio's case, lady). Conversely, it would be no enormous scandal when as great a nobleman as Lord North apprenticed his eldest son to a turkey merchant on account of his intellectual disposition; he was excessively fast, having "too much spirit" for his books or to be useful to the state.[5] Younger sons regularly entered trade. "What a gentleman is, is hard with us to define," wrote the legal historian John Selden. "In other countries he is known by his privileges; in Westminster Hall he is one that is reputed one; in the court of honour, he that hath arms."[6] Even in France, where nobility was more formally defined, a noble father would marry his daughter to a bourgeois if it meant no dowry was expected; and the commoner to whom a nobleman sold his land could assume a title, any challenge to it being legally invalid after a fixed period even if he continued working with his hands.[7] Such people claimed noble descent to avoid certain taxes from which nobles were exempt. In neither country did the heraldic expert require more than three generations on both sides (mere living memory) for a gentle line to be written down as "ancient": that is, if prompt payment of his fee did not obviate the need to trace it in the first place.[8]

Certainly there were massive complaints about upstarts and "new men." But the new man differed from the old only in the sense that whereas people had once been honoured for military service to the state, now it was also for professional services, which involved a notional intellectual component. The fifteenth-century legal authority Sir John Fortescue claimed, "There is scarcely a man learned in the laws ... who is not ... sprung of noble lineage," but that was in principle only. Judges were knighted from scratch, recruited from the sons of yeomen, merchants or even artisans.[9] Indeed, it was a stereotype of the lawyer that "his very calling writes him esquire, though his scutcheon sometimes cannot speak him gentleman, except by way of admittance" (that is, having come from outside the group).[10] Conversely, people who lost their land were not easily prised loose of their gentility. The claim to status in all its self-referentiality belongs as firmly to the social structure as any more concrete form of collateral. The Spanish *hidalgo* ("gentleman") is an abbreviation of *hijo de algo*, "son of something," recalling the complaint of the respectable English family fallen on hard times "We came from something, you know." The something in question is the title as such, rather than the long-gone landed estate. Status modes take on a life of their own when a group establishes an identity that may help it to corner some advantage which it can pass on to its descendants, hence psychology's longstanding interest in the hereditary nature of intelligence. In the shift from one mode to the other, the intelligence needed to preserve one's patrimony became intelligence *as* patrimony.

Honour and the assessment process

If honour and intelligence are similar in their relationship to social mobility, so too are they in their forms of assessment. Heraldic devices bear a functional resemblance to psychometric scores. The tensions of shifting social stratification, between society as it was and society as some of its

---

[5] Roger North, cited in Jerrilyn Marston, "Gentry honor and royalism in early Stuart England," *Journal of British Studies*, 13/1 (1973).

[6] *Table Talk*, 2031.

[7] See James Wood, *The Nobility*.

[8] Anthony Wagner, *Heralds*, 10; see also M. Bush, *The European Nobility*, 126 ff.

[9] Cited in Joan Simon, *Education and Society in Tudor England*, 13.

[10] Francis Lenton, *Characters*, B4v.

members wanted it to be, led to Canute-like attempts to preserve social difference in the existing honour mode by refining heraldry into a *scientia*, a branch of theoretically justified knowledge. This science, which patrolled the borders of the honour society, was no less specialist and complex than the psychology which patrols the intelligence society. A hobby of great interest to those who aspired as well as those who already belonged, it features in many of the behaviour guides of the period. It consisted in complex genealogical calculation, of which coats of arms were the quasi-mathematical indices. Heraldic science helped to negotiate the gulf between structural realities and the desire of the upwardly mobile for legitimation. Any mode of bidding for status, to be effective, requires public recognition and therefore external display. Honour had to be seen to be done. Its tools of authentification were exact signs that separated out-group from in-group, and grades of superiority within the latter. How the idea that heraldic knowledge is a branch of natural philosophy would have struck natural philosophers in other fields, especially in the physical realm, is unclear. Bacon thought that laws of evidence could not be applied to honour because it was all in the mind ("a satanical illusion and apparition … against religion") and therefore impossible to gauge.[11] One might criticize psychometrics from the same standpoint, since intelligence is likewise all in the mind. In fact it is often seen as all *of* the mind too, making the potential confusions even greater.

Heraldic science provided forms of assessment on which to base a jurisprudence of honour. The honour society's previous way of settling its tensions had been by private violence, which the absolute state found as threatening as private reason. Matters of honour had tended to be settled by duelling. This reached its high point in the later sixteenth century, that is, precisely as heraldic science was beginning to take shape. As the "point of honour" the duel, like the cognitive ability test, was a pseudo-legal institution in an arena where the law itself was not competent, and where the claimant to status must get himself formally authenticated by others at his own evaluation or else find that his claim is empty. Honour had to be impregnable from below, since its very premise was that inferior groups existed who lacked it. Destroying someone's honour not only reduced him to the ranks, it raised the destroyer; as the English Hymnal points out, "Conquering kings their titles take / From the foes they captive make." One recalls here the special esteem accorded to professional caregivers in segregated institutions for the disabled, or St Francis who with his pathological hatred of lepers was reborn in Christ the moment he condescended to touch one.

Decisions made by duel were deterministic, a form of necessity or fate. Sixteenth-century rulers tried to ban duelling, stood in for necessity themselves and assumed full responsibility for arbitrating all claims to honour. Whereas duels proclaimed the victor's autonomy independently of central power, heraldic signs offered the state a sanitized public equivalent which it could turn to its advantage by controlling the distribution of status. Moreover duelling, while caused by man's "natural inclination" and passions, was opposed by his "natural intelligence" (*intelligentia*).[12] Accordingly, heraldry became more scientifically rigorous during the sixteenth century: a new means of dealing with social mobility rather than the relic of an antique system about to be swamped by it. Anecdotal memory (idealized by epic poetry) gave way to precise genealogy, and previously disparate conventions to a unitary bureaucratic system. The herald, originally a tournament umpire, now analyzed armorial bearings, especially in England where the absence of clear-cut political privileges for the gentry meant that coats of arms bore the main proof of their gentility. Most of the legal "abilities" or privileges that marked out a gentleman (to hunt deer, carry weapons, etc.) had fallen into disuse, leaving only non-substantive, para-legal ones, of which heraldic display was chief. The high period of coats of arms began in Henry VIII's reign, when a permanent Commission was set up to regulate them. Republican parliamentarians were still insisting on theirs a century

---

[11] *The Charge, Touching Duels*, in *Works*, iv, 401.
[12] Giovanni da Legnano, *De bellis … et de duello*, 91.

later; only with the revolution of 1689 did the formal value of heraldic signs fade. Even then, they were still used as psychological indicators. They denote behavioural traits, for example, in the caricatures of the anonymous eighteenth-century satirist lampooning aristocrats with fake coats of arms ("two priapuses," "two virgins weeping," etc.).[13]

Heraldic science was based on three principles, each with its equivalent in the science of intelligence measurement: (1) the idea that honour and its differentials are *natural* phenomena which therefore self-evidently justify *social* distinctions, and of which the coat of arms is the external sign; (2) a theory of honour as *individual possession*, a form of property in those signs; and (3) a system of *assessment*, or heraldic visitations authenticating that possession. The elision between the signs or "tokens of nobleness" and its substance is typical of status modes in general. The sign itself becomes a substantive personal property, just as the statistical mean used in intelligence measurement, having started out as a purely numerical sign, subsequently becomes the natural phenomenon of intelligence: that is to say, what the measurer has decided intelligence is.

The heraldic Commission's freedom from state interference was a nod to the previous honour dispensation which in principle had been pluralist, the monarch himself being subject to its rules. However, the Commission was his initiative and existed for his benefit. The herald carried royal letters patent, showing that the right had been delegated to him. If some of the monarch's fellow nobles had previously held honours within their gift, now he was the fount of all honour, reinforced by his role as the earthly mediator of divine grace. Honour required state authentification as well as self-authentification. Out on the road, though, the herald remained his own master. As the honour society's informal judiciary, his quasi-forensic task was to separate the genuine from the fake. This was no simple matter. Henry's first Commission asked the heralds to assess "good honest reputation" when awarding or approving coats of arms. Men "issued of vile blood" were to be excluded. However, that was in theory; in practice, reputation meant "service done to us or another" or "possessions and riches" above a certain level. Also excluded were "heretics contrary to the faith"; religious wisdom was now a reinforcement to state power, thrusting the clergy into an honour system that had traditionally excluded them. After the first Commission, a herald periodically visited claimants to gentle status at home or summoned them to attend him. Anyone who could not justify his coat of arms had his dishonour posted up in public. The Court of Chivalry held tribunals which testify to the widespread practice of inappropriate display by those not entitled. Those who passed the test had their coats of arms entered on a pro forma, "small tickets … printed with blanks," the upper half of each page drawn with empty shields (to be filled out with the relevant emblems) and space for a brief verbal description.[14]

Before this period, it was assumed that two gentlemen meeting for the first time did not compare genealogies; all they needed (as Cicero had said) was a quick glance at each other. The new heraldic scientists thought it took a bit more than that. The social order was at stake: it was well known that "no coat of arms is more beautiful than a villein's."[15] Yet at least one manual on coats of arms, having begun with a rigorous exclusion of merchants and mechanics, goes on to qualify this out of existence by selecting "laudable" trades and crafts that might be eligible. This seems to mean any trade as long as the person under assessment could stump up the fee. The very same people who in one context might be "night-grown, mushrumps, start-ups," could in a more favourable one be "gentlemen of the first head," that is, founders of a new honourable line.[16] The latter phrase, like "meritocrat," had started out as ironic but very quickly turned positive. Goalposts moved here

---

[13] *The Heraldry of Nature*, 48.

[14] Wagner, *Heralds*, 5, 101; see also James, "English politics."

[15] Cicero, *De Officiis*, 1.30; Marois, *Le gentil-homme*, 264.

[16] Barnabie Rich, *Faultes*, 9r; Thomas Smith, "Of Gentlemen," in *De Republica Anglorum*.

and there, just as they do with intelligence when its constituent parts are selected, reselected and reconstituted even as the principle of measurement maintains its supremacy all the while.

For someone to be "creator of his own honours" in this way was justifiable because his fee contributed to the upkeep of the heraldic system, thereby improving the commonwealth. Law was at the centre of this trade. Many of the behavioural writers were at the Inns of Court, as were the prospective owners of coats of arms among their readers; this was the same professional caste which, at the opposite end of the status spectrum, was just then creating a new and antithetical caste of dishonourable "idiot" incompetents at the Court of Wards and helping to sequester their estates. Gentlemen of the first head were contrasted with "dunghill or truck-knights, whose honours have no other ... scale to rise by but only their wealth," and who pay "common scriveners" to paint their coat of arms. In principle "honourable places [are] due to great estates," so how did one distinguish between money which could buy honour and that which could not?[17] The answer seems to be that you paid through the appropriate channel. Although proofs of authenticity in heraldic science were based on lineage, an under-the-counter trade in coats of arms had always gone on, and in fact they had started out as legally alienable property. The law only prohibited this practice at the same (late) point when it confirmed the inheritability of titles.

Heraldic scientists built into their professional role an excluding jargon called "Blazon," part-pictorial, which they could use with each other, knowing that clients would not understand. Like IQ, it was an abstract code. Interest in Blazon grew sharply in the 1620s, in reaction to the Duke of Buckingham's notorious honours-for-sale policy (Peacham, the best-known popularizer of heraldic science, was tutor to the son of Buckingham's chief political rival). As the coats grew more complex and scrutinized, so did the usefulness of Blazon to heralds. It ensured that their expert services were always needed. It is impossible to convey in paraphrase the flavour of some of these texts. The minute hierarchical grading of coats, with added symbols for birth order (first, second, third son, etc.) and differentiations for the number and type of quarterings, was as complex as chi-squaring. Or the science could be disarmingly simple while equally exact: the Hall of Nobles in Stockholm, for example, displays their coats of arms with numbers running in order of their year of introduction, oldest families first.

If heraldry later came to be seen as what Voltaire supposedly called it, "the science of fools with long memories," it had critics even at the time. Some of the criticism came in the rival mode of grace. William Perkins, characteristically trenchant, says: "No man is to stand upon his gentility, or glory in his parentage for nobility and great blood, but only rejoice in this, that he is drawn out of the kingdom of darkness."[18] Erasmus mocked the air of intellectual difficulty heraldic experts cultivated and the status this lent them: people think *this*, rather than religion, is the supreme intellectual accomplishment. When gentlemen discuss it, "their forehead and upper brows [are] drawn together with very great gravity, as it were a matter of marvellous difficulty; yea and with great enforcement bringing forth plain trifles [and] think other in comparison of themselves scarce to be men."[19] Other criticisms came from the champions of honour themselves. They complained about charlatan "armorists" whose "impostures conspire in the concealing of their imagined secrets."[20] These writers feared that heraldic science might threaten the very principle of honour, because it protested too much; after all, the very call for evidence contradicts the principle behind status modes. One early seventeenth-century author for example, in a textbook description of character types, describes the herald thus:

---

[17] Markham, *The Booke*, 42; 69.
[18] Perkins, *Workes*, iii, 293.
[19] Desiderius Erasmus, *The Manual of the Christian Knight*, 93.
[20] Ferne, *Blazon*, A6.

> To the making of him went not a generation, but a genealogy. His trade is honour, and he sells it, and gives arms himself, though he be no gentleman. His bribes are like those of a corrupt judge, for they are the prices of blood. He seems very rich in discourse, for he tells you of whole fields of gold and silver, or and argent, worth much in French but in English nothing.[21]

In criticizing the heralds, this author is seeking to preserve the autonomy of country gentry, whose honour was self-evident and needed no checking. At the extreme, though, heraldic science was a "mockery," its sole aim to rake in assessment fees.[22]

When the experts defended themselves, it was characteristic of status modes in general that they did so via their opponent's psychological deficiencies: "the pride they have in their own wits and understandings, weening themselves to be very wise, where indeed they are very simple," and their "rashness, and want of judgement" (both these latter being precise terms in faculty psychology). The experts invoked a typical claim of the human sciences: to historical permanence, and hence to nature. One fifteenth-century text universally consulted through the early modern period identifies the hierarchical insignia of honour as "the nine colours in arms figured by the nine orders of angels" – medieval philosophy's nine intelligences, corresponding to the nine celestial spheres – "… show[ing] which be worthy and which be royal."[23] This demonstrated for experts the cosmological dimension of their expertise. According to this same author, "Christ was a gentleman of coat armour." A principle of nature and the cosmos thus reinforced one of socio-political order: "Bondage … began first in angel[s] and after succeeded in mankind." Practice, as well as theory, was read back into antiquity. Heraldry was traced back at least as far as the Roman patricians who put up wax images of their ancestors; and he who had none to display "was called by them … a new fellow, a son of the dunghill, fatherless."[24] Sitters for portraits wore classical dress embroidered with their coats of arms.

The perceived cross-historical validity of Blazon thereby credited honour with being a natural and permanent substance. And what was historically true had to be anthropologically true, across present-day cultures. John Gibbon, one of Charles II's heraldic officials, commented on people he had seen in Virginia with tattoos on their bodies and emblems on their shields. They proved that "heraldry … is ingrafted naturally into the sense of the human race": that is, its "internal sense" or psychological faculties. These indigenous practices proved that heraldry was universally human in the same way as, for Locke, the existence of "intelligent Americans" proved that the human understanding was universal and that they were not "mindless" as their Spanish enslavers had called them. Personality could be read off from a coat of arms as from the shape of a skull. Sign as well as substance were inalienable properties of the mind itself:

> Arms … shall be accounted … the significations, and outward marks of virtues, which have proceeded, from the soul or mind of the first bearer. And therefore … arms, are things so excellent and honourable in themselves, that they are not to be accounted, in the nature of goods, riches or lands.[25]

Honour was not concrete collateral, therefore, but an intangible principle located in a universal realm of nature where it "sympathizes with every noble and generous disposition." Not only that: heraldry meant that honour was scientifically demonstrable, indeed "the most refined part

---

[21] John Earle, *Microcosmography*, 93.
[22] William Wyrley, *The True Use of Armorie*, 7.
[23] Julian Berners, *The Boke of Saint Albans*, 15.
[24] Ferne, *Blazon*, 150.
[25] Cited in Edward Gibbon, *Autobiography*, 7.

of natural philosophy, while it taketh the principles from geometry, making use almost of every several square and angle."[26] Assessment of heraldic insignia was therefore what we now call an exact science: moreover the *ultimate* exact science, which rendered the social as well as the natural order eternal. Coats of arms, with their minutely divided orders of precedence, built hierarchical human honour into the structure of the universe. At the same time we must note that Gibbon saw nature as a modifiable set of "dispositions." On the one hand there was scientific rigidity; on the other, nurture made a difference. Hence the line between elite and non-elite remained unclear. It meant both that there could be boundary crossers (however rigorous the membership criteria), and that the sons of gentry had better shape up.

Sometimes the *scientiae* of law, medicine and heraldry unite in a single account of natural classification. Take the lawyer writing a foreword to his friend's guide to heraldic science, a textbook as meticulously positivist as anything in today's psychometrics. The author is praised for reducing "an art (much like our law), unmethodized, to … a method" and "rules."[27] He makes armorial bearings "most natural," not in the sense of faithful pictorial representation but in that of natural history: "This work, did ransack heaven and earth, / Yea nature's bulk itself, or all that is / In nature hid, before this book had birth." The author is the true heir of the great Roman naturalist Pliny. He has revealed the psycho-social laws of nature, by cataloguing the heraldic animals, plants and stars that act as their emblems and signs: "Nature's secretary we may style / Thy searching spirit …. All that honour arms must honour thee, / That hast made arms from all confusion free" – a presentiment of Pope's encomium on Newton. Turning heraldic signs into the substance of honour thus leads to a harder-edged account of nature.

The author himself heads his text with the Hobbesian declaration, "Nature is ruled by an intelligence that does not err." This strictness about nature is required because of the "confused mixture" into which coats of arms have descended. The confusion, he says, lies not in the intrusion of upstarts or fake coats of arms but in the science itself, in its present state. It needs to be made more exact. At the beginning, even Noah's despised worker-son Ham had his own armorial bearings. "In this *first* assumption of these signs, *every* man [emphasis added] did take to himself some such beast, bird, fish, serpent … as he thought best fitting his estate." These insignia were not at the outset hierarchical or exclusive but simply "marks to distinguish tribes, families, and particular persons from each other." So how did honour differentials arise subsequently? They did so first in the mind of "the ingenious beholder," who notes "after some sort [sc. classification] the natural quality and disposition of their bearers." The gradual hierarchization of the insignia of honour thus runs interactively with improvement in the intelligence of observers, so that (as in every good pseudo-science) we cannot tell whether the differentials are *ante* or *post factum*.

Another feature of this increasingly scientific approach is primogeniture, which starts to change from a legal concept into one that abstractly represents the natural order of things. With inheritable honour increasingly a possession of the individual, it became important to stress that this still did not make it a form of concrete collateral; it was not a commodity one could pass up or alienate, like one's property. The eldest son's right of inheritance was a biological definition of the person. Hence Jehan Scohier's slogan, "The eldest son never dies."[28] (It is worth noting here that "Jehan" was a medievalist affectation, sporting what the French came to know as "the heraldic h.") Primogeniture is "separate from the law of succession, and is not subject to the laws or customs of the country, but follows the order of nature alone." To establish this, the writer creates the fiction that in some countries it is the second son who inherits, "thus perverting the order of nature, with

---

[26] Henry Peacham, *The Compleat Gentleman*, 139.
[27] John Gwillim, *A Display of Heraldrie*, "To the courteous reader."
[28] *L'estat et comportement des armes*, 49.

no assurance or conformity in the office of arms, nor among heralds." Writing in opposition to the inflation of honourable titles, his tactic is to affirm the hereditary principle as deterministically as possible: "The right of primogeniture in itself cannot be prescribed, either by the sons or by anyone outside the family .... [It is] immutable ... and here is the living reason why the right of primogeniture cannot be sold." The book contains a correspondingly comprehensive catalogue of coats of arms, whose scientificity proves the natural honour of primogeniture, just as IQ scores prove natural intelligence. It is when the social need for tighter authentification arises – when there is a threat of being swamped or polluted – that one has to intrude this more deterministic sense into nature.

Virtue: mediating between honour and wit

Pitt-Rivers notes how hard it is to separate the two terms, honour and virtue. Of the things that "accompany honour like a shadow," virtue was the most frequently mentioned. It too, however, could be variously interpreted. Was virtue "blood ... conjoined with wealth," or that "which ... because it proceedeth from the mind, is true and perfect"?[29] It had long been recognized that virtuous *conduct* did not necessarily depend on one's bloodline; but the migration of virtue to the *mind* signalled a decline in the language of honour. Virtue (excellence, or perhaps "superiority") became more clearly a value term than honour itself. In the migration of status bids, it was a magic carpet on which the author could beam down from one mode of bidding to another, or mediate in the conflicts between them.

This is evident from the way heralds and behavioural writers dealt with their own dubious lineages. Cicero, who wrote about honour, was noted for having been, like most of them, plebeian by birth. Peacham (in a fictitious persona) admits, "Being a gentleman myself, I have been many times asked my coat, and except I should have showed them my jerkin, I knew not what to say."[30] To this conundrum of self-authentification, he replies that he just *knows* he's a gentleman, despite having to labour for his living by tutoring. The conundrum was solved by that value-laden slipperiness of "virtue." Heralds were needed because the king could not "pierce into every dark and obscure corner that lies hid within his dominions." And it was precisely the existence of some unvirtuous, ignorant gentlemen that created a market for the behavioural expertise of the herald. Peacham accuses heralds of "deal[ing] more bountifully with a fellow who can but teach a dog ... than upon an honest, learned and well qualified man" to advise on the upbringing of their children. The bourgeois flavour of that word "honest," as distinct from honourable, sidesteps the delicate question of his own social status being not quite that of those whom he is lecturing about their ignorant and degenerate behaviour. This mission – to rescue from itself an elite whose behavioural norms one claims to represent despite one's own dubious social origins – is another literary fixture: think Jane Austen. It typifies many of the writers in this genre and gave them career opportunities. Gibbon, who held the post of Bluemantle Poursuivant at the College of Heralds, was a shopkeeper's son with a politics that was high Tory. (Heraldic science was associated with the Tories' attachment to Royal Prerogative.) These writers read their own humble social origins back into the history of the science. The first feudal heralds, they said, had been "mechanical men" who looked after their lord's armour and were knighted in return.[31] It is worth noting here that key figures in the invention of modern intelligence and intellectual disability grew up in similarly status-ambiguous

---

[29] De Oncieu, *La précédence*, 28; Giambattista Nenna, *A Treatise of Nobilitie*, 29r.
[30] Peacham, *The Gentleman's Exercise*, 131.
[31] Symphorien Champier, *Le fondement*, 61.

positions of some kind: Baxter, the son of self-improvers; Locke, from the smallest of small gentry, bitterly dependent on patronage; Galton, from a wealthy but nonconformist family which resented its exclusion from the charmed circle of the Anglican ruling elite.

Assumptions of virtue made up for faults of pedigree. Sir Thomas Browne describes virtue as "nobility without heraldry."[32] Heraldry was "a good enough illustration of the antiquity of the race, but not the nobility of its successors; although they may be known by ... [coats of] arms, they are only noble by their virtues."[33] But the more rigorous the science, the less it could cope with such interpretive fluidity. And it coped least when virtue was reinterpreted as learning. Virtuous purity of blood had once been said to resemble the marble of a statue, and learning its surface decoration. At a certain point, however, they became man and wife: noble ancestry and "that sweet bride, good learning."[34] One encyclopaedia of heraldry points out that in Latin *ingenui*, the well born, reads almost the same as *ingenii*, the quick-witted; they must have a common etymology, since these qualities are interchangeable.[35] The same notion appears in Elyot's seminal text on how to train up a learned gentry. Though his reformed curriculum culminates (routinely for the time) in Aristotelian ethics, he recasts Aristotle's "great-souled man" as the Tudor gentleman, honourable and in grace. The continuance of a noble line depends on each generation's renewal of the virtue that existed in nobility at the outset, and renewal then comes from following his recommended philosophy curriculum. He draws no category distinction between virtue as learning ability and "ability" as the power derived from landed possessions – nor even, he hints, from upwardly mobile merchants' wealth, as long as they agree to play the game. One eye is on incumbents; the other tips the wink at any social climber who might end up being useful. The categories overlap, inasmuch as all are ways of establishing a niche for one's son in a fluid socio-economic structure where lineage may turn out to be not enough.

Honour is being framed here, in the late sixteenth century, in an increasingly abstract terminology that is civic as well as scientific. Its virtues are performed in public service. Sidney, while acknowledging the importance of heraldic science to a knowledge of human behaviour, said that he was not interested in men's pedigrees: "it sufficeth to know their virtues."[36] It is striking how often even writers with the most rigorous approach to heraldic science also credit virtue with a higher value than lineage. But the contradiction is in our eyes only. For contemporaries, one essence was not replacing another. Virtue as learning and virtue as bloodline belonged to the same class of things, or at least occupied similar taxonomic slots. If learning-based virtue was a cuckoo in honour's nest, the behavioural writers did not spot it. The moral autonomy of the individual in the old honour society had been his "franchise" (Lull's word), a form of freedom consisting in personal self-assertiveness whose ultimate sanction was violence and whose psychological location was the will.[37] During the seventeenth century this autonomy was relocated from the will to reason; freedom and the franchise came to reside in the individual's formal civic maturity, his rational ability to allow himself to be governed or (later) to actively consent to this. The behaviour guides such as Peacham's continued to be cited, but they are not a good indicator of what was going on in everyday life, since the actual practice of honour on the ground, like that of intelligence today,

---

[32] Browne, *Religio*, 66.
[33] Florentin de Thierriat, *Trois tractez*, 253.
[34] Peacham, *The Compleat Gentleman*, Introduction.
[35] Milles, *The Catalogue*, 10; see also Robert Glover, *Nobilitas Politica vel Civilis*, 16.
[36] Cited in James, "English politics," 381.
[37] Ramon Lull, *Book of the Ordre of Chyvalry*, 115.

was mundane and taken for granted, a prosaic interaction among social peers; it was a system of reciprocity and communication, and indeed of "intelligence" in this latter sense.[38]

The idea that one collateral substance has been exchanged for another is therefore illusory. In the displacement of an honour society by an intelligence-based meritocracy we can see a structural rearrangement of practical means by which power is validated, through bidding modes that are at root interchangeable. "Virtue" drew a veil over any conflictedness in the relationship between lineage and learning. Such conflicts over one's evidence base tend to be harmful to self-referential status claims; the very idea of evidence threatens the person claiming it. (This nebulousness brings to status its permanent air of crisis, and if today we talk contradictory nonsense to each other about intelligence, it is just that we do not notice our condition as one of crisis, nor do we notice the chains – social, cultural, political – in which intelligence binds us.) Once virtue, the substance of honour, began to be associated with individual intellects and their learning, the next step was its sublimation into something *made up of* intellect, thus rendering talk of honour redundant. Of course the war between excellence of bloodline and excellence of the intellect went on for a long time. A mere century ago for example, Proust's hidebound aristocrats, the Courvoisiers, still cast intelligence as the "burglar's jemmy" with which upstart commoners were threatening to break into their hallowed circle. Yet for several centuries, intellectual merit and bloodline, bride and groom, had already been advancing hand in hand.

Noble lineage and Christian learning

The identification of virtue with learning had a strongly Christian inflection. If intellectual virtues increasingly infiltrated the concept of honour, there was a corresponding halo of honour around the intellect itself, as a theological object. For the scholastics, all branches of learning were "among the number of honorabilia" because "they show that the intellect is perfectible."[39] And one branch of learning was higher on the scale than the rest: "Knowledge (*scientia*) of the soul is more certain and worthy of honour than other kinds of knowledge ... because of the excellence of its object and the certainty of knowing it." The honourable occupation of the intellect as subject is to contemplate the honourability of the intellect as object.[40] This circularity makes it proof against the corrupting influences of the body; the intellect is "more noble ... because the ability (*potentia*) of the intellect is not something organic like the senses."[41] Of course one might object that the words honourable and noble are especially loose and unspecific here, and simply mean something like "better"; but as we have already seen, this is true of all modal terms, including "intelligent."

Renaissance writers transformed Aristotle's slightly dismissive notion of honour – that it lay in the eye of the person conferring it – into a more positive theological explanation for the origins of human nature: "Honour being an external adjunct, and in the honourer rather than in the person being honoured, it was necessary to make a creature, from whom [God] might receive this homage."[42] This made honour a central principle in natural law, which is how it also came to be a species characteristic and a component of human faculty psychology. There were already inklings of this in the leading Roman educational authority Alexander of Aphrodisias, a contemporary of Galen's and a substantial influence on Arab and thence Western scholastic philosophers.

---

[38] See Marston, "Gentry honour."
[39] Buridan, *Aristotelis de Anima*, 2r.
[40] Antonius Ruvius, *Commentarii de Anima*, 15.
[41] Buridan, *Aristotelis*, 7v.
[42] Browne, *Religio*, 40.

Honour, he said, is the common possession of all men as distinct from animals.[43] On this natural history basis, the relative honour of the intellectual faculties and operations of certain groups becomes, at the lower margins, a test of their species membership. Albert, discussing half-human "pygmies," says their chief characteristic is that they "do not heed the shame resulting from what is unseemly or the glory resulting from what is noble .... No animal but the human is ashamed of doing foul deeds."[44] Honour thus marks a discontinuity on the scale of nature. As he also says:

> One property of man that makes him a man is to be shamed by the perpetration of ugly acts. This does not happen with any other animal except man. And so he is said to be a creature of inveterate shame, because when on occasion men assume the irrationality of brute nature, they are moved by the honour of reason [*rationis honore*].

The reason of human beings is thereby entailed in their honour as much as vice versa. Albert attributes honour to all humans; it is horizontal, an aspect of creaturely equality, the only exceptions being half-human or mythical. However, these exceptions are a reminder that the psychological criteria are also, and inseparably, social ones (the pygmy, for example, is unable to "maintain a perfect political system or laws" and "has no civility"), and that in this sense they mark a vertical division. Lack of reason and lack of social honour, in the out-group, are more or less coterminous: the one is not merely a metaphor for the other.

The honour of some men in relation to others has its parallel within the individual, in the hierarchy of psychological faculties and operations. The operations of the reasoning or judging faculty were seen by most writers as "more noble" than those of the imagination because the latter was linked to the external senses and hence to the material world; others thought the nobler part was the imagination because wit (*ingenium*) operated from there, and upon this depended the subsequent quality of the reasoning faculty's own operations.[45] Bodily matter too, the organic location of the faculties, reflected this hierarchy, some particles in the blood being "nobler" than others and thus more fit to receive and be directed by the soul spirits.[46]

Ingenium or wit lurked within classical concepts of honour, based as they were on public and professional office holding and its related abilities (the Roman word *nobilis* simply meant "notable").[47] The chief Christian sources for the early modern behavioural genre – Aquinas, Bartolus, Erasmus – had quoted Cicero liberally in their attempt to Christianize the military concept of honour, though without focusing greatly on professional wit. Aquinas placed honour "nearest to virtue" in the order of desiderata. Virtue was what taught the truly honourable man to adhere to a mean between the "blameworthy" extremes of "despising of honours" and "an inordinate appetite for them."[48] Bartolus identified honour with non-military virtues, but in terms of Christian character as much as learning; he divided nobility into a triad of necessity, nature and nurture/convention: "supernatural nobility" (given by and known only to God), "natural nobility"

---

[43] Alexander of Aphrodisias, *Ethical Problems*, Problem 29.
[44] Albert, *De Animalibus*, 1354; 1417.
[45] Collegium Conimbricense, *In Tres Libros de Anima*, 14; see also Gaetano Da Thiene, *Super Libros de Anima Aristotelis*, 1.2.5; Dominicus Gundisalvus, *Liber de Anima*, 31.
[46] John Banister, *The Historie of Man*, 98r; John Mayow, *Tractatus Quinque Medico-Physici*, 259.
[47] See Peter Garnsey, *Social Status and Legal Privilege in the Roman Empire*; J.E. Lendon, *Empire of Honour*.
[48] Thomas Aquinas, *Summa Theologica*, 2.2.129.

(ranks of virtue within species and across species) and "political nobility" (donated by the ruler).[49] In Erasmus, Christianization clearly does not mean intellectualization:[50]

> Let it not move thee one whit when thou hearest the wise men of this world, men of sadness endowed with great authority, so earnestly disputing of the degrees of their genealogies or lineage, ... Let other men be kings' sons: to thee let it be greatest honour that can be, that thou art called, and art so indeed, the son of God .... Take heed what manner of fellows Christ chooseth: feeble persons, fools, vile as touching this world. In Adam we are all born of low degree.

Rather than a call for equality here on earth, this is ironic advice to the gentry. Admiring the religious status of the unlearned is simply his way of warning his own social peers to cease being their own worst enemies. The reference to sadness plays on the ambiguity of melancholia, a sign of wisdom in the scholastic culture but of disability in a humanist one such as Erasmus's. "Fools" is his translator's word for *idiotae*, the word used in the Vulgate Bible for the disciples prior to their receiving the holy spirit. In this context the moral and the purely intellectual are seemingly separated: "Better an idiot untaught and well living, / Than a vicious doctor ill mannered and cunning."[51]

This humanist notion of Christian virtue fitted comfortably with the function of behaviour guides as training manuals for the career ladder. Hence their self-contradictoriness about membership qualifications. The *arriviste* could use the Christian idea of creaturely equality, suitably hedged, to penetrate the honour society. With dedications and preambles that typically address "the honourable assemblies of the Inns of Court" and "wish the reader advancement by virtue," the behaviour guides incorporate learning-based virtue in their natural philosophy of honour, in the pursuit of group interests as well as of maintaining the existing order.[52] The paradigm was William of Wykeham's famous motto "Manners maketh man" (rank me by my behaviour, not my ancestry), appended to the coat of arms he had acquired from scratch. Aspiring entrants to the in-group and established members alike complained about the degeneracy and lapsed virtue of "nobility and gentry nowadays, [whom] you shall see ... bred as if they made for no other end than pastime and idleness .... Good men and such as are learned are not admitted amongst them." Moreover, "the affairs of their estates they impose upon others"; in other words, virtuous Christian learning means having enough wit to prevent your own rapacious stewards from robbing you.[53] And when Elyot (drawing on Erasmus and Bartolus) casts learning as a form of religious humility by contrast with the arrogant military might of an unrestrained nobility, he is recommending humility towards the monarch. Knowledge is knowing your place.

Christian creaturely equality and learning-based honour therefore had their limits. While heraldic science treated the virtues of the mind with respect, its main task was still to conserve the importance of bloodline. However much the behaviour guides may have insisted that there is no honour "in hawking, hunting, hastiness, mighty power, vain vaunts, trains of horse, and servants, riot, mischiefs, bravery, roisting port, or great line" and located it instead in a Christian virtue defined by reading learned books, eminence in learning typically occurs in people who are "noble through their house and ancestors," and only incidentally in those who "are of themselves noble."[54]

---

[49] Cited in Segar, *Honor, Military and Civil*, 225.
[50] Erasmus, *The Manual*, 192.
[51] Dominike Mancin, *The Mirrour of Good Maners*, 15.
[52] Ferne, *Blazon*, A4; Leigh, *The Accedence*, A3.
[53] Peacham, *The Compleat Gentleman*, 43.
[54] Lawrence Humfrey, *The Nobles*, A4v.

One promoter of inner qualities lets the cat out of the bag. "Handicraftmen in these days," he says, "have obtained the title of honour," squatting "in the house of worthy fame ... and at this day do bear those arms which were given unto old gentry." *That* is why "noble and gentle men must diligently labour to excel others in virtue, or else there will rise comparison [sc. equality] of worthiness" – and of course social chaos.[55] In his dedication to Lord Fitzwalter he belittles coats of arms as mere externals or "coloured things"; to itemize them, as conventional dedications do, would be mere flattery. But this protestation is itself a piece of flattery, since he takes the opportunity to list instead Fitzwalter's internal, learning-based virtues. Just because we are all descended from Adam, says the writer, it does not mean there is no hierarchy. Adam was even then the gentleman. "Degree," as intellectual differentiation, has existed from the dawn of time, headed by "gentlemen ... which by their learning and knowledge excelled others, and were for that cause thought worthy of greater honour." "Nobles have the better nature," he says, but nature is inseparable from nurture and can be transformed by it through virtuous learning. The same goes for your future stock. Preserving status, in a system of landed inheritance as in a meritocracy, means preserving it for your children too. And that is why, as again in today's meritocracy, you should focus on their education: "Honour falleth to no man by descent; no man can entail honour to his heirs male, the which enfeoffeth a man in lands and possessions, [and] cannot therewith give virtue unto him, without the which no man can be rightfully called honourable." To obtain virtue requires "labour" instead, an *intellectual* labour in its broadest sense, and avoidance of "idleness." This overlaps with religious doctrines (Protestant and, increasingly, Catholic ones), in which intellectual labour is becoming a preparation for grace. Christian learning has turned into a crutch which honour cannot do without.

Definitions of virtue: the rivals to learning

The chief rival to learning in its various forms was ostensibly military virtue. But the former did not simply replace the latter. The conventional pairing of "courage and wisdom" (*fortitudo et sapientia*), ubiquitously cited in the Middle Ages as rival sources of moral authority – military and ecclesiastical – were now united in the person of the great nobleman. It was "false and ridiculous" to say that it must be arms *or* letters; there is "a double ray of honour," such that "valour and knowledge are the best parts of the virtues."[56] On the one hand, learning-based "virtue on its own does not ennoble." On the other, weapons training can be "a school of idleness," leading to the "ignorance" that is "a vice and dishonour to nobles."[57] Weaponless virtue was useful to emergent theories of absolute power because it helped to pick out compliant nobles from potentially rebellious ones; medieval tales of opposition between knighthood and priesthood nevertheless continued to be recycled, since stories about ancestral military exploits were locked into the claims of genealogy.

The rise of virtue as nobility of mind was not necessarily the decline of virtue as military valour. Both alike helped firm up the hereditary principle. The idea of *any* kind of honour being hereditary, "an exceptional quality transmitted by the blood," was recent.[58] Most behaviour guides, while they endorse inner virtue or even mere acquired professional merit, also and in the same breath insist on lineage and bravery. A textbook from James I's King of Heralds (a court office), for example, devotes its first three sections to soldiery, knighthood and duels. Only in the last section

---

[55] Braham, *The Institucion*, Epistle.
[56] Marois, *Le gentil-homme*, 509; Mulcaster, *Positions*, 100.
[57] Thierriat, *Trois tractez*, 156; Turquet, *La monarchie aristodémocratique*, 118.
[58] Cited in Ellery Schalk, *From Valor to Pedigree*, 144.

is wit discussed and virtue defined as "true perfection of reason" acquired by "habit"; by an abrupt switch, honour is then defined as what one achieves *as a result of* this latter virtue.[59] The author has trawled the entire range of contested notions of honour, glossing over their disparities in order to bring in and flatter every conceivable subgroup of gentry or indeed professional non-gentry into obedience to the state and the monarch. Strong emphasis on bloodline and its supposed association with military virtues was a reaction, not a preface, to the social and political shifts taking place in this period, which is why it appears so often alongside the appeal to learning-based virtue, usually within one and the same text. They grew up together.

The allocation of virtue to learning and professional wit was a reaction to social instability, which writers addressed by making increasingly extravagant claims for their close relationship with lineage. The ultimate destination would be nineteenth- and twentieth-century concepts of inherited intelligence. Elyot writes that "Virtue joined with great possessions or dignity, ... long continue in the blood or house of a gentleman, as it were an inheritance."[60] With this notion of virtue as a genealogy of the inner self, the self-referentiality of status could renew itself. Its rise in importance coincided with the gentry starting to claim direct blood descent from Prester John or Hector of Troy – a claim more characteristic of the late sixteenth century than of earlier ones.[61] As for the man whose genealogy was dubious, Golden Age arguments came to his rescue. His present social position was an aberration. He should cultivate his intellect so that in him "the ancient and reverend nobility may return," alongside "the glory of their wit and learning."[62] Lists of non-martial virtues could of course be moral as much as strictly intellectual in character; yet such moral claims, frequent as they are, tend to be presented as aspects or "fruits of the human understanding," which consists of "science and intelligence."[63]

A rival to learning and "the desire to understand" that was denied any claim to virtue was money, the love that dare not speak its name. Spanish writers like Cervantes and the anonymous author of *Lazarillo de Tormes* treat this satirically, comparing honour's empty self-referentiality with an empty wallet. Their satire rests on the fact that like is not being compared with like: honour is appearance, not real collateral. It will not get you a square meal. The behaviour guides, by contrast, simply contradict themselves about wealth – or so it seems to a twenty-first-century reader. "What things shall a courtier most rely upon? His God, his king, his wit, and his purse," says one.[64] In order to achieve learning-based virtue from non-gentle origins, one must already be capable of generosity, including of a financial kind. To be poor, non-gentle and virtuous is impossible. To be poor, *gentle* and virtuous, on the other hand, is not. Distinctions are made as to particular kinds of wealth: "I speak not ... in defence of all new risen men, but only of such as worthiness hath brought unto honour," says the King of Heralds quoted above: that is, the sort of worthiness that derives from some intellectual component, usually in professional learning. He contrasts these men with the "vulgar," with the "hogling ... that was but lately digged out of a dunghill, whose wit and honesty both, doth only consist but in compassing of crowns" and in "servile functions."[65] The official line was that it is *a certain type* of money grubber, the one with gold bath taps, who is to be positioned as far down the social scale as possible. Another writer, subdividing the ungentle into villeins, merchants, burgesses and servants, ranks villeins as the highest of these four because they

---

[59] Segar, *Honor, Military and Civil*, 208.
[60] *The Governour*, 111v.
[61] François l'Alouette, *Traicté*, 234; Champier, *Le fondement*, 1; Marois, *Le gentil-homme*, 223.
[62] Lawrence Humfrey, *The Nobles*, B5v.
[63] L'Alouette, *Traicté*, 173.
[64] Nicholas Breton, *The Court and Country*, in Hazlitt, *Tracts Illustrating English Manners*, 210.
[65] Segar, *Honor, Military and Civil*, 225; Rich, *Faultes*, 26v.

"minister ... necessities to man's life," unlike the merchant.[66] What seems contradictory to us (can money buy honour or can't it?) was quite straightforward to people of the time who lacked a firm category distinction between socio-economic ability and intellectual ability.

Lineage and professional skills

If, then, wit and learning – in a relationship with lineage that was part collision, part collusion – were gaining the upper hand in defining the in-group and in its closure of ranks, what exactly was the content of that learning? One author, ostentatiously favouring the inwardness of learning over the outward display of genealogical insignia, goes on to identify the paradigm of learning as knowledge of those insignia, and of the biographies of honourable men. These are, for the gentry, "the perfect mean to sharpen their wits."[67] They show us that what constitutes "learning" is often circular within any bidding mode, thus directly reinforcing it; just as the educational psychologist, in testing intelligence, tests above all the subject's potential to be an educational psychologist, so for the heraldic scientist the epitome of learning is knowledge of heraldry. One thing it is *not*, says this author, is scholarship. The mind has "more serious employments" than learning just for the sake of it. To devote one's life to scholarship is "to desert the mistress to make love to the maid" and as a result to exhaust one's soul spirits, with disastrous effects on the body's reproductive abilities and thus on the continued excellence of the genealogical line.[68]

The link between cultural representations of learning and its social practice is the professions. Giambattista Tiepolo's 1743 *Virtue and Nobility Putting Ignorance to Flight*, for example, depicts these allegorical figures in classical dress; it invites the viewer to admire and honour the profession of its commissioner, a lawyer, by embellishing it with the trappings of ancient ancestry.[69] Is this reduction of learning-based virtue to everyday professional ability essentially modern? Perhaps, but if so, its history is longer than one might think. Tiepolo got his theme from emblem books of at least two centuries earlier. Fundamental to professional learning was the ability to read and write, and many trades had long needed literacy from their apprentices. Within the honour society the need had always been there; even in the twelfth century, the philosopher John of Salisbury had likened an unlettered king to a crowned donkey. The nobility needed at least enough wit to avoid being cheated by their estate managers. It was not unusual for higher nobles to attend university, while younger sons would need to be literate for a career of service to the state. By the sixteenth century it was clearly recognized that a Master of Arts degree had "the power to create gentility," if not any actual enthusiasm for one's studies.[70]

Alongside the instant expertise of the "ingenious gentleman" noted in an earlier chapter, a contrary and once dishonourable notion began to take hold: that it had to be complemented by intellectual labour, "a sweat of the brains" as Boyle called it.[71] A gentleman needed "double honour, [to be] both *eugenes* and *polymathes*," in Peacham's words. Shirking was a sign of degeneracy. There was condemnation of gentry who "hate all things that must be obtained by industry, who most degenerately entrusting their wits as well as fortunes with their inferiors, have made them

---

[66] Ferne, *Blazon*, 7.
[67] Braham, *The Institucion*.
[68] Peacham, *The Compleat Gentleman*, 30.
[69] Dulwich Picture Gallery, London.
[70] Conrad Russell, *Times Higher Education*, 23 November 2001.
[71] Shapin, *A Social History of Truth*, 163.

master of both."⁷² In England, the demand for professional learning had grown during the early sixteenth century as a single administration of law arose out of formerly disparate legal entities loosely tied to relatively autonomous noble clans. This centralization, which required increasing numbers of officials, coincided with the state takeover of the herald's functions. For the architects of the Tudor state such as Thomas Cromwell, public verification of honourable descent as a tool of control became more, not less important. Many of the architects were of non-gentle origins themselves; Cromwell, who as Henry VIII's Chief Minister was created first Earl of Essex, was a blacksmith's son. This paradox irked the oppositional gentry: both the Pilgrimage of Grace and the engineers of Cromwell's eventual execution called for "villein blood" to be removed from the King's council.

The goal of professional learning was sound magistracy. The focusing of virtue on wit and learning, and of wit and learning on administrative skill, was made possible in England partly by the rise of secular grammar schools, of which St Paul's, set up by Erasmus's friend John Colet in 1509, was the chief example. Similar demands for a schooling in learning-based virtue as the state's response to political and religious fragmentation sprang up in France, where the first state academy for nobles was established in 1594. Promoting the image of the cultured nobleman, it was a reversal of the previous stereotype (for French noblemen "to read a good book … is in their eyes to seem like the son of a doctor or lawyer"), which in any case merely may have been a convenient fiction.⁷³ In Molière's *Le bourgeois gentilhomme*, Monsieur Jourdain's middle-class ignorance contrasts with the noble learning of Comte Dorante. Even though learning had in fact long been a part of noble life, it was presented as a novelty because only now was it a necessary mode of self-representation, formally recognized as part of the nobility's administrative role. Whereas commoners needed five years to graduate in law, three was enough for a nobleman, "either because they are more apt at understanding the sciences than non-nobles … or because it is the gentleman's desire for honour that forces him always to excel." (His superior intelligence might have also more material causes, according to this author: one of the nobility's privileges was to hunt partridge, whose meat produces "a sense and intelligence more delicate than in those fed on beef and pork.")⁷⁴ The gentleman's duty to dispense justice and maintain the common good demanded a disinterested virtue – and an administrative ability – which entitled him to honour and privileges from the community. It was his intellect and his honour together, then, that constituted "the advantage I have of the vulgar."⁷⁵

Genealogical claims were therefore only one element in the accumulated symbolic capital shoring up professional privilege, at a time when the accumulated economic capital of non-gentle but in fact highly literate and numerate merchants was increasingly vital to the state. The tensions here are clearest in France, where it led to the genealogical "nobility of the sword" being more rather than less clearly contrasted with the upstart "nobility of the [lawyer's] gown," and to a sharper distinction between honour and "merit." When behavioural writers warned against putting "honour and shame, merit and demerit, on the same rank," as if honour and merit could be of equal value, it was a sign that the vocabulary in which self-referential status bids were conceived was already changing.⁷⁶ Merit, it seemed, was replacing personal forms of authority based on ancestry with an impersonal culture enshrined in professional and administrative ability. Champions of merit defined it as ability in the "liberal sciences." One even narrowed it down as far as mathematics,

---

[72] *The Compleat Gentleman*, 28; Nathaniel Highmore, *The History of Generation*, 4r.
[73] Thierriat, *Trois tractez*, 47.
[74] Ibid.
[75] Browne, *Religio*, 14.
[76] Cited in Bitton, *The French Nobility*, 92.

the "captain" of all other kinds of learning, as long as it was "employed in the government of people": that is, civil service accounting, a precursor of the nineteenth-century social statistics that inspired the first psychometricians.[77] Conflicts over promotion to the in-group forced disputants into a consensus about the types of professional learning that were honourable; it was agreed to include anyone "dignified with the title of Doctor, or graced by some office of reputation," even if (with the rapid footwork characteristic of status modes), once "that be taken away, he shall be reputed a common person" again. Doctors should automatically have coats of arms even if born ungentle, as should lawyers.[78]

In a key move, Henri IV tried in 1604 to accommodate the bloodline concept of honour to this new outlook, by making crown offices in law and finance saleable but subsequently inheritable. The criterion of lineage turned out to be adaptable to circumstance, lubricated by the cash that passed hands in the ennoblement of both sword and gown. French and English writers accused each other's countries of instigating this practice. Peacham said that when Louis XI ennobled his Chancellor, he had "unworthily advanced [him] from a stocking-mender" for pecuniary advantage; his French contemporary said that the practice was already observable in England, "where one must have a certain income in order to be ennobled."[79] Merit was a quality of the *honnête homme*, covering bourgeois honesty as much as genteel honour. In reaction to the rise of this "new" professional, assemblies of French nobles in 1616 and 1627 showed that the existing aristocracy knew a trick or two. To resist the inflation of honours and the degradation of self-referential honour into a collateral honesty, the nobility itself began to promote "merit" – but by the Humpty Dumpty method (typical of status bids) of redefining the term. Offices should be distributed by merit, yes – as long as one defined merit as birth. Of course few in the assembly could trace their own nobility further back than two or three generations, so it was scarcely an argument against "new men" in genealogical principle, only against the numbers to be allowed in at any one point.

The threat of being swamped by outsiders could be averted by concentrating on the "cultivation" of blood, by educating your offspring: a precursor to Jean-Baptiste Lamarck's biological principle of descent by acquired characteristics. It was not enough to be well born. Parents, said the behavioural writers, had to feed the plant and "spread from the earliest age the seeds of virtues" by "honest nurture." While nurture and nature were sometimes set off against each other – Browne, for example, is grateful that his own virtue came "from the seeds of nature, rather than the innoculation and forced grafts of education" – his point was that nurture, as custom and firmly planted good advice, should *become* nature, of a type that would recur in succeeding generations. This was more characteristic of the period. The classical sources such as Pliny had looked on nature as a "nurse." The element of determinism lies not in nature but in blood. That is why blood has to be pure; hence the need for a correspondingly precise scientificity of heraldic assessment. If a noble marries a non-noble, the blood takes a hundred years to become completely "distilled" again; by contrast, the man of honour who commits a crime "nevertheless conserves his original nobility, since the virtue passed into him with the blood of his ancestors comes as much from his proper essence as from the character which nature has imprinted upon his person." Blood as internal necessity stands in contrast to "nature" as acquired characteristics.[80]

This necessity has its external, political aspect in absolute monarchy: "honours and baronies ... were [first] granted by the king," with the result that "now being so invested in our blood, and become hereditary, they cannot be revoked." The king could also "grant" a pedigree retrospectively,

---

[77] Faret, *The Honest Man*, 69.
[78] Segar, *Honor, Military and Civil*, 225; Ferne, *Blazon*, 19.
[79] Charles Loyseau, *Traité des ordres*, citing Smith, *De Republica*, 114.
[80] Pierre Dampmartin, *Du bonheur de la cour*, 47; de la Roque, *Traité de la noblesse*, 16.

or even "repair a fault of birth in those to whom nature has denied it." The idea that "none are [in] honour originally, but such as are belonging to the king" influenced the historiography too. "Nobility dative" (i.e., given by someone else) was an expression of pure necessity; it reflected the fact that the source of human honour was Adam and that it was given by God, with the king as his understudy. It was superior to "nobility native" (i.e., bestowed or acquired by nature), which was less determinate. Nobility granted by the monarch is instantaneous; it "purges the blood and the ennobled man's posterity of all taint of mechanical labour, and distils it to the same quality and dignity as if his race had been born to it."[81] In short, it can be relative and malleable (merit) at exactly the same time and in exactly the same social context as it is absolute and deterministic (blood), just as intelligence is for the modern professional who talks of intelligence in terms of constructions and discourses but nevertheless needs it to get on in the world. Bloodline combined with meritorious wit was the identity politics of an ascendant class.

In Spain, as we have already noted, the tensions between a much-discussed *limpieza de sangre* ("purity of blood") and the newer gentry's learning-based merit centred on supposed ethnic and religious difference. Professional service to the state was seen as coming disproportionately from the descendants of forcibly converted Moors and Jews, who at some point became feared more than peasant or merchant stock as the source of pollution. There were complaints about their clever "imitations" of honour. Those of Jewish blood had in fact their own self-image of inherited intelligence, drawn from their ancestors' Judaic doctrines of lineage. They were perceived as contributing significantly to the number of courtiers, magistrates and leading churchmen, as well as of lower-order professionals who complained about having to serve stupid masters of pure Spanish blood. (The myth ran that "it is a sign of noble lineage not to know how to write your name.")[82] It was these learned men of *converso* stock whom the behavioural authority Bernabé Moreno de Vargas had in mind when he warned about the subversive social effect of such imitative skill: "The commoner judges things not as they are but as they appear; and seeing that some men have the ostentation, words and title of gentlemen, he takes them for such." People "ambitious for honour" who adopted spurious coats of arms were to be punished in law, whereas nobles who lost their land did not thereby lose their nobility. Nevertheless, Bernabé did not oppose the dubbing of *conversos* or plebeians if it was done by the king, the necessary instrument of God's grace.

A classic example of this type of passage from chivalry to learning comes in the dénouement of *Don Quixote*. The man who finally cures the Don's diseased imaginative faculty is the clever "Bachelor [of Arts] Sanson Carrasco," as Cervantes pointedly always styles him. Carrasco's university qualification represents merit-based learning, against those nobles who in playing tricks on the Don "have turned into fools themselves" (the type of the "artificial fool," discussed in more detail in Chapter 9). Likewise he gets to be the Don's sidekick, replacing the peasant smallholder Sancho Panza, who may have been "a man of some standing (if a poor man may be said to have standing), but whose brains were a bit short of salt."[83] The loss of Don Quixote's foolishness, the restoration of his senses, is also the loss of his sense of honour. This fits the broader historical shift that was taking place in faculty psychology at the time. Wit (the book's ironic subtitle dubs him *el ingenioso hidalgo*, "the gentleman of wit") is relocated away from the imaginative faculty where mere appearances such as honour first impact on the mind, and towards the superior faculty of reasoning. It is not that Don Quixote's foolishness calls his honour in question; rather, the sense of honour itself is typically foolish.

---

[81] Brooke, *A Discourse Opening the Nature of that Episcopacie*, 80; Ashley, *Of Honour*, 51; Joachim d'Estaing, cited in Devyver, *Le sang*, 212; Milles, *The Catalogue*, 2; Loyseau, *Traité*, 34.

[82] Bernabé Moreno de Vargas, *Discursos de la nobleza de España*, 86v; 42v.

[83] *Don Quixote*, 1.7; 2.70.

Honour, learning and perfectibility

Virtue also plays a role in the transformation of honour-related principles of personal destiny into intelligence-related ones of group perfectibility, in service of the state. "To what end," asked a Tudor ideologue, "are so many monuments and pedigrees granted to [an] excellent m[a]n ... so much the apter unto virtue as he is of greater birth, dignity or authority ... but that by them they meant to teach posterity to be forward in virtue by imitation of their ancestors?"[84] The eugenic perfectibility of future generations, interwoven with earthly preparation for the second coming, became a central issue. "Honour," it was said, "consisteth in the perfection of kind."[85] There were three ways of doing it, in accordance with the necessity-nature-nurture triad:

> The first, antiquity of blood (by descending from noble parents); the second, nature (by the bettering of our disposition); and the third, proper virtue (by assuming and accomplishing things good and excellent).... These ... are lively roots from whence honours may grow; for we daily see that fathers, grandfathers and great grandfathers have their images and portraitures lively represented in the bodies of their children; and why not then the virtues of their minds.

Virtue here, being a matter of nurture, helps to admit "minds" into the schema and then feeds back into the determinism of blood.

In reaction to the honour-inflation crisis of the early seventeenth century, some French writers insisted that the horde of newly ennobled merchants and professionals were receiving only a nominal nobility; it was not the restitution of some real, quasi-biological superiority. But others tried to accommodate the bourgeois influx by invoking a nascent theory of development. They subdivided the in-group into a supreme *noblesse parfaite*, a developing *noblesse croissante* and a newly dubbed *noblesse commençante*.[86] This transposition of *derivation from* into *development towards* group perfection soothed the political tensions that arose from the inflation of honourable titles. Previously nobility had been the conservation of an immemorial record, within a largely spatial and steady-state cosmology; now it was an investment in staged future growth, within a temporal one. The three stages above were said to correspond with "infancy," "puberty" and "maturity," for which the author drew on the science of alchemy (lead needed three operations to be refined into gold). The three past honourable generations required for heraldic verification are now projected into the future. A static microcosm-macrocosm picture of the world was being replaced by one where the individual's development and perfectibility is that of the species: the beginnings of a Kantian universal history.

As group perfectibility became the goal, inheritance lost none of its force. Instead, the modes of honour and intellect fused and were extended beyond elite families to the nation, and finally to the human race in general. Previously, "nature" in social divisions (despite all the wild metaphor about the "multitude" being a hydra-headed monster) had been in the last resort a difference of *degree*: "Nobility announces itself in one and the same species of nature ... having in a greater degree of perfection that which is natural and proper to its species, than the other things of the same species."[87] At the twilight of the traditional honour mode, its last-ditch defenders such as Henri de Boulainvilliers turned it into a primitive theory of "natural" class struggle by asserting that social divisions follow species-like differences in *kind*, by race and class. Some of his Enlightenment contemporaries turned it into a doctrine of national honour, one branch of which fed later into fascism's "blood and honour";

---

[84] Ashley, *Of Honour*, 51.
[85] Markham, *The Booke*, 10.
[86] Scohier, *L'estat*, 62.
[87] Jehan de Caumont, *De la vertu de noblesse*, A2r.

others turned it into *égalité* and the brotherhood of man. Baron d'Holbach, for example, described revolutionary America as a "citizen nobility." The American constitution's right to bear arms, while no doubt it refers to actual weapons, might also be read in terms of coats of arms, pointing to the same thought: that every citizen has the right to be regarded as a gentleman.

Hereditary honour also fed into French republican notions of democracy and the perfection of man. The idea that honour might inhere in a universal bloodline proved compatible with meritocracy from the start. As an egalitarian of the 1770s, arguing for all children to wear school uniforms, wrote: "Uniformity favours equality. In vain has so much been written and said about genealogy, titles, coats of arms, birth; all men are born equal, of the same father. Nature has engraved that truth in ineffaceable letters on every cradle."[88] By "letters" he is implying heraldic insignia, now universalized. The 1789 Jacobins, with their claim that a fake aristocracy had filched the term "honour" from an originally egalitarian human community, were suggesting that honour could be redefined as reason; in bestowing this reconceived honour now upon all humans, they were restoring its true substance.[89] However an abstract concept of fraternity, if defined in advance of the individuals comprising it, will inevitably mean the exclusion of some of them: an exclusion upon which that concept depends for its very existence. The intimations of equality in American citizen honour still ruled out labourers and the poor, let alone slaves. Likewise with French national honour: it was "a French *gentleman* [emphasis added] that one desires to have, the habits, the manner, the grace which is truly French and not foreign."[90] If boasting about one's ancestors had come to be frowned upon, this attitude long remained ambiguous. Proust's Duchesse de Guermantes, for example (who surely knew Hippolyte Taine's *De l'intelligence*, widely read in the France of the time), was noted for choosing her friends by their intelligence rather than their birth. Judging people by their ancestry was old hat, but Proust notes that somehow the servants never forgot to address her as Madame la Duchesse.

When the radical egalitarian Thomas Paine wrote that the idea of hereditary legislators was as absurd as that of hereditary mathematicians, he little thought how he would be trumped by the absurdity of history. We did indeed come up with hereditary mathematicians. In Galton's *Hereditary Genius*, for example, mathematical abilities are the inherited intellectual property of the white race and (despite problems of regression to the mean) must be passed on to future generations. Galton came from a Western tradition which told him that humans are worthier than other animals but also, by similarly intellectual criteria, worthier than some other humans whom it might therefore be more appropriate to classify as degenerate (labourers, black people) or quasi-brutes (idiots, imbeciles). Just as control of marriage within the elite became stricter from the thirteenth century onwards in order to enhance the inheritable symbolic capital of honour, so today eugenic insemination – in line with Galton's proposal that only exam-passers be allowed to have children – is designed to enhance the inheritable symbolic capital of intelligence and the social distinctions it affords. The history of intelligence has been intrinsic to the channelling of distinctions of blood and honour into racial separateness: first English rather than French (Spanish, Italian, etc.), then white rather than black, then human rather than – what, exactly? The conceptual space certainly arises there, inviting us to fill it with something inferior or plain pathological. By "human race" we mean the rationally choosing and consenting race, with its powers of logical reasoning, abstraction and information processing. If that is the case, then from the perspective of someone deemed to lack these things the anti-racist slogan "One race, the human race" remains on an ethical continuum with racist ones: that is, until the urge to seek and fill the conceptual space with not-quite-humans is recognized as being itself the pathology.

---

[88] Cited in Jay Smith, *Nobility Reimagined*, 145; 192.
[89] Dulaure, *Histoire*, 280.
[90] Pelletier, *La nourriture*, 96.

Chapter 9
"Dead in the Very Midst of Life": the Dishonourable and the Idiotic

Here we shall be asking: who were the people that lay beyond the scope of honour, and what connection did this have with their intellectual status? Honour was a universal way of ordering social relationships, with an all-encompassing prescriptive force that justified discriminations of social class and gender and, to a lesser extent, ethnicity and religion. Intelligence too is exactly this, although its discriminations around class, gender and race and their claimed evidence base in IQ have become contentious, not to say (with certain recurring exceptions) *passé*. Only in the case of the so-called intellectually disabled does ordeal by intelligence not appear to be discriminatory or unjust.

Claims to honour, as to intelligence, are valid only if there is also a group that has no claim. This out-group can be subdivided. First, certain people are not born to the in-group. But secondly there are odd individuals who *are* born to the in-group, who therefore have a notional claim to the honour collectively ascribed to their group, but who nevertheless lack it. From the standpoint of any dominant status mode, these two types do not appear to differ from each other, since the modes generally presuppose that what it is to be honourable (elect, intelligent) is also what it is to be human. In the case of intelligence, the criterion for being human is to think abstractly, reason logically, process information, etc. There is no sense in trying to differentiate between one type of person who belongs outside the intelligence society and another who belongs in it but is incapable of meeting these criteria; the result would simply be a tautology. The same was true of concepts of honour for the sixteenth-century reader. One would not, at that time, have tried to differentiate between a type that lay beyond the honour society (labourers, shopkeepers, women, etc.) and a type that was born within that society but was incapable of exhibiting signs of belonging to it, however clear the difference is to us now. That is why, in the primary sources, we find that a single set of terms ("idiot," "fool") covers both types. Since the difference in respect of honour has been discarded and therefore *is* clear to us, we can take these types separately and in turn.

Class, race and gender: idiots before the modern stereotype

In terms of social rank, the out-group were "idiots" in the old sense of uneducated: a large sector of the population. And as Lynn Rose points out, the conceptual distance between the uneducated and the supposedly uneducable is short.[1] When Alexander distinguished between "philosophers and *idiotai*," the latter meant people naturally lacking ideas or abilities – but it also meant *ordinary* people.[2] Stoic philosophers, said Alexander, mistakenly exaggerated the importance of fate; they too could sometimes be "idiots" and so this word could, in all non-satirical seriousness, extend as far as philosophers with the wrong ideas. Conversely, *both* philosophers and idiots were capable of having the right ideas about fate; the fact that these two groups were divided in their intellectual natures did not mean that they could not be united in their response to an intellectual question.

---

[1] Rose, "The courage."
[2] Alexander, *Scripta Minima*, 171.28; 172.5; 189.12; *On Fate*, 131.

The early church fathers used *idiota* to mean someone lacking religious wisdom, and in theology up to the eighteenth century it continued to be synonymous with *indoctus* (uneducated).[3] Albert described *idiotae* more precisely as people who "do not discern the universal from particulars," i.e., those who do not make abstractions.[4] Like Alexander, he seems to have meant everyone who was not a philosopher and some of those too. The point was repeated later by Locke when he suggested that idiots (among whom he might still have included landless labourers) are like animals because they "abstract not." The deficiency is the same for Albert, Locke and today's psychologist; it is just that the number of people to whom it is attributed has gradually diminished. The abstracting skills which Albert attributed solely to those of his learned colleagues who agreed with him around the year 1200 have become, roughly speaking, the skills which psychology defines as universally human, bar a few freaks, around the year 2012.

As we have already seen, the social vocabulary of gentility and honour in the late medieval period is reflected in the theoretical vocabulary of philosophers as they order their knowledge into ranks. "One kind of knowledge is more honourable than another," says Albert in the above text; it all depends on the "incorruptibility" of the subject matter and the "certitude" with which one can reach conclusions. Lurking within this hierarchy of knowledge is the claim to honour of people who know and can demonstrate such certainties. The most certain are geometry and the existence of God, plus "the nobility and utility of knowledge of the soul." Abstraction and theoretical knowledge consist of things separated from the material world, and their highest form is knowledge of how the human soul undertakes this separation. One's place at the top of the hierarchy, natural and social, thus springs from one's ability to know one's place at the top of the hierarchy. According to Albert, souls "lose honour to the extent that they are immersed" in the images of the material things encountered in everyday life, and which themselves have varying degrees of honourability and incorruptibility. The soul's theoretical knowledge of its own theoretical faculty of knowing descends into corruption by degrees that correspond with social rankings. Recognizable modern class stereotypes emerge after this first wave of scholasticism, in the Renaissance commentaries on Aristotle. As writers inserted elements of his *On the Soul* into their commentaries on his quite unrelated theory of social rank in *Politics*, in order to support the latter with psychological explanations, so they inserted elements of his *Politics* into their commentaries on his theory of the human psyche in *On the Soul*, in order to support the latter with explanations drawn from the hard facts of social rank.

Disqualification by social rank was marked not only by deficiencies in the processes of knowing, such as abstraction, but more obviously by lack of substantive knowledge: that is, of the ideas which the processes of knowing produced. Not so long ago parents of English working-class children, on the rare occasion they might mix with those of a higher social class, would routinely warn them "Don't go getting ideas." An abbreviation of "Don't go getting ideas above your station," this became a warning against expecting too much of life or betraying one's own class. But the abbreviated version brings out its core point: ideas above your station in the early modern period were ideas *as such*, and ideas – any ideas worth the name, i.e., the abstract ones of religion, mathematics and the soul – were to be found only in the honour society. Of Stoic origin (*koinai ennoiai*), they became known in early modern texts as "the common ideas" (*communes notiones*) or more often simply "*the* ideas." They did not circulate freely among all social groups but identified a particular one: "common" in the sense of being held in common by a restricted group whose members could recognize each other by their grasp of them. Honour lay in the possession of these ideas, just as modern intelligence lies in the possession of the common processing mechanisms

---

[3] For example Pierre Poiret, *Cogitationum Rationalium*, 262.
[4] Albert, *De Anima*, in B. Geyer (ed.), *Opera*, vii, 3; 12.

such as abstraction that lead to ideas. Albert had gone so far as to say that "the common ideas are called 'honours' (*dignitates vocantur*)."[5]

The exclusions and boundaries aligning the social with the psychological in this way track the transition from early modern to modern. No clear category distinction existed between lack of the common ideas, a natural characteristic of non-gentle ranks in general, and their lack of honour. Indeed, in faculty psychology, honour itself was often presented as a constituent part of one of the faculties. This survived the breakdown of absolutism and of monarchy itself; it was an anti-monarchist parliamentarian who described honour as "that to the commonwealth which the soul is to the body," its "mind," to be kept separate from the "distempers which threaten the body politic."[6] In a slipperiness characteristic of discussions about class, the word *communes* for these ideas also evokes the commons or general population, when in fact only people of social standing possessed them. (One recalls here that English private schools call themselves "the public schools.") The inference might be drawn that only the elite are fully human, and that those who lack the ideas, in belonging outside it, might belong even outside the *communitas*, in the sense of being bestial. When "society" dresses itself up as the whole population, it arrogates to itself the definition of the human species; other groups are unnatural or deformed, in this case intellectually. Extreme social discriminations, to be justifiable, must have roots in nature. It is natural for some men to rule, not only over beasts but over bestial men.

As psychological truth (knowledge of the soul, mind and self) began to form a third set of common ideas alongside religious and mathematical truths, it too reformulated the out-group according to its own specific terms: "discussion of the soul is very obscure, and therefore God has only given knowledge of it to those who are deeply learned, and when the masses ask about this problem … it is not their concern."[7] It might be that "idiots, the unlearned and peasants can be holy without any such knowledge," but only by providence.[8] Elyot's "monster with many heads," as a threat to the gentry's "*eugenia*," would re-emerge in the Edwardian eugenicists' fear that the wrong social class was reproducing – a problem solved, some of them thought, by the slaughter in the trenches.[9] Inability to abstract and lack of "ideas" now tend to define only a small disabled out-group, though it would perhaps be over-hasty to think these other prejudices have gone away. In the words of a currently serving British cabinet minister and former educational adviser to government, "It's not only the thick but the reasonably thick part of the population, perhaps 70% or 50%, who are completely incapable of conducting a normal life in the terms in which we as the privileged elite understand it." Comforting ruminations about one's distance from the "stolid masses" (to use Michael Young's satirical formula) are, paradoxically, necessary to the meritocrat's self-representation.

Both the common ideas and the psychological operations needed for grasping them were matters of interest to the early modern professional and to the maintenance of his privileges. His subjective relation to the social order was the ascription of him to a caste whose badge of membership was not only the claim to ancestry but the "ideas" held in common with men from other professions. The intellectualocentrist ideology was related to a feeling of being under threat from the socio-economic mobility of groups immediately below the threshold: merchants, well-off artisans, yeoman farmers. When lawyers, mostly upstarts themselves, proposed barring yeomen's sons from the Inns of Court and reserving law for those "immediately descended from a nobleman or gentleman," absence of

---

[5] Albert, *De Unitate*, in Borgnet (ed.), *Opera*, ix, 452.
[6] John Pym, cited in Kenyon, *The Stuart Constitution*, 198.
[7] Averroes, *Incoherence of the Incoherence*, 333.
[8] Valentin Weigel, Γνωθι Σεαυτον, *Nosce Teipsum, Erkenne dich selbst*, 62.
[9] *The Governour*, 6r; 111v.

honour and of intellectual or professional ability alike was implied.[10] And when, conversely, it was suggested that gentlemen's sons be barred from taking up apprenticeships, it was not only because they ought not to be in trade (they often were) but because gentlemen, being "ingenious" by their very nature, ought not to be seen as needing to spend time or labour on acquiring mundane skills.

A leading early Royal Society member asserted that knowledge of the soul, let alone of mathematics or religion, was impossible for "vulgar apprehensions," but admitted that intellectual ability could sometimes be found in people outside the honour society. In their case, he said, it was "necessity" that made them wise, not their nature: either practical necessity, or the necessity implied in a divine suspension of natural laws. More usually the "common people" have "dull wits," indicative of a "brutish nature," the evidence being above all that they "have no ... feeling of honour and renown." The yokel with a comic accent, allowed just one speech at the end of an allegorical dialogue on honour, angrily denounces heraldic science as "an old smoky coat ... rotten and full of holes." He is reproved by the knight: "Thou favourest nothing but thy plough: nobility and the signs thereof is far above thy capacity." The herald moderating the dialogue asks for the yokel to be excused, because by his very nature he is incapable of knowing Blazon and cannot be held responsible for his own ignorance.[11]

Questions of social class are involved in the transition from the scholastics' general, deductive knowledge of the human soul to a modern, purportedly inductive knowledge of individual minds. The transition appears quite seamless. Wherever we find the clearest proto-psychiatric language, there we find also the clearest references to honour and social ranks, and that is because for contemporaries these two sets of references were cognate. Consider the following passage from Charron, which encompasses a wide range of textual conventions: faculty psychology, the medical theory of temperaments, species difference, the theological doctrine of idleness as living death and classical references such as the ranking of souls in Plato's *Republic* and the transmigration of animal souls in *Timaeus*:

> [The soul] may properly enough be reduced into three classes, each of which is capable of being subdivided again, and hath several distinctions and degrees comprehended under it. The lowest of these are poor and weak souls, not much removed from ... brutes. And this defect may be sometimes from the faults and imperfections of the natural constitution: too great a predominance of cold and moisture in the temperament of the brain, as fishes, whose composition is of this kind, are reckoned the lowest and most wanting of all other animals. This infirmity is born with us, and derived from our parents. Sometimes it is chargeable upon accidental failings afterwards: want of due care to awaken and exert the natural powers, and letting them rest upon our hands till they degenerate into senselessness and stupidity. Of these we can make no certain account, nor can they be esteemed a certain species; for in truth, they are not in a condition to govern themselves as men, but are minors and ignorants all their days, and ought to be constantly kept under the tuition and care of others wiser than themselves. They snore and nod with their eyes open; and while they seem to live and act, are dead in the very midst of life; moving carcasses.[12]

This could easily be taken as some transhistorical group identifiable by their pathology: an extreme deviation from the norm, with an essentialist question mark over their species membership – that is, the same tiny minority our own scientists know as intellectually disabled. But then we get the specifics. These souls are "the boors and common people, without sense, without apprehension,

---

[10] Cited in Simon, *Education*, 337.
[11] Seth Ward, *A Philosophicall Essay*, 34; Ferne, *Blazon*, ii, 27.
[12] Charron, *Of Wisdom*, i, 130 f.

without judgement ... living under subjection and management .... In a word, such as are but just men, and no more": that is, the majority of the population.

Codes defining the boundaries of the honour society, as they become rigidified, reflect the pressures of social mobility. Take, for example, the conventional employment by logicians of "Socrates" to represent any individual member of the species "man," as an illustration of how particulars relate to universals. This spread beyond the bounds of pure logic and started to be used to imply a differentiation within human nature. It became usual to pair Socrates with Thersites, representative of the out-group because he is the only non-noble to make a named appearance in Homer's *Iliad*. So in the late sixteenth century we find the syllogistic pairing "Socrates is a philosopher, Socrates is a man, Some man is a philosopher," and "Thersites is no philosopher, Thersites is a man, Some man is not a philosopher." Half a century later, as the modes of honour and wit were bifurcating, Royal Society secretary John Wilkins would illustrate the basic principles of logical dichotomy with examples drawn from what by now were assumed to be separate approaches to human nature; he casts Socrates as the illustration of the "honourable" and Thersites as its privative, "dishonourable," while "rational man" and its privative, "idiot," come under a separate rubric.[13]

As human reason and intelligence gradually prevailed over honour, rational consent theory did not moderate contempt for the out-group but did reduce its numbers. When Locke in the second of his *Two Treatises* says "We are born free as we are born rational" and goes on to mention "natural fools" as the exception to this rule, he sounds like Charron above. Charron's remark that the masses are "minors and ignorants all their days ... constantly kept under the tuition and care of others" is matched by Locke's remark that "anyone [who] comes not to such a degree of reason wherein he might be supposed capable of knowing the law" is "never set free from the government of his parents."[14] Charron has a concept of universal man just as Locke has, it is simply that his exceptions seem to be a majority of the population and to represent various aspects of a general Adamite nature, whereas Locke's are a minority "out of the ordinary course of nature." It had previously been quite usual to lump together "mad folks, idiots and old men [grown] childish, bond-slaves, and villains" as being "excepted for giving evidence" in court, on the grounds that they are all *non compotes mentis*. Moreover, that was because they "must of necessity be liars" – a classic characteristic of the dishonourable – and are therefore "bond-slaves of the Devil, whose works they will do."[15]

In the mid-eighteenth century Samuel Johnson's use of idiot terminology still mixes psychology and social class. James Boswell describes how Johnson would periodically desert "society" friends to consort with "unideaed" women; he spoke of an actress who was "in common life, a vulgar idiot; she would talk of her *gownd* but, when she appeared upon the stage, seemed to be inspired by gentility and understanding .... It is wonderful how little mind she had." Common and vulgar here stand in opposition to gentility but also to understanding; idiot stands in opposition to understanding but also to gentility.[16] The evidence for the actress's idiotism is her failure to pronounce English in the way fixed for polite society by Dr Johnson, who was only at that moment inventing the very idea of a connection between fixed pronunciation and social rank; and as the reader will by now be expecting, he too was an upstart claiming higher social connections – in William Hogarth's view "an idiot momentarily inspired."

---

[13] *An Essay towards a Real Character, and a Philosophical Language.*
[14] Locke, *Two Treatises of Civil Government*, 145.
[15] Nathaniel Wanley, *The Wonders of the Little World*, 66.
[16] *Life of Samuel Johnson*, 238.

Religion and race fed into these notions of class. The Jews were cited in debates about whether human souls differ or whether they are equal and only their "operations" different. Surely there had to be a difference between Christ's soul and a Jew's?[17] This anxiety spread to debates about the newly enslaved population of the Americas. Whereas Albert had actually added to Aristotle's list of the virtues of slaves, crediting them with the "civic intellect" (*prudentia*) denied them by his predecessor, some Spanish writers attributed to their subject peoples a permanent mindlessness (*amentia*).[18] *Amentia* till then had been a passing moment in the acute phase of disease in an individual patient, rather than a permanent characteristic of groups. In its radicalized form, it contributed to the idea of the permanence of the disabled identity, covering all individuals in the group. Spanish elites before the crisis of the seventeenth century viewed their own peasant class similarly, in whom lack of honour was also lack of mind (*mens*).[19] Later, the overlap between race and class came to be justified by interpretations of Genesis 9 which identified the three sons of Noah as the source for the first division of labour. The idea that "the descendants of Shem pray, the descendants of Japheth fight, and the descendants of Ham work" became the chief reference point for Southern whites in the nineteenth-century USA, where slaves were said to belong to the black or "Hamitic" race and their supposed psychological inferiority was still characterized primarily by an incapacity for honour.[20]

Finally there is once again the insult and its links to modern parlance. An ill-informed peer or debating opponent was characteristically dubbed "Thersites."[21] The typical insult to someone's honour, calculated to spark a duel, was to call him a villain, denying his group membership on the grounds of class (from "villein," a feudal serf). Some sense of this carries over into the phrase "an insult to my intelligence." The word "insult" here is more than mere metaphor. It does not say that you have insulted my intelligence as if it were my honour, or even my intelligence and *therefore* my honour; there has simply been a displacement of one term by the other. The structural continuity is provided by the extension of the honour society, within which (alone) there was a presumed equality of intellectual competences, into a modern, quasi-universal intelligence society. Conversely, "it's a wise man that knows his own father." In this phrase the priority seems to go to wit over honourable descent, even if the ironic implication is that such wisdom is actually impossible.

Effeminacy and mental torpor

Not only female commoners but genteel wives and daughters lay outside the honour society. Their honour lay in their bodies, a fragile private reflection of the public honour of their men. Otherwise, gentlewomen had the same psychological deficiencies as the labouring multitude. The entire sex was the natural "slave of mankind ... inferior almost in all things," hence "not so ingenious" as men; in them, speed of wit was mere rashness and produced "instability of opinion." They were advised to cultivate demureness rather than speed, and were thought incapable of abstract thinking. Writers on faculty psychology asserting that women have rational souls can seem under pressure to

---

[17] Ruvius, *Commentarii*, 92.
[18] Albert, *Commentarii politicorum*, in Borgnet (ed.), *Opera*, viii, 77 ff.
[19] Julio Caro Baroja, "Religion, world views, social classes, and honour," in Pitt-Rivers (ed.), *Honour and Grace in Anthropology*.
[20] Bertram Wyatt-Brown, *The Shaping of Southern Culture*.
[21] See Sachiko Kusukawa, *The Transformation of Natural Philosophy*, 109.

defend the point at length, though assertions to the contrary were perhaps rarely intended seriously.[22] It is true that with humanist learning dominating military valour as the mark of virtue, the way was open for some women to become participating members of "household academies" of husband-and-wife or father-and-daughter partnerships that put forward proto-feminist ideas.[23] However, this existed in very small doses. More often when women claimed a male type of honour, it was "rather some stupidity born of imitation, than true pride."[24] Huarte placed women quite outside his graded system of "callings" and its close relationship to faculty psychology: "God filling both [sexes] with wisdom, it is a verified conclusion, that he infused the lesser portion into her .... [She] is not capable of much wit," and lacks "any profound judgement."[25] Women were not entitled to benefit of clergy, the law which exempted literate men from being tried for capital offences in secular courts. They were fools not just by insult but by positive classification, in which absence of wit, common ideas or honour constitutes a unitary deficiency. Female rulers were no exception. On Elizabeth I's accession, John Knox warned that men's "hearts [would be] changed from the wisdom, understanding and courage of men to the foolish fondness and cowardice of women."[26] And when the Earl of Essex fell from her grace, he publicly complained about the "inconstancy" and "wavering opinion" that was due to her sex.

The same went for female characteristics in men. When Locke describes his intellectually disabled changelings as "unmanned," he is of course casting doubt on their species membership but gender is implicated too. Peacham warns "fond and foolish parents" against "indulgence to the corrupting of the minds of their children, disabling their wits, effeminating their bodies."[27] Effeminacy was stupidity, because it entailed idleness; mental "torpor" was a sign of "the iniquities of Sodom" that were destructive of gentility.[28] In everyday politics the masculinity of the honour elite was compromised by its members' need to be submissive to their ruler, who in former times had been their hypothetical equal; in late sixteenth-century England this was doubly unmanning because that ruler, heading up a centralized honours system, was female. Castiglione's advice was to treat honour in terms of Aquinas's mean; accommodating manners would get you further up the ladder than macho self-assertiveness.[29]

The epileptic fits of Shakespeare's Julius Caesar reflect this anxiety about feminine intellectual weakness. They are signs of both a "womanish" and a "feeble temper," at once detracting from his honour and disabling his intellect. Not just man but manliness defines reason. However, when Brutus justifies his own actions by appealing to manly honour, he has grasped only one side of a new political equation; the autonomy of the honourable male no longer consists of military valour and freedom from constraint but of a possibly hypocritical or Machiavellian reason. In despising Caesar's weakness, Brutus marks his own self-assertive honour, but he is defeated in turn by Antony's self-seeking wit. It is appropriate that Brutus's funeral oration should be in prose while Antony's is in verse; it is not just that prose is rhetorically weaker but that poetry is the higher form of reason. Antony inverts the relation between reason and honour: he convinces the mob that

---

[22] John Jonston, *A History of the Wonderful Things of Nature*, 329; Petrus Monedulatus Lascovius, *De Homine*, 103.

[23] Sarah Gwyneth Ross, *The Birth of Feminism*.

[24] De Dryvere, *Universae Medicinae Methodus*, 44.

[25] Juan Huarte, *The Examination of Mens Wits*, second proeme.

[26] John Knox, *The First Blast of the Trumpet against the Monstruous Regiment of Women*, 13.

[27] Peacham, *The Compleat Gentleman*, 30.

[28] Jodocus Clichtovaeus, *De Vera Nobilitate*, 36r.

[29] See Jennifer Richards, "'A wanton trade of living'? Rhetoric, effeminacy, and the early modern courtier," *Criticism*, Spring 2000 (BNet).

Brutus's talk of honour is mere policy and reasoned calculation, when it is Antony himself who is being calculating by talking to them in this way.

In medical terms, too, reason was male. Galen's account of brain anatomy had identified the parts of the brain by nicknames derived from their supposed visual resemblance to the reproductive and excretory organs. A sixteenth-century professor of anatomy at Padua, paraphrasing this passage, adds a term of his own which teases a near-anagram out of the pineal gland (*glandula pinealis*): "This gland is shaped like a pine cone [*pinus*] ... and very prettily reflects the form of a penis [*penis*]: thus in the brain there is the form of testicles, buttocks, anus, vulva, but of the penis no less."[30] Various reasons have been offered as to why Descartes subsequently chose the pineal gland to be the place where soul and body interact: it was hard to locate anatomically, suggesting that something in the body had departed at the moment of death; it also seemed to stand at the centre of the brain, in the middle ventricle and its reasoning faculty, rather than being duplicated in each hemisphere. Here we have one more possible reason: the appropriate gendering of the organ that houses the mind. Indeed, some Cartesian philosophers, given the problem of physical extension implicit in having the whole of Christ's body in the communion bread, surmised that only his pineal gland was there.[31] It is a modernist adaptation of the pre-Cartesian convention of "occult parallels," such as Paracelsus's selection of the phallic-shaped root Satyricon as a cure for impotence.

Conversely, wisdom itself might be a sign if not of effeminacy then of a suitable bodily weakness and above all lack of sexual *potentia*. Intellectually able fathers were said to produce foolish children, for precise medical reasons we shall discuss in Chapter 14. By the same token, not only can fools produce wise offspring, the fools themselves are hugely endowed. In Richard Turner's poem *Nosce Te* ("Know thyself," the spoof of a genre of philosophical poetry that began around 1600), he says of a female aristocrat,

> *Missa* will needsly marry with a fool,
> her reason;
> O sir, because he hath an exlent—

This convention continued into the eighteenth century, at least. Fanny Hill's colleague Louisa has sex with an intellectually deficient "changeling" whose "tool" is similarly commendable. The inverse correlation between intellectual and sexual ability has its modern heirs; there is, for instance, the eminent psychologist who currently argues that black people possess smaller brains than whites but correspondingly larger penises and sexual potency ("it's a trade-off").[32] Women's supposedly smaller brains related likewise to their immoderate sexual appetites, which could only be kept under control by the imposition of a gendered honour consisting of obedience rather than autonomy, meekness not self-assertion.

"Degenerated from his kind": the honour-disabled

So far we have looked at groups lacking ascribed status, those whose membership of the honour society was never on the cards in the first place. A further question then arises. Deficiency is not the same as degeneracy. Who were the "honour-disabled," so to speak? Who were those belonging

---

[30] Galen, *De Usu*, in Kühn (ed.), *Opera*, iii, 493; Realdus Columbus, *De Re Anatomica*, 354.

[31] Nicolas Malebranche, "Mémoire: pour expliquer la possibilité de la transsubstantiation," in *Oeuvres*, xvii, 497.

[32] J. Philippe Rushton, *Race, Evolution and Behaviour*.

notionally *within* the honour society who nevertheless lost or failed to meet the behavioural criteria ascribed to them as its members? And what were these criteria, more specifically?

Honour disability, even in its ancient form, had intellectual elements; Greek examples of the stupidity specific to the gentleman include not only wearing your cloak in the wrong fashion but Theophrastus's example of passing your accounts to someone else to add up. Some early modern writers display awareness of the conceptual kinship between honour and intelligence, and develop their notions of deficiency or *impotentia* on this basis. The reference point here is the medieval philosophical dispute between nominalists and realists. Nominalists like Duns Scotus claimed that the only things we can really know are particulars. When we sort them into categories ("universals"), these latter are not themselves real; they "are mere names and titles." The realist school, by contrast, claimed that the universal categories into which particulars are sorted have a real existence themselves, and as such are fully knowable. Robert Ashley, a late Tudor ideologue, applies this dispute to his discussion of honour: "I have heard some say sometimes that they could not skill of this thing called honour, and that they knew not what it meant because they thought that indeed there was no such thing but only a name and title which people had taken up."[33] Ashley attacks this nominalist view. His job, as a behavioural authority, is to prove that honour does have a real essence, since it was one of the official channels through which a centralized state resolved tensions over social status. However, Ashley is not a realist in the sense that he thinks honour can be reduced to concrete collateral. He denies that it consists in "external goods" and acknowledges that its reality lies precisely in its purely conceptual character, which plays a positive, mediating role in social action. Neither "riches" nor "wit" itself are "of themselves ... good, but so termed either more or less according as they draw near or decline from virtue," of which honour is the sign – "a certain testimony of virtue shining of itself." True, the comparison with wealth here suggests that wit can be a form of concrete collateral. But wit is also the main decider as to "who are capable of honour and who are not," and in this sense is conceptually compatible with the latter:

> Some [men] you shall see so heavy and dull spirited that they little differ from brute beasts.... [They] are wont to have least feeling of honour and to be least affected therewith because that the dullness of their wit depriving them of all sharpness of judgement, the worth and beauty of honour ... is unknown to them .... Such a man may be truly taken and accounted as one void of sense [that is, of internal senses or intellectual faculties].[34]

Such dullness, taken for granted in the masses, is equally threatening when it appears in a gentleman. Degeneracy is the psychological attribute of every villein, as the member of an entire degenerate social class; but when a noble bloodline "fall[s] upon a vicious, good-for-nothing, base person who is in himself [i.e., internally] really a villein," it really spells trouble.[35] The terms are naturalistic; these people are "brute beasts." They lack a theoretical awareness of their own honour – as gentlemen above other men or, in the case of villeins, as men above other animals. Not only is the desire for honour, to quote Ashley, "given us of nature, but ... the same nature hath not bestowed any better or more necessary thing upon us." Honour is not nominal but real: real, however, not as wealth is but as a "power of the mind." This "mind" is not some self-standing ability that can be defined independently of honour as such. Accordingly slow soul spirits, dull wit and lack of the sense of honour are facets of a single organic state. Any conceptual divergence

---

[33] Ashley, *Of Honour*, 31.
[34] Pierre de la Primaudaye, *Académie Françoise*, i, 78.
[35] Charron, cited in Schalk, *From Valor*, 117.

between honour and the understanding, if articulated, would have opened up social fissures by making explicit the prospect (and threat) of upward mobility.

Men "extracted from noble blood" were "commonly more prone to shame from dishonest things than others." The sense of shame was organically rooted, a "prophylactic which they carry with them from birth."[36] This explains how a gentleman who had lost his status for merely external reasons, for example through taking up "low or mechanical exercise," could regain it on leaving that occupation; the honour of inherited blood and its corresponding awareness of shame were internal.[37] It also explains why a degree of learning was important. Implicit in learning-based virtue is the notion that honour can be acquired, while implicit in the ancestral virtue of blood is the notion that honour can be mislaid. Hence virtue and ancestry are conjoined twins. In "bringing up the child of a gentleman, which is to have authority in a public weal," understanding and honour have to be combined. A child's failure to become virtuously learned means he will turn out like "the multitude" when it has "equal authority without any sovereign, never ... certain nor stable"; he will be "loathsome and monstrous," threatening the social order as well as his own future stock.[38] A contemporary of Castiglione's, widely read in English in the late sixteenth century, extends the point. Virtue necessarily exists in a virtuous object, that is, in "a man well born, prudent and wise." Nobility, however, "may be in a most vile object." When a son "capable of neither virtue nor reason" is born to "the vulgar sort," the condition is not noticed; when the son of a noble family is "out of his senses," he has to be properly identified and labelled as such. And it is a mark of the vulgar sort's own deficient wits that they, "being deceived, do hold these children in the rank of noblemen."[39]

Degenerate gentry are fools in the same way that the lay idiots of the commons are; in both cases, what they lack is knowledge of their own essence. This ignorance is at once social and natural: it is the honour society that gets to define natural states of the degenerate and dishonourable, just as it is the socially constituted group of rational choosers and consenters – the intelligence society – that gets to define the place in nature of the intellectually disabled. Doctors, with their image of the body as a microcosm of the political and social order, were on hand then as now to back up these definitions. The brain possesses honourable, "noble and princely properties" precisely because "it is the seat of the mind, endowed with the virtue of reason, which is the greatest sign indeed, to discern the difference between man and beast .... What great utility the brain proffereth, it is well to be perceived by [the existence of] idiots and foolish bodies, who having defect in this, are lame in all the rest."[40] These idiots, who do not know their own natural and social essence, are members of the doctor's elite client group, with symptoms of sloth, idleness or melancholy. The stupid gentleman is the obverse of the "syllogizing villein," each being a contradiction in terms.[41]

"Gentleman" usually excluded "fool" by definition. In Thomas Middleton's *The Changeling*, the noble Antonio masquerades as a fool in order to seduce a married woman, saying to her: "Take no acquaintance / Of these outward follies, there is within / A gentleman that loves you." Her husband is unsuspecting because he thinks Antonio is non-gentle (the woman who disguises her lover as a fool in order to pass him off in front of her husband was a stock dramatic convention). The same thing can be detected in passing uses of the word "idiot." If a writer is not clearly using it to mean the unlearned and unwashed in general, readers are to suppose that he is talking about the odd one or two of his social peers. He does not have to spell this out. For example "idiots, dolts, lunatics,

---

[36] Nicolas Coeffeteau, *A Table of Humane Passions*, 673.
[37] Lorraine, *Discours sur le congé impétré*, 5; Loyseau, *Traité*, 47.
[38] Elyot, *The Governor*, 6r.
[39] Nenna, *A Treatise*, 76r.
[40] Banister, *The Historie*, 6r.
[41] Noël du Fail, *Baliverneries*, 3.

frantics, and blockheads can no more judge right from wrong, truth from falsehood, virtue from vice, than the blind can try colours"; the result, says this author, is that they end up abusing their powers as magistrates. In other words, it is assumed they have such powers in the first place.[42]

To think that "true and perfect nobility in man consisteth ... in blood" and nothing else was itself "mere folly" and "brutal stupidity," such was the accepted place of intellectual virtues: "if nought else renown him but his wormeaten stock ... [he] is not to be reckoned amongst the noble and honourable, but rather be deemed a fool."[43] Peacham wrote about noblemen who "flatter themselves with the favourable sunshine of their great estates and ... are admired of idiots and the vulgar from the outside, statues or huge colossuses full of lead and rubbish within."[44] The mutually reflecting deficiency of the universal idiotic labourer and the occasional idiotic noble – their internal psychological rubbish – consists in their being interested only in externals. Faculty psychology enabled the point to be set in a naturalistic context. It distinguished between understanding and "apprehending," and the latter, since it belongs in the imaginative faculty, is associated with surfaces and the corrupting potential of the external senses: "The greatest part of men ... want that necessary degree of understanding which should enable them to reason as well as [they] apprehend. For reasoning and apprehending are far from being synonymous terms. They sometimes distinguish one man from another ... almost as much as they distinguish a man from a brute."[45]

Honourable status and failure to perform

There are several recurring, specific markers of failure to perform the honourable status ascribed to an individual. The simplest is failure to defend assaults on one's reputation, and particularly one's masculinity. Again this is usually a matter of externals, of readable behaviour. In Samuel Rowland's poem *The Letting of Humours*, the henpecked gentleman is recast as a "fool" for carrying his wife's pet dog: "Thus goodman idiot thinks himself an earl / That he can please his wife." "Goodman" means non-gentle; the word "idiot" plays on his betrayal of caste. Similarly, there is the nobleman who, having called in a tailor to measure his wife for a gown, asked him if he wanted to approach her from the front or from behind: "The tailor, who was more discreet than the nobleman, perceiving his foolish demand, said unto him: my Lord, I must begin to take measure on the sides."[46] This foolishness, a lack of awareness of his own (gendered) honour on the part of an ascribed member of the honour society, is offset by the manual tradesman's own "discretion," a faculty-psychology operation which by his social class he ought not to possess (the twist here being that women's tailors were stereotypically lecherous). The point is summed up by Molière's character in *School for Wives* who says, "The man of honour is he who is not cuckoo" – *cocu* meaning either cuckold or out of one's wits, but here both.

Another characteristic performance failure is deviation from the mean: absence or excess of honour. Absence of a sense of honour went with idleness and "sluggish laziness of mind"; it was one of the chief features of what doctors call "stupidity" or "stolidity," which if it prevails "destroys the powers of the mind." At the opposite end was the frenetic and intemperate abuse of honour through ambition. "Dullness," associated with melancholy, could straddle both extremes; it could take the form of slow, "stupid spirits," or of the "fury" that comes with being "puffed up with the glory of

---

[42] John Jones, *A Briefe, Excellent and Profitable Discourse*, E3r.
[43] Faret, *The Honest Man*, 69; Humfrey, *The Nobles*, F8v.
[44] *The Compleat Gentleman*, 28.
[45] Gwillim, *A Display*, Frontispiece.
[46] Nenna, *A Treatise*, 80r.

his ancestors."⁴⁷ Reason is more than just instrumental to honour here; the two categories overlap: "true honour consisteth ... in the *moderation* of the mind" (emphasis added). Of course, to be foolishly witted in the first of these senses might also mean to be holy. Yet even Aquinas had raised a caution about this. Although lack of concern about injury to one's reputation may sometimes indicate that one is above worldly things, "sometimes it can be the result of being simply stupid about everything, as in unlearned people (*idiotae*) who do not discern what is injurious to them; this belongs to folly alone."⁴⁸ In the behaviour guides, idleness and lack of motivation for honour are at once social and psychological, outer and inner. Gentlemen who "of negligence stop mustard pots with their fathers' pedigrees" are displaying the public or external face of "unsound memory," the faculty-psychology characteristic of private "idiots."⁴⁹ The very first people Dante meets in hell are those who have "lost the goods of intellect," and that is because they have led their lives without any self-awareness of shame or praise. Honour resides first in God, and there is no greater gift that He passes on to us; in this sense it is no parody of divine grace but similar to it in value. "When he maketh us blessed then are we also partakers both of his divinities," of which the divine intellect is chief, "and of his honour." Honour here is both an objective ranking system, created by God, and an internal property or "secret instinct of nature" that endows the individual with a motivating autonomy to try and match the necessary, predestined scheme. The corresponding disability is to be ignorant of all this, to be "so simply and foolishly witted that [one has] no feeling of honour."⁵⁰

A further performance failure in this respect is lack of expert knowledge of heraldic science. The herald assesses people by the criterion of his own expertise. If, as Peacham tells us, honour is a natural disposition of the soul and as precisely measurable as a triangle, then

> For these and other reasons, I desire that you would bestow some hours in the study of [Blazon]; for a gentleman honourably descended to be utterly ignorant herein, argueth in him either a disregard of his own worth, a weakness of conceit, or indisposition to arms and honourable action; sometimes mere idiotism, as Seigneur Gaulart, a great man of France (and none of the wisest), inviting on a time many great personages and honourable friends to his table, at the last service a marzipan was brought in, which being almost quite eaten, he bethought himself and said, it was told me, that mine arms were bravely set out in gold and colours upon this marzipan but I have looked round about it and cannot see them. 'Your Lordship,' said one of his men, 'ate them up yourself but now.' 'What a knave,' quoth Monsieur Gaulart, 'art thou? Thou didst not tell me before I ate them, that I might have seen what they had been'.⁵¹

This gentleman has a coat of arms, but he does not know what that means or even what it might look like. His illiteracy in Blazon is what constitutes his "idiotism." Of course it may also belong in some wider cognitive dysfunction (he is "none of the wisest"), but there was in any case no wisdom outside the honour society. The fact that he does not know his own status, as expressed in its insignia, is the primary evidence, and his eating of them expresses the symbolic confusion between outer and inner, body and mind.

Others in the honour society are not so much ignorant of its insignia as provocatively devil-may-care about its values. There is the nobleman reported as saying, "I don't care about all these ... coats of arms, crested or otherwise: I would be happy to be a villein in all four quarters as long as I still get my taxes ...; I've read no books, histories or annals of France." This "fool" is well able

---

47 Coeffeteau, *A Table*, 677.
48 *Summa Theologica*, 2.2.46.
49 Leigh, *The Accedence*, A3.
50 Ashley, *Of Honour*, 31; 48.
51 *The Compleat Gentleman*, 139.

to understand that honour and genealogical learning constitute status, but is too self-willed to attend to them.[52] In an English context, such dismissive attitudes to heraldry were perceived as politically dangerous. The ideology of heraldic science demanded a mean between the extremes of Puritanism on the one hand and Catholicism on the other. The Puritan gentleman "loves no heraldry, / Crosses in arms, they hold idolatry"; the result is "shortly, no difference twixt the lord, and page."[53] The Catholic gentleman, by contrast, devalues heraldic signs by inflation so they become "idle shows"; the result is "plebeian baseness." Both extremes are forms of honour foolishness. Puritans idealize the New Testament's unlearned but pious *idiota*, thereby encouraging Anabaptist-style revolt; the creaturely equality of souls is foolishly read as political equality on earth. Catholics lack the Word and are therefore credulous about mere externals (one type of fool was the "gull" or credulous person); their foolishness is idolatry, which was, of all sins, the only one that could be defined as "intellectual."[54] As opposite deviations from the mean, they are both forms of politico-theological disability that taint the deviators by associating them with the lower orders, against whom the social order has to be defended.

The prominence of the professional *arriviste* foregrounded another type of failure: someone who lacks the professional expertise he claims. The maverick medical authority Paracelsus refers to his predecessors as "idiots and infants"; orthodox Galenist doctors typically use the same idiot vocabulary to label the Paracelsians.[55] In these examples "idiot" clearly means someone lacking medical knowledge rather than some generalized insult in the modern sense; although it has overtones of the unlearned commoner, it targets one's fellow professionals in particular.[56] Elizabethan drama constantly plays with the conceit of the unprofessional or "idiot" actor. This is the immediate sense of the idiot tale teller in *Macbeth*; by fulfilling his ambitions, Macbeth has emptied his imaginative faculty, and the performance of this "life" is consequently void of anything except sound and fury. The idiot as professional failure is not derived metaphorically from some positively disabled person in the modern sense, since no such creature existed; idiocy is a psychological disqualification only in the sense of being a social or professional one.

Failure to perform was also identified, in faculty psychology terms, with the countryside. Country people's faculties were dull by nature. The village idiot was anyone who lived in a village, a maxim which by the end of the sixteenth century had come to encompass the country gentry. At first, it was the country gentry who "professed arms," with honour stemming from military prowess; city gentry were stereotypically emasculated because they did not fight. Tudor governments, however, urged the gentry to get out of the country, where "great rudeness" was the rule, and into the towns, where they could adopt Castiglione's ideal of a civic and professional elite.[57] The relationship is finely balanced in Shakespeare's *As You Like It*, where Corin and Touchstone, rustic fool and professional court jester respectively, debate the simple versus the sophisticated life. By the Restoration, the balance had tipped completely. One knows, said Dryden, the "fool of nature ... by his clown-accent and his country-tone"; a few years later comes Squire Western in Fielding's *Tom Jones*, who is gentleman and country clown simultaneously, with no sense of contradiction.

Fools and idiots are by definition those distant from the centres of power and ability: economic, political, intellectual. Just living in the country sufficed to make you a villein in the eyes of many;

---

[52] Monsieur d'Aubray, *Le Satyre Ménippée*, G5r.
[53] Gwillim, *A Display*, Frontispiece.
[54] Thomas Beard, *The Theatre of God's Judgements*, 418.
[55] Robert Burton, *The Anatomy of Melancholy*, ii, 209; Thomas Erastus, *Disputationum de Nova Philippi Paracelsi*, 69.
[56] For example Humfrey, *The Nobles*, R1v; John Donne, *Satires, Epigrams and Verse Letters*, 7.
[57] Thomas Starkey, cited in Fritz Caspari, *Humanism and the Social Order in Tudor England*, 95.

the behavioural writers feel bound to insist that "if a gentleman do inhabit his village, he shall nevertheless continue noble."[58] Changed relations between town and country gentry took off from existing stereotypes of the villager "who busieth himself about his plough, and ... hath his wits of no higher conceit"; the contagion of human geography had made the rural gentry "rustics" too, and all country dwellers "country clown[s]."[59] The character type of "the upstart country knight" illustrates how the stereotype appeared to heraldic experts:

> His honour [is] somewhat preposterous, for he bare the King's sword before he had arms to wield it; yet being once laid o'er the shoulder with a knighthood, he finds the herald his friend .... His father was a man of good stock, though but a tanner, or usurer; he purchased the land, and his son the title. He has doffed off the name of a clown, but the look not so easy, and his face bears still a relish of churn milk .... And commonly his race is quickly run, and his children's children, though they scape hanging, return to the place from whence they came.[60]

Indeed, fools and fields were already associated in the classical period, agriculture being the work culture that is always slowest to change – in relation to Rome's sophistication of manners as well as to the administrative sophistication of Western Europe from the late Middle Ages onwards.

Honour, wit and Shakespeare's fools

The examples above show both that the gentleman who fails to perform his ascribed honour is the disabled and degenerate person of his time, and that he is the modern intellectually disabled person in the making. Shakespeare makes the point dramatically halfway through *King Lear*, when – at the exact point where Lear is stripped of honourable status – his court jester inexplicably vanishes, to be replaced as companion by Poor Tom the beggar who is (it seems) genuinely rather than just professionally out of his wits.

In *Julius Caesar*, Antony proposes to Octavius that they sideline Lepidus, the third member of their triumvirate. They have "laid honours" on him but he has no intellectual autonomy, inasmuch as he is oblivious to the new forms of self-assertion; he is "led or driven, as we point the way." Once he has lost his usefulness, they can strip him of his honours and send him away, "Like to the empty ass, to shake his ears, / And graze in commons." He can go off to his appropriate social position amidst the plebs – appropriate because he lacks the self-seeking wit of an Antony. Octavius mildly objects that Lepidus, being a "valiant soldier," is their peer in terms of honour. But Antony sneers:

> So is my horse, Octavius, ...
> His corporal motion govern'd by my spirit.
> And, in some taste, is Lepidus but so:
> He must be taught, and train'd, and bid go forth:
> A barren-spirited fellow; one that feeds
> On objects, arts, and imitations
> Which, out of use and staled by other men,
> Begin his fashion.

The ass lacks honour of any sort; the horse does not lack valour or the "vital spirits" which all animals have, but it does lack soul spirits, that physical medium of intelligence which exists in

---

[58] Segar, *Honor*, 225.
[59] Timothy Bright, *A Treatise of Melancholy*, 52.
[60] Earle, *Microcosmographie*, 46.

humans alone. The horse is the paradigm of all non-reasoning beasts; in late classical Greek the word for horse is *alogos*, literally "non-reasoner" – hence the many satirical inversions of this theme, of which Swift's Houhnyhms are the best known. (The Yahoos, meanwhile, were probably modelled on contemporary accounts of "Peter the Wild Man," a feral outsider.) Lepidus's way of bidding for status – martial prowess rather than wit – is outmoded, channelled through the wrong mode. He is another Brutus for the taking. Antony's insult is no mere figure of speech; he does not say Lepidus is *like* a fool. Rather, Antony's reconstruction of autonomy as politic wit is highlighted by genuine absence of the latter in Lepidus. Not only are the latter's skills mere "imitations," they are by the same token behind the times; he is unaware of the change of rules, of the new bidding game exemplified in Antony's polished and cynical wit.

In *The Merry Wives of Windsor*, Anne Page's suitor Slender ("of slender wit" was a common epithet) is "well-landed but an idiot." In what sense an idiot? The word's association with commoners renders this phrase a contradiction in terms, which the audience would have grasped. The propertied but idiotic suitor is in fact a stock character in the drama: Middleton's *Women Beware Women* features one who is objectified as "The Ward" (his status makes him unworthy of a name), tied to the apron strings of an uncle whose given Christian name is Guardiano. This ward's psychological characteristics are a mix of jester-type foolery and an interest in the outmoded trappings of honour. Shakespeare's Slender varies this image slightly. He is obsessed with heraldic science, nervously responding to other characters' talk about "reason" as if it were a new fashion in hats which he is not sure about adopting. But his obsessive interest also exposes his entire ignorance of the science; that is what constitutes his idiocy. He converses normally and gives off no signs of what a modern psychologist would call intellectual disability; however, he is deficient in the performance of his own gentle status. The bourgeois Mistress Page and her daughter are well off and have no need for his land, so his recommendation as a suitor would be a mature knowledge of the external insignia that went with the landed estate and would raise mother and daughter above Windsor's prosaic middle-classness. Slender lacks such knowledge; he is a layman and hence an "idiot" in respect to the expert language of heraldry essential to his class, and this is what places him with the out-group.

In *Much Ado about Nothing*, Beatrice sets the scene for her first encounter with Benedick by way of a sarcastic pun on "difference" as a technical term in Blazon (a mark on a coat of arms) and "difference" as a term in logic and psychology (the *differentia* of rational man from other animals). In short, her witty values will prevail over his soldierly ones. And in *All's Well that Ends Well*, the fool Parolles is identified as such by his obsession with honour's external trappings; he is actually a coward who fakes retrieval of his regiment's honour (its coat of arms has been captured), and lacks a courtier's imitative grace. His friend Bertram, on the other hand, is a soldier with serious claims to valour-based honour; but he refuses to marry a woman who, despite her outstanding learning-based virtue, is his mother's ward and thus a social inferior. Just as Parolles's foolishness is defined by his lack of honour as military valour, so Bertram's is defined by his failure to recognize honour as virtuous learning. In the end he grudgingly accepts marriage, forced to admit that honour must be reconstituted as wisdom.

Halfbreeds and unsuccessful interlopers

So far we have encountered idiots and fools either as members of the out-group or as deficient, non-performing members of the in-group. There are in addition those whose original ascription to the in-group is ambiguous: for example, the offspring of class miscegenation between gentle and commoner, or those born out of wedlock to honourable fathers. Such status ambiguities were seen in naturalistic terms. "The gentle, either of blood or coat-armour, ought not to marry the ungentle," since the issue of such a relationship "should seem but half noble, nay but half a man ... monstrous and degenerated from his kind." It is as if "to tie the bodies of the quick and the dead together."⁶¹ The gentry had to be careful about marrying into non-gentle wealth for fear of producing "mongrels," just as you would conserve the breed of your dogs or as today's aspiring prospective mother is careful about the IQ and social pedigree of sperm donors. Behavioural writers cited in support Averroes's theory of an "informative power" or ability which parents transmit to the souls of their offspring. According to this, "the memorable exploits of ancestors" could recur physically in the blood of descendants; hence the "seeds of good and evil germinate over time in our souls."⁶² Gentry were warned to choose wet nurses carefully; since breast milk was thought to consist of distilled blood, it could determine the child's very identity and "make the mind more perfected."⁶³

The consequences of misalliance are as much moral as intellectual. Offspring may have no generosity or kindness, but not "no wit"; Edmund, the bastard Machiavel of *King Lear*, shows that the opposite is the case. It was for their wit that aristocratic fathers such as Louis XIV often favoured illegitimate over legitimate sons, illustrating the strength of wit in its rivalry with bloodline. It forced the diehard supporters of legitimate bloodline to recast degeneracy itself in intellectual terms; Boulainvilliers, for example, remarked of Louis that to bypass his own lineage was itself a form of stupidity or "vanity" that would corrupt future generations. Intellectual ignorance of one's own genealogy was "a perpetual forgetting of oneself which seems to amount to imbecility."⁶⁴ The cause of this imbecility (a term in which physical, moral and intellectual connotations are combined) was in Boulainvillier's view the biological "mixing" of royal blood. The idea of imbecility as a natural ignorance of one's own class culture, with dishonour as its central component, is still going strong in the nineteenth-century novel (Balzac's *The Black Sheep*, for example), where people are labelled "idiot" or "degenerate" for no other reason than that they ignore their pedigrees.⁶⁵

Another ambiguous figure was the professional fool, who was often witty enough in faculty psychology terms. Touchstone, for example, knows enough about scholastic logic to send it up, though others like the court jester of Ferrara are said not to have any rationality at all (see Chapter 13). Any supposed intellectual differences among professional fools would have been subordinate to a common element in their job description, namely their ability to mimic. Any ambiguity or threat lay rather in the fact that a gentleman born might then try to mimic the fools, thereby demeaning himself and his class. This was the original significance of the term "artificial fool": not a clever man who acts the fool to gain advantage but, rather, a gentleman who enjoys imitating jesters, finds himself stuck in the persona and then becomes the real thing – like the nobles who mock Don Quixote, or like Sir Toby Belch and Sir Andrew Aguecheek in the company of the vocational fool Feste, who in any case is much wiser than they.

Finally, there are people aspiring to cross over into the honour society: *arrivistes* on the threshold of arrival. The classic text is *Le bourgeois gentilhomme*. The very idea of a bourgeois gentleman is a comic contradiction in terms, like the mock politeness of "coloured gentleman." When Monsieur Jourdain glows with pride to learn that he speaks prose, the joke is not just that he does not know that prose is a technical term for everyday speech, but that it is an inferior medium. Like him it is vulgar, and that is because it is not poetry. Jourdain is without rhyme or, therefore, reason. When Molière at the opening of the play lists the abilities of the elite to which Jourdain ludicrously

---

61 Ferne, *Blazon*, 8.
62 Faret, *The Honest Man*, 12.
63 Jones, *The Arte and Science of Preserving Bodie and Soule*, 40.
64 Cited in Devyver, *Le sang*, 281.
65 See also McDonagh, *Idiocy*.

aspires, they are intellectual ones: "mind" (*esprit*) and "knowing how to reason." Poetry was the language of reason and thereby of gentility.

Peacham tells of a herald who visits a man claiming gentility on the basis of his newly acquired merchant wealth, and asks to see his coat. The man mistakes him to have expressed an interest in buying his overcoat. He says he can let the herald have it at a decent price with 50 percent down now. This in itself shows him to be an idiot. The lack of virtue in such "stubble curs" is their failure to understand the position in society to which they have mistakenly aspired, being "neither doers, sufferers, or well speakers of honour's tokens."[66] Peacham seeks a *genuine*, because *measurable* ("demonstrable") set of externals, those of heraldic science: "there being at this instant the world over such a medley (I had almost said motley) of coats … we should, I fear me, within these few years see yeomen as rare in England as they are in France."[67] Motley was the uniform of the professional fool; a "yeoman" was a wealthy farmer, immediately adjacent to the honour society in the countryside as burgesses were in the towns. The essential message of heraldic science, as of psychometric science, was: Repel all boarders.

Fiscal idiots: how the law invented incompetence

What do you take me for? Are you taking me for an idiot? These are strange phrases. The original phrase was to "beg" someone for an idiot, a legal expression. Guides to behaviour, nobility and heraldry were aimed at people who had studied at the Inns of Court (a frequent destination after university), and the Court of Wards was where you would "take" someone to adjudicate whether they were competent to manage their estate.

We have seen above that the disability of the gentleman who was an idiot because he did not understand coats of arms was not clearly distinguishable from that of the one who was an idiot because he could not count up to 20. However, law supplies us with the one historical context that does seem pertinent to modern concepts of intellectual disability as a marker of legal incompetence. The Court of Wards was put on a permanent footing in 1540. This was roughly contemporary with the first Royal Commission on heraldry; their trajectories coincide, and in 1542 it became the Court of Wards "and Liveries," responsible for sumptuary laws regulating the public significance of clothing as well as heraldic insignia (the two issues were thus closely linked).

The wardship jurisdiction distinguished between people who were lunatic or mad and those born fools or idiots, and it issued writs on this basis. The Roman law of the Twelve Tables, used by medieval lawyers, had said explicitly that competence to plead must be assumed in those who are "stupid" (*stulti*) – whatever "stupid" means in this context – by contrast with those who are mad (*furiosi*).[68] Their elaboration, which appears in both civil and canon law, that some people are *born* stupid is therefore a crucial element in making the category firmer and more pejorative. It appears originally in a text from Edward I's reign known as *Prerogativa Regis*. However, at this stage it seems not to have been a legal enactment but a private memo or plea; despite what has been written on this topic, the law had no standard writs of idiocy, much less separate ones for idiocy and lunacy, until Henry VIII set up the Court of Wards.[69] In this respect, too, the wardship system

---

[66] Leigh, *The Accedence*, A3.
[67] *The Compleat Gentleman*, 130.
[68] Cicero, *Tusculan Disputations*, 3.5.11; see also Theodore Mommsen, *The Digest of Justinian*.
[69] David Roffe, "'A novel and a noteworthy thing?' The guardianship of lunatics and the crown in medieval England," unpublished ms.

resembles heraldic rules: a contemporary invention dressed in feudal trappings, as if appealing to some ancient right.

A sudden upsurge in the number of writs in the 1590s, when it became a bone of political contention, gave the idiot/lunatic distinction the oxygen of publicity. We can see this from comparing Spenser with writers of only a generation later. In Spenser's depiction of the human soul in Book 2 of *The Faerie Queene*, deficiency originates in the imagination, represented here by the allegorical figure Phantastes

> That him full of melancholy did show;
> Bent hollow beetle brows, sharp staring eyes,
> That mad or foolish seemed: one by his view
> Mote deem him born with ill disposed skies.

Here mad and foolish are synonymous; at most, any implied distinction would have been subordinate to the overarching paradigm of melancholy. By the 1590s, however, professional intellectuals around the Inns of Court were employing such a distinction extensively in their literary productions, as we shall see shortly, and in so doing they helped introduce it to a wider public.

According to Richard Neugebauer, in his research into the records of the Court of Wards, the distinction between lunatics and idiots shows that professionals of the time already knew about the difference between the mentally ill and the "mentally retarded," thereby demonstrating signs of a modern psychological expertise.[70] However, there is little evidence for the "idiots" he cites from the records being mentally retarded as he, a modern neurologist, would recognize them. Conflating cause with effect, Neugebauer assumes that psychological conditions we now classify as intellectually disabled lay behind the idiot terminology used by those lawyers, when actually it was the sudden public currency of the legal terminology that fed (along with other things) into modern psychological conceptualizations of intellectual disability. Language was more fluid than now; the mutual resonances of related or even unrelated senses of one and the same word were heard more clearly than in modern English. Existing meanings for "idiot" or "fool" overlapped with those for "madman," both being dispositional rather than deterministic in a biological sense and covering a huge range of behaviours. Nevertheless, *some* sort of difference was clearly being indicated. What was it? The term "lunacy" refers to phases of the moon, which gave the mad person lucid intervals. It signified impermanence, while idiocy thus became *that which is not temporary*. It is the negative reflection, in juridical terms, of the Puritan unification of the personality that was to achieve full expression in Locke's theory of personal identity. There could be no modern idiot without the permanence of the modern "person" in this sense. However, it was only the very beginning of a process. Legal idiocy, as birth-to-death permanence, was not borrowed from some existing medical diagnosis, it came from the surface language of a professional elite, which had till now covered a broader range of oddities and social inferiors.

We need to understand how wardship applied in general, across the board, in order to grasp fully how specifically psychological categories were built out of existing social ones. As Neugebauer suggests, behind the idiot/lunatic distinction lay a fiscal crisis. Given the assumed permanence of the idiot's condition, guardians could assume greater control of his estate than of a lunatic's. The state either found these guardians or assumed guardianship itself; the finger it had in this pie explains why legal authorities and historians of the time, notably under Charles I, dated the first issuing of idiocy writs as far back in time as possible.[71] The Tudors and early Stuarts tried to finance

---

[70] Neugebauer, "Medieval and early modern theories," "Mental handicap."
[71] Sir Edward Coke, *The First Part of the Institutes of the Lawes of England*, 7v.

their state by resuscitating the minutest obligations which landholders, as "tenants in chief," had to the monarch, to whom they should in principle be surrendering the profits – though in fact this relationship was already lost in the mists of time. If a tenant died while his heir was still legally a minor, the heir became the king's ward. However, wardship rights had meanwhile become goods that could be sold on, thereby becoming the main source of royal income. This was even more the case when the first two Stuart monarchs found it hard to impose taxes. If, then, it could be proved that the heir was still incompetent after his minority ended, so much the better. The income of state and courtiers from this source increased fourfold between Elizabeth's reign and the onset of the civil wars.[72] That is how important the issue of idiocy was. An agreement not to reimpose the Court of Wards after its 1646 abolition was one of the chief conditions on which Charles II was permitted to reassume the monarchy.

The wardship system had developed out of patrilinealism. It was not entirely age related. Unmarried women and younger sons, who remained in subordination to the senior member of the family, might be condemned to a prolonged "infancy" or "youth" (both terms denoted a person of any age who had not yet succeeded to property or title) as long as that member refused to marry them off.[73] At first inheritance had been merely a frequent custom, the whim of a newly titled father, stemming from the prospective inheritor's military prowess as much as his estate management skills, let alone order of birth; only later in the Middle Ages did a formal set of rules around primogeniture evolve. Neither wardship nor indeed formal tests of competence needed to exist until the principle of a right of succession arose, and until the required prowess – military or managerial – started to be ascribed to a specific "rightful" heir rather than to someone whose outstanding performances had simply caught the eye.

Before the Tudor transformation of government, training of the elite frequently took place in great households, of which the royal court itself was simply the largest. Upbringing in these noble houses was "mainstream" education, as it were, for the wider family and other ascribed members of the honour society, plus selected children of commoners. In the late medieval period some children attended the cathedral schools, but otherwise wardship was the central pedagogical institution, a general social and educational phenomenon as well as a legal one. But when day schools in the towns became popular, those young people remaining under wardship found themselves to be a historical residue: they were a waning part of the honour society where a ward had been someone unable to succeed *to* his station as much as *in* it. Guardians controlled their estates, arranged their marriages and, in return, were supposed to educate them for their future social responsibilities; the age at which this wardship ended was a socially convenient but psychologically arbitrary point. The ward's personal and developmental maturity was neither here nor there: Shakespeare's morally and intellectually mature Helena in *All's Well* is an example, no less an inferior than Middleton's "The Ward" with his court fool behaviour. The disabling effect of tutelage and minority on any individual's sense of self-worth was as discernible in the gentry as it is in the "intellectually disabled" people created by today's intelligence society.

The governments of both Henry VIII and Elizabeth I tried to impose a centralized national curriculum ("common discipline and exercises") on the residual institutions of state wardship, in order to police the borders of honour and wit alike.[74] Archbishop Cranmer had already had to face irate gentry who, having removed their children from the educational environment of the household and set them to a humanist pedagogy in the cathedral school at Canterbury, objected to

---

[72] Christopher Hill, *From Reformation to Revolution*, 102; *The Intellectual Origins of the English Revolution*, 321.

[73] Stephen White, *Custom, Kinship and Gifts to Saints*.

[74] Cited in H.E. Bell, *An Introduction to the History and Records of the Court of Wards and Liveries*, 127.

commoners "meet for the plough" associating there with their own children and even being given preferment over them according to their talents.⁷⁵ Cranmer compromised, saying he would favour the gentleman's gifted son over the poor boy with "gifts of nature" by giving him an enriched curriculum involving lessons in how to govern, but that he would put the gifted poor ahead of the "very dull gentle-born." The state, in its demand for professional virtues, had to overlook social differences of birth, and endeavoured to tailor the curriculum accordingly. Mulcaster recommended it as the basis on which "the common and the private concur .... Neither shall the private scholar go any faster on, nay perhaps not so fast."⁷⁶ All this began to create a new kind of out-group, defined more sharply in terms of learning and intellect, across the whole education system. Legal idiocy gained a sharper focus only within this more general push towards centralization and for professionally relevant assessment criteria.

The legal idiots of the 1590s were the residue of a residue, leftovers from a once universal system. The few people who remained in wardship were those for whom the socially determined point of maturation never arrives. That is why Hooker describes his "idiots" as being in a condition that never ends. There were, nevertheless, contemporary writers who realized that it might be the system itself that created idiots. The unscrupulous guardian, it was said, would purposely "abase their [ward's] minds" so that they would never develop the ability to stand up for their own material interests. Those who remained in the wardship system were those too weak to escape tutelage. (It might explain, for example, why Henry VI's religiosity had led to his failure to assert his majority against fellow nobles, especially as he had acceded to the crown when only a few months old.) Only subsequently did they become, as in Hooker's formula, those who *needed* tutelage – the source of the conservative gloss whereby, within a liberal polity, we feel happy about forcibly segregating some people for their own protection. "Idiots" were and are those who can be imposed upon, as a result of being left behind by shifting social conditions.

Some legal experts of the time already detected a whiff of nonsense: "For the idiot, I had almost forgot him. Howsoever the matter is not great: for it is but a foolish business when all is done ... Be assured that yourself is somewhat the wiser man, before you go about to beg him, or else never meddle with him at all."⁷⁷ Many of the Court's own judgments failed to abide by the stipulated distinction, being indiscriminately entitled "Grant of Idiot or Lunatic." Butler satirically depicts a money-grubbing couple who beg their child for an idiot while still in the womb (the converse, surely, of putting your unborn child's name down for Eton).⁷⁸ More specifically, the modern-sounding "idiot" label of the legal texts is at odds with the actual symptoms of idiocy (if any) described in the court records researched by Neugebauer. A legal compendium defined an "idiot" as someone "naturally born so weak of understanding, that he cannot govern or manage his inheritance"; assessors and/or a jury had to decide "whether he be sufficiently witted to dispose of his own lands with discretion or not," or "naturally defective in [his] own discretion."⁷⁹ But that was all in theory. Mental illness, melancholy or mere failure to adapt to changing behavioural norms excited the predatory instincts of the state, guardians and close family members. These too were "idiocy."

Descriptions of behaviour or intellectual performance in the records are minimal. Neugebauer himself estimates that 80 per cent of idiot cases were not "mentally retarded" even by his own, modern criteria. Grace and honour, as well as wit, were at issue: the assessor would mix numeracy

---

75 Caspari, *Humanism*, 138.
76 *Positions*, 193.
77 Thomas Powell, *The Attourney's Academy*, 217.
78 *Hudibras*, 3.1.590.
79 John Cowell, *The Interpreter*, Nn2.

tests with questions about the meaning of the communion service or who their parents were. Several texts refer to idiots with wives and children, even though inability to beget a child was a criterion of idiocy. Counting up to 20 was not an abstract arithmetical test, as it might be in a modern developmental assessment; the ability referred to in the legislation was vocational, namely to count 20 pence. Just one case of Neugebauer's seems as if it might fit a retrospective diagnosis from today, which only highlights the general inappropriateness of the rest.[80] To judge from the records, the sheer variety of grounds on which someone might be begged as an idiot sends us back instead to issues of social class raised earlier in this chapter.

Nor did the sense of permanence in this legal definition have firm roots in nature. If the court found someone a natural idiot, it rendered null all the transactions he had previously entered into, which leads one to ask how he could have done business at all before; moreover, he was assumed competent enough to be able by himself to enter a writ directing his re-examination or an appeal.[81] And of course providence might at any time remove the deficiency. Phrases such as "naturally defective," "naturals" or "natural fools" do not refer to notions of biological cause, but they are closely linked to those of lineage and honourable status. *Nativi* ("naturals"), for example, stood for anyone outside the honour society; it translates as "bondmen," which some writers used not only for servants but for burgesses (on the assumption that they must have once been manual apprentices).[82] The law did not stand over and above the honour society, handing out judgments of competence drawn from a universally agreed "nature" in accordance with some scientific, biological or psychological script; it simply advanced that society's claims, just as the law today, in its interpretation of competence as rationality and intelligence, advances the claims of the intelligence society.

A phrase frequently mentioned in behaviour guides is the "gentleman born." From this it is self-evident that, if someone is innately gentle, his parents too are of gentle status. Not so obvious is the converse: that a "born" fool (*idiota a nativitate*, as the law termed it), being innately idiotic, is born to parents whose gentle status must therefore contradict his own. The term "idiot" could mean something precise only in relation to that social group in which it would be an anomaly (that is, in theory; in practice idiocy writs were served on non-gentry too). The peasant, by contrast, was already a born fool by social definition, and possibly by a religious one as well, since the Latin phrase evokes the state of "natural man." He did not need a competence test to work in the fields. When in *The Winter's Tale* Prince Florizel's father scolds him for being "a royal fool," it is not just because he is cavorting with country labourers but because labourers are fools by definition. The genuine anomaly is the eponymous "gentleman fool" addressed in Samuel Rowland's poem, who

> Boasts of scutcheons, arms, and high descent
> That on fool's legs even from thy cradle went.

Fiscal necessity resulted in the sequestration of idiots' estates as it did in the inflation of honourable titles. They peak in the same period. If the state could add honour to a commoner, it could subtract wit from a gentleman. They are complementary actions, enlarging the state's coffers. The first is confirmation of an achieved status: the commoner achieves what the gentleman, with his ascribed ability, already has and knows. The second is removal of an ascribed status: the gentleman is assumed to have it, and its abilities, until the opposite is proven – and that was exactly the purpose

---

[80] "Mental handicap," 29.
[81] Bell, *An Introduction*, 127 ff.
[82] Ferne, *Blazon*, 8.

of idiocy writs. Both the granting and the withdrawal of the tokens of gentility expressed a balance of socio-economic power between monarch and subjects.

In proving the heir's idiocy – that is, his dishonourable status – a certain "intellectual" deficiency might be involved, but it was narrowly defined. It might mean simply illiteracy and innumeracy. In the quite recent past, the fathers of Hobbes and Lilburne – one a priest, the other a landowner – were said to have been illiterate, at least in writing, while many non-gentles would have been fully literate because their trades demanded it. The writs indicate the extent to which illiteracy had finally become unacceptable among gentry. The point was not literacy or numeracy in themselves but their importance for the maintenance of status. Being able to count money or remember the names of your father and mother was specific to the inheritance of landed property and the administration of its profits; without such skills, the estate might leave the family. Intellectual criteria for incompetence continued to coexist for some time with older criteria such as lack of a sense of one's own honourable status. The latter remained a problem for the person's immediate family because of the dishonour and shame the loss of an estate might bring; Gracián's aphorism, "The lot of a fool, to fail in his calling," means among other things his *social* calling, his rank.[83] Intellectual incompetence *per se*, by contrast, was not a matter of shame for family members until much later, the result rather than the cause of mass institutionalization. (Charles Darwin, for example, whose last child possibly had Down's syndrome – he was born a few months before Down's invention – wrote about him with none of the sense of shame or rejection that has later been exhibited by certain eminent scientists over their own children.)[84]

Such elements as there are of a modern intellectual disability in the late Tudor and early Stuart concept of idiocy/lunacy came not so much directly from the Court of Wards itself as from men in and around the Inns of Court, the upcoming caste of professional intelligence men whose "whipping satires" and "fool sonnets" of the 1590s supplied images that entered both the seventeenth-century literary canon and the public discussion provoked by the machinations of the treasury. Henceforth the notionally deficient would routinely turn up as the pairing "idiots and lunatics" or "fools and madmen"; so too would one's intellectual opponents, for whom the word "idiot" only now takes its place in the vocabulary of abuse alongside "dunce," "shallow-brains" and so forth. When satirical poets in this period began using the word "idiot" as an insult, they were not referring to the existing psychological object "intellectual disability"; rather, they were instead helping to instigate it. A literary or otherwise popularized version of the legal lunatic/idiot vocabulary used by professionals (often about each other) was one of the ingredients in the diagnostic *foundation* of intellectual disability in its modern scientific form.

In this decade there is, in addition, a fashion for writing sonnets about unrequited love which identify love not just with absence of reason but more precisely with the lunacy/idiocy dyad. Lunacy is a metaphor for excess of passion, idiocy for its absence, or for lack of lovemaking expertise. Later in the decade, the fashion is for ridiculing the law, and the legal vocabulary itself as an affectation. A *Gulling Sonnet* by John Davies of Hereford, for example, represents the law in general as a "yoke of wardship" that "holds my wit now for an idiot." In *Vice's Anotimie*, Robert Anton warns against excessive study because it leads to recusancy in religion and discontent in politics, "Which if this be his wit to study ill, / Take my wits madman, leave me simple still" ("simple" indicating here idiocy). The very titles of Nicholas Breton's paired poems, *Pasquil's Madcap* and *Pasquil's Foolscap*, indicate the fashion. He asks,

---

[83] Gracián, *Oráculo*, Aphorism 2.
[84] Adrain Desmond and James Moore, *Darwin*, 446; 460.

> He, that of late was in a madding fit,
> Doth from a frenzy to a folly fall:
> And which is better, mad, or foolish wit?
> I think as good, almost have none at all.

The satire reflects a more general attempt across the culture to regulate meanings and vocabulary. A servant in Middleton's *The Changeling* says of the seducer Antonio, "'Tis but a fool that haunts the house and my mistress in the shape of an idiot"; hence an idiot is a *particular type* of fool, the natural one. (The servant's cash-strapped master has already asked, "Hark, is there not one *incurable* fool / That might be begged?" [emphasis added].) Although "fool" comes more often to indicate the innate type, it is also still to be found as the generic category that covers both "idiot" and "lunatic" subdivisions: "Of idiot fools I sing," writes John Marston in his *Satyra Nova* – that is, not of lunatic fools. Either way, it points towards a fixing of terms.

It was at this point that idiocy had begun to rival melancholy as the paradigmatic deficiency or absence of mind. In the 1590s, melancholy became for a while the height of fashion among leisured gentlemen, rather than a maligned disability; in Essex's verse prompted by his fall-out with Elizabeth, it expresses his emasculated *impotentia* before female power. Melancholy was an indulgence of free time, idiocy a waste of servile time. The two ran concurrently for decades. When in 1621 Robert Burton wrote his famous rejoinder to John Lyly's *Anatomy of Wit*, he entitled it *The Anatomy of Melancholy*, not of idiocy, in which he expressed little interest despite the noise it was making around him in the legal and political spheres. On the other hand, idiocy of the legalistic type was beginning to acquire significance in the burgeoning genre of philosophical poetry. Here it starts to be inserted within the schema of faculty psychology. The purpose of these long didactic poems, their themes derived from De Mornay's *De la verité*, was to equip the mind to know the mind in order to defend the soul's immortality against notions of its materiality and corruptibility. They include Fulke Greville's *Treatie of Humane Learning* (a title echoing Bacon and foreshadowing Locke) and Sir John Davies's influential *Nosce Teipsum* ("Know thyself"). Both authors had been at the Inns of Court during the 1590s, and both use the idiot/lunatic dyad in support of religious and psychological argument. Davies, defending the purity of the rational soul, puts these words into a sceptical opponent's mouth:

> What? Are not souls within themselves corrupted?
> How can there idiots then by nature be?
> How is it that some wits are interrupted,
> That now they dazzled are, now clearly see?

Idiots and lunatics, in this dyadic form, are now starting to be the paradigmatic exception to the rule of "man is a rational animal." De Mornay's idea of possible exceptions had been "madmen," "lunatics" and "melancholics," but not any permanent category. Davies himself, elsewhere in the poem, writes about an "idiot, which hath yet a mind, / Able to know the truth, and choose the good." Yet the above stanza citing the idiot from birth ("by nature") marks a point at which the language of wardship becomes involved with that of grace and reprobation – and it is to these topics that we now turn.

PART 5
Intelligence, Disability and Grace

Chapter 10
From Pilgrim's Progress to Developmental Psychology

Our examination of the relationship between grace and human reasoning will lead eventually to the examination of a different in-group/out-group division, this time between the elect and the reprobate, and of the ways in which modern notions of the intelligent and the intellectually disabled emerge from this distinction. Both themes can be traced through any number of religious texts whose concerns often overlap with those of the behaviour guides just discussed but which articulate a separate set of status anxieties relating chiefly to inner states, and initially to one's status with God.

The philosophical poem of Sir John Davies with which we ended the previous chapter is characteristic. In a section entitled "Of human knowledge," he asks:

> Why did my parents send me to the Schools
> That I with knowledge might enrich my mind?
> Since the *desire to know* first made men fools,
> And did corrupt the root of all mankind.

The Reformation's insistence on the privacy of faith and its exposure of Christianity's public, worldly failures brought the problem of intellectual curiosity to the forefront of discussion. Aristotle's "desire to understand" was equally Adam's disobedient curiosity. Davies's reference to "fools" here suggests he disapproves of Aristotle's desire, and of scholastic philosophy ("the Schools") in general. Yet the poem's very title exhorts us to know *something*: ourselves. A cure for Adamite corruption might be to make the individual himself the object of his own quest for knowledge. The empirical approach which anatomists had begun to apply to the human body might be applied also to the mind, and to one's own soul in particular. And the most important thing to know in this respect was, am I saved?

This question of status in the afterlife, of who was elect and who not, affected earthly behaviour. Huldrych Zwingli, who claimed political authority for religion, and the Anabaptists who revolted against him; Charles I who sought absolute rule, and Oliver Cromwell who had him beheaded: all did so secure in the knowledge that they were in receipt of divine grace. But this same doctrine also made for anxiety: Luther veering between self-transcendence and self-abasement, or Cromwell again, sure that his military victories were a sign of his election but plunging into gloom once his political leadership stalled.

Reason, faith and the will: a shifting balance

Grace, according to Marcel Mauss, belongs to that which lies beyond mere obligation and is therefore extraordinary or "sacred."[1] It retains, however, a sense of exchange. When Jesus took the punishment originally due to humans, he was giving his life in exchange for God's gracious gift of salvation to us (or some of us). The gift comes through the sequential process of regeneration,

---

[1] Pitt-Rivers, "Postscript," 217.

faith and justification (a quasi-legal pardon for Adam's sin). Some saw the gift of grace as one-sided and unmerited by humans; others saw it, once given, as enabling the individual to change his nature or disposition. This latter suggestion, that humans themselves have something to contribute, posed a problem about the will. Grace was the will of God. The human will could not by itself achieve salvation. But if individual wills are so insignificant, God's will appears to be a kind of determinism; and if man is a sinner then God, in withholding grace from some, seems to be the determiner and author of sin – an evident absurdity.

The elevated profile of wit and reason – a specifically *human* reasoning – partly arose from attempts to solve this conundrum, and the concept of disability was bound up with it from the beginning, as we shall see later. The individual's ability to enter into a quasi-juridical act of exchange with God was expressed as His side of a legal contract. This "covenant theory," initially a reaction against papal diktat, did not sit easily with the idea of God's omnipotence. The parties were so unevenly matched. How could such a relationship be mutual? One answer was that the individual pays a "peppercorn rent" in return for his possible salvation. His side of the bargain is an effort of will, even the smallest effort being acceptable. By 1700 this had largely been replaced by an effort of reason, of which the smallest amount was not at all acceptable. "Ability" would no longer be the simple ability to be saved but the intellectual ability to *understand that* one was saved, and how. The principle of exchange in this form – of intelligence for salvation – is buried deep within the modern mind-set.

How did human reasoning rise to this position? Our modern narrative tells us there was a battle between reason and faith, which reason won. However, in early Christianity human reasoning did not even occupy the same arena of discussion – not even by way of antagonism – as grace, or individual faith (the proxy for grace). They were brought together by late medieval philosophers who distinguished between what we can know by reason without faith and what we can know only by faith. Thus the two became strands in a single overall theme, if not yet oppositional. For Luther, human reason was a "stinking whore" when it broached things due to grace alone but "the great light of nature" in the everyday world, which was a "kingdom of reason" enabling humans to rule over beasts. For Calvin, "natural reason would never direct men to Christ"; it was not so much contrary to faith as secondary to it ("unless you have believed you shall not understand," wrote Isaiah).[2] In "studying to approach God," reason is a hindrance or at best a by-product; it is only valuable because it deprives us of the excuse that we are ignorant of sin. On the Catholic side, Pascal would write that "reason's last step is to see that an infinite number of things are beyond it," natural as well as supernatural; and Vives had matched Calvin's image of the mind as a labyrinth with his "man is a difficult animal," "most arduous and difficult" to get to know.[3] This launched a tradition of studying how to place human reasoning and emotions within nature that went through Huarte, Francisco Suárez and Hugo Grotius to Locke. Recognition of the mind's complexity provoked investigations into how it worked, its operations and actions. Studying to approach God through the literal truth of the Bible led to studying God's creation through the literal truth about nature on an inductive basis, and that included human nature.

The first Reformers' humanist interest in the law of nature increased with the second generation, and threatened to dilute the primacy of faith. In natural law theory, the complement to revelation, reason was a common thread uniting the realms of providence, human action and the workings of the external world. Heinrich Bullinger, Zwingli's successor at Zürich, unwittingly endowed reason with its own discretely human dimension: "The law of nature is not called the law of nature because in the nature and disposition of man there is of or by itself that reason …. But because God

---

[2] Cited in W. Stevenson, *Sovereign Grace*, 15.
[3] Blaise Pascal, *Pensées*, 56; Vives, *De Anima*, 50.

hath imprinted or engraven in our minds some knowledge, and certain general principles ... which, because they be grafted in us and born together with us, do therefore seem as if they are naturally in us."[4] The history of ideas is littered with cases where people have woken up one morning to find that "as if" is now the literal truth. The notion that *divine* reason occurs *naturally* within human beings was to blossom in later writers of broadly Calvinist persuasion, such as Baxter and Locke. It is not just that natural human reasoning is erected to a higher, less corrupt level; in their work, it has already, at its very root, an investment of divine light and of the "spiritual intelligence" of grace.

The relationship between faith and reason, once established, was always more than one of simple antagonism. In any case, neither functioned independently of the will. Before the Fall, man's reason had been compatible with his will; it was only his corruption that led to conflict between them. The English civil wars gave the will a bad name, following which the balance of power swung towards reason. Men like John Owen, Cromwell's chaplain and later a friend of Locke, continued to assert that men would be judged for "the obstinacy of their wills," not of their understandings; he was wary of any calibration of concepts in which "the natural man is allowed to be the rational man."[5] However, his contemporaries had already dispersed into sects, an "army of ten thousand wills" as Locke put it, with catastrophic results for society and religion.

A plethora of attempts to cure this anarchy ensued, with constant fine-tuning of the necessary balance between reason and will, reason and faith. But human reasoning ran out the winner. The idea of instant regeneration through faith, in preparation for an expected imminent rule of the saints, gave way to policing the *means* to regeneration, within the individual. The Cromwellian regime's political failures signalled postponement of that rule. The means would now primarily be reasoning ones, partly because they were optimistically thought to have a socially calming effect. Formerly the word "means" denoted a single act of God, His pardon or "justification," to which any effort of the human will was purely reactive. Now that word began to denote the constant self-perfection of one's own understanding, offered as the human contribution in the act of exchange that was grace. Within the overall scheme of natural law, as refurbished by proto-Enlightenment humanists such as Grotius and Samuel Pufendorf, human reasoning began to acquire a more grown-up relationship with divine reason, reserving for the latter the role of first cause. Among its products would be Newton's theory of gravity. No such lasting success would attend human reason's theory of itself, however.

Predestination and grace

Divine, saving grace is deterministic: it arrives of necessity. In our modern, nature-nurture pairing it is nature that is deterministic and necessary. We are never offered a rationale for there being *only* nature and nurture. Why just two? Why *these* two, exactly? Who chose them? This pairing is not in fact a historical constant. It is the late nineteenth-century's reduction of a previously tripartite formula. On one side stood nurture, covering also custom, convention or sheer hard work. On the other side stood necessity: "fate" in secular terms, "predestination" in religious ones. Nature stood somewhere in the middle, between nurture and necessity, somewhat overlapping both (but often closer to nurture): multifaceted, soft-edged, negotiable.

If a time-travelling doctor from this period were to hear our cognitive geneticists talking about DNA as the cause of intelligence or disability, he would bracket them with the proponents of fate or predestination rather than nature. When Aristotle drew a distinction between natural and acquired intemperance, he meant by "natural" a *disposition*, not a determination; human character

---

[4] Heinrich Bullinger, *Decades*, i, 194.
[5] *Pneumatologia*, 310.

was not ultimately innate. It was subject to the necessities of fortune. Cicero and Alexander placed a clear boundary between fate and nature.[6] In medieval philosophy, the nature in "natural law" was not infallible. According to Aquinas, natural causes in this world were "indeterminate": subject to planetary influence or sheer luck.[7] God could in any case suspend their operation, this being the point of the Old Testament story about the Israelites who did not burn when thrown into a fiery furnace. Human behaviour was a matter of disposition (*habitus*), which is in the last resort changeable; when changes in the individual are described as happening "by disposition and nature" (*per habitum et naturam*), these are complementary rather than opposite.[8] Fate, providential decree and the predestination of souls, by contrast, were all forms of a necessity that was impenetrable to fallen man. Law was likewise a threefold system: unchangeable divine law at one end, the malleable positive law of the courtroom at the other and natural law in the middle. When we come across an apparently dyadic formula – Mulcaster, for example, writes about wit being "by nature implanted, for nurture to enlarge" – it is on the premise that some prior, necessary force has implanted nature in the first place.[9]

Seventeenth-century theologians and natural philosophers continued to keep this soft, dispositional nature separate both from nurture and (more sharply) from the preordained necessity of the soul's after-life destination. Salvation was possible only because "for his elect God hath altered the course of nature." Anyone attributing necessity to nature was a Hobbesian atheist; in Hobbes's state of nature, if the sequence of events in the external world follows an inevitable, determinate pattern as billiard balls do, then so may the inner nature of the human being. Opponents protested that "the world was not caused by the necessity of nature," meaning that necessity lies somewhere other than in nature. The danger of Hobbes's view, for this author, is that allocating the role of necessity to nature turns it into a form of blind chance, thereby denying its openness to divine intervention (as for example in the regeneration of the elect). Nature can never be a "first cause" or "sustain and direct" all second causes.[10] The decline of the doctrine of election later in the century led to a more distanced perspective, in which fate and predestinarian grace came to be seen as subcategories of a single determinism. Whereas predestinarians had disliked "fate" because of its pagan, Stoic associations, the post-Calvinist religious establishment saw an equivalence between "fate [and] Calvinistic predestination as it is called." So eventually no difference was perceived between the *arbitrary* fatalism of predestination (you are saved because of some unknowable divine necessity rather than your good behaviour) and Hobbesian *natural* fatalism (behaviour x necessarily leads to behaviour y).[11]

The tripartite formula withstood the decline in beliefs about election. One's nature was still something one might acquire. Doctors saw bodily nature as changeable by nurture.[12] Political theorists – even a seeming modernizer such as the Leveller Richard Overton, for whom equality of political rights was a "principle of nature" – nevertheless represented this nature as a midwife, her feminine pliability contrasting with the strictness of God, the necessary and all-determining father of that principle.[13] In the eighteenth century, closer to modern life sciences, the Enlightenment

---

[6] Aristotle, *Nicomachean Ethics*, 7.5; Christopher Gill, "The question of character development," *Classical Quarterly*, 33 (1983).

[7] *Contra Gentiles*, 92, cited in Pietro Palazzini, *Dictionarum Morale et Canonicum*, ii, 563.

[8] Da Thiene, *Super Libros*, D7v.

[9] *Positions*, 25.

[10] William Bates, *The Whole Works*, i, 20.

[11] Henry More, cited in Howard, *The Life of the Pious and Learned Henry More*, 59.

[12] For example Gian Filippo Ingrassia, *In Galeni Librum de Ossibus*, 61.

[13] Richard Overton, *An Arrow against all Tyrants*, A2.

naturalist Buffon continued to think of nature in tripartite vein, quoting his predecessors with approval on this point: "'Natural' is spoken of in man concerning that which is not fixed, nor general, but which changes with temperament or education."[14] One might extend the tripartite framework as far forward as Freud, with biology as necessity, civilization as nurture and the unconscious as nature.

God's saving grace was deterministic and necessitarian, and precisely as such was *distinct* from nature. St Paul claimed that no two things were more opposed. Aquinas kept them separate, but added that nature could not attain its own ends without grace, while grace could not exist without natural matter for it to work on. Nature and the necessity of grace had been compatible before the Fall, it was said, and – here is the importance for us – they might be so again. From the mid-seventeenth century onwards, the autonomy of nature came to be seen not so much as alien to grace but as something the free gift of grace could "reform and perfect."[15] A new optimism about nature extended across political and religious divides. The nonconformist Baxter attacked those who "can never speak bad enough of nature" just as his Catholic contemporaries were conceding that "grace acts according to nature and does not pervert its order."[16]

There was also a blurring of the originally sharp distinction between "special grace" – the grace that was divine and led to salvation – and "common" grace, which was shared out among everyone in the form of their individual "natural" graces. Everyone possessed these latter regardless of their elect or non-elect status, and human reasoning featured prominently among them; the first Reformers thought that these natural graces existed only to equip civic and religious authority with the ability to prevent civil society from descending into a chaos of sin. Over the next two centuries, their positive aspect was increasingly emphasized. The natural graces became constituent parts of honour and gentility, God-given powers which compelled the admiration and assent of social inferiors. Baxter noted with dismay how the idea was beginning to creep in that "saving grace differeth not *specie* [in kind] but *gradu* [by degrees]" from natural grace.[17] But the horse had already bolted. In the political changes that provoked the elevation of human reason, the distinction between natural graces (earthly status) and special or saving grace (after-death status) risked being lost. The modern usage "a saving grace" is itself an example, since it has come to indicate some quality personal to the individual, a natural grace in someone who otherwise might be reprobate and *lack* divine, saving grace. The temptation is to think that modern psychology has universalized, as general intelligence, the individual and secular human reasoning formerly regarded as a natural grace. However, it could not have done so without universalizing, within this, some element of predestinate divine grace too. Grace, like honour, defines an in-group (the company of the elect) and an out-group; it has border controls, verification and assessment systems, and a protective apparatus against pollution. The faculty of "human understanding" rode to the rescue of grace when its immigration levels reached crisis point, and ended up entirely redrafting the policy. It extended the denomination of the in-group until they were a majority (the possessors first of a reasoned faith, then of reason without faith), thereby creating a new, much smaller out-group.

The *necessity* of grace, in the form of predestination, had been invoked to explain both the causes of everyday behaviour here on earth and of status in the hereafter. In the case of earthly behaviour, such a strong degree of determinism would mean there was no rationale for civil government, when in fact we are constantly having to hold back a tide of social chaos. The very

---

[14] Antoine Furetière, cited in Michel Bouvier, "Le naturel," *XVIIe siècle*, 39 (1987).
[15] Ralph Cudworth, *The True Intellectual System of the Universe*.
[16] Baxter, *The Cure of Church Divisions*, 138; Jacques-Bénigne Bossuet, cited in Bouvier, "Le naturel."
[17] Cited in Norman Keeble, *Richard Baxter*, 72.

idea of "human laws presupposes the lapse, or disablement of man."[18] Calvin had denied, on these grounds, that one's earthly behaviours were predestined. However, he valued the fear this notion induced; it was a way of humbling people before earthly authority, showing that there was no point in taking one's destiny into one's own hands. This in turn gave rulers the idea that they might coerce certain behaviours, since they themselves were earthly transmitters of God's grace. Henry VIII, for example, switched his favours from the previously dominant doctrine of free will to the predestinarian school because he identified the former with the personal autonomy of the honour society's leading nobles whom he was trying to tame.

In the case of the afterlife, strong predestination theory claimed that God had already determined, before the beginning of time, whether an individual soul was saved or damned, elect or reprobate. This rigidified existing notions of religious status. Honouring certain people for their worthy behaviour – and thereby preserving their memories, as the genealogies of the honour society did – had begun informally and was at first conducted by local Christian communities. It was then taken over by local bishops, and around 1200 came under the control of the papacy, which formalized it as sainthood and codified it as canonization. The Reformation replaced this posthumous sainthood with the living company of the elect, establishing the idea of a "rule of saints" that would prepare for the second coming. The doctrine of election, marginal before the Reformation, *internalized* sainthood and made the faith of the individual its supreme criterion, thereby opening up sainthood to ordinary believers.

The central reference point for debates about predestination was the fifth-century quarrel between Augustine, who had emphasized the prior necessity of divine grace, and Pelagius, who credited individual human beings with their own abilities, chiefly those of the will. (Without free will, said some, it would be impossible to judge people for their actions.) The Reformation largely sided with Augustine. People were not free except to sin, so they were certainly not free to work at their own salvation. The Counter Reformation likewise anathematized Pelagius; some Catholics, notably the Jansenists, went on to agree about election and reprobation too. The notion of a predestined in-group matched state directiveness about honour; rulers saw the company of the elect forming a bulwark against factious nobles on the one hand and social inferiors on the other. With their enthusiasm for predestination theory, however, came the need to keep controversy on a tight leash. Even the Swiss Reform elites, whose brainchild the strong interpretation was, banned sermons on the topic. The Church of England, despite many opportunities, always avoided adopting any final position on such matters, from its 1553 Articles of Religion through to the political climax of the predestination dispute at the 1618 Synod of Dort. Rulers feared that over-insistence might rouse sleeping plebeian dogs. James I, banning preachers from raising the issue, said it should be left to "learned men, and that moderately and modestly"; an Italian visitor to London agreed, complaining that "here the very women and shopkeepers [are] able to judge of predestination."[19]

While every Calvinist was a predestinarian of sorts, the strong version of it had become increasingly popular and rigid after Calvin's death, he himself having been unsystematic about it. "Double predestination" turned reprobates into a strictly defined group symmetrical with the elect. This rigidification and codification of grace came from Calvin's Genevan successor Beza, the Dutchman Francis Gomarus and the Englishman William Perkins. What Calvin had called a mystery they turned into dogma and orthodoxy. Nevertheless, the idea that individual effort might count refused to go away. To the idea that the elect are robots who "of necessity" yield assent and obedience, the objection arose: "Whosoever holdeth man's will and election to be subject to the necessities of destiny, destroyeth utterly ... all that appertaineth to human prudence ... for if it

---

[18] W.M., *The Middle Way*, 40.
[19] Izaak Walton, cited in Cummings, *The Literary Culture*, 281.

were so, ... what difference were there between the wise man and the fool?"[20] Predestination is not false, says this author, but should not discourage us from reasoning as far as we can.

The loudest opponents of double predestination were Jacob Arminius and his disciples. For them, salvation came from belief and, as it seemed therefore to their orthodox opponents, from a Pelagian-type effort of the will. Gomarus accused him of promoting the idea of a "universal grace." Arminius appeared to suggest that salvation might be within reach of anyone who belonged to the Church: a meritocracy of the will. All humans *can* be saved, he said, by responding freely to the divine call, but only if they *will* it. In fact this was not a universalist position, since it still involved election secondarily, on the grounds of God's prescience ("God foresaw what good courses I would take out of my free will, so did elect me"). God bestows a "sufficient grace" on everyone: sufficient, that is, to save anyone as long as they persevere. Special grace is not, as his orthodox opponents saw it, "effective," that is, fixed absolutely from before the beginning of time for a limited number of individuals. For the Arminians, "to be able to believe is in nature, to believe is of grace."[21] In other words, anyone can progress from ability or potentiality to the actuality of belief, if he has the will. Human depravity only began at a certain historical point, with the Fall, and hence cannot have been preordained in some individuals before the world began. If God had ordained before the creation that certain individuals were not to be saved then He, not they, would apparently be author of their sin.

The Arminians were ejected from the Reformed Church at the Synod of Dort. A watershed political event of the century (delegations attended from all over Europe), the Synod again illustrates the strong link between grace and honour. The dispute between Arminius and Gomarus had originated in the theology department at the University of Leiden where both men worked; each was engaged by rival factions in the Low Countries in a power struggle between pragmatic, decentralizing urban oligarchs who supported Arminius, and a nobility whose centralist, coercive policies were well suited to predestinarian doctrines like Gomarus's.

Give me a sign, Lord: grace and the assessment process

The critical problem for the company of the elect, as for the honour society, was how to authenticate their membership. Am I saved? The answer was a sealed book which God does not permit us to open. Grace gave the elect regeneration (the start of a new life), justification (removal of guilt) and sanctification (sustainability). But were there *signs* of membership? Was there a religious version of heraldic science? The question was crucial in respect of oneself because one's everlasting future was at stake, and crucial in respect of other people because they had to be made ready for the rule of the saints. Whereas Calvin's remarks about predestination were merely a warning to everyone to pull their socks up, later divines could not escape the urge to probe their own and others' individual status: this despite the maxim that in allocating grace God was not responding to "circumstances inherent in the person" (to use the modern phrase that derives from it, he was "no respecter of persons").[22] But divine arbitrariness only heightened the anxiety. The individual was unable to call upon anything within himself to alter his destiny, but this made signs more, not less, of an issue. After all, it was incontrovertible that *some* of us are elect.

Any bid for membership of the company of the elect was more hope than claim. Because the decision was God's alone, and mysterious, the very existence of signs was disputed. William

---

[20] Bryskett, *A Discourse*, 168.
[21] "A declaration of the sentiments of Arminius," in *Works*, i, 551.
[22] Perkins, *The Workes*, i, 10.

Tyndale warned against guilty speculation, against those "unquiet, busy, and high-climbing spirits" who "bring hither their high reasons and pregnant wits, and begin first from on high to search the bottomless secrets of God's predestination, whether they be predestinate or not." He contrasts such people's quick, "fleshly wit" with Jesus's "idiot" disciples, unlearned men whose modicum of understanding was nevertheless authentic. His criticism tars wit with the same brush as honour; it is a natural grace of the courtier, couched in terms of faculty psychology ("a sharp wit and a quick apprehension, a smooth speech, and a sound memory"). Later critics, in similar vein, identified these self-proclaimed elect who "exclude all others" with the episcopacy itself, which for them was just papal authority under another name.[23]

Anxiety about membership, as with all self-referential status modes, was objectified in the detached, scientific form of statistics. This too had its medieval precedents. In the early fourteenth century William of Ockham had been prominent among a group of scientifically inclined Oxford philosophers, whose studies of extension and acceleration led them to draw an analogy from the primary qualities they were dealing with (light, heat, colour, etc.) to the growth of qualities such as grace and charity within individual human beings. Every continuum was divisible into parts and therefore ought to be measurable: why not grace? These speculations, cut short in any case by the plague, were confined to a minute avant-garde.[24] The Reformation, on the other hand, led to grace becoming an obsession with the entire massed ranks of the literate, their anxiety all the greater because of the small number of the elect (the 144,000 mentioned in the Book of Revelation was a popular figure). According to the English church in 1595, the elect were "a determinate and certain number, which can neither be increased nor diminished," a view echoed on the Counter Reformation side by the Council of Trent.[25] The notion of a limited number then led to that of a predetermined Grace Quotient or order of precedence among them. Bishop Lancelot Andrewes attacked mere mortals who try to second-guess God; they think "they have sounded it to the bottom and ... can tell you the number and order of them just[ified] with 1.2.3.4.5."[26]

Signs of grace had their own dialectic within the individual. This began with the sense of "assurance" said to accompany faith. There followed the thought: how do I know this is not mere smugness? As Perkins complained, "Many in their own thinking shall be predestinate, even though they can never be truly persuaded." Self-knowledge had to be a genuine "inward testimony of the spirit ... in the heart of everyone that believeth, that he is elected." Some people, however, might reach this stage and then doubt their status. They would combat their doubts with strenuous piety. But then, this could not alter their fate; it might in fact be mere acting. So some of them went on to exhibit this internal wrestling externally, so that it was precisely *lack* of assurance that was the sign of being elect. Then again internal wrestling too might be counterfeited, by hypocrites or "wicked histrionical professors" who "tread those twisting paths so as to seem to approach the God from whom they flee." The sign therefore had to be "doubt interspersed with momentary windows of overwhelming joy," including visitations by the holy spirit and the power of prophecy.[27] People began to record daily accounts, quantifying these inner signs of election.

There was also the sign as it appeared to others. Anne Hutchinson was accused at her trial of terrorizing people, particularly pregnant women, by suggesting that they had fooled themselves

---

[23] Tyndale, *Doctrinal Treatises*, 505; Brooke, *A Discourse*, 13.

[24] J.A. Weisheipl, "Ockham and the Mertonians," in J. Catto (ed.), *The History of the University of Oxford*, i, 639.

[25] Dudley Fenner, *The Artes of Logike and Rethorike*, C1v.

[26] Andrewes, *XCVI Sermons*, 548.

[27] Perkins, *A Briefe Discourse, Taken out of the Writings of Her. Zanchius*, 19; John Beverley, *Unio Reformantium*, 71; Jean Calvin, *Institutes*, 1.5.51.

into believing they were in grace when they were not and thus questioning the religious status of their unborn children (she duly received the divine punishment of miscarrying a physiological "monster" herself). She allegedly claimed that "if she had but one half hour's talk with a man, she would tell whether he were elect or not," volunteering her own spiritual state as the baseline assessment.[28] More usually, though, the doctrine of divine inscrutability prevailed. Signs could only be indirect, "given off" by certain secular abilities in each individual. Hence the catechism. Invented by the early church fathers to screen out pollutant individuals from church ritual, the catechism subsequently developed into a measurable indicator of ability – part of a general tendency to reduce religion to whatever could be taught and learnt. The Reform theologian Jerome Zanchius wrote about the "deeper learning" that comes "by rehearsal and catechism, which is done by mutual questions and answers of the young beginner." Although a "deeper divinity" still lay untouched beneath the catechism, questioning might at least elicit something. Even if we cannot "look into the rolls of eternity ... election makes itself evident, and declares itself in our sanctification: for sanctification is, as it were, a temporal election."[29] Sanctification became for members of the company of the elect particularly important in this context. During the early Reformation it was very much the junior partner to regeneration and justification. These latter were complete and instantaneous, whereas sanctification, which would eventually come to dominate, had a temporal character; it was that aspect of grace which "once begun, daily increases" and "is continually at work in us."[30] It was therefore open to development, as well as to human intervention, in the form of training and curricula. It became an opportunity for members of the company of the elect, like those of the honour society, to know exactly who they were: a form of mutual recognition which doctrine had at first forbidden, and which was facilitated by its gradual transmutation into secular intelligence. In this way it acquired a "stereotyped, programmed corporateness," helping the godly "to survive in the face of the reprobate."[31]

Correct answers to catechical questioning gave evidence of sanctification, in the form of a reasoned understanding of one's religion, and could be taken as a proxy sign of election. The catechism was already a "science," as people of the time understood the word.[32] At some point the intellect, the psychological faculty of "human understanding," would cease to be a proxy and became election's substantive replacement, thus putting the cart before the Calvinist donkey. Grace might not be achievable through earthly merit or ability, but the search for *signs* of grace and election ushered human intelligence in by the back door, giving it room in which to grow and to become "effective" or determinate, like grace. The focus on signs helped to pin down the human understanding as a psychological object. Asking *whether* one was elect led to asking *how one knew*. By what experimental evidence did people obtain both psychological validation of their election and a sense of membership of a wider community?[33] This question was the stimulus for the epistemological issues being raised in philosophy that culminated in Locke's *Essay concerning Human Understanding*, replacing elect and reprobate with "moral man" (a regenerate universal reasoner) and "changeling" (a prototype of the modern intellectually disabled person).

---

[28] Winship, *Making Heretics*, 15.
[29] Jerome Zanchius, *Confession*, 331; Bates, *The Whole Works*, iii, 7.
[30] Martin Luther, *Werke*, xxx, 191.
[31] Ian Green, *The Christian's ABC*, 209.
[32] Adrian Velicu, *Civic Catechisms*, 30.
[33] Green, *The Christian's ABC*, 387 ff.

How faith became "an act of reason"

Descartes wrote that human reasoning, in the form of the *cogito*, is itself a "permanent act of grace." As such, it indicates a birth-to-death personhood rather than a one-off event. Spinoza, too, wrote that "reason is the saving grace" in human beings. But the great philosophers are not necessarily thereby the pioneers. Before Descartes or Spinoza, sixteenth-century religious texts foregrounding grace had already, if unwittingly, triggered a process that would elevate the status of human reasoning in relation to grace and faith, challenging the oft-cited injunction from the Book of Proverbs, "Lean not on thine own understanding."

To grasp this, we need first to analyze the terms involved. Reason (*ratio*) was at least three things: reason as the binding principle in the law of nature, an entire cosmological reference-frame with a divine core; "right reason" (*recta ratio*), that which human beings possessed before the Fall or will one day possess in their perfect regenerate state; and an everyday, practical human reasoning that is potentially corruptible. The understanding, on the other hand, was the *intellectus* of faculty psychology: the divine *intellectus* itself and/or its human embodiment ("intelligence" too was sometimes used in this sense). Reason and the understanding were separate concepts. If a primary source makes them seem interchangeable to us, that is not because they were growing closer (though they were) but because writers simply assumed their readers knew the difference. Finally there was knowledge (*scientia*), which had objective and subjective forms, knowledge and knowing, the confusion between them in matters psychological being no less than it is now. The one clearly objective body of knowledge to which humans might aspire was "Godly learning," which came from scripture rather than reason, and its Counter Reformation equivalent "Godly thinking." There was also a Faustian "devilish learning," and devilish thinking. What there could not be was *neutral* thinking of any kind. Even such a subordinate and apparently neutral concept such as "calculation," when employed in the scientific study of nature by Bacon or the Royal Society, had a divine element inasmuch as its goal, like that of today's geneticists, was "remaking Eden" (as in the title of Lee Silver's well-known futurological/eschatological tract).

Renaissance Christianity attempted to recuperate and turn the increasing elevation of specifically human reason and understanding to its own uses. The attempt was entangled in the much-debated issue of whether pagans could be elect. The elect experienced regeneration, justification and faith because at a certain point in history Christ had come along and died for them. So what about those ancient philosophers who had contributed so much to present knowledge (including theological knowledge), but who had predeceased him? Were their reasoning abilities no more than mundane natural graces? Erasmus tried to insist on the status of Aristotle, the epitome of this type. However, predestination seemed to rule out the very possibility of saving grace even for him, because he was already dead before the atonement took place. Calvin was said to have asked, "Shall we say that they had no wit, which by setting in order the art of speech, have taught us to speak with reason?"[34] The answer was clearly no. Nevertheless, these learned pagans could not have been elect; God simply willed that "we should be holpen by the travail and service of the wicked in natural philosophy." For Calvin it was self-evident that wit could be no sign of election.

His doctrine was undermined by his successors. By the start of the seventeenth century, a substantial group of humanist theologians was trying to weave a way between the twin dogmas of orthodox predestination on the one hand (elect and reprobate are mere pawns) and Arminius's disciples on the other (the elect are those with the will to persevere, already known as such to God). The first attempts at compromise arose in France, among students of De Mornay; his fame in

---

[34] Cited in A. Bergvall, "Reason in Luther, Calvin and Sidney," *Seventeenth Century Journal*, 23/10 (1992).

the history of political ideas as a pioneer of contract theory is significant, because the intellectual autonomy and ability he imputed to human beings as political subjects he imputed to them as religious and psychological subjects too.

This group remained within the Reformed church after the Arminians were expelled, but between the alleged universalism of the latter and the "special" grace of the orthodox church leadership, the group forged a middle way, known as "hypothetical universalism."[35] This was not so much a separate doctrine as the orthodoxy of Dort with one crucial alteration. The Synod had agreed a five-point platform. Fallen man in his natural state lacks the ability (*potentia*) to believe; God has decided already which sinners he will elect, so they do not have to fulfill any subsequent conditions; grace, when it comes, is irresistible; once the elect believe, they remain in faith and grace without any lapse; and Christ came to earth to save the elect alone ("limited atonement"). The last of these was what the middle way found objectionable, because it was unjust. Christ's love expressed through the atonement was surely universal; it went out to every individual human being, even though it was unrequited by many. Alongside this French attempt at a middle path, a comparable doctrine arose in the English church known as "conditional universalism," which deemed that "rationality is a necessary condition always presupposed in the subject whether predestinate or reprobate."[36] To these we can add others who pursued a moderate line mainly out of political fear that debate might get out of hand. Richard Hooker, for example, mindful of the damage that competing dogmas had done to the church and to fellow churchmen's necks since the Reformation, wove his way between the extremes by his frequent appeals to the socially calming effects of what he dubbed "sweet" reason.

The French middle-way theologians were particularly disposed to place value in the human subject. Human beings were not just "blocks of wood" determined by the blind forces of predestination, any more than by arbitrary edict from an infallible Pope. This line, in the wake of Dort, provoked hostility from their own orthodox church leaders. It could be taken as implying, first, that reason and the will are free to do good independently of God's grace (the Pelagian heresy), and secondly that salvation is achieved not through faith imputed in the elect alone but through meritorious works undertaken in this life (the Romanist heresy). In opposition to their orthodox colleagues, who believed that Christ died only for the elect, these middle-way compromisers argued that Christ's act of atonement was a separate matter from God's preordained choice of the elect. It was not paradoxical to think that Christ died on everyone's behalf while election itself was limited to a few; his task had been to make salvation possible for all *hypothetically*, even if God had made it actually possible only for certain elect individuals. In opposition to the Arminians, on the other hand, the compromisers followed their orthodox colleagues' line that salvation is conditional on faith, not on works. However, they did give this an unorthodox twist: faith required the prior co-operation and activity of the intellect here on earth. In other words, faith itself was a work. At the same time, human reason was repositioned *within* faith which, like the will, came to depend on prior intellectual components. Using human reason as a probe in groping their way through the dark of competing dogmatisms, the middle-way theologians triggered an erosion of category boundaries. The limited company of the elect, defined by their faith, would in a few generations become the near-universal company of the intelligent.

In any case the Reformation, despite itself, had from the very start allowed human intellectual ability to insinuate itself within faith, through its recommendation of personal gospel reading. Its insistence on the literal truth of the Bible turned literacy into the highest of the natural graces. Special, divine grace had become the fulcrum of religious debate and reached the common people

---

[35] See F. Laplanche, *Orthodoxie et prédication*; B. Armstrong, *Calvinism and the Amyraut Heresy*.
[36] John Davenant, *Dissertatio de Morte Christi*, 114.

through the invention of printing, itself described by Luther as "God's highest and extremest act of grace" and "the last flame before the extinction of the world."[37] This nexus between grammar and grace helped to enlarge the godly in-group, previously closed to lay, unlearned idiots. The arguments about grace had to be known by all, and one had to be literate in order to advance the correct line that had been standardized by print – even if grace itself was unknowable and beyond reason.

The middle-way theologians tried to free human reasoning of its corrupting taints. They tackled, for example, the orthodox dogma of a simple opposition between learning ("human") and understanding ("spiritual"), like that expressed in the title of a widely disputed Baptist text of 1640: *The Sufficiency of the Spirit's Teaching without Human Learning. Or a treatise tending to prove human learning to be no help to the spiritual understanding of the word of God.* A middle-way critic asks the author to "bewail your ignorance that you had no more of human learning, that you might have the more easily understood by the help of the holy spirit that divine learning which is revealed in the holy scripture." In other words, human and divine learning can be compatible or even intermingle.[38]

The question of whether pagan philosophers could be elect was revived for this purpose. Pre-Christian Greeks with enough wit to know "necessary truths" (i.e., mathematical ones – those which even God cannot temporarily suspend) must surely have had some sort of uncorrupted knowledge of God too, since necessary truths are "sovereign and uncreated" aspects of the divinity himself. And even those writers who disapproved of Aristotle could always appeal instead to a Baconian concept of human reason as experimentally embedded in practical things; this could then be a bulwark *against* the wishy-washy, "corrupting philosophy" of Aristotle and the scholastics and therefore compatible with faith, even enhance it. Either way, it became possible to say that it was not human reasoning abilities in themselves that are corrupt, only how they are used. Sidney's friend Fulke Greville, simultaneously a Baconian and a strict faith-based Calvinist, had already suggested that the status of our subjective reasoning abilities is guaranteed by the objective ones enshrined in experimental method; the latter "supply the natural defects" of "wit" in the former.[39] Godly learning, then, having begun as an objective body of biblical knowledge opposed to the corrupt human sort, expanded to become the basis for a scientific knowledge of the natural world, to which might be added a scientific knowledge of human nature and of the subjective processes of knowing.

Baxter, a champion of the middle way, had been forced as a chaplain in Cromwell's army to cope with in-fighting sectarians who believed the mere intensity of their faith meant they were elect. He warned such people, "If you overthrow your reason, you will be a reproach to religion …; it is an ill sign when your zeal is beyond the proportion of your understanding."[40] Baxter was trying to redress a balance that had tipped too far towards the will and instantaneous faith during the civil wars. In his baroque ramification of divisions and subdivisions between will, faith and reason, we can see a desperate attempt to maintain parity among them. But we can also see, with the benefit of hindsight, that the very need to maintain parity caused him unwittingly to highlight the autonomy and positive value of human reasoning in particular.

Even the opposing orthodoxies on either side of the middle way, forced to engage with the centrality of reason, tacked towards it and were eventually forced to endorse it. Their new course then became permanent. Following the reshaping of the political landscape for Protestants in the mid-seventeenth century in both France and England, orthodox Calvinists came to look on the path

---

[37] Cited in Cummings, *The Literary Culture*, 50.
[38] Immanuel Bourne, *A Defence … of Infant-Baptism*, 8.
[39] Fulke Greville, *A Treatie of Humane Learning*, in *Poems and Drama*, 157.
[40] Baxter, *The Cure of Church Divisions*, 123.

to grace as "rational conviction of the mind," while Arminians ceased locating the primary human ability in perseverance of the will and sought it instead in the reasoning faculties that differentiate one individual from the next.[41] As one of them put it, "The divine essence or nature of God is one thing, and that virtue that he was pleased to put forth to give being to the reasonable soul of a man, are ever distinct .... The essence of God is one thing, and that radical virtue or potency is another thing" and varies in each of us.[42] The very drawing of such a clear distinction between divine and human reason helped in this changed political context to promote the latter. By the 1670s it was clear that "the loud outcries ... against reason" now only came from "sects" and "fanatics." It was "sober use of our faculties," by contrast, that should be the aim. Even if the premise remained that reason in humans was corrupt, sobriety would make up for its shortcomings. Hence "faith itself is an act of reason." Moreover, "to disgrace reason, is to strike up religion by the roots, and prepare the world for atheism."[43] After 1660 it was usual to add "and reason" to any mention of revelation or scripture in support of a theological argument, where previously the author would either have omitted such a phrase or sounded defensive about it. Intelligence could only ever have come to dominate our views of human nature by being socialized in this way, and can only do so still: that is, by demonstrating a superior claim to divinity. Once human reasoning was identified as a positive means to divine grace, the way was open for that outcome which earlier disputants had explicitly warned against. Mundane "natural" grace no longer knew its place. Instead, it had absorbed elements of the "special" grace formerly confined to the elect.

"Soul-experiments": testing the rational conscience

What, more exactly, was the relevant content of the knowledge that lay in the human intellect or understanding? Three interlinked components predominate, all of them pointing inwards: first, understanding of the understanding itself, in a theoretical sense; secondly, the practical aspect of self-understanding known as conscience; and finally, the concrete application of conscience by self-examination at holy communion. All three went with an extension of human reasoning (and its status) down the social scale.

A thirteenth-century clerk, trader or peasant on the make might have been surprised to hear a present-day historian say, as many have, that "self" and "individual" are modern concepts. Their practical manifestation is well in evidence from the social history of the earlier period and has already been well covered in Alexander Murray's *Reason and Society in the Middle Ages*. Our concern here, however, is with the value accorded to them at a doctrinal level, which grew in a rather piecemeal fashion. Godly learning was increasingly supplemented with "learning about humanity" (*studia humanitatis*). Calvin, for example, began his great work with the sentence, "The knowledge of God and that of ourselves are connected." This led to attempts to know the mind, and later its perfectibility. The critique of this project, that it is circular, gradually emerged. Could the cure for a corrupt human understanding be effected by the understanding itself? "A disease in the body is perceived by the mind; but when the soul is the affected part, and the rectitude of reason is lost," as it is in fallen man, then "there is no remaining principle to give notice of it."[44] To think that the understanding can understand the understanding, says this author, is to dream of union with the divine essence, just as an unreasonable enthusiast or sectarian does. One met this critique, then as

---

[41] Flavell, *The Method*, 71; 73.
[42] Francis Duke, *The Fulness and Freeness of Gods Grace*, 105.
[43] Glanvill, "Anti-fanatical Religion," 17, in *Essays*.
[44] Bates, *The Whole Works*, i, 219.

now, with studied avoidance. Baconian science's attempt to clarify the relation between objects of knowledge and subjective abilities of knowing and understanding did not extend to that discipline in which the object of knowledge is the human understanding itself.

The problem in religious terms was the Roman church's admiration of surface images, perceived through the external senses and the faculty of imagination. One had to look inwards: "though ... a man's self be not the only object of his own care, yet himself ... in the first place must be looked into. Our charity must begin at home."[45] The easy descent of the imagination had to be abandoned for the steep climb of introspection. How might one reach an understanding of the understanding? One option was Platonism. Its theory of the intellect encouraged circular thinking since it was premised on the compatibility or even, potentially, the unity between understanding as object and understanding as subject. For Greville's adopted son Robert Brooke, this unity represented the perfect human reason of the afterlife, where "the understanding and the truth-understood are one." The existing Aristotelian convention that drew distinctions between "a soul recipient, a being [sc. a substantial truth] received, and a faculty which is the understanding," was over-complicated nonsense. All three are the same thing, and comprise a single act of divine grace: "However the understanding be enriched with this treasure of truth ... then is it, itself that truth, that light .... Thus the understanding and light are different in names, may be different in degrees but not in nature." Such an ideal reasoning might even be possible on this earth. "Who shall tell us what is *recta ratio* [right reason]? I answer *recta ratio*," he continues; any other answer would be "most papal." The idea of "us" (the putatively elect) establishing human reason, in perfected form, as its own psychological object, came partly from the refusal to let popes, bishops and absolute rulers tell us and thus also, in Lord Brooke's case, from his honourable status.[46]

If a Platonist reduction of terms was one route towards understanding of the understanding, another was the proliferation of terms typical of middle-way doctrines. Baxter wrote to Boyle with proposals for another suitable piece of Royal Society research. The core ability of the human understanding was a "waking, working knowledge" of itself, and of the "faculties and capacities" distinguishing us from other animals. Boyle agreed: men must "make themselves part of their own study."[47] Where early modern wit starts to lift itself from the corrupting mire of original sin, its first topic for study is itself. Our knowledge of this reasoning human nature, writes Baxter, is like our knowledge of the existence of God or mathematical truths: human nature is itself demonstrable *a priori*. Locke would a few years later call himself "bold" for saying that the place of the human understanding in the natural order is a universal truth as "capable of demonstration, as well as mathematics"; but Baxter had already submitted psychology's bid for scientific status.[48] He situates the understanding's understanding of the understanding in the realm of natural history. Renaissance writers had wondered vaguely whether it might not form part of natural philosophy. Baxter goes further by proposing it as an exact, inductive science, which (as he wrote to Boyle) the Royal Society should position within "the alphabet of physics," to be investigated by means of "soul-experiments."[49] These latter were the direct descendants, in a new natural-philosophy context, of the "experimental predestinarianism" recommended by earlier Calvinists for assessing the signs of grace in oneself.

---

[45] Martin Blake, *The Great Question*, 88.
[46] Brooke, *The Nature of Truth*, 53; 5; see also James, "English politics."
[47] Baxter, Letter to Robert Boyle, 14 June 1665; Boyle, cited in John Howe, *The Reconcileableness of God's Prescience*, 7.
[48] Locke, *An Essay*, 43; 516.
[49] Baxter, *Reliquiae Baxterianae*, i, 124.

Baxter's circular definition of the understanding was linked to a circular definition of the species: to be human is to possess the intellectual ability to know what it is to be human, which is to possess the intellectual ability (to know what it is to be human, which is ...), and so on. Yet it was still an understanding that knew its earthly place. It was the distinguishing mark of the human from other natural species: a *preparation* for the rule of the saints, but not the ensuing enlightenment itself. Adam before the Fall had this enlightenment. He knew the essence of the rational soul "far more then we do ours ...." However, "he knew it not by its effects"; he saw a unitary "selfness" in "the souls of all creatures with himself," such that their "specificating forms" were to him invisible.[50] Once the "reasonable soul" is in its ultimately perfect state, any knowledge about the place of the human understanding in nature becomes redundant because it is no longer needed; the prelapsarian Adam's participation in divine reason meant that he was "clouded to perceive his own nature." Understanding of the understanding was therefore only an intermediary step, towards perfection.

If we look more precisely at individual minds, of what did this understanding consist? Baxter, in the same year (1671) as Locke first conceived the need for the *Essay concerning Human Understanding*, gives us rare chapter and verse:[51]

> 1. That you understand who Christ is, as in his person and his offices; 2. That you understand the *reason* of his undertaking; 3. That you understand, what it is that he hath done and suffered for us; 4. That you understand the nature and worth of his benefits, and what he *will* do for you; 5. That you understand the terms on which he conveyeth these benefits to men; and what is the nature, extent, and condition of his promises; and 6. that you understand the *certain truth* of all this. [emphases in original]

The model for this understanding, as Baxter makes clear, was reflexive: it was *his own sense* of election. Discovery of one's inner self complemented the external, objective workings of the transmission of grace. It was experimental, an application of Baconian science to the soul; in the words of Baxter's colleague Gabriel Firmin, "Great is the work of the spirit upon the understanding .... God hath given man a rational soul, set up his candle and light within him, made able to reflect upon it self, try and know what is in himself, it is able to draw conclusions from premises: hence when the Lord sets him upon examination, he sets him about a rational work, to which he hath fitted and enabled him."[52]

We find such increasingly detailed and systematized psychology in another of Baxter's colleagues, a certain W.M. He ignores the formerly crucial question of how grace arrives in the elect, in favour of how one's own mind works to combine with it. He writes about the importance to religion of "hav[ing] a right understanding and due conception in our mind, touching the notive power of man, in or unto the specifying and determining of his own acts or actions."[53] God does not determine the detail of individual human actions and is therefore not the author of sinful ones; the only thing he determines is the one-off act of conversion. This then stimulates the soul to regenerate its natural faculties by itself, "rendering them capable of taking in a new impression ... to which the soul was disabled before." If God works any other direct changes on the individual, it is "objectively, also by offering reason to it," on the grounds that "faith [is] the most solid understanding." Knowing the self and the mind thus involves both divine determination and human reasoning. On the one hand we are responsible for our own actions and God does not determine or

---

50 Duke, *The Fulness*, 3.
51 *Directions and Perswasions to a Sound Conversion*, 192.
52 *The Real Christian*, 291.
53 *The Middle Way*, 8 ff.

predestine them; on the other, there is His "offer" of right reason. To make the two work together, some third thing has to mediate between them: not intuited intellectual ability as such ("notive power," *nous*) but a separate "understanding," a conceptualization of that ability. The human mind has, of necessity, something in it that thinks about its own thinking.

Whether this human nature was a universal one remained an open question. For the medieval philosophers, self-knowledge meant "Know your essence," where "you" is the broad category "man." For Protestant humanists, it increasingly meant "Know your *individual* self," and again this raised the hypothesis not only of differences among individuals, but of a hierarchy of difference, and perhaps of exceptions to the entire rule. An exasperated pastor like Firmin thought the very category "man" was rendered unstable by the mass ignorance he encountered in "trying and knowing" his parishioners – that is, in assessing them with the catechism. Any hypothetically universal human category continued to exist in tension with the restricted one of the elect. Were reprobates really human? W.M.'s teasing out of the multidimensional workings of grace within individuals, in terms of their psychological faculties, was a fix for the problems grace was encountering in the political sphere. Authority, threatened by sectarian rashness and enthusiastic self-assertions of elect status, sought in active, reasoned and reflexive internal examination the kind of self-policing it would much prefer from its citizens.

In medieval philosophy the faculty of understanding had been mainly static and meditative – with some significant exceptions. One can see small changes starting in the thirteenth century. For example, iconic church art previously designed to be adored, began to demand an active response. The Madonna now inclines her head as if to provoke thought in the onlooker, even among the illiterates in the nave. Subsequent humanist art poses its philosophers to point vaguely at their books, though Titian's ecclesiastics still stare contemplatively into space even when they have books on their laps. It was only the debates about election that gave the human understanding its fully active profile. By the seventeenth century we find contemplation being redefined as "deliberate research" and contrasted with "those vulgar heads that rudely stare about, and with a gross rusticity admire [God's] works" – admiration having formerly been contemplation's main purpose.[54] The evidence obtained from self-examination was self-knowledge in action, and ultimately a verification of the individual's in-group membership.

Aside from the immediate emotional signs of election mentioned above, evidence could be sought in two further aspects of this Christian self-understanding: conscience, and participation in the eucharist. Beza, a hardline codifier of predestination, acknowledged that all forms of evidence for one's membership in the company of the elect had their limits. Revelation and visitations by the Holy Spirit had occurred only to a few prophets and saints; right reason, as a complete and accurate knowledge of the natural world, was only available to natural philosophers, and in any case its truths were not hard and fast since nature was incomplete without grace. Most ordinary human beings had no signs to go on but their own everyday wit, which operated by "practical syllogisms." Beza took this form of second-order, *a posteriori* or evidence-based judgement, and applied it to personal conduct. From observing one's own external behaviour, one could reach logical conclusions about one's "sanctified" state; but one had to bear in mind that such conclusions did not necessarily reflect one's afterlife status, which God kept hidden. Or, to reverse the emphasis, one could not know one was elect; but one could make a good stab at it by examining oneself for authentic signs of grace. And the supreme sign was conscience. Amidst the corruption of the Fall, just this one spark of divinity remained.

For Calvin, conscience was pre-rational; it was distinct from the understanding and from the will, though it coloured both by enabling them to distinguish between good and evil. But Perkins,

---

[54] Browne, *Religio*, 15.

widely read across Europe's Protestant communities and another hardliner on predestination, went much further. For him conscience was the "essence" of the human soul, primary evidence for its immortality. It was the one trait that differentiated humans from other animals. Unlike his predecessors, he found a place for conscience, this one fragment of the divine image, within the individual's faculty psychology; it was "*part of* the understanding in all reasonable creatures, determining of their particular actions …. Conscience is not placed in the affections nor will, but in the understanding: because the actions thereof stands in the use of reason" (emphasis added).[55] Here we see the start of an unwitting demotion of the will in definitions of what it is to be human; not just conscience but faith too was in the "mind of man, not the will." This was a crucial move. It was impossible, said Perkins, for conscience to be "partly in the mind and partly in the will," because the grace from which it derives is "single" and therefore cannot "be seated in diverse parts of faculties." Grace, when it arrives, lodges in the understanding. Conscience, as one of its components, is "a supernatural gift of God in the mind." The mind, however, has two parts, "theoretical" and "practical." The theoretical part goes no further than contemplation. Conscience is essentially *practical* understanding, actively seeking to know the goodness or badness of a particular action. As conscience is located in the understanding, so, too is the emotional assurance of election; feel-good conscience authenticates membership of the in-group. Perkins takes something which is (thus far Calvin would have agreed) "of a divine nature … placed of God in the midst between him and man," but places it categorically within the sphere of everyday human reasoning, as part of a "natural faculty." It is not quite true then to say, as some have, that with the decline of religion intelligence has *replaced* conscience as the defining property of the human species.[56] Rather it was the fact that reasoned conscience was the membership qualification for the company of the elect that opened the way for intelligence to become the qualification.

The conscience's decisions, said Perkins, proceed by practical syllogism. The "property" of conscience is to take the "conclusions of the mind and apply them, and by applying them either to accuse or excuse." The terms are at once psychological and juridical. The "two assistants" of this logical reasoning are "mind and memory"; the mind keeps the "rules and principles" like a law book, presenting to conscience the rules of divine law "whereby it is to give judgement," while the memory brings to mind "the particular actions which a man hath done or not done, that conscience may determine of them." Enter syllogistic reasoning: "Every murderer is cursed, saith the mind. Thou art a murderer, saith conscience assisted by memory. Ergo, thou art cursed, saith conscience, and giveth here sentence." Conscience is also consciousness; they have a common basis in self-examination and reflection. It is the job of conscience not to conceive a thing in itself but to reflect on what has been conceived: to "know *what* I know" (emphasis added). Perkins agrees with Calvin that man's reason is corrupt, owing to worldly temptation. Nevertheless, his novel focus on conscience highlights man's unique place in the scale of nature because this essential, uncorrupted spark of divinity is now something *specific to him*, the core of his own individual reason. (God and the angels have reason but not conscience, having no need of it.)

This intellectualization of elect status can be seen not only in the position of conscience within faculty psychology but in self-examination at the eucharist. Although Reformers such as Zanchius denied that the bread and wine were Christ's body and blood, this did not mean they were "simple marks, or bare signs." Rather, they were "instruments," by which Christ's atonement is "called to our remembrance, his promises are sealed, and our faith stirred up." The ritual was not empty. On the contrary, it was even more intense, since it required the communicant to knuckle down to intellectual labour. The basic principle was that "Every man descending into himself do

---

[55] Perkins, *A Discourse of Conscience*, 1 ff.
[56] Erica Fudge, *Perceiving Animals*, 9.

prove himself, that he eat not and drink not thereof unworthily unto his condemnation." Now the average Catholic's understanding was not taxed by his asking himself whether he had fornicated that week, and he could grasp in some vague mystical way that Jesus's body actually is the bread and wine. To grasp the ritual as metaphor, however, or by any other of the contortions whereby the Reformers distanced themselves from Rome, was another matter. It required and generated a complex cognitive act.

Reformers wrote about the need for communicants to "understand what is signified and offered to us ... to be understood in the mind, and received by faith."[57] Zwingli called the relation of sign to signified an "analogy." This doctrine, held also by Baxter, was the hardest of all to grasp intellectually because it relied on a series of inferences occurring within the communicant's mind. It was in exactly this context that Zwingli complained about lack of ability in "the feeble multitude, which is ... in general pretty stupid."[58] Here the modes of grace, honour and intelligence are one. Zwingli's view of the eucharist as something to be grasped cognitively arose at the height of his rift with the working-class Anabaptists in the 1520s. Having led these apprentices and *idiotae* of the urban commons into battle against the Roman church and its learned *doctores*, once in power he sought to civilize them and make them see reason. Not all of them appreciated his efforts. So they had to be reprobate. Not members of the honour society, they formed an out-group in terms of election too, and the combination of these elements led to their being recast in terms of their intellectual stupidity – in spite of the fact that they were literate and could read all the arguments.

Grace remained the centrepiece. "Come warm your hearts all intellectual capacities, at this fire," was the call.[59] Nevertheless the intellect was developing a presumptuous autonomy and giving out some heat of its own. This was happening across doctrines. Some Counter Reformationists were now saying that the supernatural grace of the eucharist has to be accompanied by the individual's own "congruous" reasoning processes.[60] While both Protestant and Catholic churches continued to emphasize the corruption of natural man and his reason, certain theologians of both stripes were trying to detoxify not only human reason but also the human nature in which it was lodged.

This sprang from their criticism of the orthodox Calvinist doctrine that grace was irresistible and human beings completely determined. Surely the individual must have some degree of autonomy in his contract with God, and if so, it must be of an intellectual kind. "No grace that any man hath, but it passeth in through the understanding," said Firmin. Understanding had primacy over the will: "God in conversion or drawing to Christ, works upon a rational creature .... He calls the will and affections off from the objects to which they are glued, to close with other objects: a reason for that, saith the will, ... therefore doth the spirit set up this light in the understanding first."[61] And that was because "in order of *nature*, the work upon the understanding precedeth, which agreeth with a reasonable creature" (emphasis added). Now there may be less to this than meets the eye. There is the usual nod towards the old universal category of man as rational animal ("reasonable creature") but the restricted category of the elect was the more important one, and nature was still subordinate to it. As he goes on to say, "The light depends not upon the strength of men's natural parts .... We shall observe among Christians, that are weak in understanding compared with others, yet the notions of God, of sin, and creature, which they have, are more clear ... than are the notions of other Christians (really such I mean) that have greater parts and natural abilities." Nevertheless the outlines of a natural science of the mind are already visible, adapted to the framework of election.

---

[57] Zanchius, *Confession*, 106.
[58] *The Defence of the Reformed Faith*, ii, 367.
[59] Samuel Rutherford, *Christ Dying and Drawing Sinners to Himselfe*, 13.
[60] W. Craig, "Middle knowledge," in C. Pinnock (ed.), *The Grace of God and the Will of Man*.
[61] *The Real Christian*, 29.

They pose the very question which Firmin simultaneously tries to close down: might not the human understanding or even just plain "learning" be signs of grace?

The idea of a natural history of man, fusing divine with natural grace and spiritual with natural intelligence, created a more fundamental role for the contrasting category of emotion, with which intelligence is often paired. A seminal eighteenth-century educator like the American Jonathan Edwards placed great value on "the affections" because he had noted a feedback loop in his concern for reason, which excluded many of the population. Understanding leads to regeneration, and regeneration in turn produces understanding and the capability for "abstraction"; hence "the more rational any gracious person is, by so much more is he fixed ... and satisfied in the grounds of religion." While only God knows for sure about my salvation, I can observe my own behaviour and form practical syllogisms about it, on a rational basis. Emotion was in some sense an afterthought. Practical syllogizing could not be the sole basis for convincing oneself of one's elect status, because it was not available to uneducated, i.e., non-syllogizing Christians. How might they too have conviction? Since the view now prevailed that rational conviction was a continuous internal state rather than a single act of regeneration, it followed that this conviction had parallel bodily states, "motion[s] of the blood and animal [soul] spirits." These congregate especially round the heart and arouse affection, which can "effectively" stimulate a blessed state in the uneducated.[62] Affection enabled anyone, by "various degrees" from "babes in Christ" to the most godly, to receive special, saving grace, and allowed the "use of means" to be proportionate to one's intellectual abilities. In short, Edwards inserts election fully within a natural history of the individual mind, even though mind is differentiated across a spectrum of those individuals' abilities. "There is no distinguishing," he concludes, "between the influences of the spirit of God, and the natural operations of the faculties of our own minds."

"The economy of human nature": early notions of psychological development

We have already noted the growing tendency for grace to be seen as a continuous process rather than a lightning bolt, and the consequence which writers like Baxter drew from this, that grace is a coalescence of ends with means: not the longed-for gift alone but the continuous working of a reasoned faith towards it. "Wit's pilgrimage" – the satirical title of John Davies of Hereford's 1605 poem attacking just such tendencies – now became the central preoccupation, in all seriousness. This turned reasoning into something temporal, a series of moves from a to b to c, etc., out of which came what modern psychology calls developmental (dis)ability: "growth of grace" or "growth in grace," to use the terms of the era. The modern concept can be traced back to those attempts to rescue predestination from its own excessive rigidity. The idea of process was common enough among non-Calvinists, but only in a very broad sense; it was rather from Calvinist writers who had once insisted so much on the suddenness of grace that a more exact description of process grew, mainly because for them it was tied to self-examination and self-development.

In medieval philosophy, the terms ability and ability – *potentia* and *impotentia* – were applied across a huge referential range, from the cosmos to the individual soul. They could also apply to individuals in a legal sense; a villein was disabled from pursuing his landlord in the courts, a penniless tenant was disabled from paying rent. Theologians adapted this legalistic language to the subject's relationship with God, creating an interplay between religion and jurisprudence in which ability was individualized, and intellectualized, as "competence." The rigidly Calvinist view, however, had been that when God justifies the elect, it is not because of anything they have

---

[62] Edwards, *A Treatise concerning Religious Affections*, 24 ff.

done to deserve it; faith *precludes* ability and competence. "God made man with abilities to fulfill his commands," and that was it. Ability therefore consists in "obedience to his law ... not by setting himself upon the exact fulfilling of it by his own feeble strength but upon considering the impossibility of the thing."[63] Just as Hegel (in Bertrand Russell's paraphrase) defined freedom as freedom to obey the police, so Calvin defined ability as the ability to be determined by God. Natural ability amounts only to that. The elect may indeed be "able to all things," as the above author puts it – but only because theirs are *spiritual* abilities. The abilities possessed by the regenerate man just so happen to be those of the holy spirit regenerating him. In that case how could man have abilities of his own at all? One solution was to differentiate more carefully among different categories of ability. According to Wilkins there were "*spiritual* abilities ... infused from above," a form of necessity, and "*artificial* abilities ... acquired by our own industry."[64] Writing in the 1640s, he would now have associated reliance on spiritual abilities alone with the sectarian enthusiasm and rashness of the commons. Nor, of course, were artificial abilities enough on their own. Room had therefore opened up for *natural* ability, situated between the spiritual and the artificial. Its status was raised. There were even rarefied instances where a man "could turn nature into grace," if only by means of being able to keep his soul spirits in his brain and to prevent them from abandoning it for his genitals – this was said of the reputedly virginal Boyle, for example.[65]

In fact natural ability very much resembled a non-instantaneous and therefore politically acceptable version of spiritual ability (one that could be predicted and monitored). As we have already noted, the compatibility between spiritual and natural grace which is at the root of modern psychology arose in part from the need to resolve corresponding tensions between the honour of gentility and the honesty of the bourgeois. Being drawn out gave it a flexibility which emerges in the doctrine of "preparedness." For orthodox Calvinists, the prepared state of an elect individual was not a result of his own intellectual striving but something God had already done to him in advance, and in any case it amounted to no more than an acknowledgement of his own wickedness. For the Arminians, preparedness did come by individual effort, but the effort was one of belief rather than reason. The middle-way authors redesignated preparedness as a state of constant stand-by for the receipt of grace, in which everyone was to be primed for an impending rule of the saints. After the waning of these millenarian hopes in England in the 1650s, and with reason seeming less dangerous than the plethora of wills that had proved so unruly during the revolution, preparedness began to be seen more often in terms of natural intellectual merit. And because it was now clear that glory was further off than expected, room opened up for further observation, nurturing and continuous assessment of the individual's inner intellectual state. "There is a husbandry of the soul, as of the estate, and the end of the one, as of the other, is the increasing and improving of its riches," wrote the Anglican Richard Allestree in the 1680s. "Now the riches of the soul are either natural, or divine. By the natural I mean its faculties of reason, wit, memory, and the like; by the divine I mean the graces [which] are given immediately by God, and both these we are to take care to improve."[66] Or more starkly: "It is said the elect of God ... are passed from the state of nature into a state of grace: and what difference is there between the two? Are they not both one and the same thing?"[67]

In England the trigger for this shift was the desperate dissolution of the Barebones parliament at the end of 1653, which dispelled hopes for an imminent godly political regime that might prepare

---

[63] Dudley Fenner, "A defence of the thirty-nine articles of the Church of England," 10.2, in *The Artes*.
[64] Wilkins, *Ecclesiastes*, 3.
[65] Shapin, *A Social History of Truth*, 165.
[66] *The Whole Duty of Man*, 165.
[67] Edward Lane, *Du Moulin's Reflections Reverberated*, 65.

for the second coming. A new way of talking about reason took hold across the politico-theological spectrum from this point onwards. If at the Restoration bishop and king went back in the bottle, the old reservations about human reason did not. As well as the Anglican Bishop Henry Hammond, who wrote of "the reasonableness of Christian religion" as the resolver of "doubts of all sorts ... by the dictates of nature," the Congregationalist Owen, the Platonist Glanvill and the maverick (because moderate) Baxter were all caught up in this shift.[68] The common ideas were coming to be seen as the outcome of prior, micro-mechanical reasoning operations, the "aids and assistances" of ability which Locke would further expound in the *Essay*, as part of an ever more complex timetable for the kingdom of heaven on earth. The dystopian fantasy consequently arose of certain people who might lack these natural developmental abilities and disrupt the schedule. The fantasy gained ground in proportion to the fading of utopian visions of a rule of the saints. Preparation was clearly going to be a longer, harder haul than had so far been envisaged.

The idea of development also sprang from the much-debated distinction between *moral* and *physical* ability. The "moral" was the domain in which God has a continuing, malleable relationship with man; the "physical" was the domain he has already irrevocably ordained. The categorization of people into elect and reprobate, for instance, was physical. The eucharist on the other hand was moral, a conversation with God. (That was precisely the papists' error: they thought it was physical, conveying grace into anyone receiving the sacraments.) Baxter complicated matters as usual. Defending himself against the charge that his middle way was not in the middle at all but just another name for universalism, he begins by protesting that "for predestination I go higher than the Synod of Dort," in other words that he is more Calvinist than Calvin. But, he continues, suddenly switching to an Arminian vocabulary: "As for that point of [all men being capable of] moral suasion .... I know God useth external suasion, and whether he so manage not objects as thereby he may be said internally to persuade I know not well: but I think he doth."[69] That is, Baxter posits a dynamic interactivity between the physical and the moral. God has created a world where our ability for "internal" moral persuasion, for a flexibility of regeneration and inner development, also contains mechanisms ("managed objects") that have the same determinate character as external, one-off "physical" causation and the predestined gift of effective grace.

This is not the old, vague talk of God combining external "means" of grace with "inward enlightenment."[70] Nor is Baxter talking about the predestination of individual behaviours. Rather, he imports a deterministic element into the detailed *workings* of the individual mind that lead *to* those behaviours. This seems to interpolate a fresh tier of causation; the detailed workings are located in the intellect, as the condition *sine qua non* of moral ability, urging the will too in the right direction. He equates the physical with the natural ("not nature as corrupt" but "nature as nature")[71]. The physical, necessary force of predestination thereby comes to have its own embedded components within the subject himself, and particularly within what Baxter calls elsewhere his "natural intellectual ability." God has created a situation where the individual's moral ability, his ability to be internally influenced by sound arguments, belongs at the same time to an external, preordained and objective system. As a colleague of Baxter's put it, "God knoweth how to reach the reason, and elective faculty, the main springs of the soul, and how to fasten a nail there."[72] Human reasoning, while it is the individual's responsibility, has a quasi-divine mechanism within it. "Physical determination," formerly the antithesis of the "convincing reason" that may or may

---

[68] Hammond, *The Miscellaneous Theological Works*, ii, 7.
[69] Letter to Peter Ince, 21 November 1653.
[70] William Pemble, *Workes*, 553.
[71] Cited in William Lamont, *Richard Baxter*, 139.
[72] W.M., *The Middle Way*, 8.

not persuade, inserts within that reason certain processes with a life of their own. The defensive loquacity of middle-way authors such as Baxter against the doctrinaires on either side thus threw up a modern hypothesis: the existence of a specifically human intelligence as a natural phenomenon controlled by necessary laws which operate on a person-by-person basis.

The notion that physical and moral abilities might be interactive raised a further possibility: they might be susceptible to ongoing improvement. Baxter's friend Howe, another of Cromwell's chaplains, wrote to Boyle claiming that although God intervenes providentially through regeneration to determine a person's understanding and behaviour, his intervention has to be already "agreeable enough to the nature" of that person.[73] It was unreasonable to suppose that the inner nature of "intelligent creatures" was dictated entirely by external, automatic "impulses," or that they were incapable of "motions" of their own; this would mean that God's precepts "whereof their nature is capable" would all be irrelevant, "and that [men] should be tempted to expect, to be constantly managed as mere machines that know not their own use." Howe's insistence on the relative flexibility of the individual psychology is a conscious echoing of Boyle's denial that chemistry was a mere machine (Newton made a similar denial about physics). Nevertheless, it was equally unreasonable "to suppose that God should have barred out himself, from all inward access to the spirits of men." Instead, "divine government, over man, should be (as it is) mixed or composed of an external frame of laws ... and an internal effusion of power [sc. ability] ... which might animate the whole, and use it, as instrumental, to the begetting of correspondent impressions on men's [soul] spirits," thereby influencing physical motion and behaviour. Moreover, the necessity of God's grace is not instantaneous. It acts "*gradually*, and with an apt contemperation to the subject upon which it is designed to have its operations"; moreover it is "*constantly* put forth ... upon all, to that degree" (emphases in original), echoing Boyle's principle of constancy in nature. The topic is still, palpably, God's favour to the elect and their steady, ongoing sanctification. But as Flavell's self-conscious book title of 1681 shows, grace now has, or even is, a "method."[74] And what were once providential *instants* (regeneration, justification) in the life of the elect have become developmentally progressive *phases*.

Development in the elect soul aimed at an eventual perfection, at "being with Christ," as Howe puts it; and our present understanding of our own natures is that of an embryo by comparison with what it will be when we join the elect in heaven. This suggests a change of relation between ends and means. When means consisted in an entirely external or "effectual calling," as it did in the core texts of high Calvinist orthodoxy such as Perkins's, even infants dying at birth could be "inwardly, in a certain peculiar manner ... called, and justified, and glorified," as long as they were already elect.[75] Perkins too, though, had come to believe that there were "some certain means annexed" to this effectual calling, "which albeit they have no place in infants, by reason of their age, yet they belong to all other elect, howsoever they are found in some [adults] more plenteous and lively, and other some more slender and weak." In a sense, he was positing the idea of gradations within the elect state. A specifically intellectual gradation and development were subsequently inserted in this template (Calvin, and Perkins himself, would have been horrified). Moreover, space was created not only for individual differences but also for the concept of someone in whom "annexed" means never arrived: an infantile adult. Once means became defined mainly by the individual's reason later in the seventeenth century, a context arose in which the end is not to be with Christ but to be with Intelligence – an end achievable on this earth, following a process of intellectual maturation. In Richard Fenn's words, "If the Puritans had disenchanted the spiritual world of the medieval

---

[73] *The Reconcileableness*, 141 ff.
[74] Flavell, *The Method*.
[75] Perkins, *A Briefe Discourse*, 37.

church, divines like Baxter [and Howe] re-enchanted this world with the residues of heaven."[76] Modern intelligence as conceived by cognitive psychology and transhumanism is just such a re-enchantment – a spiritualized natural grace – and these divines were their direct ancestors.

We can trace the roots of this developmentalist tendency at least as far back as the educational policy recommendations of Lodowick Bryskett, a member of the Sidney circle. He calls human reason "the means to perfection," a temporal process in our life on earth; perfection is "so peculiar to reason, that not only unreasonable creatures can be no partakers thereof, but young children [and] ... the young man ... are excluded from the same." Adopting the terms of faculty psychology, he associates the vegetative soul with infancy, the sensitive soul with the concupiscence and irascibility of youth and with maturity the intellective soul "whereby we understand and make choice rather of one course of life than of another."[77] Catholicism had apportioned means to this life and ends to the next. The first Reformers brought ends and means closer: if the end of election is to be with Christ, the means of it is Christ within us. By 1660, the downturn in prospects for a Calvinist political establishment and the accompanying postponement of the kingdom of the saints had led to a renewed separation between means and ends, but with the ends now situated partly on this earth. And so middle-way preachers would write, in a way largely novel for the period, about a "*transition* [emphasis added] from the infant state to the age of discerning .... The first step to our cure is begun in the knowledge of our disease, and this discovery is made by the understanding when it is seeing and vigilant, not when it is blind" as it is in childhood.[78] The rational soul's supreme virtue, *contemplatio*, is no longer static and timeless but has become itself part of a veritable "economy of human nature," as Glanvill called it, a household management of the mind. It follows an inner journey, progressive and measurable (in this sense replacing Catholic doctrine about the stages of purgatory), as well as a physiological path around the body via the soul spirits and the circulation of the blood.[79]

The increased importance of human reasoning as intrinsic to faith and as a manifestation of grace was not merely the triumph of one particular doctrine. Many orthodox diehards had by now capitulated, accepting as *fait accompli* the elevation of reason and the upgrading of human nature. The fact that it found its way into the rival orthodoxies as well as the middle way points to a deeper cultural shift. The physical element of special or effective grace is now said to act "gradually with several steps," and by degrees that vary from one individual to another in proportion to the need to supplement their natural graces. The Calvinist notion of an individual response to grace has become "a real *internal* efficiency" (emphasis added), a necessity within the human subject himself.[80] William Lamont's *Richard Baxter of the Millennium* has shown us how after the decline of millenarian aspirations, in which the perfection of the elect was regarded as imminent, writers like Baxter channelled their energies into supervising the means to perfection instead, foreseeing a whole period in which people would need to continue developing their intellectual abilities. Locke's *Essay* continued this task, but with more focus on the concrete detail of the means. If Baxter and Locke differ, it is in their estimate of the pace at which perfection would arrive. Both held a doctrine of postponed intellectual perfection (which in some sense is what modern psychology's doctrine of child development is too). Neither envisaged the postponement as being that long. Howe, too, wrote on the assumption that "this world shall continue but a little while."

---

[76] Fenn, *The Persistence*, 81.
[77] Bryskett, *A Discourse*, 34.
[78] Bates, *The Whole Works*, i, 219.
[79] "Of the modern improvements of useful knowledge," 3; 5, in *Essays*.
[80] Flavell, *The Method*, 71; 73.

By the eighteenth century, predestination, espoused by Priestley as "necessitarianism," had made its peace with gradualist notions of progress. The arrival of a concept of psychological development coincides with the arrival of concepts of social and economic development. They all share a new emphasis on time over space, illustrated by their transformation of two core themes in metaphysics: microcosm and macrocosm, and potential and actual.

In medieval cosmology, the macrocosm-microcosm relationship between individual and society was spatial and static. There was debate about the development of the rational soul, but only in the foetus; once born, the soul was already complete. The concretization of purgatory as a space in the cosmos around 1200 had from the beginning contained a crude temporal element, as demonstrated by the selling of indulgences to reduce one's time there.[81] From the mid-seventeenth century onwards, macrocosm-microcosm turned into a relationship between individual development and societal progress; that is, it became temporal and progressive. Jacob's Ladder gave way to Pilgrim's Progress: to give it its full title, *The Pilgrim's Progress from This World to That Which Is to Come*. This temporal model creates the cut-off point we have already noted between cognitively complete human beings ("adults") and cognitively incomplete ones ("children"), and hence between proper adults and childlike (because cognitively incomplete) adults. A type is created who is unredeemable because he plateaus at a certain developmental point, provoking a social anxiety for which the old spatial model had not possessed any conceptual basis. The Puritan notion of "backwardness" is likewise transposed into a secular educational psychology.[82]

Secondly, and similarly, the key medieval distinction between "potential" and "actual" (active) human intellect was spatial: the latter had closer *proximity* to the divine intellect than the former. This has since given way to a temporal distinction, in which potential intellect precedes its actual performance. In this model the child has potential, the completed adult human has potential *and* actual intellect (the distinction between these two having been elided). And the childlike adult lacks both: if you cannot actually perform the extended catechism or its descendant, the developmental test, you obviously do not have potential in the first place.

"Trains of ideas": the intelligence gym

Time, once cyclical, now became linear and irreversible. The tempo of individual intellectual preparedness and development had to be calibrated with the tempi of everyday life, where rhythm (natural, fluctuating) was being replaced by pulse (calculated, regular) along with new practices in the division of labour.[83] Psychological and socio-economic development depend alike on the maturation of the individual's natural faculties. Bunyan's Pilgrim frets endlessly about making up for time lost on his journey. Regular development of the human understanding is a social obligation, says Baxter. And so, in the words of a fellow nonconformist around 1670, one has to "set a just value upon time, and consecrate it to those things that are preparatory for the future state of blessedness.... How should we redeem every hour, and live for heaven? .... The neglect of it for a day, is of infinite hazard."[84] Everybody, says Baxter, should set aside time each day for "heavenly thoughts." This was more than the standard daily self-contemplation recommended by earlier Puritans. The very idea of compartmentalizing time, its measurability and its commodification, belongs (as Weber pointed out in a related context) to a market culture. It is socially structured: meditation "will not

---

[81] Jacques le Goff, *The Birth of Europe*, 227.
[82] Baxter, *The Reduction of a Digressor*, 138.
[83] James Tully, *An Approach to Political Philosophy*, 245.
[84] Bates, *The Whole Works*, i, 103.

prove every man's duty" because "all cannot allow it the same time .... Such are most servants ... and many are so poor that the necessities of their families will deny them this freedom. I do not think it the duty of such, to leave their labours for this work, just at certain set times." Locke similarly developed the convention of exempting certain people in whom "the croaking of their own bellies" denies them the time to develop definitively human "abstract thoughts."

At the same time, what Baxter means by meditation reveals a shift from scholastic contemplativeness to something more like the "trains of ideas" which were the basis for Locke's model of logical reasoning and human identity. These basic units of rationality consist not in single syllogisms, where one or at most two mental leaps need to be made, but in whole sequences, extended in time and divisible into phases. Descartes had written of a chain or "order of cogitations," but its temporal aspect was concealed by the person's apparently intuiting the whole chain at once. Hobbes wrote about "trains of thought," importing from physics into psychology his billiard-ball analogies about the causes of movement. Baxter's preferred term was "methodical meditations," which should be in "right order, not wrong."[85] The 1670 Conventicles Act, banning even the smallest congregations of Nonconformists, was the last nail in the coffin of a church unity which both they and the Anglican hierarchy, each on their own terms, had continued to try and re-establish because without it a stable social order was inconceivable; it was a sign of final breakdown that the goal of "order" as previously conceived, now an impossibility for the nonconformists, became displaced from the ecclesiastical realm to the minds of individuals, and to the micro-processes of intellectual ability which Locke was to catalogue in the *Essay concerning Human Understanding*. "It is every man's duty," said Baxter, "to exercise his thoughts or meditations in the most clear, methodical, practical way that his abilities and opportunities ... will reach to." The psychological and socio-economic aspects of ability – development and opportunity – are not fully separable here. Both extend downwards through a class-based hierarchy of the cogitations (diluted as one descends) required for certain social and religious duties.

Even Baxter's friends baulked at the idea of a set, timed duty. It seemed to point reason in the direction of Hobbesian calculation, emphasizing achievable and assessable merit at the expense of the divine grace that comes only by visitation and "without measure," as Milton had put it in *Paradise Lost*. It also looked suspiciously like the Romanist idea of counting the hours in purgatory. (Baxter's reply was a typical shuffle: "We wait for his grace in the use of those means, which tend to prepare us.") Firmin had warned Baxter, as one might warn the IQ tester, "Let that which measures be able to contain the thing measured"; methodical meditations implied something like a Grace Quotient and smacked of the "spreading heresy" of Socinianism, which claimed there was nothing in religion that could not be understood by reason. He pointed out to Baxter the existence of "gifted" children, whose gifts of grace and regeneration have been bestowed on them regardless of any need for chronological maturity or systematic reasoned preparation. Baxter replies that although such children learn their catechism quickly, they do so by the same suspect skill of mimicry that reprobate hypocrites use: "They scarce understand the sense and matter of any of the plainest words which they have uttered. And we find it is just so with too many of the aged [sc. adult] also."[86] As with Locke, a reconstruction of childhood is implicated in the reconstruction of the adult out-group.

Preparedness as measured intellectual exercise was the curriculum path to salvation. It expanded to fill the time available, in proportion as immediate prospects for a rule of the saints receded. Baxter's first text focusing on "rule and pattern," a methodological concomitant to Locke's "trains of ideas," appeared in 1671 at the point where Locke was embarking upon the *Essay*. Both men

---

[85] *The Duty of Heavenly Meditation*, 4; 11; 19.
[86] Baxter, *The Cure of Church Divisions*, 320.

link order, uncorrupted human nature and understanding of the understanding in a novel relation dominated now by sequences and allocations of time. Many religious writers by this stage would have agreed with Baxter that "the light of nature is not contemptible," but he adds here the more radical claim that "if scripture had never spoke it, yet by the law of nature it had been a duty to do all things in *order* and to *edifying*." This model of orderly thinking "requireth that the understanding go first." In making personal destiny and perfectibility depend on method and intellectual preparation rather than instantly bestowed light, Baxter was putting nature (disposition and habit) at par with election (necessity and permanence) in estimating human value. Method and preparation belonged to a theory of identity based on the whole life rather than on a single instant of regeneration: "Men are to be judged godly or ungodly according to the ... operation of their souls, and the bent and courses of their lives, and not by a particular act: because no act will prove us holy indeed, but what proveth a habit; and a predominant habit."[87]

Alongside his repeated formula concerning the "*time* and *labour* ... necessary to maturity of knowledge" (emphasis in original), Baxter claims that religious knowledge can be acquired in the same way as mathematical or medical knowledge – except that it is not a training for some particular profession or calling but incumbent on everyone.[88] In this quasi-egalitarian shift, what has happened to election and reprobation? After the waning of millennial hopes in the 1650s, Baxter does reassess the doctrine, but in a quantitative rather than qualitative sense. Early on, Puritans such as Baxter assumed the elect to be very few. This was partly because they realized that a large number of the population resented them, with their snooping on everyday behaviour and their apparent harshness towards children, which lay people found shocking.[89] By the 1670s, Baxter's receding optimism about an immediate rule of the saints correlated with an increasing optimism about the numbers of the elect, so that he could write: "It's very probable that ... the number of the damned will be very small in comparison of the blessed." He hoped this might persuade melancholics to shed their despair, since it pointed to the falsity of claims that "God condemneth the great part of his intellectual creatures."[90]

The external, public face of internal trains of thought was their performance via the catechism. We have already discussed the changing role of the catechism, from a mere prompt to the means of verifying the evidence for election in this or that individual, and its extension down the social scale. Thus in some sense it was also a framework for assessing intellectual ability. As the role model for an entire generation of pastors, Baxter during the critical period of the 1650s is known to have gone systematically through his parish spending an hour with each family; he was also (like Locke) a physician, ministering to their integrated bodily and intellectual states. Anxious about families too poor to buy books, he solicited the charity of the local elite, as illustrated by the full title of his 1684 text *The Poor Man's Family Book: Teaching him How to Become a True Christian ... with a request to landlords and rich men to give to their tenants and poor neighbours either this or some fitter book*. This shelf-busting primer of daily religion is a one-sided dialogue between the effusive, regenerate Paul and the tongue-tied, struggling Saul. Poor Saul is already complaining on page 62 – he has another four hundred to go – "Alas, sir, when shall I ever be able to understand and remember all this?" Paul, alias Baxter, replies: "It is all but your common catechism ... a little opened," a crammer to test worthiness for membership of the company of the elect.

---

[87] Cited in Laurence Womock, *Arcana Dogmatum Anti-Remonstrantium*, 517.
[88] Baxter, *The Cure of Church Divisions*, 5.
[89] See Frank Luttmer, "Persecutors, tempters and vassals of the devil," *Journal of Ecclesiastical History*, 51/1 (2000).
[90] Baxter, *Gods Goodness, Vindicated*, 45; *Catholicke Theologie*, 1.2.368.

Trains of ideas became staple fare both in the philosophical psychology of David Hume and Thomas Reid and in the everyday culture. Popular religious writers like Watts, Edwards and John Wesley grasped the value of method. Watts, like the psychometricians, thought that any programme of preparation and training for the receipt of grace should consist mainly of mathematics, this being the best and most abstract example of "a perpetual chain of connected reasonings, wherein the following parts of the discourse are naturally and easily derived from those which go before."[91] Edwards recommended accountancy ledgers as a model for making lists and enumerations of "arguments," "evidences" and "proofs," which he calls the "practice" and "exercise of grace." The very act of practicing is itself "a sign of grace." If people do not do their daily practice, it is a sign they are reprobate; conversely, it is a work that is necessary *even if* we are already in receipt of grace. Grace itself was now, at least in part, experientally learnt; in this sense, one sanctified oneself. Calvin would not have been amused.

In the "exercise" of grace we find one of the deep roots of the modern psychology of intelligence. Much of the early state education curriculum in England has its origins in models provided by the Dissenting Academies, which provided men such as Watts and Priestley with their schooling. In this curriculum "your common catechism," designed to verify your sanctified state, opened wide enough to become a complex assessment of all things intellectual, secular as well as religious. It was meant to be extended to the lowest social classes, and to servants whose catechism had previously been "answered for" by their masters. It played a large part in the moral revolution of respectability in early Victorian Britain; a similar language appears in Walt Whitman's famous picture of American presidential democracy ("What Best I See in Thee"), in which the masses "were all so justified" as to be equal with Europe's feudal monarchs. The idea of grace as belonging to the elect alone was not jettisoned, it merely became politically incorrect. Election was sublimated within the idea that grace could exist in anyone, the price for this concession being to exclude from "anyone" those whose deficiency was reinterpreted along intellectual lines. The only proviso was that one worked at one's state of grace, with order and method.

In charity schools, teaching not just of morals but of literacy and the general curriculum was often done directly through the catechism, typically using *The ABC with the Catechism* which sold at least 25,000 copies per decade from the 1560s until the early eighteenth century.[92] Then came the famous *New England Primer*, launched in the year of Locke's *Essay* and at the core of the American school curriculum for the next two centuries, which bears a remarkably close resemblance to Baxter's *Poor Man's Family Book*. The first school inspectors emerged, around 1700, in the person of the local clergyman who would observe the teacher or do his own assessments of the children. The word became a general term for any short textbook or crammer, as in the nineteenth-century set of mass publications "Pinnock's Catechisms," which included *A Catechism of Arithmetic*, *A Catechism of Geometry* and so on, not to mention *A Catechism of Heraldry*. The first professionally administered psychological assessments and prototype intelligence tests in schools were not imported from some separate, already existing clinical setting or from beyond the educational sphere at all, but devised on the basis of early psychologists' observation of existing methods of classroom assessment, themselves derived from catechical routines. The practice of psychology thus precedes its pure theory.[93] And from very beginning there was a considerable focus on tackling the moral/intellectual degradation of those repeatedly described as having the "weakest" and "meanest capacities" or, if you prefer, on disciplining the underclass.

---

[91] Watts, *The Improvement*, 150; Edwards, *A Treatise*, 334.
[92] Green, *The Christian's ABC*, 53; 173; 558 ff.
[93] Theodore Porter, *Trust in Numbers*, 209.

In France, similarly, a line extends from the Jansenists' doctrine of election and reprobation through to the deified reason of the Jacobins and to the psychiatry of Philippe Pinel and Jean-Etienne Esquirol, who were major contributors to nineteenth-century theories of idiotism. The Jesuits too wrote of the "sacred science of the catechism," though in an inclusive way that covered "those that do not have the use of reason," and tried to replace imitation and memorizing with a technique that might "instill intelligence" (*intelligence*).[94] Revolutionaries rewrote the catechism to suit a quasi-egalitarian national honour (for example "What is baptism?" "It is the regeneration of the entire French people begun on July 14, 1789"), and to inculcate civic duty.[95] Condorcet, tasked by the revolution with setting up a state education system, insisted that catechical routines should also be used to inform a secular and neutral intellectual training. In fact a "catechism of human reason" had already been employed for some while in the primary school curriculum generally, and during the revolution it was central to the setting up of the Lockean-inspired *écoles normales*.[96] It is in this national context that we need to situate Binet's mental age tests, which arose from the needs of the French state education system as it closed the church schools a century later. Further investigation might well be able to track a continuity, via a change of terms, from reprobation to mental defectiveness.

The Calvinists above all among Protestants discovered in the catechism a substitute for the Catholic mass as the way of identifying value within the individual, and of enhancing that value with intellectual means. At least it seemed an improvement on mumbling some uncomprehended Latin.[97] But it also assumed a different kind of human personality: one that can develop towards a goal of perfection in this world, religious at first and then (from the mid-nineteenth century onwards) secular. Our prospective intelligence is there, just ahead of us, to hold our hands in the dark night of the soul. The catechism and its successors reconfigured the out-group too. "Intellectual disability" can be seen as an adaptation of testing and segregating practices that date from as far back as the early church, which feared its holy ritual being polluted by incompetent catechumens. But while this points to a historical continuity of method, there have been major discontinuities in the way we conceive who is to be kept out. As one seventeenth-century theologian put it, what defines certain people as "ignorant" is that "they do not in a due manner understand and comprehend the doctrines of the gospel; and so perish for want of knowledge."[98] Who more precisely the ignorant may have been, and the manner of their perishing – soteriological and social – are questions to which we now turn.

---

[94] Henri-Marie Boudon, *La science sacrée du catéchisme*, 43.
[95] Patrice Higonnet, *Goodness beyond Virtue*, 310 ff.
[96] Velicu, *Civic Catechisms*, 34.
[97] Motley, *Becoming a French Aristocrat*, 55.
[98] Owen, "The nature and causes of apostasy from the gospel," in *Works*, vii, 133.

Chapter 11
The Science of Damnation: from Reprobate to Idiot

Claims to grace, like those to honour or intelligence, depend on the existence of an out-group. There must be some people not qualified even to advance a claim in the first place. In respect of grace it is the reprobate who fill this role, and we examine now the historical transition from concepts of reprobation to modern ones of intellectual disability. The characteristics of grace do not at first sight overlap with those of honour and social rank. For one thing, all the divisive talk about election and reprobation sits side-by-side with an equally fundamental hypothesis of creaturely equality. In the honour mode, the idea that everyone of whatever social rank has his own smattering of honour was either a routine piety, easily ignored or more often flatly denied. But the idea that God created each individual human soul, and that – since He could not be the author of imperfection – all souls were equally divine, ran throughout Christianity, Calvinist and Jansenist included. Sir Thomas Browne, writing in the early 1640s, thought the difference between himself and a beggar was "accidental." He could not "forget that common and untouched part of us both: there is under these … miserable outsides … a soul of the same alloy with our own … and in as fair a way to salvation as our selves." And conversely, the Fall affects everyone: "We all are monsters."[1] Counterbalancing this sense of equality, however, the elect-reprobate divide rested on a decision made before the beginning of human history or time itself. God, the great cognitive geneticist in the sky, has already decided who is to be saved and who not.

"The natural weakness of their brains": labourers, women, melancholics

One dealt with this contradiction by studied avoidance. It was, said Browne, "folly in man … to pry into the maze of [God's] counsels." Even angels were not allowed to know. Nevertheless, the curiosity of pastors, those psychotherapist-guardians of private behaviour, led them to suspect they knew who were the "visible saints" and who not. And there was a tendency, if no more than that, to demonize as reprobate the usual crowd: labourers, servants, women. The revolutionary ferment of the 1640s in England spawned increasing horror at the multitude's "grace-destroying and land-destroying opinions."[2] Correspondingly, the fit between the company of the elect and the honour society could often be seamless. The Anglican church, even when it inclined towards Calvinism, was also the honour society in one of the latter's particular manifestations. Usually doctrinal contradiction was avoided by restating it as a mere contrast, between the posthumous equality of souls and the earthly social divide, so that the same Browne who put his own rational soul at par with a beggar's continued in the same breath:

> If there be any among those common objects of hatred I do condemn and laugh at, it is that great enemy of reason, virtue and religion, the multitude …. One great beast, and a monstrosity more prodigious than Hydra. It is no breach of charity to call these *fools*.

---

[1] Browne, *Religio*, 81; 67.
[2] Cited in Hill, *The Intellectual Origins*, 341.

Admittedly, he qualifies this by saying that he does not mean here "only ... the base and minor sort of people," and that conversely there may even be "a nobility without heraldry, a natural dignity." Yet the masses set the tone. The "rabble [that is] even amongst the gentry" have an over-active imaginative faculty that puts them at "the same level with mechanics."[3]

In terms of establishing an out-group, then, reprobation broadened the criteria of disgust but did not always denote a different class profile. Early sixteenth-century Reformers like Zwingli, especially in the humanist urban milieux in which they operated, routinely despised the stupidity of the countryside they had left, either as sons of peasants themselves or of undistinguished country gentry tainted by proximity to the soil; their own bids for religious status relied directly on their contempt for the residual poor peasant and his absence of both grace and intellect. The low-born Bunyan's autodidactic search for a higher "calling," at once social and religious, led him in *Grace Abounding* and *The Pilgrim's Progress* to chart the path to self-improvement. Conversely, those born to high social status whom economic chaos had forced downwards doubted and despaired of their elect status. If the world was against you, so was God: hence the search for a religious calling to validate your status, in place of the social one from which you had fallen.[4]

Prior to the 1590s the word "idiot" applied to grace similarly as to honour: it signified a lay person, inexpert in the knowledge appropriate to that mode. According to Bullinger, God "did not choose learned men but simple and idiots to be his apostles." He feels bound to add that by this he does not mean "fools and dizzards, which be indeed ignorant in all manner of things .... He is called a simple man, not he that is without wit, without reason and wisdom, but he which is plain and sincere ... else it would come to pass, that every man should defend his error by ignorance" (the "ignorance" of the fool suggests Romanism).[5] The decisive distance of *both* the fool/dizzard *and* the plain or simple idiot from our modern disabled person is clear. In any case, the labels were multivocal for contemporaries too, since "idiot" could also sometimes be used to denote the Catholic idolater.[6] And even where it does signify the virtuously unlearned, its negative psychological connotations in respect of the person's social class remain clear. For example, Bullinger says he wants his thoughts "to be perceived [not] only by the wit and true judgment of learned heads, but also to be seen as it were with the eyes, and handled as it were with the hands, of very idiots and unlearned hearers."[7] The superior, internal senses – wit and the faculty of judgement – belong with the common ideas and therefore with the honour society, while the inferior, external senses – the eyes (proxy for the imaginative faculty) and the hands that do manual labour – are associated with idiots, however virtuous. Catholic idiocy was the abuse of an education, class idiocy the lack of it.

The inferior social ranks were considered particularly prone to melancholy, a symptom of mental weakness ("imbecility") especially when manifested in a lack of assurance about one's salvation. The same was true of women of whatever rank. Melancholia, the paradigm of problematic mental states, is depicted in art sometimes as menial, sometimes as female (often a witch). Initially it was fast or slow, clever or foolish, restless or pensive. Then in Protestantism, where faith was seen as a mental activity, pensiveness came to suggest salaciousness (Cranach's *Allegory of Melancholy* depicts her as the tempted Eve), and melancholia acquired the sense of sloth as opposed to mania – a position later to be occupied by idiocy as opposed to madness. When Baxter describes labourers and idiots as being at the bottom end of his hierarchy of "ability and opportunity," he illustrates this

---

[3] Browne, *Religio*, 66.
[4] See John Stachniewski, *The Persecutory Imagination*.
[5] Bullinger, *Antidotus against the Anabaptists*, F2v.
[6] See Peacham, *The Art of Drawing with the Pen*.
[7] Bullinger, *Decades*, ii, Introduction.

with characteristics of the old melancholia paradigm. To lack the ability to form trains of thought, he said, is to be "disabled by melancholy and other weakness of brain." Such people should avoid overzealous mental training regimes. He urges "most women and all melancholy persons, to take up more with shorter and occasional meditations ... and not to over-stretch their brains, by striving to do more than they are able, and so disable themselves yet more." Women, because of the "natural weakness of their brains, and the strength of their passions, are unable to endure ... serious deep affecting apprehensions." Royal Society members such as Glanvill recommended "real, experimental philosophy" as the cure for "effeminate fears" and for developing a "strong and manly temperament."[8]

Order had always, since Plato, been the supreme value in intellectual activity. The classic image is Dürer's 1514 *St Jerome in his Study*, whose ordered state is neither laborious nor fast but contemplative and timeless; *Melencolia*, in the engraving usually paired with it, is a slothful female figure sprawled amidst a chaos of unrelated activities. Baxter's order, however, is now temporal rather than spatial. Timed regularity was a therapy for the universal disability of the Fall, a cure (in Baxter's medical language) for the "lazy humour." The profitable *suspension* of time which medieval psychology sought in human reason, re-emerged in the Protestant ethic as profitable *use* of time. The contemplation that by definition was timeless might now be criticized as slothful and lazy. It led melancholics to excesses of repentance, to despair of their elect status and as a result to become "unreasonable, and useless." When Baxter says "to be deprived of the use of reason, is a ... dishonour to the Gospel," it is melancholy he is talking about. The cure is for people to be up and doing, in "a lawful calling" – though this advice was somewhat rich coming from a writer who had spent a lifetime dabbling in "furious curiosity, needless speculation, fruitless meditation about election, reprobation, free will, grace," and thereby helping to stoke up more melancholy.[9]

Children and childlike adults

The reconstruction of childhood, along with the invention of the childlike adult discussed earlier, is a prominent feature of the disputes about grace. One might think that the idea of a childlike adult came from the Anabaptists. After all, it was they who made competence an age-related issue by insisting that only adults be baptized: "Infants do not have the ability to hear, they cannot believe, and because they do not believe, they cannot be born again."[10] Nevertheless, the Anabaptists did not ask whether there might be adults who lack this ability. That is because the ability they had in mind was not a development at all, but an instantaneous regeneration; it was this that could not occur in childhood. Moreover the anomalous adult was not an intellectual defective but one who "walks still in the unclean, ungodly lusts of the flesh.... Where there is no renewing, regenerating faith ... there is no baptism." Anabaptists, unlike the modern psychologist, were still at the stage where, as they put it, "What is meant by 'children'?" was an open-ended question. The Bible, they said, speaks of children in many different ways.[11]

Baxter on the other hand, to be followed by Locke, defined adults in this context as "Men of years that be not idiots." He has to create the disabled identity (men of years that *be* idiots) in order to set a boundary to the category of those able to "grow in grace," their understanding

---

[8] Baxter, *Directions and Perswasions*, 161; Glanvill, "The usefulness of real philosophy to religion," 14, in *Essays*.
[9] Baxter, *Gods Goodness*, 7; Burton, *The Anatomy*, iii, 421.
[10] Menno Simons, *The Complete Writings*, 131.
[11] John Spilsbery, *A Treatise concerning the Lawfull Subject of Baptism*, 2; 10.

being something that grows in the process. With Baxter, the term "idiot" thereby came to denote childhood extended beyond a chronologically inappropriate age. The concept of a *retarded* adult cannot exist without that of psychological *development*; it is what allows the World Health Organization, for example, to define mental retardation as "a state of arrested or incomplete development of mind." But also, without the childlike adult, the real man of modern intelligence and rational autonomy could not exist. Furthermore, we cannot have childlike adults without first having modern "children." Youth had formerly been a loose category, defining anyone who had not yet inherited his father's property. Conversely, creaturely equality was often attributed to children; "the circumstance of age is a thing altogether impertinent," since the spark of regeneration could come at any point in life.[12] But the Puritan notion that the human personality is a unity formed over a whole lifetime, together with that of "preparedness," gradually helped to turn religious status into a matter of chronological age and maturity. Some writers could see where all this was heading, like the critic of Baxter who complained that he "seems to make infants a distinct species."[13]

Deficiencies of grace in adults had always been described as a form of childhood: "naturally we are all children of darkness," just as spiritually we are children of the "immortal God" and politically of what Hobbes called the "mortal God," the state. If only in this very broad sense "children of years" often had "children of understanding" bracketed with them.[14] But the gradually sharper conceptual separation of the child, and of pathologically conceived childlike adults, were to play formative roles in the creation of modern intelligence. In this separation, not only is an idiot a chronologically inappropriate child, a child is a chronologically provisional idiot. (Piaget's "mental logic," for example, seems to be defined as whatever does not occur in children.) Anabaptists were accused of asking, "How can infants get good by baptism, when they have not the use of reason?" and although these were in fact straw Anabaptists (real ones were interested in children's faith, not their reason), we can detect here a growing general anxiety.[15] The old defining property "man is a rational animal" was at crisis point. The new reason was more a property of aggregated individuals than of some overall species entity. The disappearance of the ancient formula's protective shield over deviations and deficiencies, which were mere "accidents" of matter and did not detract from the form or essence of being human, opened the way to *comparing* and *ranking* those individuals by a developmental principle: how far (if at all) along the road to perfection is this one as opposed to that? Anxiety on this score affected children and childlike adults in the same way.

With these chronological approaches to personality there came also a complete reworking of the idea of the capable subject. In Aristotle there was a huge metaphysical gulf between *having* a capability like reason and *using* it; the first of these was ascribed to the human subject *qua* human and implicitly included children, while the latter related to one's social function. Theories of development have muscled aside this distinction between having and using. Use now results directly from and indicates possession; hence the often-heard parental desire for children to "fulfill their potential." Reformation theology took the old capable subject, which had notionally covered the whole species, and restricted it to the elect, to "subjects capable of glory." At the same time, the distinction between spiritual and natural intelligence was starting to evaporate, with the capable subject being redesignated as capable not only of glory but also of reason, and moreover of *developing* that reason as the *means* to glory. These shifts rendered the formula less universal than Aristotle's.

---

[12] Womock, *Arcana*, 405.
[13] John Tombes, *Anti-paedobaptism*, 199.
[14] Pemble, *Workes*, 529; Green, *The Christian's ABC*, 255.
[15] Thomas Hooker, *The Covenant of Grace Opened*, 11.

They also cast doubt on the religious status of children. When the blessed Governor of Connecticut in the 1640s included "both men of years and children" under the heading of "subjects capable" of his godly commonwealth, by the very act of putting them on the same developmental plane he was emphasizing the contrast between them. "Children are capable of baptism, men of years of the supper .... To make a person capable of the supper of the Lord, a man must be able to examine himself; he must not only have grace, but *growth* of grace: he must have so much perfection in grace, as to search his own heart" (emphasis added). What is required is a developed intellectual grasp of eucharistic metaphor, as opposed to a static and idolatrous gawping.[16] Furthermore "growth," as a drawn-out internal and rational process, has the potential to solve the problem of whether pagans can be elect. By "subjects capable" of profiting from communion, says the Governor, "I speak of men of years; because if any blackamoors, or of other nations should come and offer themselves, they must be thus admitted." In short, they should be assumed to be already hypothetically regenerate – unlike children.

In this proto-developmentalist doctrine, the child – half-capable and incomplete, just like the individual adult who constantly grows in grace – was a microcosm of the wider society that was just then emerging from "the infancy of the world itself."[17] Reprobates are those who fail to participate in this otherwise universally human development. They too are a type of childlike adult. The idiots Locke cites in his second *Treatise of Civil Government* are, like reprobates, in a state of permanent infancy. They are disabled from joining the next stage of universal human history that Locke was projecting out of biblical history here, or – which amounts to the same thing – from contributing to the progressive accumulation of knowledge. If the political part of Locke's script was already suggested by the Levellers, its psychological part was suggested by the altogether more establishment figure of Hooker, who in the 1590s had envisaged that in future "if there might be added the right helps of true art and learning ... there would undoubtedly be almost as much difference in maturity of judgement between men therewith inured, and that which now men are, as between men that are now, and innocents" ("innocence" implying both childhood and disability). So too Bacon, who had made Kantian predictions about "the understanding [being] emancipated – having come, so to speak, of age."[18]

Could children, then, belong to the company of the elect? Regardless of whether grace were instantaneous or developmental, the question remained: what happens to people who die before their religious status is confirmed? The problem was that although status is determined before birth, regeneration and the infusion of God-given grace can only occur at some point in the actual life of an individual. There were several possible answers. One was to assume, as Zwingli did, that *all* children who die in infancy, pagan or Christian, go to heaven. Anything else would be unfair: "children because they are children" are elect. That is because they have not yet had a chance to sin, or to reason about "eternal rewards and punishments."[19] For the stronger predestinarian, it was the other way round. Having no faith, children are saved only if elect. "They must be *capable* of grace, or they are not elected" (emphasis added).[20] The language is deterministic and psychogenetic: "some infants have faith and repentance seminally" while others have "unbelief and impenitency seminally."[21] It was also possible that *no* infant dying before baptism is saved. Gomarus, whose doctrinal duel with Arminius had provoked the split at the Synod of Dort, claimed that all such

---

[16] Ibid., 21.
[17] John Cotton, *The Grounds and Ends of the Baptisme of the Children of the Faithfull*, 13.
[18] Richard Hooker, *The Lawes of Ecclesiastical Politie*, 4.17; Bacon, *Works*, iv, 247.
[19] Owen, *Of Infant Baptism and Dipping*, 8.
[20] Spilsbery, cited in Thomas Hooker, *The Covenant*, 24.
[21] Firmin, cited in Grantham, *The Infants*, 27.

children are dead in hell because they have not had access to the means to grace, earning him the sobriquet "Dr Fry-Babe."

It was the middle-way writers who once again came up with the necessary ramifications. One of their answers was that as long as the child is elect in the first place, God performs the appropriate subjective and internal operations on the child's behalf, since "infants do not ... nor cannot exercise their understanding, ... therefore all such power upon their actual apprehensions, signification, taking, and working, of abilities of their own, it is only to men of years, it is beyond the rank and order of infants, and the means cannot work in this regard."[22] The author does not say that children do not *possess* understanding, only that they cannot *exercise* it: its objective foundation is already imputed to them. If they die early, the requirement for them to grow is waived. At death, God puts into elect infants, directly, the faith and spirit which the living and regenerate only acquire as adults. Another answer was to consider parents as proxies for their children – a kind of religious genealogy, in imitation of the honour mode: "as the children are brought into covenant by a parental right and not a personal, so ... all infants, may be imputatively called believers."[23] Their parents had to be "visible church-members," i.e., those whom one could at least guess might be elect.

The problem of whether idiots are among the elect first arises out of this controversy about whether children are. Catholic doctrine consigned dead infants to limbo. The *limbus infantium* at some stage became an entire *limbus fatuorum* (the original of our "fools' paradise"). Arminians, using Noah's Ark as their allegory, pointed out that not everyone who drowned would yet have sinned, and so "all in this flood who perished being infants or in childhood or natural idiots or the like, passed through ... to eternal felicity."[24] Idiots and children here are default members of the elect. However, the increasing status of human reasoning required more elaborate explanations. The widely read middle-way theologian William Pemble claimed that adults are "called both inwardly by the work of the spirit, and outwardly by the voice of the word .... Now a voice presupposing ears to hear, and an understanding to perceive, infants cannot properly be said to be called by any such voice." In children, God bypasses the need for faith, and "this which hath been said of infants may be also applied to ... deaf or fools, having such natural defects as make them uncapable." If infants sometimes prove to be elect, so then may idiots.[25]

But Pemble also thinks that individuals vary in the ability of their understandings to respond to grace. This differentiation by degree starts to compromise the stark black-and-white necessities of predestination. It interpolates faculty psychology into the mode of grace, attributing to the corruptible, "sensitive" soul and its faculties a role in the achievement of perfection that had previously belonged only to the soul's immortal part:

> You must put a difference between men's abilities .... All men are not alike qualified with inward abilities; there is not the same fastness of memory, quickness of apprehension, soundness of judgement in one, that is in another, nor have all the like benefit of outward helps in their education, for the perfecting of such good parts as nature hath lent them .... Where [God] gives little, there he requires but little. He that naturally is slow of wit, dull of concept, short of memory, weak in judgement, such a one would be pitied and lovingly helped forward, so far in knowledge as his weakness will give leave.

And so, in exactly this context, Pemble recommends barring from the eucharist "all such as through natural or casual impotency are not able to examine themselves: as children, fools, madmen,"

---

[22] Thomas Hooker, *The Covenant*, 26.
[23] Baxter, *The Duty of Heavenly Meditation*, 240.
[24] Duke, *The Fulness*, 55.
[25] Pemble, *Workes*, 34.

regardless of whether they are elect. It is characteristic of such doctrines, as indeed it is of modern intelligence measurement, that difference by degree (the "slow" and "dull") and a hypothetical difference in kind (the "idiot") are co-dependent.

In Pemble's "idiots" and "fools" we should note the continuing dominance of the melancholia paradigm, in which a central symptom is the doubt of the "weak Christian" about his elect status. Moreover there are "many a hundred [who] can show wit enough in other matters, and have all abilities of mind to serve their turn in inferior employments, to apprehend, discourse, plot and contrive matters as they list," yet who in religious matters are "as much the better for all, as the pillars of the church against which they lean ... [and] very children in all Godly knowledge." There is no clear category boundary between these people and those "born stark naturals or idiots," and the association between the two categories carries no satirical undertones.

Intellectual disability and the psychology of reprobation

Reprobation was defined as a "disability to supernatural good."[26] Did this mean that all the non-elect were bound for hell as surely as the elect for heaven? The harsh logic was often fudged. "Single" predestinarianism, in which election was sure but reprobation unsure, was widespread. When Baxter expressed anxiety about non-elect souls, it was because he thought he could improve them. Fudging had in fact been the norm among the doctrine's originators. Augustine had simply said of the non-elect that God abandons them, leaving them to experience the consequences of their own sin. Calvin went further and said, if only in passing, that "God has once for all determined both whom he would admit to salvation and whom he would condemn to destruction." Christ's atoning sacrifice was "sufficient" for all, but "efficient" or "effective" only for the elect.[27] Reprobation was chiefly a useful scare story designed to humble believers and remind them of the limitations of their own reasoning abilities, but it was not central even for Calvin.

It was certain second- and third-generation Reformers who asserted that anyone not bound for heaven was bound, by an equally determinate decree, for the other place: that election and reprobation were symmetrical. Even then, they often distinguished between those who are called but relapse and those not called in the first place. By Perkins's time the doctrine had become a systematic "double" predestination, supported by the rise of new forms of logic that had strictly dichotomous approaches to classification. It was as fierce a science of damnation as modern psychology's doctrine of intellectual disability. Many preachers felt uneasy about making reprobation as certain as election, but few denied reprobation as such. Just as the honour elite did not stand in simple opposition to the undifferentiated whole of the *communitas* but rose organically within it like cream to the top of the milk, so the elect belonged to a whole reprobate species and were simply the ones who had been let off. Single predestinarians assumed that once baptized, you were also elect; only if you rejected the covenant later or failed to stick to its conditions might your essential reprobation be revealed. They allowed room for dealings between man and God and for the individual to connive somehow at his own destiny. Double predestination, on the other hand, was unchangeable.

Short of obvious external signs such as sleeping through a sermon, what was the reprobate's internal psychology? The central ingredient of reprobation is hypocrisy, and its companion mimicry. A hypocrite is someone who repeats the words of the ritual but does not feel or understand them. Parrots are the recurring image of repetition, while the garrulousness is borrowed from the social

---

[26] Bates, *The Whole Works*, i, 226.
[27] Calvin, *Institutiones*, in *Opera*, i, 861.

role of the occupational jester: "The prating parrot that licentiously thus speaketh ... is always like the fool, a consonant when he should be a mute: and a mute when he should be a consonant."[28]

Pastors wanted to know whether Christ was present, if not in the bread and wine, then in those at the altar rail. If they were secretly leading wicked lives, they were to avoid communing. The scrutiny of such people exhibits a balance and interpenetration between moral and intellectual elements. The Westminster Assembly, which the English parliament convened in 1643 to plan a role in government for the church, allowed people to be excluded for pure "brutal ignorance" as well as their sins, though the relationship between ignorance and hypocrisy was close and sometimes the former is a secondary aspect of the latter.[29] One of the Assembly's core tasks was to establish strict criteria for the public identification of those to be excluded from communion. People who see in grace, honour or indeed intelligence the one lifeboat that can rescue them from drowning in a sea of nonentity will do their utmost to beat off those clutching at the sides. Guarding against pollution from reprobates was, explicitly, more important than reassuring the elect: "We say that the elect alone may be, and indeed are, sure of election, that so we may exclude the reprobate hypocrites," as Perkins had put it.[30] "Reprobate" translated a New Testament word (*adokimos*) that meant not just unworthy but unexamined. The disability entailed in hypocrisy, therefore, was lack of sound examination of the inner self, as much as conscious pretence. As one of the Westminster divines put it, "Let King Solomon be the interpreter, who, everywhere, by a *fool*, understands a *wicked and reprobate* person" in communication with Satan (emphasis in original).[31] He also had pre-natal diagnosis up his sleeve: the reprobate foetus could sin in the womb like Esau, Jacob's reprobate twin who "unreasonably kicked and punched in the womb of his mother, beyond the rate of ordinary infants."

Calvin had originally said that *all* human minds are in a state of "dullness ..., sunk in stupidity and destitute of understanding." Human reasoning is itself a disability, and "it is not merely from the intrinsic insufficiency of wealth, honours, or pleasures to confer true happiness that the psalmist proves the misery of worldly men, but from their manifest and total incapacity of forming a correct judgement of such possessions." Disablement from grace manifests itself in an excess pride, deviating from the mean just as it does in the honour mode: "we are erected into a stupid and empty confidence" about our ability to achieve immortality by pulling on our own boot-straps.[32] The specific characteristics of the reprobate's disability show it to be part of a long-term history of practices surrounding defilement and pollution, social segregation and incurability, that overlap with modern eugenic ones about intelligence. According to the character type of the reprobate, "His wit is always in a maze, for his courses are ever out of order; and while his will stands for his wisdom, the best that falls out of him is a fool." Like Galton's feeble-minded who cause general regression to the mean, he is dangerous because "he marreth the wits of the wise, and is hateful to the souls of the gracious .... He is an inhuman creature, a fearful companion, a man-monster." Not only is he "born for the service of the devil," he is "a devil incarnate" himself.[33] The solution is obvious: "They which being taught and admonished will not amend: to let them be made known to the whole congregation openly, and separated from the holy assemblies and from conversation with the other faithful, least by their contagion others should also be infected."[34]

---

[28] Thomas Walkington, *The Optick Glasse of Humors*, Foreword.
[29] Westminster Assembly, 20 October 1645, 791.
[30] Perkins, *A Briefe Discourse*, 19.
[31] John Lightfoot, "Matthew, Chapter 5," in *Hebrew and Talmudical Exercitations upon the Gospels*.
[32] Perkins, *Workes*, i, 109.
[33] Breton, *The Goode and the Badde*, 35, in S. Brydges (ed.) *Archaica*, i.
[34] Zanchius, *Confession*, 32.

The fact that the human understanding was assuming a more active role in grace might seem to exclude most plebeians from the company of the elect, since they lacked the common ideas and so any ability for abstraction or logical reasoning (which in any case, as psychological phenomena, were largely restricted to religious matters). The political movements of commoners grasped this; it led them either to interpret their lack of social status in this life as a sure sign of their elect status in the next (the Anabaptists), or to reject predestination outright and espouse Pelagian-style free will and social mobility (the Levellers). In theory, however, reprobation was classless. Creaturely equality was equality of sinfulness. God "estated all mankind alike" with its original damnation, as "a company of lost men." Just as he is not the author of the sins of this or that individual, so in the act of justification he removes a "general, imputed guilt" rather than actual sins. *Everyone* is born reprobate, but *anyone* can be earmarked for salvation. God has singled out a few; for example, He gives faith, in the form of an ability to perform miracles or "the gift of prophecy, [to] some doctors."[35] But these special cases are a mere token, to demonstrate the existence of grace; he does not elect learned men especially.

Special, token cases can be found at the bottom end of the scale too, in the form of a divinely and purposely created deficiency. A good example is the *moriones* mentioned by Augustine. I leave the word in Latin to highlight the foreignness of the concept, since it has sometimes been mistakenly used as evidence for the existence of a modern type of intellectually disabled person in ancient history. (Paul Cranefield's standard English translation of the relevant text entitles it "The case of certain idiots and simpletons," but this mock-archaic heading is Cranefield's own.)[36] Augustine describes *moriones* as "fatuous," "little different from beasts." Again, we have to ascertain what exactly the fatuity consists of, their actual psychological characteristics. They display nothing like a modern, "intellectual" disability. In fact Augustine explicitly says that he is not talking here about those who are "stupid" (*stulti*) or slow of wit: "that is said of others." Their chief psychological characteristics are inappropriate social behaviour and a penchant for dressing up, both of which are drawn from the household jester whose deliberate foolery enhanced the honour of his supposedly wise master because of its entertainment value for guests. In Augustine's Rome that was what the word *morio* meant, its normal usage.

Augustine's *moriones* too have a "vocation," albeit a "wondrous" one: they are here for the higher purposes of assisting in doctrinal dispute. One such purpose is to refute the transmigration of souls: the idea that human intellects vary because of sins committed in a previous life was nonsense, since no one can have behaved so badly as to end up being a *morio*. A second is to challenge the Pelagian view that earthly abilities improve one's chances of salvation: if that were true, one would not come across *moriones* who, though lacking abilities, seem as if they might be elect, such as the one Augustine knew who could not bear hearing Christ's name abused. A third purpose is to rebut the doctrine that children are innocent: they are not, and so we should not laugh at childish misbehaviour any more than we should at the behaviour of *moriones*. Finally, he uses *moriones* to assert the spuriousness of all claims to infallibility: Cicero, for example, claimed never to have said anything in his life to cause him shame or dishonour, and if it would be absurd to hear a *morio* say such a thing, how much more absurd a supposedly wise man.

Calvin took up Augustine's *moriones* in this general sense, as an instructive and divinely appointed special case. However, he recast them as people lacking natural graces of any kind. Each natural grace corresponds with an earthly vocation; *moriones* lack any vocation, even Augustine's "wondrous" one. Instead, as Watts was later to put it, God has created them to remind the rest of us "to derive lessons of thankfulness to God" for our own natural graces: there but for the grace of

---

[35] Duke, *The Fulness*, 47; Flavell, *The Method*, 568.
[36] In J.-P.Migne, *Patrologiae*, xliv, 127; xxxiii, 728; iii, 143.

God go I.[37] Calvin's creatures are deficient in morals and manners, but they are not reprobate. They may lack natural graces, but what reprobates lack is special, saving grace. Indeed, one clear sign of reprobation is the claim to be above *moriones*, to which one must reply "Whosoever shall say thou fool, shall be in danger of hellfire." To claim superiority is to express a total confidence in one's own state of grace and understanding, and this is not only a moral error but an intellectual one, stemming as it does from "Adam's tree of knowledge" which "made him and his posterity fools."[38]

Ambivalence about the relationship between election/reprobation and human reasoning occurs also in covenant theology, which was popular across doctrines. Borrowed from jurisprudence and the law of contract, the idea of a covenant between God and man threw up ideas that were compatible *both* with the emerging value placed on human reasoning *and* with a strongly necessitarian position on grace. In *The Pilgrim's Progress* Mr Feeble-Mind (the name is significant, though the substance not at all modern) "was true of heart, though weak in grace": his initial gift of grace is small, but he works at his side of the bargain. According to Bunyan,

> Eternal reprobation makes no man a sinner .... Not God but sin hath made him unreasonable; without which, reasonable terms had done his work for him: for reasonable terms are the most equal and righteous terms that can be propounded between parties at difference; yea, the terms that most suiteth and agreeth with a reasonable creature, such as man .... Here lieth the point between God and the reprobate .... God is willing to save him upon reasonable terms, but not upon terms above reason; but no reasonable terms will [go] down with the reprobate, therefore he must perish for his unreasonableness.[39]

Although reason and lack of it are still expressed here in terms of a universal contract rather than of individual psychology, the latter nevertheless plays a part. Grace does not originate from individual abilities (hence the possibility that an idiot may be elect), but the insertion of legal terms helps to introduce an element of *non compos mentis* into reprobation.

This threatening, psychological-cum-legal unreason of the individual reprobate was part of a tighter classification of reprobate types, which encouraged the infiltration of elements of necessity into the individual's nature. A reprobate, for example a covert Romanist whose "stupidity lies in titles and images," may have a recidivist "nature" or "disposition" which is set and cannot be "forced" to change.[40] To begin with there had simply been "resistance to grace." Middle-way theologians then began to insert a quasi-necessitarian component within what they still viewed as natural, that is dispositional, characteristics. At the root of this increasing rigidity of definition lay anxiety about pollution of the in-group and its rituals by people who "dote upon carnal outward ceremoniousness."[41] Pemble divides "the stupidity of [the] many" into "either popish or clownish." In the latter case, there was an enemy within: "ignorant Protestants, of whom there be thousands that understand nothing at all." What they do not understand is the complex symbolism of the eucharist. They come to communion "because they are now at years of discretion and must do as others do. But ... examine them, they cannot tell you what a sacrament is, what the outward signs are, what the graces thereby signified are .... They understand you no more than if you spoke in an unknown language." They *think* themselves capable of grace, since "they will scorn to be questioned" – a characteristic, noted in Chapter 5, of all three of our self-referential in-groups.

---

[37] *The Improvement*, 36.
[38] Thomas Brooks, *A Golden Key*, 168.
[39] *Reprobation Asserted*, 34.
[40] Brathwait, *The English Gentleman*, 59.
[41] Bates, *The Whole Works*, iii, 206; Pemble, *Workes*, 495 ff.

However, they have "a disability in [the] understanding." Just ask them about "common points in catechism and mark their answers; you shall see them ... so hack and hew at it, that you may almost swear they speak they know not what ... though they be the wisest and craftiest headed men in a parish ... in other matters." What partly defines hypocrisy is thinking that the outward behaviour is enough, without "due examination of one's self." Hypocrisy, the chief pollutant of communion and community, thus shares a metaphysical basis with the new idiotism of wardship law: a sense of *absence*. Hypocrisy of the deliberate as well as of the ignorant type led in the same direction: "an hypocrite, or dissembler, or double-hearted man, though he may shuffle it out for a while, yet at the long run he is discovered ... and betrays very much folly."[42]

As I suggested in Chapter 5, the change from one bidding mode to another is the unwitting outcome of attempts to stipulate more exactly the terms of the original mode. The importance of a specifically human reasoning in election, and of unreason in reprobation, arose from the need to devise a tighter authentification system. The problem had always been that while it would be presumptuous to try and know who is and is not in grace, we desperately *need* to know in order to avoid pollution. Covenant theology, with its part reliance on jurisprudential reasoning, held out the promise of an improved positive method for sizing up the aspiring communicant. Among other things, it contributed to the fusion between the legal language of idiotism and the religious one of reprobation, playing a direct part in early modern psychology's reconstitution of human difference along intellectual lines.

"Natural intellectual disability": France, phase one

The orthodox Calvinist story of limited atonement, in which Christ died only for the elect, was harsh. The opposing Arminian story did not credit human beings with much intelligence, only with stubborn perseverance. The seeds of these respective doctrines hibernate in the mainstream of modern culture, whence they can be translated into our attitudes to the people we call intellectually disabled. In that Calvinistic fable *The Lion, the Witch and the Wardrobe*, the children are advised (oddly enough, by a faun) "When you meet anything that ought to be human and isn't, you keep your eyes on it and feel for your hatchet," whereas in *Lord of the Rings* Frodo Baggins agrees to save the whole of humanity "even though most of them are completely dull and stupid." In this context the middle-way story, in which Christ died for everyone but only the elect are actually saved, looks a lot closer to the orthodox doctrine in its harshness. Nevertheless, it was out of the narrow negotiating space between these two doctrines that the idea of a "natural intellectual disability" sprang.

The middle way was represented in this debate by John Cameron, Moise Amyraut and other members of the French Reformed Church who influenced Baxter. Dates of the important texts are clustered around major political events: the 1618 Synod of Dort, the 1629 annulment of French Protestant political rights, the failure of republican government in early 1650s England and the attempt in 1670 to suppress the Dissenters. The idea leads us through to Locke's account of the changeling, who is the clearest precursor of the modern intellectually disabled person. While the names of Cameron and Amyraut will be obscure to historians of psychology, they are only too well known to today's surviving double predestinarians, since they are the answer to the disappointed utopian's question "Who has betrayed us?" The regrettable dominance of universalism today (everyone is saved if they try hard enough) is directly due to these fifth columnists; it was they who stripped grace of its discriminatory force, by confusing it with the earthly merits derived from

---

[42] Cited in Shapin, *A Social History of Truth*, 80.

reason. This paranoid expression of what is actually a historical truth misses the essential point: that at the core of this "betrayal" lay a novel concept of disability.

"Natural intellectual disability" came from the middle-way theologians' attempt to refute the orthodox doctrine of limited atonement while making tactical concessions to it. Cameron, a Scot, was professor of divinity at Bordeaux during the Synod of Dort and later at Saumur, where Amyraut worked. To avoid implicating God as the author of man's sin, Cameron maintained that the unregenerate have rejected God of their own free will. This indicated that there had to be a contractual element in regeneration. At the same time, however, they are precisely those people whom God has himself already chosen to reject. So predestination is determinate as well as contractual: the determinism consists in God's foreknowledge of who these people rejecting the contract will turn out to be. Letting God off the hook created room for an element of human responsibility and free will that looked to Cameron's orthodox critics suspiciously Pelagian. In order to develop a reply, Cameron probed the question of what went on within the individual, elect and reprobate, in more detail. How did God move him? "Physically," that is deterministically? Or "morally," by interacting with him in a mutuality that required the individual to fulfill certain obligations? Cameron's answer was both. He applied metaphysical concepts of ability and disability (*potentia*, *impotentia*) to the question. He drew these from scholasticism, but he also applied a new and anti-scholastic form of logic, Ramism (invented by Pierre de la Ramée, who had taught Cameron's own teacher Johannes Piscator). This simplified system, in contrast to Aristotle's, consisted in a continuously proliferating subdivision of terms which was perfect for sidestepping criticism; the tactic was, roughly, "When I said x just now, I meant x_1 rather than x_2." This procedure was said to obtain ever closer approximations to the truth. And that is how, with Cameron, disability came to be first "*natural* disability" (subdivided from moral disability) and then "natural disability of the *intellect*" (subdivided from natural disability of the will).

Cameron's orthodox opponents were always under pressure to say how they could square the gloomy divisiveness of their double predestination doctrine with the idea of an all-loving God. How can he be loving or just, if he demands belief from all humans when he has already determined most of them will not believe? And how is the irresistibility of God's grace compatible with the idea of personal responsibility? If humans are unwilling and unable to cast aside their unbelief other than by receiving God's grace, how can the reprobate non-receiver be personally to blame? Cameron recognized both the validity of the charge that double predestination assumed a malignant God, and the inadequacy of the usual orthodox response, which was that the distinction between elect and reprobate is beyond our knowing. At the same time he had to avoid the charge of Arminianism, which the orthodox school in France saw as politically dangerous because its supposed universalism might have weakened the defensive ghetto which the company of the elect had built up in their semi-autonomous Reform communities; it pointed in an ecumenical direction at the very moment when the Catholic French state was threatening to gobble those communities up.

Cameron steered through the middle. The orthodox position was that reprobates lack grace "not because they cannot (though they cannot) but because they will not …. Your cannots are your willnots"; readers familiar with behavioural disorders as described in educational psychology textbooks, or old enough to have been weaned on Charles Kingsley's *The Water Babies*, will recognize such language.[43] Against this, Cameron promotes the individual's possession of an active reason that might respond to grace. The Arminian line, on the other hand, was that everyone is able to be saved "if they will." Against this, Cameron insists that the case has been altered by the Fall: "by nature man is able but because corrupt he will not."[44] His route through the middle

---

[43] William Fenner, *Wilfull Impenitency the Grossest Selfe-Murder*, 4.
[44] Cameron, *Opera*, 332a; 333b; 649a; 340a.

then proceeds as follows. It is true that our wills are determined by God's special grace, but once inside us the motions of this grace are "moral" (negotiable and contractual) rather than "physical" (determinate). He immediately qualifies this by saying that the motions are nevertheless "*as if* physical." This quasi-physicality of grace he calls "intelligence" (*intelligentia*). Intelligence is a force that enables faith to "travel around" the body, instructing it how to behave and instilling the "demonstrable" truth of the common ideas. But in the last resort intelligence is still only *quasi*-physical; it operates not by coercion but by "persuasion," convincing us that scripture is true. This is a delicate balancing act. Intelligence is not some blind predestinate force activating the elect alone (as it would be if it were *merely* physical). Nor, however, is it a Pelagian-type ability equally possessed by all. It still sorts sheep from goats.

Since these intelligent motions of grace are in the last resort moral, their *absence* too is a moral disability, making the individual responsible for his own fallen state. However, this does not in itself absolve God of some responsibility, since the moral relationship between man and God is a continuing and interactive one. The Arminians' charge about turning God into the author of sin would not have been solved, merely displaced from the physical to the moral realm. Cameron's typically Ramist way out of this dilemma was to subdivide his terms. Disability, he said, is dual (*duplex impotentia*). One type is the moral disability we have just mentioned, a culpable one. A clue to the second type of disability comes with that idea that the motions of intelligence are "as if" physical. Cameron modelled his idea of these motions on the soul spirits, the highly rarefied material substance said by physicians to ferry the soul around the body. The "physical" – in theological terms, that which is necessarily predetermined by God – overlaps in this medical analogy with the "natural." Nature itself thereby takes on a certain determinism. In this realm of deterministic nature there may be a *non*-culpable disability, distinguishable from the culpable "moral" disability of hardened unbelief which is mere second nature. Humanists had traditionally distinguished "essential," *a priori* nature from an "accidental," *a posteriori* one, but Cameron takes a further step and identifies the first of these with physical necessity. If moral disability is *a posteriori*, a second nature which the hardened unbeliever has a personal responsibility for changing, then space remains for a more fundamental disability, existing *a priori* and – this was the novelty – unchangeable, even by providence. Unlike reprobation it is caused "by infirmity, not by malignity." Like bodily impairments it deserves pity, not blame.

Cameron then maps this duality of natural disability/moral disability on to that of intellect/will. Taking the first term from each pairing yields a "natural disability of the intellect." This was an entirely novel category. All he was trying to say was that unbelievers do not inhabit this realm of *natural* disability, and thus have *moral* responsibility for their own depravity. But in saying this, he raised the possibility that such a realm might exist. What kind of creature would inhabit this so far empirically empty category? He was not under pressure to reply. His followers at the Saumur Academy however, under fire from the orthodox leadership for their allegedly universalist tendencies, were provoked into attempting a concrete illustration of who these naturally intellectually disabled people might be. Orthodox church leaders thought that this shifted attention away from the division between elect and reprobate and towards something monstrous.

"Natural intellectual disability": France, phase two

Amyraut, coiner of the phrase "hypothetical universalism," took Cameron's thoughts a stage further, in an uncertain political atmosphere. The 1620s saw much conversion to and from Protestantism among the French nobility. In 1629 the Peace of Alès withdrew the clauses in the Edict of Nantes which had granted Protestants some political autonomy. Amyraut first proposed his doctrine not to the Academy but in the vernacular, to a Protestant aristocrat whose convert husband was threatening to reconvert to Catholicism because he could not stomach the gloominess of double predestination.[45] Some people, Amyraut told her, were different because their place in *a priori* nature made them incapable of any moral or contractual relationship with God; therefore they were excused from fulfilling the obligations entailed on them by Christ's act of atonement.

This inevitably provoked questions. How are you defining these people? What is the specific make-up of the naturally disabled intellect? Another of Cameron's Saumur pupils, Paul Testard, probed the issue in more detail. "Moral disability," he said, is like natural disability in that it is an "error of the mind" and "a disability of the intelligence and judgement," but it differs from natural disability in being "pragmatic, deliberate, voluntary" and therefore inexcusable.[46] The hardened impenitence of the morally disabled – the reprobate – has not been created in *a priori* nature, they have simply failed to fulfill their side of the covenant. God is not therefore to blame for having created them. Testard, steering between the rigidity of orthodox Calvinist doctrine and the Arminian principle of "everyone can be saved if they will," says instead that everyone is hypothetically capable of benefiting from Christ's atonement *if they can*. This is a crucial move. The universal applicability of the atonement now becomes conditional upon that word "can." Beyond that disability which is merely moral and in some sense willed, there is one that consists in "deprivation of the natural faculty of intellect." Out of Cameron's hints emerges a natural psychological phenomenon unconnected with original sin. Earlier accounts of faculty psychology had speculated that in some individuals an injury to a particular faculty might incapacitate the whole, but not permanently – whereas the absence of a whole "faculty of intellect" is clearly more than temporary or accidental.

The element of determinism and permanence in reprobation, which Calvinism had located beyond time, in a metaphysical realm, was thereby shifted into the realm of nature. Calvin's own historical scheme had been simple and twofold: first there was the covenant of grace, then the covenant of nature. In any case, the latter simply referred to man's obedient state before the Fall. Cameron subsequently divided the covenant of nature itself into two: first Adam's prelapsarian state, but then a second, postlapsarian one in which everyone was obliged to continue keeping its promises, as a means to their redemption. In short, the idea of predestination was not incompatible with that of mutuality between man and God. By locating the covenant and its promises in a historically evolving nature, Cameron had created the conceptual space for a type naturally incapable of promising in the first place because they lacked a whole "natural faculty," as Testard put it.

Amyraut began to ask what were the concrete symptoms by which they should be excused, or indeed excluded. He found an analogy in physical and sensory deprivation. His orthodox critics like Pierre du Moulin, a leading figure in the French Reformed church, and André Rivet and Friedrich Spanheim at Leiden, had no time for such analogies. Blindness was not a fault, since "no man is by natural obligation bound to see," whereas "impotency and disability of believing ... is voluntary."[47] If a purely "intellectual" disability really existed, it could not be *analogous* with sensory or bodily disability because, in a Galenist view, intellect and body were just two facets of the same thing.[48] Amyraut replied that the natural intellectual faculty is itself "physical," in the sense that is created once and for all in an objective realm. Having a defective intellect is "like" physical disability inasmuch as both are "a defect of the faculty," but the two kinds of faculty are entirely different. (His analogy here rests on the *a priori* character of each, rather than on Cartesian dualism.)

---

[45] Laplanche, *Orthodoxie et prédication*, 89.
[46] Testard, *Synopsis Doctrinae de Natura et Gratia*, 17.
[47] Du Moulin, *The Anatomy of Arminianisme*, 80.
[48] Amyraut, *Speciminis Animadversionum Specialorum*, 10.

So where might Amyraut go to borrow a descriptive framework for this natural intellectual disability? In the embryonic anthropology of the time, the French Protestant Isaac la Peyrère was shortly to publish his proposal that the Jews be classified by their separate origin in nature. (He was also interested in Spanish doctrine on the permanent mindlessness of first nation Americans.) Consequently a crude idea of natural divisions among the human race may have been at least conceivable for Amyraut. However, his inductive approach led him to think about nature in causal terms. Existing legal and medical frameworks he found inadequate. Although deprivation of a faculty might excuse someone from fulfilling legal obligations, legal "categories of impediment" did not explain the "constitution of the faculty."[49] Incompetence might exist in infants, adults "driven out of their minds" by some accident, or old people. These, says Amyraut, are not examples of mindlessness (*amentia*) as such but merely resemble it; someone in this state does not use his mind, so "it is *as if* he did not possess one" (emphasis added). What would be real mindlessness, then, where lack of use really does imply lack of possession? (We should note here that any such implication would have been unusual for the time.) It would certainly be a deprivation "in the natural make-up of the organs." In this sense it would resemble defects in bodily organs: Lazarus's paralysis, the Ethiopian's skin colour, or madness and "the melancholic humour," this too being an organic condition of bodily elements. Amyraut would also have entertained the influential proposal of De Mornay, a former mentor, that the new anatomy described by physicians should be used as a model for dissecting also the faults of the mind. But if the legal categories were inadequate, so too were medical ones. To fit the criteria of Amyraut's natural disability, *amentia* had to be not merely organic and temporary, like madness, but to circumscribe the whole person by being both congenital and incurable, beyond providence. "Whoever *really* is *by nature* destitute of mind because of the unfortunate make-up of their organs, is *never* in control of himself" (emphasis added).

The idea of a human difference marked by the permanent, non-accidental absence of the whole intellectual faculty and therefore exempt from natural law solved one problem but raised another. If God cannot be responsible for imperfections, how can we include such people in the category "man"? Pressure for an answer came from the orthodox leadership. Amyraut claimed he was furnishing them with better and more robust arguments against their Romanist and Arminian opponents, who complained that the God of the Calvinists seemed to have given human beings a law they were unable to obey while still demanding perfect obedience. Amyraut's argument was that inability to obey was "moral" and inexcusable only when it was an *abuse* of the appropriate faculty; natural intellectual disability was not abuse but *absence*.[50] Du Moulin accused Amyraut of challenging the fixity of species: creatures in whom the intellectual faculty was absent, in this natural, *a priori* sense, would by definition be non-human.[51] Amyraut would then have to say where in species terms he would categorize them. Moreover, said Du Moulin, it was pagan (that is, Stoic) to imply that nature might have physical or deterministic properties, equivalent to fate.

Friedrich Spanheim, another orthodox critic, said that Amyraut's distinction between *a priori* natural ability and *a posteriori* moral ability led to the Pelagian heresy; if moral ability, the source of faith, is *a posteriori*, then surely Amyraut must be saying that faith is dispositional, thus changeable and unstable. Amyraut denied the charge. It is true, he concedes, that in one sense bad moral habits are so ingrained as to be effectively incurable; and where moral disability is incurable it just *is* a natural disability, as Spanheim asserted.[52] However, the converse does not follow. Natural disability cannot be fully assimilated with moral disability. People naturally disabled by intellect are different

---

[49] Amyraut, *Fidei circa Errores Arminianorum*, 55 ff.
[50] Amyraut, "Eschantillon de la doctrine de Calvin," 14.
[51] Du Moulin, *Esclaircissement des controversies Salmuriennes*, 215.
[52] In Amyraut, *Speciminis Animadversionum Specialorum*, 99; 10.

from others at an *a priori* level, just as the absence of limbs or senses is *a priori*. Spanheim teased out the implications. If absence of the intellectual faculty sums up the whole person from birth to death and is more than accidental, and if there is a subtype of such precariously human creatures incapable of using their intellects, then God's authorship of imperfection is back in the frame. On this account not just moral vices but "defects of the intellect," says Spanheim, would have to be due to God withholding grace, just as in the case of the reprobate – for surely he would have created "no one in such a bad condition as to have no intellect or will at all by nature." For Amyraut, the creature whose congenital nature is defined by incurable permanence and total absence is still a man. Spanheim tried to force the issue: "If natural disability is a privation of the intellect *qua* intellect, then he is deprived of that with which he was made a man .... Whoever is a man who does not possess intellect?"[53] A creature disabled in this sense, lacking the essential core of his humanity, is inconceivable. For Amyraut, those whose humanity by this criterion is open to challenge are not beasts but excused humans. His opponents nevertheless pointed out the alternative and heretical consequence of his position: that it might allow for a separate species in natural history *between* beast and man. Locke was to seize on this opportunity.

Over time, Amyraut wavered between the position described above and a more conventional one in which natural disability is merely a difference of degree within the universal disability created by the Fall. Perhaps the strong concept only applied to defective members of his own social class; he was also the author of works on honour and genealogy, and may well have taken lack of a natural intellectual faculty in labourers for granted.[54] Be that as it may, the idea that natural intellectual disability rendered people different in kind rather than in degree only came up when his orthodox critics pressed him for clarification. The quarrel was a temporary by-product of the crisis in the French Reformed church provoked by the restrictions placed on them in 1629. The pathological type that Amyraut describes was the upshot of his attempt to break out of the politically unviable narrowness of Reform orthodoxy while avoiding assimilation into a state doctrine of universalism and free will. Once that crisis temporarily subsided, in the late 1640s, Amyraut's references to natural intellectual disability revert to impermanent or non-congenital examples, such as "phrenitis" or "wounds to the head."[55] During the crisis period, however, he unwittingly invented new terms of natural classification for human difference, which were to influence English writers. His orthodox colleagues actually challenged him to do so, because that was their only way of forcing him on to a terrain where they could point to the absurdity of such a position; it meant they could reaffirm election-reprobation as the dominant and determining classificatory difference among human beings, over and above differences in their intellectual nature. In fact Amyraut never arrived at the Lockean paradigm of a separate, natural realm of human intellectual ability. However, it is easy to see why his critics thought he was heading in some such direction, since he certainly sought to classify a natural intellectual *dis*ability.

"Natural disability of the intellect": England, phase one

English theologians dealt with Amyraut's startling doctrine of natural intellectual disability by adapting it to their own purposes. Some took the phrase "natural disability" or "impotency" and began using it as a synonym for the lapsarian "weakness of mind" in reprobates, thereby reinvesting

---

[53] Ibid., 58.
[54] Amyraut, *La vie de François, seigneur de la Noue*.
[55] *De Libero Arbitrio*, 59; 77.

it with traditional orthodox resonances.⁵⁶ Others did identify natural disability with "stupidity," "distractedness" and that "peculiar sin" which is a "disease of the body" or the phlegmatic bodily temperament, different from the general moral disability which is "disease of the soul" in all of us; but this natural type too remains merely unamenable, not actually incurable.⁵⁷

Whereas the French synods ended up charging Amyraut with heresy, the Westminster Assembly, which was in a much stronger political position, could afford to be more tolerant of its own Amyraldian faction. The Assembly's first Speaker, William Twisse, conceded that there might indeed be a natural intellectual ability, separable from the moral. However, he said, in the end it was just verbal acrobatics. Things impossible by nature, as for example intellectual ability in disabled individuals, are possible by God's grace; unlike the amputee's limb, natural intellectual ability can be restored, at least in the elect, because it partakes of divine influence.⁵⁸ The conflation between the natural and the moral makes up what Twisse terms "moral man" (*homo morale*). There was an ambivalence to this phrase. In secular terms it denoted Aristotelian virtue, the ability to restrain one's desires; in religious ones, it denoted Adamite moral weakness. Twisse's moral man is an elision of this ambiguity: he is *both* someone "who can discharge his [moral] duty to God by the proper use of the faculty of will" *and* a being "created by God in nature," hence morally weak. By the time Locke came to use the same phrase in the *Essay concerning Human Understanding*, his more optimistic conflation of the natural with the moral would amount to a psychological definition of the human species.

From the mid-1650s, Baxter introduced natural intellectual disability into his discussions of election and reprobation. Cameron and Amyraut topped his list of recommended authors for students; this was significant in view of his huge and lasting influence on popular Christian literature in Britain and New England.⁵⁹ As we have seen, Baxter was full of protestations that he was ultra-orthodox about election. But he also set great importance on natural ability. It could seem, then, as if his claim to believe in election is just a way of covering his exit; he senses that it is on the way out and has covertly abandoned it for the proto-scientific idea of an intellectual ability whose detailed workings, following implantation by the Almighty, are thereafter the responsibility of individuals. However, this presupposes that the doctrine of predestination had begun at its dogmatic "height" with Calvin and was in decline in Baxter's time. In fact the reverse is true. Calvin had been uncertain about it. It became a dogma only with time, in reaction to the rise of Arminianism; even the Synod of Dort avoided being too strict about it, for fear of alienating waverers. It reached maximum rigour only just before its *rigor mortis*. Already sidelined from public debate in the late 1650s, its most dogmatic English text, Owen's *The Death of Death in the Death of Christ*, dates from as late as 1648. When Baxter toed the line on predestination, he was sincere; this classification of human types was no less fundamental to him than that of ability and disability. When he started to call election and reprobation "these dangerous doctrines," it was not because he opposed them but because they threatened to provoke social unrest from lumpen religious sectarians claiming to be elect. He neither sought to replace election and reprobation with intellectual ability and disability, nor saw the two pairings as mutually contradictory. Eventually, however, the first was to become sublimated within the second.

The invention of natural intellectual disability saved Baxter, like his French predecessors, from the charge that he was an Arminian who imputed ability (i.e., the ability to be saved) to absolutely everyone. Accused of being "Amyraldus' proselyte," he was more original than the

---

⁵⁶ Owen, *Pneumatologia*, 224.
⁵⁷ Bates, *The Whole Works*, i, 226.
⁵⁸ Twisse, *De Vindiciis Gratiae, Potentiae ac Providentiae Dei*, 754; 768.
⁵⁹ Keeble, *Richard Baxter*, 42.

label suggests.[60] However, we also know that in the mid-1650s he was halted halfway through his writing of *The Universal Redemption of Mankind* either by a Damascene encounter with Amyraut's most radical work, the 1646 *Specimen*, or simply by the discovery that Amyraut had already said there what Baxter himself was going to say. In this and concurrent texts, Baxter probes the moral/natural distinction. Moral ability is a "disposition" or habit, he says, second rather than first nature; therefore something more fundamental is needed to set it going. A separate space thus exists for some prior, purely natural ability: "infused habits ... are not of the same quality as the *potentia naturalis*" or natural ability. By way of illustration Baxter criticizes the stock Calvinist view of the unregenerate sinner as being "dead in Christ." An illiterate man, says Baxter, can no more read the Bible than a corpse can; but while illiterates lack the disposition or habit, a corpse lacks not only the habit but also the natural ability or faculty. Sinners are like illiterates; their moral disability makes them unable to change their spots, but not to the extent of being "equally distant from an actual change as a dead man." Therefore "morals [pre]suppose naturals, and constitute them not." There are many morally disabled, "dull Christians, ignorant and injudicious," like Baxter's own "silly chambermaid," about whom one is pessimistic but whose corrupt human nature is ultimately ameliorable. They should be distinguished from naturally disabled people, whose incurability somehow helps along the thought that everyone else may be improved and illustrates the importance of reasoning to that improvement: "We do not use to reason men out of a *natural impotency*, nor to *persuade* them to do that, for which they have no faculties or object; but it is the very means of overcoming a *moral impotency*," and of "making men willing of the good which they rejected." Natural disability is not coterminous with moral disability, or with a mere lack of natural graces as exhibited by Calvin's *moriones*. It is a lack of the intellect's "working, waking knowledge." Since this knowledge was constitutive of faith, the lack of it, in Baxter's terms, might mean not to be human.[61] Who is not just "dead in Christ," abusing his second-nature moral disposition, but in addition lacks the natural faculty that instigates such dispositions in the first place? Who are the *living* dead?

The answer, specifically, is the legally *non compotes mentis*: "infants and idiots." They are naturally disabled in terms of faith because they lack its reasoned substructure and their redeemability is therefore questionable. In infants the disability is temporary; in some adults, though, it is permanent. They continue to experience the infantile state. Amyraut had already dealt with this point. Asked how new-born infants still unaware of sin could be responsible for their own moral disability, he had replied that their "disability of believing" was dual even at this early stage, since some infants might have "a natural, already existing imperfection of the organs" that would extend right through their lives. Baxter, instead of using these medical terms, reaches for the legal "idiot" vocabulary of wardship law. He wavers about whether idiotism is difference of degree or difference in kind. True, he says, there is some overlap between the moral and the natural, and in this sense the "moral difference [among men is] grounded but in a gradual natural difference."[62] But sometimes they do not overlap. In that case, i.e., where the disability is purely natural, does it imply that such creatures are a different natural species?

Baxter hesitates. On the one hand "God can ... save men ... without letting them once know that Christ satisfied for them, else he cannot save an infant or an idiot."[63] This thought is compatible with hypothetical universalism: everyone (even idiots, whoever these are) can expect that Christ's

---

[60] Cited in Baxter, *Certain Disputations of Right to Sacraments*, Preface.

[61] Baxter, *Apology*, 128; *Of Saving Faith*, 39; *Apology*, 291; Anon., *An Antidote against Mr Baxter's Palliated Cure of Church Divisions*, 14.

[62] Baxter, *The Universal Redemption*, 477; Amyraut, *Fidei*, 28; Baxter, *The Right Method for a Settled Peace of Conscience*, 142.

[63] *The Universal Redemption*, 477.

atonement applies to them, that they *may* be saved. True, it is on condition that they have the natural intellectual ability to understand this; but if they do not have that ability, they are excused. Excusal suggests they do not need an intellectually structured faith; hence some "idiots" may even be elect. This was certainly the implication, as we have seen, in other middle-way writings; it occurs also in the more orthodox Twisse, who wrote that if "as a result of some natural disability a man's abilities do not correspond to his will," this does not diminish his status with God.[64] But on the other hand, Baxter's wariness about trying to guess whom God has chosen to exclude sometimes gives way to a more decisive tone when the topic is idiots. It may be that "universal redemption is not to be tried thereby," because "it hath pleased God" to leave it uncertain, but there is nevertheless a slippery slope. Could you be elect if you had heard only two or three sermons, or how many? Could you be a lifelong sinner, converting only at the moment before death, and still reach salvation? Idiotism is a category even further down this slope, threatening to fall off the edge. The doctrine of hypothetical universalism inevitably led probing minds to ask whether there might not be individuals who are not even hypothetically redeemable, and by what criteria.

The concrete examples suggested by this legalistic "idiot" language are the people Baxter would have encountered in his pastoral office as administrator of the local poor law. His anxiety about incurables sprang from their unproductive state of idleness and their being "kept without parts and gifts, next to useless, if not burdensome."[65] Flesh appears on the theological bones when fiscal concerns are uppermost. These concerns reflect the Reformation's insistence on the industrious pursuit of an earthly vocation. All such vocations were particular examples of a "general calling" that corresponded to common grace, "a necessity of vocation enjoined of all, of what rank or degree soever." Lack of a calling of any kind put one entirely outside the social order; since it must entail idleness, it "maketh of men, women, of women, beasts, of beasts, monsters."[66] Baxter's idiot belonged in this latter group. Moreover, while one's calling was a rank in a vertical, hierarchical order in which one was assumed to remain for life, the idea of a *general* calling had a horizontal dimension (it justified the adoption of coats of arms by the guilds, for example). The Levellers took this to its logical conclusion, transforming the idea of the general calling into something like a universal, abstract human right in a more modern sense.

Baxter did not like this, and used his "idiots" to attack its appearance in James Harrington's quasi-democratic utopia of 1656, *The Commonwealth of Oceana*. He accuses Harrington of advocating "the ploughmen's vote." In so doing, Baxter gives us a prime example of the necessary interdependence between concepts of pathological absence beyond the law of nature ("as a man is not man without an intellect and will"), and those of inferior reasoning within the band of normal. There are, says Baxter, "gradual" natural differences in active intellectual ability, which warn us against extending the franchise below a certain point; it is the existence of a species in whom there is no ability at all (the new, legal idiots) that best illustrates the absurdity of giving a parliamentary vote to labourers (idiots in the old sense), or even to the "majority, who are ... scarce able to talk reason about common things."[67] Indeed, it may have been the latter anxiety above all, a political one, that finally provoked from him these hints about idiots' difference in kind, in which "species" of human society are differentiated "analogically, even no more than an idiot is a reasonable man."

---

[64] Twisse, *De Praedestinatione, Gratia & Libero Arbitrio*, 37b; see also James Ussher, *The Power Commanded by God*, Preface.
[65] Baxter, *The Universal Redemption*, 427.
[66] Brathwait, *The English Gentleman*, 31.
[67] *The Holy Commonwealth*, 232; 52; 318–23; 60 ff.

It should be added that similar anxieties existed in Catholic cultures. More than a century earlier Vives, a pioneer of welfarism, had complained about the many people whose disability forced them to live by begging, "regardless of where or when, even during celebration of the mass." Such people, subdivided between the furious (*furiosi*) and the stupid (*stupidi*), polluted the sacraments. Their proper place was in hospital, since "this is the way it is done by the human body …. All filthy matter is collected in a sewer so that it will not harm the rest of the body." Fear of pollution is displaced from reprobates to a new category of person and a new model of social segregation. As ever, we do not know exactly who it is that the author has in mind by "stupid." His general disability heading of *impotentia*, as a category of public administration, makes no clear distinction between impairment and poverty. A single entity, the "lost and useless" alike, are the supreme threat to the "purity and honour [*dignitas*] of knowledge."[68]

"Natural disability of the intellect": England, phase two

The first historiographers of the Amyraut dispute are the English Dissenters following the Restoration of the monarchy in 1660, to whom we now turn. This was a period of decline in religious optimism and consequently in the disputes about grace, election and reprobation – if not necessarily a decline in their tacit importance. The Restoration bishops held a new variant of Arminian universalism that promoted reason alongside belief and endowed the monarchy with "a monopoly of reason as well as honour."[69] They claimed that the Dissenters lacked reason, with the result that the latter were forced to insist on its place in their own doctrines and the absence of it among the bishops. Thus the reasoning human subject became the focus of religious dispute.

In 1671 Baxter's protégé Joseph Truman weighed in against the church establishment on this issue, in his *A Discourse of Natural and Moral Impotency*. Truman defends the middle way not so much against the old Calvinist orthodoxy as against the opposite flank, the universalism of the "Protestant papists" in the Anglican hierarchy. Truman's book, attacked for being "taken from the writings of Amyraldus and supported by Baxter's authority," continues the intellectualist trend we have already noted.[70] The "understanding" is now unproblematically compatible with faith. It is "irradiat[ed] with reasons as to cause [the] choice" between good and evil; the will makes its moral choices only after considering "suitable objective evidence" obtained via the prior workings of this "intellectual medium."[71] Truman "dare not yet say … how" this medium works in detail, but it was beginning to become obvious that the "how" was exactly what the Dissenters needed to specify, in order to defend the reasonableness of their own position. The bishops had called their bluff. Truman's book was published in the same year as Locke committed himself to detailing the "how" in his proposal for what would become the *Essay concerning Human Understanding*. Anglicans and Dissenters alike were by now comfortable with the notion that reason was intrinsic to faith. But for the Anglicans reason was absolute, its ideas innate; its specific content was whatever the bishops, as the mediators of God's will, said it was. The Restoration meant that "we are now *rasa tabula* and your honours may write what you please upon us."[72] For the Dissenters, reason was the act of intellectual labour in each individual by which he responded to Christ's atoning sacrifice; therefore it could not be politically dictated by others. In their attempt to answer the Anglican

---

[68] Vives, *De Subventione Pauperum*, 59 f.
[69] *A Modest Plea*, 25; see also Richard Ashcraft, *Revolutionary Politics*.
[70] George Bull, *Examen Censurae*, 155.
[71] Truman, *A Discourse of Natural and Moral Impotency*, 80.
[72] *A Modest Plea*, A2.

charge that this labouring intellect, being individual, was Antinomian, self-willed and incapable of reaching the absolute truths of the "common ideas," some of them tried to relocate the absolute away from the ideas and towards what they thought might be quasi-deterministic, innate working mechanisms of the "intellectual medium" itself.

Disability was crucial to the dispute. According to Truman's Anglican detractors like George Bull, hypothetical universalism was not universal at all but a disguised version of the old sheep-and-goats orthodoxy of double predestination. In fact, *everyone* is disabled by the Fall, and *equally*. Anglicans like Bull redefined "natural disability" as this universal inability to obey; the universal grace that cures it comes from the church hierarchy's own ability to obtain "universal submission," religious and political. Truman, coached in hair-splitting by Baxter, responds by subdividing natural intellectual disability into three types: not knowing what is required of you, as in pagans; external hindrances to religious observance, as for example poverty, blindness, deafness, or "a body [not] rightly disposed"; and total absence of "the natural faculties of understanding and willing," as in "natural fools."[73] Truman only invents these natural fools in order to depict what we might *all* be like if we were naturally disabled as Bull says we are, and hence the absurdity of his position.

At the same time, however, Truman's idea of natural intellectual disability and natural fools is more discrete and specific than Baxter's. So much so, that it is only a short step from here back to the original orthodox dogma that the moral and the natural are the same thing – but with the new proviso that humanity contains some *un*natural exceptions, even to this rule. Where Bull calls "natural impotency" a universal characteristic caused by sin, Truman makes the cause specific to certain individuals and groups. Sin causes "natural dullness of understanding and blindness, and lameness of body."[74] The idea of disability being a result of sin was not in Amyraut or even Baxter. It invokes the guilt-ridden divisiveness of election and reprobation, under a new guise. It focuses sharply on the question of whether people with a natural intellectual disability differ from the rest of us in kind or by degree. Where Baxter had at least hesitated, Truman turns "kind" and "degree" into a positive distinction that foreshadows the one made between "idiot" and "imbecile" categories by Edouard Séguin and John Connolly in the nineteenth century and between "severe" and "moderate" in modern psychology. "Total natural impotency" is one thing, he says, but "degree of it" another:

> If a man be ... blockish, something dull, it is some excuse for his not understanding difficulties in religion which he might yet possibly, with great difficulty, understand; but if quite a fool, so as to have no more use of reason than a beast, it is a total excuse from any command to learn or understand ... for, he cannot if he would.

The "excuse" for total fools is no longer benevolent, as it had been in Amyraut. They are in a limbo created by Truman's shrinking of the circumference of the human species to what he calls the "moral man," which he defines in opposition to the Arminians' "whole lump of mankind." Where Twisse had effectively restricted his concept of "moral man" to the putatively elect, Truman conflates it with that of "man the rational animal," so that it becomes the logical essence of the species. Neither phrase, says Truman, adequately defines us without the other. But the *whole* species? Whoever lacks "natural power" or ability is "no rational creature," because rationality consists in the individual's "power and knowledge to choose" good over bad. The identification of moral ability as something natural, implicit in his "moral man," may paint a veneer of humanist

---

[73] Truman, *A Discourse*, 6; 47.
[74] Ibid., 44; 6.

optimism, but only by excluding a natural intellectual idiot who lacks rational choice and without whose separate classification moral man could not exist.

Truman resumes the scientific aspirations of Baxter's psychology. The fusion between moral man and rational animal, says Truman, can refresh the old formula of the "capable subject" with a new content. Whereas for earlier Calvinists it had meant a subject capable of passive receipt of the holy spirit, here it signifies his active ability to reason about truth and falsehood. The causes of this ability, and of its absence, now lie in human nature.[75] His Dissenter contemporary John Ray was just then reinforcing the definition of biological species in natural history; the difference of Truman's natural fool lies not only in *kind*, in the old sense, but more precisely in natural *species*, in Ray's sense.

As for the doctrine of election, this had finally become, if not redundant, an embarrassment. Bull asserted that "God doth love and will the conversion of everyone." Truman's entire background would have led him to object that God willed conversion only for the elect. Instead he simply says that God wills conversion for some more than for others, "and take notice once for all that I exclude the case of infants and idiots out of this discourse, as being alien and of less concernment in religion, and also difficult."[76] Whereas Baxter saw no contradiction between ability/disability and election/reprobation as criteria of differentiation, Truman senses that there might indeed be one. While no doubt sticking to the "dismal ... fierce and churlish reprobatarian doctrines" increasingly dismissed by contemporaries, he sounds palpably evasive.[77] Tacit hints of election remain lodged within "moral man," however.

There are similar strands in the historical treatment of the Amyraut dispute by Robert Ferguson, Truman's Dissenter contemporary and politically close to Locke at the 1671 gestation point of the *Essay concerning Human Understanding*. Ferguson published several texts in this period which discuss "rational choice," then (it seems) a neologism – though at this stage a choice between heaven and hell rather than Coke and Pepsi. The Lutherans had foregrounded choice, starkly represented in paintings of the crucifixion that divide the people at the foot of the cross into mourners on one side and dice players on the other. "Reason is but choosing," says Milton in the *Areopagitica*. Baxter situated choice at the juncture between the two main subdivisions within human nature, natural intellectual ability and natural free will: "It is as natural to a man to be a free agent as to be reasonable …. The gain or loss must be their own."[78] At the hands of Ferguson and others, "rational" choice became the *sine qua non* of faith. As he put it, "there can be no act of faith without a previous exercise of our intellects about the things to be believed."[79] And it was the necessary detail of this previous exercise that Locke had in mind when he offered himself as an "under-labourer" to "examine our own abilities."[80] Rational choice, linked to free will, was still compatible with election. The elect made use of their labouring intellects, rationally weighing evidence and probability; they could not fail to do so, since any failure would defy the intentions of their creator. According to self-styled "politico-theologians" such as Ferguson, the Calvinist law of perfect obedience that unites religion and government was now, in this current and final stage of Biblical history, a "law of rational subjection" (an adequate description, one might think,

---

[75] *A Discourse*, 39; 43; Truman, *The Great Propitiation*, 20.

[76] *A Discourse*, 115.

[77] Glanvill, "Anti-fanatical Religion," 22, in *Essays*.

[78] Baxter, *The Cure*, 104.

[79] Ferguson, *A Sober Enquiry into the Nature, Measure and Principle of Moral Virtue*, Epistle; *The Interest of Reason in Religion*, 21.

[80] *An Essay*, 7; 10.

of the link between psychology and the political and social order today).[81] The supreme model of regeneration and grace offered here, as one might expect, is Ferguson himself.

His comments on Amyraut's doctrine of disability reveal the same reductionism as Truman's. "Moral impotency," he says, is not "a deprivation of any essential power or faculty of our rational being; this Spanhemius as well as Amyrald, Twisse as well as Truman, are at an accord in .... So that whether it ought to be styled a moral or natural impotency is for the most part but a strife about words." For Ferguson, moral disability is not "as if" natural, as it had been for Amyraut; they are downright identical. Disability is "natural" because "entailed on us by the Fall," "moral" because it is redeemable through "industrious improvement" of the individual intellect, without a need for the mediation of bishops. This is a disability that reveals the fallen humanity of everyone. But that is because we are already led to understand that in "mere idiots," who are "under no sanction," not only ability but even the *dis*ability naturally specific to fallen man is absent.[82] These exclusions belong in an implicitly non-human natural realm, since absence of intellect is absence of something essential to "being." Idiots, like reprobates, have a "physical disproportion" as deep and determinate between them and the rest of us as between the rest of us and God. Thus Ferguson's concept of disability, far from being Amyraut's, reverts to crude orthodox Calvinism, inasmuch as it denies Amyraut's partial disjunction between "moral" and "natural." At the same time, though, it introduces a category that is morphologically human but entirely lacks a reasoning faculty – a move against which the orthodox had explicitly warned. Ferguson has cut his idiots off from his hypothetically universal humanity far more decisively than Amyraut or Baxter did theirs.

Idiots and access to holy communion

The categorization of idiots in a realm of intellectual nature was aided both by developments in the doctrine of election and by the increasingly strict gatekeeping that accompanied it. Aquinas had laid down rules of competence for participation in church ritual and the ability to examine oneself, and these did indeed include a category lacking the use of reason from birth, one which he associates implicitly with the category of people "possessed by unclean spirits."[83] However, this was set at an abstract level, and it is more likely that the people whom the Dominican Aquinas has in mind are atheists, heretics and those exhibiting disruptive behaviour. The reassertion of the exclusionary principle in the mid-seventeenth century draws more concretely on concepts of reprobation. Bunyan's identification of reprobation with lack of reason is a case in point. It is tied to the power of local ecclesiastics: a form of exclusion responding to a more marked and immediate urgency (social as well as doctrinal) than the pontificating of scholastic theologians. It therefore focuses concretely on the individual, and on the detailed condition of his intellectual operations.

Reformers of a few decades earlier had in fact maintained that at communion "the hypocrite hurteth himself and not others." Even the double predestinarian Perkins wrote that "every man of years ... is bound in conscience by God's commandment to use the Lord's supper"; only self-doubters were a problem, or those already publicly excommunicated for scandalous sins.[84] Divines around the Westminster Assembly deemed that "that ordinance which is profaned by admitting infants and idiots, who can make no good use of it, is much more profaned by admitting abominable

---

[81] *The Interest*, 234.
[82] Ferguson, *A Sober Enquiry*, 148; *The Interest*, 264; 112.
[83] *Summa Theologica*, 3.80.9.
[84] Bullinger, *Decades*, iv, 425; Perkins, *Workes*, 81.

and known profane persons, who make a very bad use of it."[85] And on a wider scale, well into the seventeenth century, the problem might be tackled by programmes of positive discrimination. There were idiots, of "crass wit and dull intellect" (the author also includes deaf people here), who were to be lovingly helped through the practice of communion. Who exactly were they? These were of course the "stupid serfs," "peasants" and "rustics, ... more suitable for perceiving the spiritual gifts of God than those who are puffed up with knowledge, swollen with honours." God does not require more from anyone than they are capable of. Even this Catholic author, though, seems on the defensive by now.[86]

Meanwhile Joseph Mede, an early figure in the secularization of the Devil, drew on the legal distinction between "him that is mad but by fits and hath his lucid intervals" and "him that is continually and always mad," like the idiot, who might "by his indecent actions and foul miscarriages of his own, or by his daemoniacal clamours disturb the people of God and the church service," though again it may well be that we are meant to understand this latter group as "melancholics."[87] It was the question of power, of who controlled the service and in particular the altar rail, that led to increasingly strict assessments of ability and preparedness for grace, and so to keeping certain people out on a permanent basis. In England it was the loudest ecclesiastical dispute of the mid-seventeenth century, threatening the church's political unity. The emphasis on assessment, in face of the dangers of pollution by an out-group, went with the view "that one unworthy receiver being admitted to the sacrament would draw down damnation on all the rest."[88]

In the dispute about open versus restricted access to communion, the sides did not correspond exactly to those taken in the dispute about universal grace versus limited atonement. Rather, they corresponded to a dispute about church government between Erastianism (control by the civil authority) and strict Presbyterianism (control by church elders). The first wave of this dispute came in the 1640s. At this point the Erastian view was that only those unable to examine themselves – children and "idiots" (here, the unlearned and illiterates) should be barred – while Presbyterians were mainly concerned about abuse of the intellectual faculties rather than their absence. Although texts about ability to receive the sacrament deal massively with "ignorance," this bears no relation to modern intellectual disability.

The administrative dispute flared up again a decade later, during the republic. One side was led by John Humfrey. Humfrey thought one should admit all communicants without assessment, since God alone knew who was elect or reprobate. Only infants and mad people should be excluded, chiefly because of the pollutant effects of their disruptive behaviour; their religious status nevertheless remained unknown. Opposing him were mainstream Presbyterians such as Roger Drake, who agreed that only God knew but who thought the pastor could at least guess which individuals were not regenerate and could therefore screen them out.[89] Anticipating those psychologists who were to prioritize measurement of intelligence over its actual definition, Drake and his colleagues maintained here that "the judgement may be false, but the rule of judging infallible." They accused Humfrey of contradicting his own principle of open admission by excluding infants and mad people. Humfrey's reply was that their conditions are not permanent; infants grow up, mad people (subsuming "fools") have lucid intervals. Excluding them therefore did not contravene open

---

[85] George Gillespie, *Aaron's Rod Blossoming*, 256.

[86] Gregorius Teretius, *Confessio et Instructio Idiotae*, Preface, 1 ff.

[87] *Works*, 48; 30.

[88] Cited in Martin Ingram, "From Reformation to toleration," in T. Harris (ed.), *Popular Culture in England, c.1500–1800*, 119.

[89] Humfrey, *An Humble Vindication of a Free Admission unto the Lords Supper*; Drake, *A Boundary to the Holy Mount*; Anthony Palmer, *A Scripture-Rale to the Lords Table*, 79.

admission in principle. They were temporarily excused from self-examination. Drake countered that by invoking non-permanence, Humfrey was implicitly overriding the distinction between elect and reprobate, these being by definition permanent and predetermined states. So through the dialectic of debate and, it seems, on Baxter's advice, Humfrey was forced into specifying in subsequent texts a disqualification that would be permanent but would not contradict his own doctrine of open admission. In order to be permanent it had therefore to be a category which (a) exists in nature, and (b) encompasses the whole creature from birth to death. This category Humfrey calls "idiots," a term not discussed in either side's original position. And it seems to involve him and his accomplices acknowledging what they would otherwise like to deny to their Presbyterian opponents, namely a right "to determine of the lowest degree of what is necessary to receiving or excluding in respect of *every* member" (emphasis added), and to make discriminations among "different subjects" a matter of "church administration" rather than leaving it up to God.[90]

There was an element of anxious complicity here. Surely there was *some* category of person who, we would all agree, will never be admitted to communion? Surely, it is asked today, there must be *some* category of disability so severe that the person cannot be part of mainstream life: school, workplace, social relationships? The exclusionary principle, emanating from fear of pollution, precedes any concrete historical content such categories may have. This tacit agreement among ecclesiastical adversaries sprang from the need for a united front against an encroaching tide of doctrinal relativities exacerbated by civil war. The underlying need for all sides to maintain church unity preceded and actually created the thing itself, a common and absolute exclusion. Excommunicates, like mad people, are still technically "church members," albeit "under cure"; pagans, like infants, are capable of being baptized and eventually of taking communion; even reprobate hypocrites, the initial source of anxiety, merely exhibit a difference between inner and "outward man." Beneath any such concrete distinctions lies the underlying metaphysic of a level of *absolute* exclusion. Who or what exactly constitutes it? Disputants in the gatekeeping debate were driven to conceive a creature that has *neither* curability *nor* potential, nor even any "inner" man: a last-resort exceptional case.

The debate about who was in charge of exclusion also involved practical problems at parish level, concerning the administrative duties of churchwardens and clerical deacons. These experts in the minutiae of discrimination, who had the job of ensuring that certain people did not physically get beyond the chancel screen, were also social security officers whose job was to apply the Poor Law, and it may well be that the new ecclesiastical category of idiots still encompassed the labouring poor. Daniel Defoe's 1697 *Essay on Projects* contains a passage often cited as prefiguring later efforts to make a clear institutional division between mad people and idiots. A great plagiarizer, he took most of these projects from pamphlets of the early 1650s, and this one may well come from the same period as the pastoral debates discussed above. Defoe wanted to prove that having a clearly separate institution for "natural fools" would reduce the fiscal burden of relieving poverty. One had to discriminate in order to prevent "idle drones," beggars and scroungers, from milking the system; genuine idiocy, properly assessed, was "natural" and so could not be counterfeited, whereas madness could.

The element of permanence in this ecclesiastical concept of idiocy corresponds with the Puritan unification of the personality. It has two ingredients: *congenital incurability*, drawn from legal accounts of wardship, and *determinism*, drawn from religious accounts of election and reprobation. Humfrey's opponents claimed that by positing idiocy as the one fundamental category

---

[90] Baxter, Letter to John Humfrey, 20 June 1654; Humfrey, *A Second Vindication of a Disciplinary, Anti-Erastian, Orthodox Free Admission*, 20; John Timson, *The Bar to Free Admission to the Lord's Supper Removed*, 303; 322.

of exclusion, he was elevating "natural intelligence" over "spiritual intelligence."[91] In fact the two were merging, and any opposition between them was secondary to the need to authenticate and exclude. Admission to Presbyterian communion was based on a close assessment by the pastor, on the evidence of which he would issue the aspiring communicant with a ticket. We have detailed records of Baxter's examination of his parishioners' catechism, which show us how complex and "intellectual" an exercise it had become, in a recognizably modern sense.[92] Until now long and detailed catechisms were the preserve of ecclesiastical elites; all the masses had needed were easy-access idiot's guides. Humfrey, in drastically reducing the numbers of people he excluded, also pathologizes them. John Collinges, one of Drake's allies, warned him that by pressing the "Amyraldian" Humfrey too hard to concede that *some* category at least should be barred from communion, Drake was unwittingly "creating monsters": "I remember the ill influence learned Spanhemius [in] his answer to Amyraldus had upon him to this purpose," meaning that it seemed to posit some separate, non-human species.[93] Collinges knew that theoretical disputes like that between Amyraut and Spanheim could produce real-life problems. In debating these conceptual categories, Drake was playing with fire.

Humfrey's goal was church unity and thus the maintenance of social order. Drake, he said, risked driving the many people he excluded on "spiritual" grounds into separate congregations. Even worse, people denied a ticket would react by withholding their tithes.[94] Humfrey sought to minimize this potential for social disintegration by maximizing the pathology of the few he did exclude; idiots may have been *non homo legalis*, as he calls them here, but their shift from the courtroom into nature and natural law made them seem simply *non homo*. No longer were idiots with "natural disabilities" merely "suspended" as before, they were assumed to be "as much delivered over to Satan as any scandalous persons" – and permanently so.[95]

---

[91] Drake, *The Bar*, 174; see also K. Weintraub, *The Value of the Individual*.
[92] Lamont, *Richard Baxter*, 48.
[93] John Collinges, *The Preacher (Pretendedly) Sent, Sent Back*, Preface.
[94] Ann Hughes, "The frustrations of the godly," in J. Morrill (ed.), *Revolution and Restoration*, 81.
[95] William Prynne, *A Vindication of Foure Serious Questions*, 7.

PART 6
Fools and Their Medical Histories

Chapter 12
The Long Historical Context of Cognitive Genetics

Our object of study, as we perceive it today, rests on a scientific and more particularly a medical description of human types. This medical model of "intellectual disability" draws its validation from a wider and specifically modern mélange of biology, psychology and ethics (to be examined in Part 7). In narrower, diagnostic terms, it is validated by empirical evidence. Without such evidence, all talk of intelligence or disability and its identification of in-group and out-group remain stuck in the realm of mere values. In modern society there is only one social institution that might be able to recognize this dependence on values, and to adhere instead to a principle of unconditional acceptance, and that is the family. Beyond the family are mainstream social institutions – school, workplace, everyday social life – entitled, often by law and certainly by moral consensus, to say Keep Out, while pre-natal testing means that families' own values are themselves sometimes eroded by medical ones. The medical profession, once the very lowest rank of the honour society, has risen to become the arbiter of what it is and is not to be fully human, acting on behalf of other professions and social institutions in this respect. To use a phrase of Baxter's, it is Keeper of the Keys of the House of the Lord. For the medical profession, therefore, unconditional acceptance is not so much an alternative set of values as a doctrinal heresy. In the face of heresy, the separate identity of the pollutant out-group must be secured all the more tightly, by a system of external verification and the re-education of waverers (especially families) which forces them to internalize the medical profession's own systemic bias as to the value of certain people.

The medical history of intelligence: absolute presuppositions

In order to uncover the historical connections and disconnections in the medical model of intellectual disability (which are entirely distinct from those of the physical model that dominates "disability studies"), we need to look first at its most deeply rooted assumptions, at the various bits of the modern conceptual apparatus that inform it and act as obstacles to our understanding. Earlier we saw that honour and grace were given facts of the era to which they belonged. They were, to use historian R.G. Collingwood's phrase, "absolute presuppositions," constituting the farthest horizons of that era's world-view. It is our job as historians to get round the back of our primary sources' presuppositions. Otherwise we have no hope of understanding them. Intelligence is as absolute in our own era as honour and grace once were. How did it become not only a given fact of nature but so firmly embedded in medical science? How do we stand outside it?

The first barrier to understanding, dominating the rest, is mind-body dualism. In the pre-modern era, no separately "intellectual" form of ability existed. Identifying Greek *psyche* with the Christian "soul" or the modern "mind" can lead to gross misinterpretation of the texts. *Psyche* was, rather, the principle of growth and movement in all living things, animating their material existence. In early Christianity this role was partly taken over by the understanding (*intellectus*), with soul (*anima*) being reduced to something less active. As categories broke down and re-formed, the Latin "mind" (*mens*) came to be synonymous with both, and completely separated from the body.[1]

---

[1] See Katharine Park, "The organic soul," in C. Schmitt and Q. Skinner (eds), *The Cambridge History of Renaissance Philosophy*; David Claus, *Toward the Soul*.

Yet even among the pioneering scientists of the Royal Society, who knew their Descartes, the old conceptual schema hung on. Alongside dualism a distinction continued to be made within the disembodied soul itself, between a spiritual and immortal super-nature and the mortal faculties and their operations. Ordinary doctors hung on to this picture well into the eighteenth century.

As for the body, the assumption was that it would be reborn at the Last Judgement, in as perfect a condition as the soul; after all, they were inseparable aspects (matter and form) of a single entity. Michelangelo's fresco depicts bodies that are sublime in their own right; they are not just tokens of the soul's perfection. Only later was the body excluded from personal identity and relegated to an anonymous agglomeration of matter. One does not need a body in order to be resurrected, says Boyle; correspondingly, the "person" was now distinct from the physical "man," and described mind alone. The person became that part of us which, when judged, expects the good or bad deeds performed over a whole lifetime to be tallied up. Separation of the person from the body turned it into a potential object of pathology in its own right. In this Cartesian sense, the mind is a solipsistic self "sitting at its console in its windowless tower communicating with other, similarly secluded diamonds by signals run up between towers and relayed to these beings by a perpetual miracle."[2] And this creates room for the idea that there might be some towers that fail to send or receive signals, in a way that could not previously have been imagined. Dualism led to the quasi-biological notion of what the preacher Jonathan Edwards termed "a natural history of the mental world," which fed into modern medical classifications of disability.[3]

A second barrier is the idea that there are laws of human nature. Like mind-body dualism, this is of fairly recent origin. For the Greeks, law (*nomos*) was simply a set of conventions invented by human beings themselves for their own daily affairs; they would have been baffled by the idea that there are "laws" of nature of any kind, let alone human ones, and even more puzzled by the idea that there are laws of the mind with uniform external descriptors indicating the same thing to everyone. Medieval philosophers subsequently attributed law to nature, but only in a very broad sense. According to Aquinas, natural law has three strands: God's providence, the external world and the human understanding. Yet each was inseparable from the other, since there was a divine element connecting them all, and only on the threshold of the modern period did the connections begin to loosen. The idea of a discrete set of laws pertaining to a specifically human nature first arose, controversially, in the seventeenth century. It was founded on the belief that our world originates in a steady "state" of nature and functions by laws we can discover for ourselves. According to Hobbes in Chapter 14 of *Leviathan*, nature can be divided between an external nature – verifiable by the size, shape and velocity of measurable, material things – and an internal nature within human beings consisting of that which occurs in our own minds as a result of our cognitive grasp of external nature. Human reasoning in this sense is a mundane "calculation"; it reflects the arithmetically ordered external nature from which it has been separated, and operates by correspondingly mechanical rules.

This repositioning of our place in nature had a partly political motive. It meant our behaviour was predictable. Hobbes's vision of human nature as a set of ordered stimulus-and-response mechanisms matched the perceived need for a renewal of absolute authority over a society that had disintegrated into a factious pit of "masterless men" and their competing individual wills. His contemporary Grotius, followed by Pufendorf, asserted by contrast that human beings are naturally capable of governing themselves, even in situations where the "positive," everyday law of the state has broken down. Locke then claimed that human nature is a state of liberty where individuals are untrammelled by the will of others: the source of political liberalism. These highly

---

[2] Mary Midgley, *Science and Poetry*, 86.
[3] Cited in Fiering, *Jonathan Edwards*, 363.

disparate state-of-nature arguments sprang from a shared recognition that the idea of natural law as a divine force had lost its political clout, its ability to coerce from without. New forms of coercion had to be sought within the individual. Specifically human nature, separated from its previous interconnectedness with divine nature, now had cognitive operations at its core. Thus the underlying properties of the human intellect came to match those of the world outside it and the study of both to resemble each other. Now that human behaviour was, like external nature, predictable and therefore governable, there was no longer a need to insist that humans answer for it directly to an omnipotent God. An earthly authority might assess and manage it instead, whether directly as in the absolutist conception or indirectly as in the liberal one.

Thirdly, the idea of laws of human nature has led to our modern emphasis on the minutiae of internal psychological operations. "Intellect" (*dianoia*) for the Greeks was a succession of temporary states, not a stable psychological object open to detailed investigation. For medieval and Renaissance writers, the *intellectus* was structured by soul into its various faculties; the analytic focus was on these broad, static entities, and any sense of operational detail was to be found rather in the soul's bodily matter such as the "soul spirits." Only subsequently was this sense of detail transferred to the mind, as a separate entity. This shift coincided politically with the loss of power of kings and ecclesiastical authority to dictate a uniform political and religious doctrine. Since the supposedly universal "common ideas" had in fact been the property of an elite with the authority to prescribe them, typically human psychological operations such as abstraction or logical reasoning occurred only in such people. But the civic disorder of the mid-seventeenth century, especially in England, was an omen: the lower orders were "getting ideas," of their own and on their own. When Locke recommended toleration for this diversity of political and religious views among the general population, he was not indulging in relativism. Quite the contrary: he threw the principle of uniformity a lifeline, by disengaging it from the innate ideas prescribed externally by church and state doctrine and applying it instead to the micro-mechanical internal operations of the mind. He did not so much get rid of uniformity and absolutism as re-establish them somewhere else, in a discipline where the out-group no longer consisted of labourers or heretics but of people with faulty operations: a near-seamless transition from religious uniformity to psychological uniformity. The problem of intellectual heterodoxy now lay not in the common ideas themselves but rather in the mechanisms by which one reached them. And this has been the founding metaphysic of modern psychology.

Fourthly, there is the modern habit of separating cognitive states from moral ones. This was not fully achieved until the late nineteenth century; and if today it is still possible to talk about "wisdom" as combining moral with intellectual judgement, this does not occur within psychology. The Greek philosophers seemingly subdivided the four cardinal virtues into moral ones (bravery, justice, temperance) and an intellectual one (civic intellect), but the core principle was that none of these could exist without the others. Aristotle appears to draw some sort of distinction: for example, the person at the bottom of the scale in his *Ethics* (someone lacking moderation) bears little resemblance to the slave at the bottom of the scale in *Politics* (lacking deliberation and forethought). However, this difference is not fundamental, since ethics and politics were for Aristotle the same area of enquiry; it simply reflects different social functions. The first person is someone who ought to be honourable because of his social station but is not; the second is engaged in manual work. Aristotle's underlying criteria for what it is to be human are multifaceted; they are not *either* moral *or* intellectual. This held good beyond the onset of Christianity. When the early church fathers call man "rational" on the grounds that "he is discerning about the true and the false, the good and the bad," these phrases are in apposition, not opposition; Aquinas's principle that "the good and true each include the other" echoes through the Middle Ages and Renaissance, accepted by theologians and medical humanists alike.[4] Conversely there are "fools," intellectually limited, who for that very reason are wicked, like Cloten in Shakespeare's *Cymbeline*; and there are clever people, like Edmund in *King Lear*, whose cleverness entails wickedness and so leads them to a sticky, unclever end.

In the proto-psychiatric texts of this period, carnal sin is synonymous both with atheism and with the general intellectual disability of the masses, who are "so weak and ignorant touching the faculties of nature" that they "little differ from brute beasts .... Divers men (or rather monsters) are of the same condition with those, whereof the prophet David speaketh, saying, the fool hath said in his heart, there is no God."[5] The atheist, in his cleverness, is vulgar, plebeian and beastlike because he only follows his pleasures. The label "Epicurean" was frequently used for this condition; it was a characteristic insult, employed to describe both his doctrine and his appetites, as well as his urge (like the Greek *idiotes* with whom he was associated) to seek happiness in a purely private sphere and avoid his public responsibilities for ruling over the masses. Typically, "stupidity" is a "spiritual lethargy" or "insensibility of mind" both to moral feelings *and* to understanding. It might also be a defence against wisdom's own enemy, "passion," but more often it meant "not having the body at [the soul's] command."[6] First Locke and then Kant with his "moral imperative" subsequently set such a priority on rational processes that anyone who never refers his passions and appetites to his reason was not so much a bad person as not a person at all. Only in the late nineteenth century did science finally separate the moral from the cognitive. However, they have been separated only to reconnect as a pair of opposites. Langdon Down already seems to have been on the defensive when he insisted that the "mongols" he identified were fully ethical beings despite their intellectual primitivity. In the age of amniocentesis, any suggestion to the biotechnology industry about the moral (let alone cognitive) worth of someone with "intellectual disability" goes against an even stronger tide: it is at most a private choice, and more often a doctrinal heresy.

Fifth comes the notion that intelligence and its disabilities are specifically human properties. Some account of previous applications of the word "intelligence" will be useful here. Central to *intelligentia* was always a sense of activity or transmission. Medieval philosophers conceived of a cosmos ruled by nine intelligences, each of which was a function of its first cause, the divine *intellectus*; angels were also, as their Greek etymology implies, messengers or "intelligenc*ers*." Humanist discussions of faculty psychology used *intelligentia* for the movement of the rational soul around the body; the soul was "entirely perfect" and "freed from the body" but had to communicate to it somehow.[7] If "intelligence" could be still used in the larger cosmic sense, so too could disability; universal disabling forces passed through the individual – melancholy, for example, was represented in this way.[8] We can also find *intelligentia* used in a prototypically modern sense. Already in the mid-sixteenth century complaints were voiced about its misuse as a synonym for *intellectus*, the "understanding."[9] Medical textbooks, tending to overlook philosophical niceties, often use the two interchangeably.[10] Intelligence was also sometimes conflated with mind (*mens*), which itself could cover a multitude of things: from "a general faculty in the universe as a whole" to the human individual's organic, "sensitive" soul, the one that remained in everyday contact with

---

[4] John Damascenus, *De Fide Orthodoxa*, cited by Albert in *Summa de Creaturis*, 516; Aquinas, cited in Voak, *Richard Hooker*, 62.

[5] De la Primaudaye, *Académie*, 869; 427.

[6] Charron, *Of Wisdom*, ii, 8; Thomas Milles, *The Treasurie*, 898.

[7] Bryskett, *A Discourse*, 274.

[8] Michael Schoenfeldt, *Bodies and Selves in Early Modern England*, 11.

[9] Elyot, *The Governour*, 239r.

[10] Akakia, *Galeni Ars Medica*, 105.

the material world. Baconian experimentalists used *intelligentia* to denote the specific knowledge content of *intellectus*, the latter being a mere shell. The seventeenth-century genre of psychological poetry discussed in Chapter 10 throws up examples such as "Intelligence (supreme pow'r of the soul) / wherein alone w'are like the deity"; in this sense it has become an elevated version of "wit," a specifically human reason that in its own modest way can be compared with divine reason, rather than being suspect as in Augustine or Calvin.[11] Locke reproduces this range of meanings, transmitting it to his eighteenth-century followers. At times intelligence is for him something merely human: "intelligent Americans," he says, are the Englishman's equals in their cognitive ability. At other times he uses the phrase "intelligent being[s]" in the Platonist sense, to cover the whole spectrum from humans to angels and God.[12] Behind these many adventures of the term, then, the axiom largely held that intelligence was attributable to divine as well as human beings. If by the early twentieth century Pearson and Spearman had transformed intelligence into a possession of the mass individual, as if it were a material property like height or eye colour, beneath this runs a deeper historical continuity with respect to the *goals* of intelligence: the aspiration to a transhuman perfection, whether divine or earthly.

Sixth is the cast-iron scientificity provided by statistical method. The scientific accreditation and social power of the dyad "normal/abnormal" was reinforced in some cases by evident physiological difference, which suggested an empirical verifiability for a cognitive difference akin to racial difference. In the mid-nineteenth century, Britain built its first large segregating long-stay institution (the Royal Earlswood), whose chief physician from 1858 to 1868 was Dr Langdon Down himself. Asked to come up with some system for classifying the unwieldy numbers of inmates, his intuition was to separate them by physical appearance. Physiognomics was already popular among "mad doctors."[13] The upshot was "mongols." The visible difference between mongol and non-mongol was only evident because the mass scale of the new social incarceration made numbers important. Statistics spread as a way of looking at the social world; they were "state" numbers, devised to serve administrative purposes. And the result of looking at people in the mass was that where *difference* was observed, the question of the *numbers* in each group suddenly struck the observer as never before. In Langdon Down's case, the fact that 599 out of every 600 people belonged in one group and only 1 in 600 in the other suddenly became, in itself, significant. "Normal" was originally, and for the pure statistician remains, a scientifically neutral term. But in human terms, something about the numerical disproportion of that 599 as against the 1 adds or subtracts social value and promotes labelling of the 1. And that something is, in the first instance, an artefact of institutionalization.

Langdon Down borrowed the mongol label from his contemporary James Hunt, whose "recapitulation" theory stated that each (white) human embryo individually recapitulates the development of the human race from primitive to civilized. Non-white groups were relics stuck at more primitive levels of intelligence; consequently a mongol born to white parents was a throwback to an earlier stage of species development. Hunt's theory seems drawn in part from earlier faculty psychology, with its theory that the vegetative, animal and rational souls arrive at successive stages in the growth of the foetus which correspond with infancy, youth and maturity in the living individual. But whereas faculty psychologists had denied that the foetus could already have "an intelligent or stupid mind," Down's 1 in 600 was already an intellectually inferior subspecies at some point of arrestation in the womb.[14] This enhanced the racial and cognitive superiority of

---

[11] John Davies of Hereford, *Mirum in Modum*.
[12] *An Essay*, 265.
[13] Sharrona Pearl, *About Faces*.
[14] Bryskett, *A Discourse*, 274; Otho Casmann, *Psychologia Anthropologica*, 51 ff.

the 599, and drove the notion of cause further back into a deterministic "nature" of the individual. It is a prime example of how, in the human sciences, "normal" has come to connote value, and of how from being a neutral term it has come to be an everyday term signifying "good."

Last but not least of our absolute presuppostions is the importance we place upon cause. This all-pervading and (in the case of disability) thoroughly modern obsession *derives from* our desire to root out "intellectual" monstrosity; the fact that it also *leads to* a scientific knowledge of that monstrosity is secondary. True, as far back as the ancient Greek physician Hierophilos there is evidence of an interest in causes; it led him to vivisect slaves, and for this reason he is said to have "hated men so that he might know." Nevertheless, he vivisected them in order to learn about human anatomy in general and because their social status allowed him to, not because he thought the inferior intellectual features of this group were biologically caused by the peculiar formation of their bodily material. Far from it: Greek doctors explicitly denied that intellectual inferiority was the province of medicine; their mythical patron Asclepios made the blind see and the lame walk but, it was said, could not make a fool wise. In Aristotelian and scholastic accounts of nature, causes were inseparable from "goals." In the explanatory apparatus of Galenist medicine, causes were subordinate to a more general of theory of "signs," from which they were not always distinct. Bacon's natural philosophy was the turning point. His inductive method, proceeding from empirical observation to general truths, led to a focus on the underlying causes of the detailed processes of knowing, which became the stuff of modern psychology. The mind was not to be left to take its own course but "must be guided at every step; and the business done as if by machinery."[15] By the eighteenth century, it was a type of mechanical and irremediable deficiency the physiognomist Johannes Caspar Lavater would have in mind when he modernized the Asclepios reference into his widely quoted saw, "The idiot born can never without a miracle become a philosopher."[16] The equation which modern medicine draws between explanation and cause is thus historically specific. Physicians, concerned as they normally are with cure, have developed a strong interest in that which is defined by its incurability, perhaps not so much because cures are in prospect (the track record is negligible), but because it affords them a fundamental social role, one might say a priestly or "necessitarian" role, in the verification and ostentation of difference.

Whereas modern medicine divides causes into two, normal and abnormal, early modern writers divided them into three: natural, unnatural and praeternatural. The unnatural was simply the unusual, an exotic manifestation of the natural itself; monstrous births involving (say) androgyny or conjoined twins, though unnatural, did not thereby *contradict* the natural. "There are no grotesques in nature," says Browne.[17] A praeternatural cause, on the other hand, was one that lay outside the patient. For Greek and Roman doctors this meant things in the external environment. In early modern medicine, external explanations usually boiled down to God or, more often, the devil. In the latter case the praeternatural cause was not only outside but *against* nature. Modern concepts of disability were born partly out of the collapse of the distinction between the merely unnatural and the demonically praeternatural within an originally tripartite conceptual framework. It was reduced to a dyad, natural/unnatural, which merged with that of normal/abnormal under the influence of statistics and nineteenth-century social policy. Behind this displacement of monstrosity from exotic nature to anxious pathology lay the threat which the cognitive monster posed to religious doctrine, and subsequently to secular development and progress. The preferred proof of God's existence during the eighteenth and early nineteenth centuries was the Argument from Design; a natural world whose operations dovetailed so perfectly had to have been created by a supremely

---

[15] Cited in Shapin, *The Scientific Revolution*, 90.
[16] *Essays on Physiognomy*, 231.
[17] *Religio*, 17.

intelligent being, and to be progressing towards a divinely ordained goal. Idiots appear to be a design fault in this picture, an obstacle to progress. Their existence might be used to disprove that of God, or alternatively as a sign of the reality of the devil in people's lives. Either way, it was the same problem: as Diderot, Kant and Darwin were all to ask in their various ways, how could such creatures contribute to God's purposes for the world?[18]

And so the fear associated with praeternatural causes was attached to the monstrous human consequence as well; the term "abnormal" to describe the statistical incidence of disability carries subliminally these demonic overtones. People bearing labels of intellectual monstrosity cease to be merely an unusual or alternative expression of the natural and become instead objects of a utilitarian anxiety about consequences. Eugenics is in this sense merely a secular expression of the Argument from (Intelligent) Design. Abnormality and intellectual disability are thus not so much the *motive* for eugenics, as is usually supposed, but its conceptual *product*. "Abnormality" is the kind of thing that happens when fear of pollution, at a certain historical stage and in a fresh social and economic context, reconceptualizes its target population. It expresses in a social form (fear of the representative other) what psychiatry's *Diagnostic and Statistical Manual* lists as a specific phobia. In this phobia about dirt and pollution we at last find our genuinely long-term mental disorder, whose symptoms are, if perhaps not transhistorical, then visible across much of recorded history: far longer lasting than the short- and medium-term disabilities we have so far discussed. Most research is effectively focused on expanding and exacerbating a negative image of these historically provisional kinds of difference, when it could instead be focusing on enabling people who are "intellectually" disabled by the modern era to be part of ordinary life. A successful cure would be one that touched the deepest root, the long-term phobic disorder, and thus would operate on the principle "Physician, heal thyself."

Behaviourist, behave yourself: the behavioural phenotype and its inventors

Having examined the largely unchallenged value presuppositions that lie behind the modern medical model of intellectual disability, we need now to define that model more sharply. With the entry of mind-body dualism into medicine, a philosophical conundrum about how mind intersects with body became a practical one. Adjectives from two entirely separate realms of nature, "intellectual" and "physical," were attached to one and the same noun, "disability." In intellectual disability, today's primary research focus is on the behavioural phenotype, which scientists define as a pattern of somatic and psychological characteristics with a corresponding pattern of genes. In reducing the body to certain ultimate entities in this way, they are following age-old convention. Skull shape, soul spirits, "elements," humours and genes have all filled this slot over the centuries. But whereas in Galenist medicine "stupidity" consisted simultaneously in slow soul spirits, slow somatic features (the muscles, for example) and slow psychological and behavioural ones, with no clear separation among these various categories, in modern medicine genes run a quite separate, if parallel, course with the mind. The problem of dualism is that whereas DNA exists in material nature, changing at the pace of biological evolution, intelligence and disability are purely conceptual and can therefore change with great rapidity. To try and map one on to the other creates muddle. It is as if a cartographer were to confuse lines formed by political entities, which change every few years, with those formed by physical geography, which change at the pace of continental drift.

---

[18] Denis Diderot, *Letter on the Blind*, 68; Immanuel Kant, *Critique of Teleological Judgement*, 84; Francis Darwin, *The Life*, ii, 311.

In defining cognitive or behavioural characteristics, let alone classifying them, what is our starting point? We begin inside our own heads. Psychological phenotypes consist of views we human beings have of each other; they originate in the realm of appearances. Of course appearances are in their own way real, and from Aristotle onwards have been regarded as the proper point of departure for scientific investigation. For this reason too, it may be proper in a medical context to speak of "cognitive impairments," to the limited extent that they relate to the particular historical and social conditions that render them impairments in the first place. Nevertheless a psychological phenotype – not just the concept but the actual stuff of which it is made – has its roots in human consensus alone. Attention Deficit Hyperactivity Disorder (ADHD), for example, exists because in the 1980s the American Psychiatric Association disputed and then elected a list of symptoms, eventually agreeing – it went to a second vote – to abide by the result. The selection of symptoms of autism was through a similar process. Private thinking, lack of empathy, monotropism, lack of eye contact, oppositional defiance, repetitive behaviours, flat intonation, a triad of impairments: any of these? All? Which ones? How many? Who decided? One can shuffle the pack, remove or add certain cards, even invent new and more sophisticated suits, but some common denominator is always presupposed; the existence of autism is something that everyone just knows, just as once upon a time the existence of the devil was something that everyone just knew. The stuff of every psychological phenotype originates in a social consensus reflecting the values of a particular time and place. It consists of behaviours which contemporaries – parents, social institutions, professionals – find problematical. The stuff of genes, by contrast, originates in the material realm, which exists irrespective of what people of any time or place might think. Although a consensus has to be reached among human beings working in laboratories about where to partition DNA sequences and thus about what is called a gene and how it is separate from some other gene, the basic stuff, DNA, is not something that only goes on in our heads.

Genotype and psychological phenotype belong to realms of existence so unalike that something freakish, and historically specific, is bound to happen when we try to link them. It is not just that genetic causes are by and large "not known" (fragile X) but simply "being sought" (autism), or "thought to exist" by some psychiatrists while flatly ruled out by others (ADHD); nor is the simplistic notion of "a gene for x" improved by that of "a complex cluster of genes for x." Even in the commonest assumed link of all, between sex chromosomes and gendered human behaviour, a pathway from one to the other eludes researchers once they get beyond broad-brush statistical correspondences and reach the laboratory stage. Hopes are then scaled down, and redirected to male and female transgenic mice. The supposition here, that there is no essential distinction between human and other animals, points to one possible solution to dualism: behaviourism. Typically, behaviourists deny experimental usefulness to the notion of mind and analyze the directly observable entity, behaviour, alone; mind, unlike behaviour, is not an observable phenomenon. But behavioural phenotype theory does not describe human subjects in general, only those deemed to be disordered. Knowledge of their behaviour is a substitute for the knowledge normally available from subjective communication, knowledge which one *can* experimentally obtain from most individual human minds but which is lacking in disabled ones. Behavioural phenotypes presuppose the existence of an invisible but normally observable cognitive ability which lies deeper than behaviour, and whose resistance to observation is mere pathology in certain individuals. Today's theory is as uninterested in distinguishing between the cognitive and the behavioural as it is between ability and performance. Does intellectual disability exert such "a profound influence on ... psychiatric and behavioural disorders" that this disability should be seen as prior? Or is it that intellectual disability is equal with motor, linguistic and social abnormality under a "behavioural" heading? Or is it simply that intellectual disability *is* behaviour, and hence subsumed under the latter?[19] The question is not thought to be worth pursuing.

Unlike pre- and early modern medical theory, which explained the relationship between mind and body as an organic interaction, today's doctrine is nothing but causal. In the relationship between genes and psychological characteristics, genes are prior. True, the environment may act back on them, somatic entities such as enzymes may work backwards to influence gene expression, and natural selection makes behaviour ultimately responsible for genetic change. And one can retreat when under attack into modest disclaimers about a multiplicity of risk factors, only to sally forth once again with a deterministic claim once the coast is clear. But in the behavioural phenotype, causes are ultimately one way. And the long historical perspective teaches us that this preoccupation with cause is itself a cultural bias. Causes only matter where elimination is needed or enhancement sought.

Furthermore, the association between genotype and psychological phenotype lends the latter an air of stability when actually it belongs to the unstable realm of consensual appearances and values. Its stability is established purely by association. The language used suggests that *psychological* phenotypes are the same order of things as *somatic* phenotypes. Nevertheless, this is mere wordplay. In earlier textbook biology, a phenotype simply *is*, by definition, somatic. Things such as size or eye colour have no trouble corresponding with a genotype. But to expand the range of the noun "phenotype" by replacing the adjective "somatic" with "psychological" is to smuggle in a metaphor.

We owe the genotype/phenotype formula to the botanist Wilhelm Johannsen, who also coined the word "gene." From around 1900 onwards he conducted experiments that matched the somatic appearance or "phenotype" of peas to their genotype. In the 1930s, the term started being used to describe behaviour in animals. Psychiatrists subsequently applied it to humans, following a much-referenced 1972 article by William Nyhan.[20] Biologists, in a pincer movement, have extended the "somatic phenotype" to cover psychological categories.[21] But mere metaphor is not sufficient to manoeuvre the psychological into the same realm of being as the somatic. From peas to minds is a big jump. The strictness of the mind-body divide is belied by the ease with which experts traverse the disciplinary boundaries. Nyhan, for example, despite his espousal of psychiatric terminology, was a geneticist. Johannsen too was a double agent, who built his theory of the somatic phenotype upon notions covertly supplied by psychology. As the "pathbreaking" inspiration for his formula "phenotype = genotype + environment," he cites not Mendel's work on botany but Galton's on human genius. He was seeking, he said, a verification of Galton's nature-nurture idea from the biologist's perspective. Statistical representations of "environment" had so far been speculative, but now its relationship to genes could be made concrete. A pure line of peas resembled a racially white and thus intellectually pure human population; it had its own "racial hygiene."[22] Historically, then, human differences in intelligence – a cultural matter of status differences – have gone into the very making of statistical biology, as well as the latter finding explanations for the former.

Johannsen's Reformed church background, like Galton's nonconformist one, may well have subliminally predisposed him to rethink the divine predestination of souls as the biological determination of intelligence. There is nevertheless one point on which modern psychiatry can

---

[19] G. O'Brien and W. Yule, "Why behavioural phenotypes?" in O'Brien and Yule (eds), *Behavioural Phenotypes*; J. Flint and W. Yule, "Behavioural phenotypes," in M. Rutter et al., *Child and Adolescent Psychiatry*; R. Plomin, "Behavioural genetics," in P. McHugh et al., *Genes, Brains and Behavior*.

[20] Nyhan, "Behavioural phenotypes," *Pediatric Research*, 6/1 (1972).

[21] Richard Dawkins, *The Extended Phenotype*.

[22] Wilhelm Johannsen, *Elemente der exakter Erblichkeitslehre*, 232; 703.

claim to be more robust than its pre-modern ancestor. Galenist medicine attributed the soul spirits' invisibility to the ultra-refined material of which they were composed, but actually they were a figment of the Galenist imagination. Soul spirits did not exist. DNA strings do. Modern psychiatry presents itself as an exact science because it deals with things that really are there to be measured. This is an inadequate claim, however. It was skull-measuring phrenologists who first advanced it, from whom there is a historical link through to genetics and psychology. Galton tried out physiognomics and phrenology as a young man, while Binet's first, unsuccessful experimental attempts to measure intelligence involved craniometry; conversely, nascent ideas about inheritance and eugenics flourished first among phrenologists.[23] The ultimate bodily entities in phrenology were the parts of the skull; the size of these, an indicator of the cerebral mass they contained, was correlated with degrees of ability or "mental power."[24] The intuition, then as now, was entirely fortuitous: that the bodily entity we are capable of measuring (formerly skulls, now genes) just happens to be that which can be correlated with whatever psychological feature we (one society in one era) decide is important to measure – and that therefore we can infer intellectual abilities from bodily ones.

Nyhan's article highlights this weakness. Despite his reputation as the pioneer of the behavioural phenotype, he makes not a single mention of this phrase in his paper. It only occurs in the title. The paper itself discusses not *phenotypes* but something far more mundane, namely *stereotypy*, or repetitive behaviour. Nyhan's point, his actual "first," was that stereotypies enable us to look at behaviour "in a quantitative sense." The title phrase was a mere verbal flourish, expressing his optimism that this fresh quantitative approach would at last make psychiatry a genuine science. What was more, scientific status would mean that behavioural disorder would have its own "specificity" and thereby cease to be just some sub-specialism under mental retardation. Indeed, it would replace the latter as the main area of study. And it is true that a stereotypy can be counted, measured and chi-squared. Take hand flapping: interested researchers find statistical significance in its "bout frequency," "mean bout length" and "bout length variability."[25] But interest in hand flapping comes only from the realm of our views of each other, from human consensus. There are many possible motives for isolating a particular behaviour. An experimental researcher thinks that *because* it is countable, *therefore* it is interesting. A teacher may dislike teaching a certain child, so Oppositional Defiant Disorder is diagnosed and the child removed from class. Parents in need of practical support with a family member might need a label that points to a genetic cause, thus triggering an allocation of funds. Admittedly Nyhan himself was more person centred, since his main concern was self-injury. But this is an exception. In most behaviours linked to disability, the suffering is not physical and so is usually imputed and/or value laden.

When Nyhan egged his study of stereotypy with its grand new "behavioural phenotype" heading, he was making a power bid. He wanted to give behaviour at least equal status with intelligence and retardation, an equal claim to be an exact (measurable) science. Of course, empire building does not in itself make the science questionable. The real problem is that two and two cannot make four if the first "two" exist in a different ontological realm from the second. Just because repetitive behaviours and DNA strings are both measurable, it does not mean they can be correlated.

---

[23] Fancher, "Francis Galton and phrenology," in *Proceedings of Tennet* IV; V. Hilts, "Obeying the laws of hereditary descent: phrenological views on inheritance and eugenics," *Journal of the History of the Behavioral Sciences*, 18/1 (2006).

[24] G. Combe, *Elements of Phrenology*, 21.

[25] S. Hall et al., "Structural and environmental characteristics of stereotyped behaviors," *American Journal of Mental Retardation*, 108 (2003); M. Lewis, "Ultradian rhythms in stereotyped and self-injurious behavior," *American Journal of Mental Deficiency*, 85 (1981).

This fallacy has been compounded as the psychological phenotype expands to cover such things as "social cognition" or "flexibility and responsiveness in social interactions."[26] The very existence of the idea of correlation rushes researchers into assuming that collecting evidence about genes is the same kind of activity as collecting evidence about social interactions, even though one is done in a laboratory, using pipettes, and the other in a social and verbal intercourse with human beings, using questionnaires. Genes that impair social cognition and responsive interactions in Turner's Syndrome, it is claimed, are expressed only from the paternal X chromosome; yet the evidence of impairment comes from interviews with people already imbued from their child's early infancy onwards with the idea that Turner's syndrome has a genotype impairing social cognition and responsive interactions – which may well have affected their upbringing of the child and fed back into the parental responses. And that is before we have all debated what "social interaction" is and submitted to the provisional consensus of the times we live in, and to the more powerful among the debaters. Hacking has noted such feedback loops in the conceptualization of autism, though he clings to the thought that they do not necessarily compromise its underlying reality.[27]

Because psychological phenotypes originate in the unstable realm of social consensus and anxiety, their boundaries cannot be drawn with the quasi-logical precision of biology. Once a pathological phenotype has been suggested, ever milder forms of it are observable, to the point where these forms cease and merge into the normal; and since the decision about where that point lies is likewise consensual, it too is arbitrary. Or a phenotype may sprout near-replications of itself with infinitesimal degrees of difference; the shading of specific psychological features is then thought to mirror the shading of specific genetic ones, and "shading" to be therefore the same kind of thing in both cases. It is not. It cannot be, because the assumed link is between unconnected orders of reality. There is also blurring between a phenotype and merely *analogous* behaviours or "behavioural phenocopies."[28] All this leads to phenotypic borders expanding to cover more and more individuals. ADHD, with no known genotype, is only the most startling example of this. Autism, where studies of dizygotic twins show that one of them can have certain distinctive genetic and behavioural traits while the overall category to which he or she belongs remains soft-edged, is another phenotype in the middle of a diagnostic epidemic.[29]

It is not only the phenotypes themselves but the theory as such that has these imperialist tendencies. There are people (with Down's syndrome, for example) whose distinctive biology has been in no doubt for a century and a half and who are now said to "have" a behavioural phenotype; or even, the syndrome just "is" a behavioural phenotype.[30] This pulls the rug from under the theory by eliding any distinction between known and assumed cause. Once the behavioural phenotype becomes a routine category, one can say that not only Down's syndrome but autism or attention deficit "is" a behavioural phenotype, regardless of whether or not a corresponding genotype in these latter cases has been or will ever be found. "Behavioural phenotype" then becomes so loose as to mean just unusual or worrying behaviour. And that is how one society will find itself justifying practices which another finds abhorrent. Take drapetomania for example, first diagnosed by the nineteenth-century American physician Samuel Cartwright, which undoubtedly would have been marked as a "behavioural phenotype" had such a phrase been around then. Its symptoms consisted,

---

[26] D. Skuse et al., "Evidence from Turner's syndrome of an imprinted X-linked locus affecting cognitive function," *Nature*, 387 (1997).

[27] *The Social Construction*, 119.

[28] Berrios and I. Markova, "Conceptual issues," in H. D'haenen et al., *Biological Psychiatry*.

[29] Morton Ann Gernsbacher, "Three reasons not to believe in an autism epidemic," *Current Directions in Psychological Science*, 14/2 (2005).

[30] Berney, "Behavioural phenotypes."

exclusively, in the urge to escape; its victims consisted, exclusively, in black slaves. Is/was this objectionable? If drapetomania, why not oppositional defiance? Or private thinking? Both of these, under some name or other, have likewise been pathologies with respect to the maintenance of social order. Kanner's 1943 reinvention of autism was conjured up at a major turning point in the world development of techniques of mass coercion over private thinkers in general; and his particular, autistic types do more than oppose or defy Big Brother (d.o.b. 1948), they are innately and genetically incapable of responding to him.

All the above exposes how indissoluble the behavioural phenotype is from social stereotypes and from its own underlying eugenic motives. At the same time, our knowledge of the biochemistry has outstripped our knowledge about what it is we are trying to eliminate. Henry Goddard invented "morons" a century ago as a way of demonstrating that the destitution and fiscal burden of certain families was due to (or simply was) an inherited psychiatric disability. In so doing he launched a generation of moral panic about racial hygiene; moronism was the core myth of first-wave eugenics. Goddard felt a need to nail a social anxiety to the reality of material facts, demonstrable by an exact science, so that the anxiety could be eliminated. Once a rule of correlation has been established, one can then go out and search for people who will fit it. A consensually reached psychological category generates a social identity, a receptacle into which the observer already primed with knowledge about the relevant phenotypic features can place individuals. The key point about morons was that they could not be distinguished by their appearance, pointing to the panic about imitators – people who may look normal but are not (a modern variant of the reprobate hypocrite). Similarly, coinciding with second-wave eugenics, today's cognitive geneticists have revived concern about "low intelligence within the band of normal" or "mild mental retardation," a category that had become almost obsolete between the two waves.[31]

In seeking a genetic basis for psychological categories, one may be aiming at cure, although this is plausible only in a tiny number of much-touted cases such as phenylketonuria (one in 15,000 births). And one may be aiming to alleviate the distress of parents, although the distress is imparted by the values of the medical model itself and the social institutions it inspires. Early modern doctors, too, held ambitions about cure, achievable by diet and training, for the plebeian intellectual deficiencies they detected in families of the gentry. But prevention has been and remains the far more frequent aim; and the result of attempts to explain psychological patterns by ultimate bodily entities – whether genes, skull shapes or soul spirits – has tended to be the denigration, segregation or elimination of some aspect of our common humanity. Good faith is not usually in doubt, but good faith for a scientist also involves going back and rechecking one's premises.

---

[31] For example Michael Rutter, "Genetic influences on mild mental retardation," *Journal of Biosocial Science*, 28 (1996).

Chapter 13
The Brain of a Fool

The idea of a behavioural phenotype sets off in two diametrically opposing directions at once. In terms of pure theory it starts from the natural phenomenon of genes, which give rise to psychological classifications that in turn give rise to a social phenomenon, anxiety. The investigative sequence is the reverse. It starts from a social phenomenon, anxiety, which gives rise to psychological classifications that in turn give rise to the discovery of the natural phenomenon of genes. The doctrinal basis of cognitive genetics and behavioural phenotypes is unidirectional, seeking precise causal links from genes to intelligence when in fact intelligence is an artefact that covertly imports (social) causes of its own into the calculation.

In this broad sense, Renaissance medicine and behavioural phenotype theory are alike, even if their respective biological and social components differ. Where we place genes, our predecessors placed soul spirits, humours and qualities of elements. The social group to which they attributed the familiar modern characteristics of disability – inability to think abstractly, reason logically, process information or maintain attention – was not our small pathological one but a huge section of the population: the lower social orders, women and ethnic or religious minorities. What these doctrines share is that a given feature of the social world, the inferiority of certain population groups as perceived and feared by their betters, has been converted into a feature of the natural world. The social inferiority of these population groups is then represented as a *consequence* of their natural inferiority.

Despite these shared long-term characteristics, we cannot disregard the medium-term but deep conceptual differences. Medieval and early modern medicine invoked a general "foolishness" which it described in very disparate terms of Adamite degeneracy, infancy, old age, bodily disease, deaf mutism, eccentricity, drunkenness, the simulated foolishness of the jester, mental illness, melancholy. Most of these were seen as dispositional rather than a personal possession, none with a clear separation between the psychological and the physiological. A reader who searches the index of a Renaissance medical compendium for the various Latin terms translatable as foolishness (*stultitia, stoliditas, stupiditas, fatuitas*) and then looks up the referenced passages to check the corresponding symptoms will mostly find things quite unfamiliar to modern medicine – unlike historians of madness, who will often find symptoms that resemble a modern condition when looking up terms such as *mania, phrenesis* and similar designations. Modern, Renaissance and Hippocratic doctors might agree, if only in the broadest terms, on something we now call bipolar disorder, as they certainly might on physical disability. One has to draw the methodological consequences. Even the most radical historians have only ever treated "intellectual disability" either as a footnote to the history of *mental* pathology dominated by mental *illness*, or of *disability* dominated by the *physical* disability. But as J.L. Austin warns us in *Sense and Sensibilia*: whenever we see the first concept in an antithetical pair crumbling beneath our critical gaze (in our case, madness versus intellectual disability), be sure the other will be crumbling too, but that this will have escaped our notice.

Another significant historical difference lies in the doctor's relationship to his patients. In order to find a long-term theoretical context for the medical model, we need to study up, as the anthropologists say: to assess the minds of doctors as well as the disabled. For any doctor, thinking about disease partly involves imagining oneself in the patient's state. But in the case of *intellectual* disability, even though it follows a disease model, the doctor's diagnostic approach does not start from imagining him- or herself in this state. Modern doctors cannot vicariously experience the intellectual state of a creature they deem innately and incurably incapable of the abstract thinking and logical reasoning which is the premise of their own intelligence and expertise. Foolishness, however, was something a Renaissance doctor could and did empathize with. If he could perceive certain brain states in himself – "dullness," "excessive languor" and "sluggishness of the internal senses," to be found in stolidity, lethargy, drunkenness, the after-effects of intense emotion, the curable "stupidity" of melancholy, the "stupor" or "mindlessness" that heralds the resolution of a bodily illness or for five minutes after a nap (all these examples are drawn from contemporary medical accounts of foolishness) – then he could know such things in his patient.[1] The empathy of such learned doctors extended to a "foolishness" that was in some sense general and (as it were) normal.

A third historical shift is from slowness to absence as the dominant model. In this sense medicine was no doubt influenced by the legal model described in Chapter 9, which highlighted absence and removal. The fool's intellect is (so to speak) sequestered, like his property, in perpetuity. This is a key moment. The Renaissance model of intellectual health as a mean (either between slow and furious melancholy, or between melancholy defined as slow and other mental states defined as furious) began to absorb the legal and fiscal controversies over idiocy and lunacy of the 1590s. Absence, in addition to slowness, came to characterize the legally incurable idiot, in contrast to the excess activity and speed of the lunatic with lucid intervals. John Donne's *Elegy: the Dream* demonstrates this when he debates with himself whether it is better for his lover to be present in reality or only in his imagination. His final couplet resolves in favour of the first: "Filled with her love, may I be rather grown / Mad with much heart, than idiot with none." Donne's language fuses a medical explanation (excess/deficient mental activity) with a jurisprudential one (curable/incurable absence); lunacy takes over the first characteristic in each pair, idiocy the second.

Specifically medico-psychological usages of the latter word had till now been very rare. One general guide to health of 1579 places idiots under the heading of "defect" and absence, alongside mania under the heading of temporary "sickness," but it does not present a clear dyad since other headings are involved.[2] James I's physician Helkiah Crooke writes in 1615 about people who lack certain parts of the brain and its corresponding faculties, and who are "esteemed foolish idiots ... even by the common people," that is, by those who simply by virtue of being common would usually be termed idiots themselves. Crooke was also Keeper of Bedlam, which would have placed him at the centre of legal controversy over the sequestration of incompetents' estates, and the hospital's records show that its governors were taking increasing care to weed out "idiots" because they were not deemed to be curable.[3] It took another two centuries for the medico-legal brew to be fully digested, however.

Physiognomics

The advanced medical teaching centres of the Renaissance at Padova, Leiden and Paris eventually located intellectual problems in the head and the brain. The importance of the brain depended on the activity of certain ultimate atomistic components of matter. These medical men shared

---

[1] Felix Platter, *Praxeos Medicae*, 2; Girolamo Cardano, *Opera Omnia*, ii, 265.
[2] Jones, *The Arte*, 93.
[3] Helkiah Crooke, *Microcosmographia*, 505; Patricia Allderidge, "Management and mismanagement in Bedlam," in C. Webster (ed.), *Health, Medicine and Mortality in the Sixteenth Century*.

with their modern successors the urge to break the important physiological features of intellectual difference down into its smallest entities. Whereas today the features consist chiefly of genes, in pre- and early modern medicine they consisted of the soul spirits, the four humours (blood, yellow bile, black bile, phlegm) and the balance of qualities (wet, dry, cold, hot) associated with the four elements (water, fire, earth, air).

However, there was nothing like the modern neurologist's assumption that your brain is who you are, that death is brain death.[4] The ancients had located thought in the heart or diaphragm rather than the head. Renaissance doctors admitted, like Shakespeare, that they could not tell where "fancy" – the imagination, the entry point into the reasoning faculty – was bred: in the heart or in the head? Donne's idiot has no "heart." Theologians tended to think of the heart as the source of our intellects, the evidence being that the latter are dominated by our private passions. "The fool hath said in his heart, there is no God" meant "said to himself" – that is, in secret, in the privacy of his own body. William Harvey at times locates the soul in the blood, and in dedicating his book on the circulation of the blood to Charles I, he refers to the heart as the place whence, in addition, "all power and grace flow[s]."[5] But in the main text he demotes it, both socially and physiologically. "Blood is not the natural vehicle of honour," he writes. "Nobility ... civil and political" belongs to the organ at the top of the body, and of the body politic. The head stands above and separate from blood and the passions, and is the vehicle for both honour and wit. Brain theory emerges with a new theory of public reason, though with competing emphases on brain structure (its division into ventricles, their corresponding psychological faculties and operations) and brain function (the motion of soul spirits around the brain, and their animation of the rest of the body).

While physical medicine was going through these realignments, the very premise of faculty psychology was the existence of a link between the human intellect and cerebral anatomy. Now the idea that such a link is possible suggests (a) a clear conceptual distinction between thinking states and their bodily organ, and (b) some degree of causality in their relationship. Furthermore, an impaired brain is surely the one organ that might be thought to fix a permanent psychological identity. Perhaps, then, a Renaissance doctor might have recognized something like a modern disability of the intellect? His source texts would have come from physiognomics, the reading of character from the body and especially the head – an ancient body of knowledge that had found its way piecemeal into Roman medical textbooks, Galen's among them. Early modern writers therefore had two separate textual traditions to draw on: one a "pure" physiognomics in its own right, the other strictly medical and Galenist with embedded physiognomic elements. Physiognomics provided a theoretical link from the realm of nature to that of intellect and behaviour, and a practical guide for policing them. Roman social elites used it to appoint new colleagues to public office and private salons, to prove the stupidity of opponents and to select wives, servants and wet nurses.[6]

A formal branch of the curriculum in the first universities at Bologna and Paris, physiognomics was viewed as the bridge between the study of nature (*libri naturales*) and morals (*libri morales*), in which role modern psychology has replaced it. As a diagnostic instrument, it was employed to accredit the professional and administrative skills necessary to the expansion of papal and state power. Its chief scholastic advocates such as Michael Scotus and Jean of Jandun saw physiognomics as the branch of knowledge that would at last enable philosophers to integrate with society, because it gave them a practical role in supplying the elite with reliable recruitment tools. The humanists likewise saw it as a form of sophistic or "useful" knowledge that would help civic leaders assess

---

[4] See Michael Gazzaniga, *The Ethical Brain*.
[5] Hill, *The Intellectual Origins*, 244.
[6] See Jole Agrimi, *Ingeniosa Scientia Naturae*, 235 ff.

the citizens in their charge.[7] Countless physiognomic textbooks were published, often laid out in tabular form as briefing notes, supplying shortcuts to certainty about people in public life and raising the social status of their authors by associating them with the civic intellect or *prudentia* of ruling elites. Its scientific method paralleled the methods used in heraldic science to assess honour. Children were said to resemble their parents physiognomically for three or four generations, the same requirement as for the authentification of a family's gentility.[8] Biological and social concepts of group continuity modelled each other.

Pure physiognomics drew inferences directly from the morphology of the head to human character and behaviour; medicalized physiognomics dealt also with what was going on *inside* the head. A certain shape might be an external sign of "stupidity," a condition at once physical and behavioural, reducible to laziness and inertia. It was on this basis, for example, that Erasmus and a fellow countryman, the popular medical writer Levine Lemnius, attributed stupidity *en masse* to the peasants of Batavia in the Rhine delta, whose external environment and inner constitutions were excessively wet (this led to "Boeotians," as the classical exemplars of stupidity, being replaced in medical textbooks by "Batavians"). Stupidity led to melancholia, unbelief and ultimately mindlessness (*amentia*), whose symptoms these authors listed as hypocrisy and an incapacity for sincere faith.[9] Both writers had been born in Batavia, and were thereby distancing themselves intellectually and socially from its generally boorish reputation – though far from attacking the folly of honourless peasants, Erasmus's actual target was his peers in the local ecclesiastical elite, for their arrogant intellectualism and lack of understanding of the egalitarian quality of grace.[10]

Physiognomic signs referred primarily to *actions*. Lazy or stupid behaviour was a source of anxiety because it impacted on the person's allotted social calling. In this sense physiognomics was the external form of what later became, as psychology, an internal science of control. From its very debut in the curriculum, well before the rise of humanism or the Reformation, it alerted medical observers to the possibility of a creaturely equality among princes, citizens and servants, since physiognomic and anatomical types palpably did not always correlate with social roles. However, in the texts on physiognomics these egalitarian hints are mere rhetoric, a safety valve allowing room for any renegotiation of status boundaries that might be demanded by political pressures. Physiognomics remained hierarchical in the sense that it created a scientific *typology* of physical appearances and gave them appropriate labels as Adam had done for the beasts, and one of which, of course, displayed the morphological difference between "philosophers" – experts on physiognomics, for example – and "bestial men."

Despite this, physiognomics was by no means deterministic. In interactions between body and mind, the body too was changeable. Physiognomic signs loosely indicated material conditions in the important somatic sites, among which the brain was merely one among several, and particularly the balance or "complexion" there of the four elements and their qualities, and the four humours. (Some of our present-day usages hark back to this: both "crass stupidity" and "coarse wit," *crassum ingenium*, originally referred to a coarseness of the brain's material constituents.) In Galenist textbooks, an imbalance of material qualities in the brain is *as such* a cognitive impairment. In a classic passage, at the core of the medical curriculum for centuries via its reproduction in Avicenna's *Canon*, Galen itemizes the intellectual impairments: coma, apoplexy, paralysis, catalepsy, vertigo,

---

[7] Voula Tsouna, "Doubts about other minds and the science of physiognomics," *Classical Quarterly*, 48 (1998).

[8] Devyver, *Le sang*, 167.

[9] Levine Lemnius, *De Habitu et Constitutione Corporis*, 17; Thomas Willis, *De Anima Brutorum*, 506.

[10] Erasmus, *Familiarum Colloquiorum*, 245; *In Praise of Folly*, 100; see also Erika Rummel, *The Confessionalization of Humanism in Reformation Germany*, 55.

lethargy, fainting, melancholy, epilepsy and phrenitis.[11] Thinking states (*dianoia*), cerebral matter and the size and shape of the skull are all taken together in this passage as signs of a patient's health and particularly of the physical health of the brain, where "health" carries a moral inflection. It consisted in temperament and balance, and "balance" may seem to imply fluctuation: transience rather than permanence. True, a defective mixture of elements might not be of short duration as in fevers, but something much longer term; nevertheless, tenacious as the mixture may have been, the imbalance was ultimately just dispositional. Explanations of a chronic condition did not differ essentially from those of an acute one, and this held true even for the structure of the skull. Now while common sense says that imbalance may be transient, to say that anatomical structure is transient seems curious, at least to us. What could be more permanent about our bodies than the shape and size of our heads? But pre- and early modern doctors saw things otherwise.

First, as we have already noted, the fact that a human characteristic is permanent, even if it belongs to each and every species member, is not enough to qualify it as an essential property of that species, since the very notion of permanence suggests a need to keep checking that the characteristic is still there. As Aristotle put it, the "essential property" of what it is to be human must *a priori* lack any incompatible elements and therefore does not require checking.[12] Moreover, divine acts of grace and regeneration affect not only the soul and its faculties but "must as well reach the body too, the ministerial and organical parts, which are also said to be sanctified"; conversely, "to be deprived of the use of reason, is one of the greatest *corporal* calamities in this life" (emphasis added).[13] Neither in Galen's Rome nor in early modern Europe did *permanence* indicate *identity*, as it does for us. Despite a gradually increasing interest in certain causal aspects of behaviour and intelligence, no theory of medical necessity arose that could rival the religious one of predestination. In fact determinism of a biological or natural type was explicitly refuted:

> The reasonable part of man ... depends, in all its ordinary and natural operations, upon the happy or disordered temperature of those vital qualities out of whose apt and regular commixion the good estate of the body is framed .... Yet this dependence on the body is not so necessary and immutable but that it may admit of variation .... The toughest and most unbended natures by early and prudent discipline may be much rectified.[14]

For doctor as well as theologian, necessity could be nothing other than divine; it transcended any medical nature. The "unbended natures" here are still *within the sphere* of nature – not within that of reprobation, which was indeed determinate and unbendable. Conversely, predestination theologians themselves distinguished between the "medicinal [sc. therapeutic] excommunication" of waverers and the "exterminative excommunication" of reprobates; in this we can see foreshadowed the terms of nineteenth-century debates about the curability or incurability of various types of idiot.[15]

Secondly, physiology and psychology were not simply juxtaposed; they jointly inhabited the same explanatory realm. Body and soul interact, so the body too undergoes change. As a widely read textbook put it, "When there is a change in the disposition of the soul, it simultaneously changes the shape of the body; conversely when there is a change in the shape of the body, it

---

[11] Galen, *De Locis Affectis*, 3.5, in Kühn (ed.), *Opera*, viii, 76.
[12] Aristotle, *Topics*, 482a.
[13] W.M., *The Middle Way*, 8; Baxter, *Directions and Perswasions*, 161.
[14] Edward Reynolds, *A Treatise of the Passions and Faculties of the Soule of Man*, 4.
[15] W.M. Hetherington (ed.), *Notes and Debates of the Proceedings of the Assembly of Divines at Westminster*, 88.

changes the disposition of the soul."[16] Admittedly, this writer confines his examples to "grieving people with gloomy faces and happy people with cheerful ones." But he was not making the point that grief *causes* a certain facial expression. Rather, he was demonstrating their *synchronicity*, as evidence of sympathetic interaction between soul and body. In Renaissance medicine, intellect and head shape both belonged on the same side of the signifier/signified divide; what they signified, jointly, was the material (im)balance or temperament of a bodily organ, the brain.

Cranial sutures and their psychological symptoms

Such were the founding principles of physiognomics. We now need to look at some of its recurring themes. First of all the individual's physiognomy was linked to his cranial sutures, the cracks along which separate sections of the skull are aligned. Aristotle claims that humans have more sutures than other animals, his absolute presupposition being that more "parts" means better.[17] One Hippocratic author writes similarly that four sutures are healthier than three, without saying why. A second author describes a variety of arrangements of sutures.[18] Neither Aristotle nor the Hippocratics discuss thinking states, behaviour or character in this context. In *The Art of Medicine* Galen proposes a "suitable" shape for the healthy brain: it is an elongated sphere "slightly depressed at the sides."[19] There are also unsuitable shapes, he said, associated with sutural deficiencies (in this sense it is a discussion about values).

The second Hippocratic author had depicted each sutural arrangement as a letter of the alphabet, and Galen, followed by dozens of Renaissance Galenists, adopted this schema. The healthy brain, he wrote, sits in a skull where one suture (the coronal) runs across the front of the skull from one side to the other, down to just in front of the ears; another suture (the lambdoid) runs parallel to it across the back; and the third (the sagittal) runs down the middle of the skull from front to back, joining the other two sutures at their respective midpoints. Viewed from above, this arrangement of sutures resembles an H (capital η). In one type of unsuitable skull the coronal suture is missing, and so too the skull's frontal projection; the resulting arrangement is a T-shape. In another type, the lambdoid suture and thus the skull's rear projection are missing, in which case the arrangement is T again. In a further unsuitable type, both the front and rear projections are missing; the sagittal suture is in place, but is intersected by a single transverse suture running across the middle of the skull. Viewed diagonally, this arrangement resembles X (capital χ).[20] Galen labels these unsuitable types "pointy heads" because of the appearance created by the missing projections, though he mentions no intellectual impairment in this context. He then adds:

> It is possible for a fourth type of pointy head to be imagined, albeit not to exist, which measures longer from ear to ear than from front to back. If this type were to exist, it would not accord with nature and would be the opposite of spherical: its length would become its depth. Now so great a deviation from the natural could not exist; it would be a monstrosity rather than just a pointy head, and would not be capable of life .... Either the front or the rear eminence might be absent, or indeed both at the same time, but not to such an extent that some of the brain itself is missing.

---

[16] Aristotle (attrib.), *Physiognomics*, 808b.
[17] *On the Parts of Animals*, 653a.
[18] Hippocrates, *On Injuries of the Head*, in E. Littré (ed.), *Opera*, iii, 182; *Places of Man*, in ibid., vi, 284.
[19] In Kühn (ed.), *Opera*, i, 751.
[20] Galen, *De Usu*, in *Opera*, ii; *De Ossibus*, in *Opera*, xvii.

Galen criticizes his Hippocratic predecessor for not mentioning this other type, even though it is merely hypothetical ("missing some of the brain" meant it was unviable). This monstrosity is again purely anatomical; thinking states are not mentioned. He does, however, refer here to the pointy head of Thersites, Homer's "private" soldier who steps out from the ranks to attack the warmongering nobles. Like a medieval jester-fool, Thersites speaks truth to power. His physical deformity (he has bandy legs) is therefore a sign of his oppositional politics, and his other characteristics too are external and behavioural, rather than intellectual; he merely "plays" the fool.

Pointy heads and head shape turn up in two further Galen passages. One of these, which remained unknown to most Renaissance readers, does link head size to intellect: "Thinking states (*dianoia*) are clearly impaired in those whose head is too large or too small."[21] In a large head, thinking states are usually but not always faulty; Pericles, despite his famously large head, was "an extremely alert thinker." In a small head, thinking states are defective without exception. At the same time they are merely one sign among others (for example, "small eyes, stuttering and irascibility") of the main medical concern: the overall physical health of the brain and its proportionality to the rest of the body. A large head means a weak neck, so the upper and lower jaws do not fit: "Such people have constant headaches and ears that weep with a thin and watery or purulent and stinking matter producing much evil superfluity," the function of sutures being to evacuate fluids from the brain. The difference between excessively large or small heads was that in a large head "the brain and medulla being bigger, there is a larger flow of spirit (*pneuma*) and room for it; the opposite is the case with small brains."

Here as elsewhere Galen had been reticent about the neurology. Thinking states were affected by the quality and mixture of "spirit" (*pneuma*), but only in very general terms.[22] He was interested in the health of each main bodily organ; thinking states were important only as a secondary indicator of the health of this particular organ, the brain. In early modern medicine physiognomics became more closely involved with intellectual states, mainly via the numerous commentaries on *The Art of Medicine*. Actually, of the four texts of Galen's quoted above, this has the least to say on head shape; but the commentators tended to bring in elements from the other texts. Although these commentaries arrived in distinct historical waves, I deal with them here as a whole, since they do not differ essentially in their approach to our topic.

Size was as important for these writers as shape. The optimum size was usually a mean. Aristotle was quoted as saying that small heads were intellectually superior, but in fact he had merely been talking about dwarfism, where the head seems too large for the rest of the body.[23] And whereas Galen, who wrote about small heads being invariably defective, had not done so in terms of their relationship to thinking states (apart from one or two vague mentions of "spirit"), later Galenists speculated more about the links between head size, the condition of the soul spirits and the cerebral material through which these spirits move. Ibn Ridwan in the tenth century wrote that "smallness is the essential sign of a bad brain composition" because it "constricts the channels and ventricles ... [and] the soul spirits do not have enough space in the brain to let them move on freely to complete their operations." Avicenna's ubiquitously read *Canon* repeats the point. The spirits get compressed, so they dry out and "burn up." Conversely, large heads are excessively moist. In a small head there is "smallness in the nerves connecting to the [external] senses; all the senses are weak and the operations of motion are weak." The problem of constriction is insoluble. A large brain, by contrast, is not necessarily faulty; it "has the merit of good composition, with open channels in which clear spirits pass freely without much confusion of images." The problem

---

[21] Galen, *Commentary on the* Epidemics 6 *of Hippocrates*, in *Opera*, xvii, 818.

[22] Julius Rocca, "Galen and the ventricular system," *Journal of the History of the Neurosciences*, 227.

[23] *On the Parts of Animals*, 686b.

is that "it is far from well-tempered, because it accommodates an over-abundance of material." It may well signify "disability [*impotentia*] of nature, which cannot produce material" because it has so much room that the soul spirits get lost.[24]

Faculty psychology played a part in these discussions. In Fuller's character type of the "natural fool," for example, "their heads sometimes [are] so little that there is no room for wit; sometimes so long, that there is no wit for so much room."[25] The cerebral substance was said to contain certain chambers or "ventricles" that housed each of the faculties separately. The allocation of separate cognitive functions to specific parts of the brain helped reinforce the idea of "intellect" as a psychological object, something more than just a passing series of thinking states. Galen had made occasional reference to imagination, judgement/reasoning and memory, but nowhere did he match these particular faculties to particular ventricles. He merely said that a general psychic spirit is stored in the ventricles as a whole, whence it is distributed through the brain and the rest of the body. The identification of specific faculties with specific ventricles had to wait for the fifth-century Galenist Nemesius, a Christian writer whose account of the soul was the chief source text of early modern faculty psychology.[26] From this account arose the idea both that variations in ventricular capacity could be externally verified by the shape of the individual's head and that there must be an association between shape (together with the consequent state of the cerebral substance) and the intellectual faculties.

This idea, first elaborated by Ibn Ridwan and Avicenna, then by Renaissance doctors, gave rise to various disputes. One was about whether it was the size of the head or its shape that should take priority as an indicator of the condition of the faculty. Some thought size was more important because it had to be proportionate to the size of the other bodily organs; others thought it was better for the head to be perfectly shaped but on the small or large side than to be proportionately sized but imperfectly shaped. For example, although imagination is housed in the front ventricle, a large frontal eminence would not necessarily indicate greater powers of imagination; in fact, the opposite might be true.[27]

A second dispute concerned whether the functioning and cerebral substance of the brain, or its shape and size taken together ("structure rather than temperament") were primary. One school claimed that "the cause of [differences in] civic intellect (*prudentia*) is a variety in the structure of the brain," while another claimed that, on the contrary, balance is prior: "the bad structure and pointy head ... have their origin in a bad mixture" of soul spirits, "narrowness of the brain" being merely a trigger or "proximate" cause. Even though the head "must have symmetry with the rest of the body," this external structure may not be decisive: "brain substance [in a small head] is necessarily very little, the ventricles narrow and the soul spirits few and insufficient for their functions ... [but] while [the functions] are imperfect, they are not necessarily faulty, as long as the soul can properly apprehend and render intelligible the images of things and pay attention." It is just that where "cogitations are long and drawn out, more spirits are expended than the brain ventricles can supply," and so the faculty gets tired more quickly.[28]

Another frequent dispute was about whether an injury to one ventricle affects the rest of the mind, or only the faculty corresponding to that ventricle. If injury did affect the whole cognitive process, did that mean it impaired the rational soul, which links the individual to divine

---

[24] Ibn Ridwan, *Galeni Liber*, unpaginated; Argenterio, *In Artem*, 215; Oddi, *In Librum*, 118; Galeazzo di Santa Sofia, *Libellus ... in Artem Parvam Galeni*, 102; Riolan, *In Artem*, 41.
[25] Fuller, *The Holy and the Profane*, 4.12.1.
[26] Moreno Morani, *Nemesii Emeseni De Natura Hominis*, 68.
[27] Giovanni Sermoneta, *Quaestiones Subtilissimae*, 53.
[28] Argenterio, *In Artem*, 219; Santorio, *Commentaria*, 214; Akakia, *Claudii Galeni*, 101.

reason – and could it do so without making it seem as if the Almighty himself were responsible for creating impairments? (This question, as we have seen, was also central to theological disputes about reprobation.) Moreover, the *lack* of an eminence, caused by lack of one of the cranial sutures, might create the same impairment as an *injury* to it. Some claimed that the absence of one or another eminence, or of a section of it, did not necessarily indicate "weakness" of brain matter. Others assumed it did. For the advocates of size, small-headed people were dispositionally "foolish and inattentive," "inconstant" and also "fearful" (a reference to the melancholia paradigm). Big heads, being humid, were "foolish," an indicator of the "leaden wit (*ingenium*)" of "the lazy, somnolent man." They were also colder, "thus actions are blunted .... Big heads are dull (*hebetes*), mindless (*amentes*) and full of catarrh."[29]

The word for "dull" here originally signified a defect in the five external senses, its intellectual significance coming only with the arrival of the intellect as a separate psychological object. We need to keep asking: what was the actual content of all this stupidity and foolishness? An extra-large forehead, for example, "indicates a ponderousness extending to foolishness, and when it is broad, paucity of discretion," but the illustration here is "the pointy head of Thersites the fool": the reference is to commoners in general. Furthermore, doctors do not distinguish between cognitive failings that are cognitive *per se* (a distinction that can only be modern) and those that accompany physical disease. Imperfect shape points to a general impairment "in all the principal actions of reason such as imagination, reasoning and memory," but the concrete illustrations then tend to be things like apoplexy or epilepsy.[30] Medical writers claiming that "people who are fatuous, stolid or mindless have a deficient head structure" reach by way of illustration for Galen's list of coma, apoplexy, lethargy, and the rest. Either fatuity, stupidity, mindlessness, etc., are mere "symptoms and effects" of these, or there is no clear distinction between physical and mental ("this apoplexy is, as I take it, a kind of lethargy, ... a kind of sleeping in the blood," says Falstaff). Their moral aspect is exemplified again by the lazy, "ridiculous behaviour" of Thersites, evoking the occupational behaviours of the jester.[31]

We today may see the physical and the mental as self-evidently distinct dimensions of the human person, but Renaissance writers drew their distinctions elsewhere. External behaviour and cognitive operations, and internal (material) mechanisms such as the soul spirits, complemented each another. Or intellectual rubrics might actually be subordinate to physiological ones; "learning difficulty" (*dusmathia*) is important chiefly as the sign of a cold brain, and "stupid spirits" as the sign of a wet one. A phrase such as "too much stupid, or stirred" (failure to keep to the mean) might refer without distinction to cognitive and moral faculties, soul spirits and the movement of the muscles, in respect of one and the same human activity. The terms translatable as "stupid" or "foolish" (*stultus, stupidus, stolidus*) describe a moral type – in this case, the lazy person.[32] Descartes used *stupidus* to describe exactly that characteristic which marks the body off from the mind. Often it is also an expression, not just a metaphor, for spiritless atheism.[33] Moreover, unlike modern intellectual disability, all the impairments were treatable. The Stoics had the idea of a "medicine of the mind." Once Galenism became Christianized, divine providence was another possible cure. And if temperament and complexion could influence morphology, then even something as seemingly determinate as head shape might be rectified. One Hippocratic author, much cited in the Renaissance, mentions a tribe

---

[29] Ugo Benzi, *Expositio super Libros Tegni Galeni*, 21; Riolan, *In Artem*, 41; Da Monte, *In Artem*, 132.
[30] Sermoneta, *Quaestiones*, 53; Oddi, *In Librum*, 118.
[31] Argenterio, *In Artem*, 218.
[32] Franciscus de le Boe, *The Practice of Physick*, 373; Dryvere, *In Τεχνην*, 108; Giovanni Manardi, *Annotationes in Artis Medicinalis Galeni*, 195; Riolan, *In Artem*, 41, 54; D'Abano, *Conciliator*, 119.
[33] For example Cudworth, *The True Intellectual System of the Universe*, 3.

of *macrocephali* ("bigheads") who customarily performed cranioplasty on their infants because elongated heads were valued more highly. Ali ibn Abbas recommended the binding of malformed heads. In this therapeutic sense, custom or nurture could *become* nature, it was said. Even the monstrous sutureless skull could be cured, if "with great difficulty."[34] Such ideas contrast with the determinism and incurability that dominate our own notions of disability.

Collectively, to the extent that they can be separated from the body at all, these "foolish" states tend to be secondary symptoms of melancholia. Pieter van Foreest, founder of the medical school at Leiden, noted two diametrically opposite constituents of foolishness (*stultitia*). One was excess phlegm, his example being a young boy whose symptoms consisted of stammering and dressing up; the other was an excessively dry brain, the example here being goitrous Alpine peasants.[35] According to Van Foreest, whereas foolishness can be either wet or dry, melancholy is only dry. The dryness of the Alpine peasants shows that foolishness can be confused with melancholia, and that only a clever doctor like Van Foreest can tell them apart. In short, foolishness was only worth discussing to the extent that it said something about melancholy.

We occasionally come across a description of symptoms that does not relate back to melancholy but sounds more modern, such as the inability to think abstractly; however, this latter will probably have strayed into medical texts from its more usual place in theology, and in any case it will have been used to describe an entirely different population. Luis Mercado, for example, claimed that congenitally deaf people cannot grasp essences, that is, the kind of knowledge that comes from sorting concepts and the ability to abstract. That was because the images that stimulate wit (*ingenium*) can only be aroused by the spoken word. People who cannot hear perceive the world as a mass of unsorted "accidents," because they are unable to gather concepts, let alone knowledge, from words. (In the Spain of Mercado's day, a deaf son could not inherit his father's estate unless he could speak.) Where he does mention foolishness (*stultitia*, *fatuitas*), on the other hand, it is dispositional, rather than developmental as in the case of the incurably deaf.[36]

Instability of opinion and attention deficit

Out of Galen's brief comments on physiognomy in *The Art of Medicine*, Renaissance doctors teased another wide-ranging condition which is almost as important as melancholy: "mobility" or "instability of opinion" (*mobilitas opinionum*). People with this condition were unable to make firm judgements or concentrate on one thing at a time. It touched a raw social nerve similar to attention deficit today. Giambattista da Monte, professor of medicine at Padova, noted that there are people who "persist sometimes in one thing, then another and then another."[37] Vives remarked on the rapidity and infinity of mutable particulars to which our attention is constantly drawn, which constitutes an "obstacle to the intelligence."[38] The original condition was a wavering about religious and moral beliefs, rather than (as for us) about morally neutral objects of attention – though people of the time would not have made any such distinction. Its moral focus, and its link

---

[34] Hippocrates, *Airs, Waters, Places, Hippocrates I*, 110; J. Wiberg, "The anatomy of the brain in the works of Galen and Ali Abbas," *Islamic Medicine*, 40 (1914/1996); Ingrassia, *In Galeni*, 61; G. Aranzi, *Hippocratis Librum de Vulneribus Capitis*, 15.

[35] *Observationum et Curationum Medicinalium ac Chirurgicarum*, i, 354a.

[36] *Opera Omnia*, 164; 172.

[37] *In Artem*, 135v.

[38] *De Anima et Vita*, 94.

to questions of social and religious status, can be seen in the 1631 trial of the Earl of Castlehaven, who had handed control of his purse to a male household menial with whom he was having sex. Apart from erasing "the difference between a servant and a son" and thereby disturbing a political order based on lineage, an important symptom of his libertinism was the fact that "in the morning [he] would be a papist and in the afternoon a protestant."[39]

Unstable opinion was a defect of the will. The will, like reason, affected the body via the strength and supply of soul spirits to and from the brain.[40] If a patient's opinion simply followed his appetites, it showed that his will was divorced from his reason. Constancy and steadfastness of the will were characteristic of the social elite, of the man of honour who remained faithful to his freely given promise; this in turn was a worldly equivalent of the grace obtainable by the Christian for whom, in the words of Bunyan's hymn, "There's one will constant be." The paradigmatic mind changer was Eve, when she listened to the serpent. It went with her gullibility, a frequently cited medical symptom of unstable opinion. Instability undermined the patient's knowledge of what was true and (the same thing) what was good for him: "People who keep changing their opinion not only go from true to false and vice-versa, but change their minds about what they want and don't want."[41]

Mutability was an ever-present theme in the behaviour guides too. Stability meant being "armed … against the change of times, and mutability of fortune, for nothing in this life is steadfast and permanent."[42] Mutability was a threatening feature of the external world, and one had to guard against its invasion of the self. To become "profitable members of the commonwealth," it was necessary "to leave these wandering wits (which are constant in nothing but uncertainty)." In the early seventeenth-century's moral panics about inconstant behaviour, people with unstable opinions were labelled "changelings" – probably by extension from "worldlings," those seduced by earthly rewards. In 1650 John Bulwer, author of what historians have seen as pioneering texts on psychiatry and deaf education, published a long poem, *Anthropometamorphosis: Man Transformed; or, the Artificial Changeling*, which satirized religious and political waverers. He likens them to people who frequently change their style of clothing in order to conceal their reprobate character or their social inferiority (class cross-dressing was still technically illegal), or who cosmetically "alter [their] bodies from the mould intended by nature." Civil war sermons warned the worshipper how easy it was to become a "changeling" with a fickle will, a credulous "weather-cock, carried up and down with every wind."[43] Reason was a constant. It came from God, not from individuals who might each arbitrarily will their own separate, shifting beliefs. English congregations would have experienced the effects of intellectual and behavioural instability at first hand, in the social and doctrinal disintegration around them. Bunyan uses the word "changelings" to attack time-servers in the priesthood (Baxter calls them "opinionists").[44] Within a few years the psychological resonances of the word were to coalesce with its other existing meaning (till then quite separate) of a child exchanged in the cradle for another; the upshot was a concept much closer to modern intellectual disability, as we shall see in Chapter 16.

---

[39] Cited in Rictor Norton, *The Homosexual Literary Tradition*.
[40] Akakia, *Claudii Galeni*, 101.
[41] Argenterio, *In Artem*, 221.
[42] Haly Heron, *The Kayes of Counsaile*, 84.
[43] Jeremiah Burroughs, *Irenicum*, 139.
[44] Bunyan, *Holy War*, 42; Baxter, *Directions and Perswasions*, 345.

Social biases in the medical model of intellectual disability

The soul spirits consisted of a material so refined that no anatomist could claim actually to have seen them. But they had to exist. How else could one explain the varieties of human behaviour? (Their behavioural role survives in everyday expressions such as "Keep your spirits up" and "In good spirits.") Any specific cognitive or moral dysfunction simply *was* in the last resort the specific material fault and vice-versa: an excess mobility or sluggishness in the patient's soul spirits. But who, more precisely, were the stereotypical groups thus impaired? The social dangers they represented can be put under three headings: melancholy (thinking slothfully or despairingly), changeableness (thinking rashly or variably) and heterodoxy (thinking for oneself). These cognitive impairments, and the respective condition of the soul spirits, typified certain populations who corresponded closely to those excluded from the honour society and from the company of the elect. They are the usual suspects: women, children, racial or religious minorities and the lower social orders. There was only one Reason, consisting of the common ideas fixed for all time by God and expounded by bishops and gentry – just as now there is only one set of normal cognitive operations, fixed for all time by a determinate genetic "nature" and expounded by psychologists, psychiatrists and doctors. Beyond the category of fee-paying gentry, who ideally if not exclusively formed his client group, the doctor saw foolishness and instability of opinion not merely as the psychological symptoms but as the very identity of his social and religious inferiors *en masse*. "Difficulties in learning" were simply their everyday condition, since it was well known that their soul spirits were made of a less refined matter.[45] Medical writers were not greatly interested in them. Torrigiano, for example, mentions them only inasmuch as they throw the normative characteristics of the elite into relief: "He who exhibits instability of opinion and rapid changes of plans and desires is *like* a child," and thus like a woman, Ethiopian or labourer.[46] In other words, an elite male patient in this condition bore a merely temporary resemblance to such groups, whose fixed degenerate identity was a reminder of the Fall.

According to Ali ibn Abbas, women kept their hair as they got older because their brains were excessively humid, which impaired their intellectual functions; their cranial sutures were narrower than men's and so had poorer drainage. Renaissance medical writers followed him, commenting that "people who have narrow sutures, women for example, are somewhat crazy." Noting Aristotle's remark that women not only have smaller brains than men but fewer sutures, the author claimed that this deficiency gave women harder skulls, though there were also writers who insisted that they were no different from men's.[47] As for size, unnamed (and possibly nonexistent) ancient authors were cited as saying that women were "wiser and more prudent than men" and that since women also had smaller heads, smallness could therefore not be a defect. This gave the commentator the opportunity to establish the opposite point: that women's "wisdom" and "prudence" are just a devious, imitative cunning, not the real male thing. And if (as Aquinas had said) small-headed men are impetuous and aggressive, then the smallness of the female's clinched the point.[48]

Instability of opinion, in a male patient of social standing, was not the sign of degeneracy it was in his social inferior. Medical writers have in mind someone who, when healthy, reaches an opinion, turns it into a judgment, then enforces it on the rest of the population; instability of opinion in other social groups refers to people whose job is to *follow* judgements handed out by their superiors.

---

[45] Akakia, *Claudii Galeni*, 105.
[46] Torrigiano, *Plusquam*, 46v.
[47] Ali ibn Abbas, *Liber Totius Medicinae*, 12; Oddi, *In Librum*, 122; Aristotle, *On the Parts*, 653a; Aurelius Celsus, *De Re Medica*, 468; Andreas Vesalius, *De Humani*, 15.
[48] D'Abano, *Conciliator*, 114; Tozzi, *In Artem*, ii, 28.

This was particularly true of women, universally regarded as fickle and mobile. A typical Dutch portrait shows the astronomer Huygens with a female companion; both have their hands on a sheet of music, but while it induces him to contemplate the music of the spheres, her inquisitive glance strays sideways towards the viewer and is distracted from the main business, the common ideas.[49] There are the inevitable sartorial references: "'Tis strange, that women being so mutable, will never change in changing their apparel."[50] Being a male of rank, in itself, constituted privilege, of which the making and enforcing of firm judgements was one particular expression. If an eighteenth-century bluestocking had asked whether a woman might not claim the same privilege, the answer would have been no: a woman's privilege is to change her mind. This familiar saying may well have started life as an ironic inversion of elite male norms of intellectual and behavioural constancy.

As one physician put it, "women are somewhat unstable when it comes to taking advice: they waver between this and that, as if navigating without oars or sails. Being stupid, they find it hard to recognize what is advisable and profitable."[51] A man displays the symptoms differently. Being a man – that is, a gentleman – he makes up his mind quickly. His job is to give advice, not take it. If his opinion turns out to be wrong, says this author, he swaps it immediately for the right one. He is not like the stereotypical woman, it is just that he has jumped to his first conclusion too quickly; he then stands his ground before belatedly arriving at the one and only true conclusion. This view of women proved adaptable to Cartesian dualism. A late commentary on Galen's *Art of Medicine*, in which the mind is now seen as a domain for analysis in its own right and detachable from the material make-up of the brain, discusses these same cognitive impairments and criticizes earlier texts for explaining women's unstable opinions by the unbalanced temperament of the female brain. The real cause was not material or organic, but the fact that women are intellectually null: "It is women's *ignorance* that endows them with the utmost credulity, hence they are easily persuaded about whatever is put in front of their minds, and they turn out to be unstable and changeable" (emphasis in original).[52]

With religious and racial minorities, the stereotyping is less obvious in this period. Polygenism, the theory of the separate natural origins of races, mainly concerned bodily difference, and in any case (the notorious case of La Peyrère aside) was not in evidence before the late seventeenth century. The fully "scientific racism" which held that black people's inferior intellects resembled those of intellectually disabled white people did not flourish until the early nineteenth. Previously there was a less systematic view of ethnic difference, both in medical and in broader cultural terms. Renaissance painters intentionally positioned black people among the travellers on the way of the cross, highlighting their creaturely equality. The initial discriminatory model was that of the Jews, who had demonstrated their changeableness by deviating from the New Testament path. Jewish intellectuals were barred from office in many of the first universities, not because of religious affiliation alone but specifically because they were incapable of grasping abstract and thus stable truths.[53] "Ethiopians" (black Africans in general) were sometimes said to exhibit violent changes of mood and thought. A sixteenth-century Galen commentator, writing about unstable opinion, gives as an example their characteristic "rashness of counsel"; they were prone to hasty judgements. In Spain after the reconquest, original Christians were repackaged as typically calm people, those with Jewish or Moorish blood as "unquiet and turbulent."[54] Shakespeare reaches for the same stereotype.

---

[49] Jacob van Campen, "Portrait of Constantin Huygens with Suzanna van Baerle," Mauritshuis, The Hague.
[50] Thomas Tomkis, *Lingua*, 12v.
[51] Dryvere, *In Τεχνην*, 129.
[52] Tozzi, *In Artem*, ii, 42.
[53] Roger French and Andrew Cunningham, *The Invention of the Friars' Natural Philosophy*.
[54] Oddi, *In Librum*, 132; Castro, *Le drame de l'honneur*, 92.

When Iago's companion Roderigo doubts their chances of provoking Othello to jealousy, Iago reassures him that "these Moors are changeable in their wills." Shakespeare links this changeability, and its associated credulity, to Othello's outmoded sense of self-assertive honour. When Othello says he murdered "all in honour," it sounds not so much like a self-justification as a belated realization that the honour mode is itself foolishness when confronted with the Machiavellian wit of an Iago; the latter, like Falstaff, knows that "honesty's a fool." Othello himself, once he learns the truth, concurs that he is a fool because he has been "rash."

The Roman medical authority Aurelius Cornelius Celsus had claimed that monstrous crania, lacking sutures and hence abnormally shaped, occur oftener in hot climates; Ethiopians showed the same tendency to impetuosity as women, and the same hardness of the cranium. Celsus's suggestion was taken up by Renaissance anatomists who sought to establish that the "impossible" type of sutural deformity might really exist, and located it in places where the inhabitants were exotic and different, such as the Indies.[55] Nineteenth- and early twentieth-century anatomists still noted that in "Negroes and the lower races of mankind" sutural closure occurs earlier. (The street myth that black people have hard skulls survived to the twentieth century and may still be circulating today.)[56]

Links between unusual physiognomy and impaired cognitive faculties were drawn most starkly in terms of social class. The masses were the touchstone of deformity, physical, intellectual and moral. The Galenists' most frequent illustration in this respect was again Thersites, whose foolishness was identified directly with the shape of his skull: "In Homer the head of Thersites, because it is pointed and badly shaped, is called *fatuus*."[57] He could also be described as having a *small* head, indicating "rash and heedless judgement, on account of the paucity of spirits," or as having a skull of Galen's unsuitably sutured X type which led to him being "not so much stupid as useless in all things, having neither an anterior nor a posterior eminence."[58] Da Monte added several more skull types to Galen's list, linking them to various types of imbalance among the elemental qualities and soul spirits that occurred in certain social groups. One was typical of labourers, in whom the rear eminence may be present but some or all of the frontal one missing. This damages the psychological faculty belonging to the front ventricle, the imagination, whose task is to "apprehend" the information that comes from the five external senses and to combine particulars into universals. Lack of the frontal eminence and its corresponding faculty impair in turn the middle ventricle's operations of *discursus* and "reasoning." Another of Da Monte's types is the slave. Aesop, for example, had the rear eminence missing entirely, but the frontal eminence only partly. Hence he was "lazy and of weak motion" but at the same time "clever and very astute" (*ingeniosus et prudentissimus*). Then there was the jester, whose cognitive and moral characteristics induce a tone of disgust:

> The ninth [and lowest] grade has a small head, misshapen on both sides, lacking any eminence, and so in all operations they are the worst; foul and deformed, they are the most disproportional, and have bad inclinations [*mores*]. Of these Ianelus, the Cardinal of Ferrara's fool, had less wisdom than a dog. He was a mimic, with a crippled hand and a large head resembling a vegetable. He was quick to anger and always looking for a fight, now with one person, now with another. He did not

---

[55] Celsus, *De Re Medica*, 468; Ingrassia, *In Galeni*, 65; Alessandro Benedetti, *Historia Corporis Humani*, 242; Caspar Hofmann, *Commentarii in Galeni de Usu Partium*, 216.

[56] In Todd and Lyons, "Endocranial suture closure," *American Journal of Physical Anthropology*, 7 (1924).

[57] Santorio, *Commentaria*, 191.

[58] Riolan, *In Artem*, 41; Da Monte, *In Artem*, 130 ff.

know anyone's name or anything at all, and I think he did not have a rational soul, since all his operations were like a dog's.

People like Ianelus ("Little Johnny," a historically documented figure whom Da Monte would probably have known) had a formal slot in the landed household economy, probably from the same entertainment budget that paid painters, musicians and actors, alongside whom jesters honed their skills. Little Johnny was presupposed to have the characteristics appropriate to his jester's occupation.

As for instability (*mobilitas*) of opinion, the masses were "in all things mutable, but mutability."[59] Shakespeare gives us a classic description of the lower ranks as a changeable, unreasoning mob. In *Julius Caesar*, when the plebeians are easily convinced of Caesar's guilt by Brutus and then equally quickly convinced of Brutus's by Antony, the intellectual instability of the crowd provokes social instability and civil war. The word "mob" was a recent coining, an abbreviation of the Latin phrase *mobile vulgus* ("the seething crowd"). The common herd was fluid intellectually as well as physically. Elyot describes his much-cited "monster with many heads" as "never certain nor stable." In the Galenist tradition, instability of opinion in a gentleman was due to excess heat, but in male commoners and all women to an excess of damp; it was the "phlegmatic" type, with their moist brains, among whom one found a large concentration of "such as have had … no better education than their trades."[60] Da Monte on the other hand remarks that in the brains of labourers, the soul spirits and consequently the opinions are hyper-mobile, so that they overheat and "burn up": this, he says, is the chief reason why people of this class are incapable of meaningful intellectual activity.

---

[59] I.M., *A Health to the Gentlemenly Profession of Serving-Men*, K1r.
[60] Anon., *A Modest Plea*, 120.

Chapter 14
A First Diagnosis? The Problem with Pioneers

Historians of our topic tend to start by searching for a "first." Who, for example, made the first scientific diagnosis of intellectual disability? The very question makes the mistake of supposing that there is such a condition (under whatever name), with an objective, permanent and cross-historical existence just waiting to be discovered. The label of pioneer has been pinned notably on Paracelsus, Felix Platter and Thomas Willis, but can only be justified if the symptoms of "foolishness" and "stupidity" in their work bear some relation to those of modern "intellectual disability." And they do not. Nevertheless, close examination of the symptoms these doctors wrote about reveals something further about the wider social and religious questions raised above, and about the groups of people that the symptoms describe.

Foolishness, medicine and theology: Paracelsus

"Alternative medicine," for any Renaissance doctor, would have meant Paracelsus, the Swiss polymath who represented the main alternative to Galenism. Paul Cranefield calls his *On the Generating of Fools* "one of the most remarkable documents" in the history of "mental deficiency," and sees it as the start of a modern diagnosis.[1] But Paracelsus's medicine is intricately bound up with his theology, and it is the latter that dominates this text. He "greatly wonders" at the fact that fools are redeemable. Why, he asks, "when God has redeemed man supremely and so dearly by his death and blood, does he allow him to be born unwise?" Foolishness here is obviously the general human condition, a consequence of original sin: "medicine has nothing to do with it." Hence it is incurable in nature, that is to say by doctors, even if it can be cured by divine providence. The mad and "possessed," however, *are* curable in nature. In other words, the medical or disease model is appropriate to madness (a minority condition) but not to foolishness (a ubiquitous one). Paracelsus's wonder is not therefore, as Cranefield suggests, that fools are redeemable in spite of their disability, but that we are all redeemable despite the fact that we are all fools simply in view of our humanity.

Paracelsus does, however, go on to single out some more restricted characteristics. The first is "inability to recognize or understand religion." This might have covered the newly encountered peoples of the New World, or virtuous pagans such as Aristotle. The universal possibility of redemption shows us that God is even-handed towards people who "cannot recognize or understand his name, his death, his law, his signs, his work, his goodness shown towards man." They cannot be held responsible for their own ignorance, and so surely cannot be predestined for hell. Inability to understand religion is also characteristic of the Christian laity in general, inasmuch as their faith has to be prescribed for them by a learned elite.

Paracelsus's foolishness is so far of the allegorical type, influenced by Erasmus's *In Praise of Folly* and Sebastian Brant's *Ship of Fools*. Erasmus, who spoke for many with his belief in the salvation of virtuous pagans, was attacking supposedly Christian elites foolishly seduced by power and worldliness. As for Brant, historians of psychiatry have debated whether fools at that time were

---

[1] Paracelsus, *De Generatione Stultorum* (translated by Cranefield and Federn as "The begetting of fools"), in K. Sudhoff (ed.), *Sämtliche Werke*, xiv, 74.

really cast adrift on boats, when their question should be whether we ourselves would recognize any of them as fools. Brant's passenger list includes most members of the human race; none of the 110 types listed in his table of contents remotely indicates our own disability model. A *trompe l'oeil* effect in Bosch's painting of the same name encapsulates the point, since what looks at first like the ship's mast turns out to be rooted on the bank, with apples growing on it: it is the tree of knowledge of good and evil.[2] All this begs a question, however. Even if Paracelsian foolishness were in some way universal and allegorical, a metaphor for the human condition, surely metaphor only works by pointing us to some positive referent that already exists in the real world – to some small, pathological intellectually disabled group, for example? Paracelsus does go on to discuss a small group which is, if not pathological, then odd, as we shall see. But the intellect and behaviour even of this group bear no resemblance to the modern disability model; they are a metonymic expression of the more general human folly. Metaphor in ancient and early modern literature can be explanatory, not just a literary device; the narrative slips from universal foolishness to more specific states and back without any sense that somewhere reality ends and metaphor begins.

In his preamble Paracelsus hints at some such smaller group when he separates certain types of fool from "wise" men, albeit only to emphasize that they are "brothers ... before God." After discussing pagans, he gives a long list of types of natural corruption: "fornicators, gamblers, robbers, crippled children, the blind, the deaf, the mute, the lame, the timorous [sc. melancholic], fools, monsters, the malformed." It is tempting to assume that these fools correspond with our "intellectual disabled." However, the premise underlying the list as a whole is that man no longer reflects the divine image; there are no grounds for supposing that "fool" refers here to some distinctly cognitive impairment in a modern sense. In order to suppose so, one has to read what is not there.

Cranefield also claims that Paracelsus "discovered" a connection between goitre and intellectual disability in Alpine peasants; he calls this "the earliest mention of cretinism," though Paracelsus himself does not use the term. Modern medicine found a link between intellectual disability, thyroid hormone deficiency and the iodine deficiency of Alpine spring waters; sixteenth-century medicine, on the other hand, placed goitrous deformity in an organic domain where no clear line is drawn between the physiological, the cognitive and the behavioural. Paracelsus himself observes that goitre is not a *propertium* or defining element of foolishness, since not all goitrous people are fools. Modern medicine too came to acknowledge the unreliability of the links between goitre and the mind. But for Paracelsus even this representation of foolishness was designed to show simply that "we are no longer in the image of God but have had it taken away": a general Adamite incurability in which neither goitre nor foolishness are separate from universal human corruption.

On the Generating of Fools has undercurrents of the scholastic philosophical doctrines from which this self-proclaimed rebel had ostensibly distanced himself, and which would have been as familiar to his readers as his biblical references. Writing about the defectiveness of the "internal instruments" in foolishness, he comments that although there are conditions which deprive people of some faculty or other (that is, some organic impairment means that they do not seem to be operating rationally), the rational soul nevertheless remains present throughout. However, he also refers here to a contrasting, theological doctrine of St Paul's, which defined the highest part of man as "spirit" rather than any philosophical abilities. Like Luther, Paracelsus was wary of "fleshly" or "animal reason," the corrupt reasoning of fallen man. True reason was inspired, not rationally worked out. So philosophers, too, were a type of fool, "stuck in their own wisdom and not progressing to God's."

---

[2] Hieronymus Bosch, "La nef des fous," The Louvre, Paris.

But if there are no elements of modern psychological characteristics of disability in Paracelsus's fools, not even in those who might be of a discrete type, then what exactly *is* the precise content of their foolishness? Two characteristics are mentioned. One of these consists in being holy. Here the familiar notion of the holy fool needs closer examination. The original narrative said that if you are supremely contemplative, a "prophet," then other people, who are mostly corrupted by earthly desires, will think you foolish; your foolishness is precisely your lack of such desires, not some transhistorical pathology. The Islamic sources of the narrative bear this out.[3] The original representation of the contemplative prophet as a fool was later employed in the *invention* of the holy fool as akin to a modern, intellectually disabled type, albeit in one of its more optimistic variants. A narrative that described intuiters of divine reason as fools turned into a narrative that described fools as intuiters of divine reason. The medieval prophet was a philosopher whose contemplations were occasionally so perfect that he accessed the divine intellect directly rather than by a laborious apprehension of the connecting terms of syllogisms. The more usual philosopher reasoner, who had to labour at his syllogistic expertise, was only one rung below this ideal state. Paracelsus, however, ranked him near the bottom, because earthly reason was suspect. He values his own "fools" precisely because they do *not* deliberate in this way. Syllogisms lie in the temporal realm and so have time to be "fashioned," using "lies and deceit."

The other symptom of Paracelsian foolishness is playfulness and tricks, evoking the social occupation of the jester. In the popular drama which featured prominently in the didactic literature of the Reformation, various kinds of foolishness can be distinguished: fool as intellectually deficient, fool as morally deficient, fool as unbeliever, wise fool, pure fool, fool as man in general, all of them overlapping to a considerable extent.[4] The main symptoms of "intellectual" deficiency are laughter-inducing tricks and an eccentric loquaciousness which nevertheless uses normal syntax and grammar. Audiences laughed not at any disability we might ourselves recognize as such but at the characters' *uninhibited* speech and behaviour, which Paracelsus associates with children and drunks. This image is a relic of the medieval Feast of Fools, which earlier ecclesiastical authorities had only partly succeeded in reining in, and in which foolishness cannot be distinguished from general unruliness. Any "intellectual" deficiency is more or less indistinguishable from a lack of socially appropriate inhibition, whose modern form as a psychological category is, as Roger Smith has shown, a socially and historically contingent phenomenon.[5]

The uninhibitedness of licensed fools and jesters who tell home truths to their master is a constant literary theme. In Paracelsus's time, jesters still had paid employment in noble households. The literary and socio-historical sources are Roman; *moriones*, as we have seen, tended to be *kept* fools, with behaviours that corresponded to the jester's job description. They had, as Langland put it, the "wit to work."[6] Don Francesillo de Zúñiga, for example, jester to Charles V of Spain, was a hereditary gentleman who wrote his memoirs in perfect Spanish and was competent to leave his estate to his family.[7] When Fuller defines the jester's "office" as one "which not but he that hath wit can perform, and none but he that wants wit will perform," it is easy to overlook the first of these two clauses. Some jesters did come to the job possessing some natural difference as their prior qualification: short stature, spinal curvature, or unusual physiognomy. Peasants, too, were recruited

---

[3] See Dols, *Majnun*.
[4] Heinz Wyss, *Der Narr im Schweizerischen Drama des 16.Jahrhunderts*.
[5] Roger Smith, *Inhibition: History and Meaning in the Sciences of Mind and Brain*.
[6] *Piers Plowman*, Prologue.
[7] Zúñiga, *Crónica*; see also Mans, *Zin*, 52.

as professional fools simply because of their rustic personae. Otherwise, and irrespective of any natural differences, fools learned and acquired their prescribed behaviours.[8]

To sum up, Paracelsian foolishness is sometimes the fallen human condition in general, and sometimes an eccentric but positive condition marked by the overlapping behaviours of holy or intuitive insight and of the jester's licensed truth telling – positive because it bypasses the hypocritical deliberations of human reasoning. The closing paragraph of *On the Generating of Fools* returns to an interweaving of the two, within a single image. Paracelsus's aims in this text are thus instructive ones, about all of us. This is clear from his successor in the German mystical tradition, Valentin Weigel, who begins the key section of his book *Know Thyself* with a similar description of foolishness; only from this starting point, he says, can one proceed to establish what human wisdom is.

Foolishness and brain substance: Felix Platter

Another medical authority often held up as a pioneer of psychiatry is Felix Platter. Scheerenberger, for example, places him among "the first to offer a multi-level description of mental retardation."[9] And certainly Platter deals with impairments of the faculties, among them "foolishness," on the very first page of his compendium of medical practice. He was also one of the first physicians to examine disease in terms of its "syndromes," or sets of related symptoms. Like the Galenists, Platter still sees cognitive impairment as a subset of bodily injury; but the syndromic approach means that he describes and classifies such impairments in relation to each other first, only later relating them to their organic, material aspects.

This distances them relatively from the body. It also leaves the door open for praeternatural causes. If Platter is a pioneer of modern psychiatry it is partly because of, not despite, the reality he allots to the devil. Historians who think they have found a "first" modern psychiatrist have tried, in defiance of the texts, to ignore the presence of the devil in Platter's aetiology of mental states, but it is there for all to see.[10] Moreover, he passed it on to his successors. Caspar Bauhin for example, Platter's heir as head of the medical faculty in Basle, was (as we shall see) a contributor to the theory of demonically conceived, mindless "changelings" that would feed into modern accounts of intellectual disability via Locke's *Essay*.

Platter puts cognitive symptoms under four headings: consternation, defatigation, weakness and alienation.[11] "Consternation" is about absence, but he makes no mention of foolishness of any sort under this heading. "Defatigation" is about sleep. The third heading, "weakness" (*imbecillitas*), describes a generic "dullness (*hebetudo*) of mind" and impairment of the faculties: "slowness of wit (*ingenium*)" in the imagination, "imprudence" in the faculty of judgement and "memory loss." Weakness and dullness, however, are facets of bodily disease and sensory impairment; they are not distinctly intellectual in a Cartesian sense. While slowness of wit may seem to relate to a modern model of disability, Platter's specific examples are old age, concussion, loss of blood, injuries to the sense organs, under- or over-use of the faculties, and melancholy. There is a

---

[8] Thomas Fuller, *The Holy and the Profane*, 182; see also Beatrice Otto, *Fools are Everywhere: the Court Jester around the World*.

[9] *A History*, 29.

[10] For example Raymond Battegay, "Felix Platter und die Psychiatrie," in U. Tröhler (ed.), *Felix Platter in seiner Zeit*; Heinrich Buess, "Basler Mediziner der Barockzeit," in *Beiträge zur Geschichte der Naturwissenschaften*.

[11] Platter, *Praxeos*, 1 ff.

brief reference to hereditary conditions; but his examples ("clever and industrious people have children like themselves," while "the ignorant beget the torpid") evoke a Reformation concern with spiritual self-development rather than intellect *per se*. Also under the heading of weakness comes a reference to people who "barely learn how to speak, and apprehend letters and skills with difficulty." The Latin phrase here (*discunt literas*) is a conventional phrase that refers to the formal school curriculum; we should infer "barely learning to speak" as describing the unschooled and the lower social classes in general. The cause of slowness is "imperfection of the instrument," and above all of the cerebral substance (an over-moist texture, for example); even if inherited, it can be improved upon by industrious "exercise," a form of nurture that can become "second" nature.

It is only under the fourth heading, of "alienation," that the vocabulary of foolishness appears (variously *stultitia, fatuitas, moria*). This embraces drunkenness, hypochondria, melancholy (again), mania, devil possession, hydrophobia and frenzy – a taxonomy of conditions that would hold no coherence for today's psychiatrist. All of them are equivalent examples of an overarching "alienation or hallucination" that consists of "judging and remembering things which are not, as if they were; or things which are, wrongly and irrationally." And this latter is simply the Galenist description of delirium. The symptoms of the alienated mind occur across a wide range of human types, all of whom come under the one heading of "foolish" (here, *stulti*): infants, old people, "all men in every age inasmuch as all their actions seem to be foolish as Erasmus and Brant have elegantly shown" (that is, virtually the whole human race), "fantastics" who excel in wit (*ingenium*) but whose attention-seeking turns them into buffoons with asses' ears, and people seized by strong emotions. Halfway through this (to us) highly disparate list come people "born" foolish:

> They show signs of foolishness straight away as infants, by a habit of mimicry exceeding that of other infants; they are not submissive or amenable, so that often they do not learn to speak, much less to take on functions requiring industriousness. This evil is frequent in particular regions, as cited … in the Valesian village of Bremis where I have seen it myself, and in the Pinzgau valley of Carinthia; many tend to have, as well as foolishness, a poorly shaped head and a goitre, are dumb, with a huge swollen tongue, and present a deformed sight sitting in the streets gazing at the sun, putting sticks between their fingers, writhing about, mouths wide open, moving passers-by to laughter and amazement.

Goitre had been associated with poor head shape and dwarfism long before this, as the iconographic record shows. The sticks between their fingers seem to invoke a pre-existing convention about melancholics idly building models out of sticks and clay, while their lack of industriousness points us again towards the Reformation's urban values. These Alpine peasants turn up again in Platter's account of deafness, where alongside the elderly they illustrate the cognitive element involved in an excess of humours and catarrhs.[12]

To the reader who may be looking for a juicy primary source, please note: any supposed intellectual disability in the above is not conceptually separate from the other items on the list. Cranefield describes it as a pioneering diagnosis of cretinism; but this label arrived only in eighteenth-century medicine, which regarded Alpine peasants in their entirety as "little better than senseless beasts."[13] The symptoms Platter lists are physical and behavioural as much as intellectual. What unites the seemingly disparate list of people in which these people "born foolish" are embedded is the arousal of wonder in the onlooker. The category is therefore religious and symbolic, like Augustine's *moriones*. Paracelsus, too, who had seen goitrous peasants drinking the "metallic and mineral

---

[12] Véronique Dasen, *Dwarfs in Ancient Egypt and Greece*, 247; Henri Beek, *De Geestesgestoorde in de Middeleeuwen*, 113; 96; Platter, *Praxeos*, 250.

[13] Albrecht von Haller, *Elementa Physiologiae*, 570.

waters" of the Pinzgau, focused in this context on their bodily symptoms, bar a passing comment that people with goitre tend "more towards foolishness than to skilfulness." The symptoms belong to an indivisible physical-intellectual-behavioural-moral defect marking fallen man as a whole.[14]

Platter's comment that he had seen these peasants himself refers to the visit he made when young to the Valais with his father Thomas, who had grown up there. A shepherd born to poor peasants, Thomas Platter had learned to read and write only as an adult, while running dispatches for the Zwinglian reformers. He eventually became a teacher of classical languages and the printer-publisher of Galen, Calvin and Vesalius. As an autodidact, he viewed his own intellectual development in terms of an escape from the ignorance of the countryside and its people, who Zwingli had said were fit only for herding cows. In this sense Thomas was following a common humanist tradition, like Erasmus when he promoted the public image of himself as a refugee from the notably stupid Batavia of his birthplace. In insisting that *their* yokels were more stupid than anyone else's, the intellectuals of Basle and Leiden were advertising their own intellectual superiority.

Thomas's suppression of his own social and, as it were, unintellectual self was essential to his Christian rebirth, and this helps perhaps to explain his son's horror stories about the stupidity of the local population. The Alpine foolishness described by Felix was the polar opposite of the new urban Jerusalem of the humanist academy, and his portrayal of it was tinged by a vicarious recollection of his father's great escape. The idea that slowness (*tarditas*) of wit and the peasant condition (*rusticitas*) were synonymous was in any case already a stock convention of classical Latin literature.[15] The Valesians with sticks between their fingers were a social and intellectual distillation of the poor peasantry in general, who subsisted within the father and threw into relief the son's identity as a great professor of medicine. Paracelsus, too, had grown up in an Alpine valley where there were silver mines; goitre was to be found, he said, wherever mining went on, and his own birthplace was another region whose peasants were deemed exceptionally foolish (perhaps because they were mostly Slavs). In Paracelsus's idiosyncratic Christianity, just as in the Platters' Swiss Protestantism, knowledge came through spiritual self-development, for which landless peasants lacked even a potential. In both, the medical foolishness of the goitrous is the wider social idiocy of the village. Research would later reveal in fact that iodine deficiency was no greater in the Alps than in many other regions of the world where no prevalence of mental deficiencies has been noted.

Platter divides the causes of general "alienation" of the mind into internal and external, or natural and praeternatural.[16] Head size and shape are not necessary causes or even signs of impairment, because sometimes a fault in the brain is only detectable within: ideally one should "open it up after death" and inspect its internal nature. Even then one may not arrive at any ultimate, fixed cause of cognitive symptoms. Although Platter does talk about some things as "incurable," he also says that "custom changes nature." Nature is the acquired as well as the innate, the imitative as well as the original. The "imitative" type is drawn from the Roman jester model; men from noble families grow up enjoying the antics of professional fools, "acquiring a habit in it which later becomes irremovable, so that they become permanent and genuine fools themselves." The "original" type, by contrast, exists from birth, and is due to "the seed of the parents." Platter subdivides this latter, original type between parents whose seed is defective because they themselves are foolish, and parents who are not foolish but whose "seed has acquired some fault." Whatever it is that has caused

---

[14] Cranefield, "The discovery," 489; "Paracelsus on goiter," 463; Paracelsus, *Von Apostemen ... am Leib*, in *Werke*, iv, 222.

[15] Platter, *Observationum in Hominis Affectibus*, 1.

[16] Platter, *Praxeos*, 89; 98; 105.

the foolishness causes the soul spirits too (which it must be remembered are material entities) to be impaired, in which case people may be born "deaf, or dumb, or crookbacked, or with goitre." All these causes are secondary, however. The paramount type of cause is praeternatural – from God or the Devil – and so not a suitable topic of study for the physician.

Foolishness and brain function: Thomas Willis

Willis was founder in the 1650s of the Oxford Anatomical Club, its lectures attended by medical innovators such as Thomas Sydenham and his future collaborator, the young Dr John Locke. Whereas Willis's predecessors had written about the structure or substance of the brain, he himself placed greater emphasis on its *function* and on the activity of the soul spirits within it. He thus gives greater centrality and power to the invisible. It is this aspect of his work that has led to his being seen as a precursor of modern medical thinking on our topic. Cranefield calls Willis's account of foolishness in *De Anima Brutorum* ("On the soul of animals") "not the earliest systematic discussion of mental deficiency known, but ... an early one"; his psychology is "primitive" but "far more subtle ... than Descartes."[17] Now it is true that Willis was influenced by Descartes, as well as by other radicals of that generation, notably Gassendi (hence his inclusion of human beings and their souls under the heading of "animals"). Yet he retained in many respects an organic, pre-Cartesian mind-set. The soul, or its rational part, is an incorruptible substance, the body alone is capable of defect, and the brain is the material domicile of the soul: "the health of the soul begins with the health of the body."[18] He brings in a range of unreferenced sources from the previous century (Platter among them). Samuel Pordage's 1683 English translation, on which historians have based their interpretations, obscures this strong element of conservatism in the texts. Willis did not provide a precise terminology for foolishness, and Pordage interpolated his own as we shall see in Chapter 16. Furthermore, whenever Willis writes about foolishness (*stupiditas*) in his other works, it is clearly a symptom of melancholia. These things must be borne in mind when examining *De Anima Brutorum*.

Located in the imagination, foolishness impairs the "corporeal" soul (Gassendi's refurbishment of the "sensitive" soul of faculty psychology). This impairment "eclipses" the non-corporeal faculty of intellect and the rational soul. Willis's analytic procedure follows the traditional pattern of his predecessors. He starts with immediate causes (brain size, shape and substance and the quality, amount and activity of soul spirits), proceeding thence to antecedent causes, and ends with cure. Immediate causes are of the conventional Galenist type: the "natural and optimum" state of the brain is medium size, spherical shape and balanced temperament. These are important because they affect the brain's task of producing soul spirits. Deviations from this morphological ideal are a "natural" cause of foolishness but not a necessary one: "although not always the case, that is very often the way it turns out." Antecedent causes, meanwhile, are of two types (in this he follows Platter). Either they are "original ... hereditary ... as when fools give birth to fools" and thus "*connate*": the product of an ancestrally foolish line. Or they are "*congenite*": caused by poor sexual performance at conception, and thus "accidental and individual." That is, born fools are either hereditary or non-hereditary. Each of these two types of antecedent cause comes with a corresponding social stereotype.

---

[17] Cranefield, "A seventeenth-century view," Willis, *De Anima*, 357 ff.; Willis (trs. Samuel Pordage), *Two Discourses on the Soul of Brutes*.

[18] Akihito Suzuki, "Mind and its disease in Enlightenment British medicine."

Original, "connate" foolishness (*stultitia*) is typical of the "offspring of village and country people frequently liable to poor brain texture, [in whose] families we may trace back many generations and find scarcely one bright or clever person." Their internal nature is an indicator of their class stupidity, that of country people beyond the honour society and the learned doctor's professional remit. The model for this is biblical: original foolishness (*stultitia*) is a reflection, socially differentiated, of original sin.

By contrast, the individual, "congenite" foolishness (*stupiditas*) caused at conception is typical of the offspring of Willis's client group. It is a defect of brain function rather than of original brain texture. It is an accident, occurring not as the result of some hereditary class taint but precisely *because* the father is wise and has "a supreme wit" (*ingenium*). One may also infer that he is at some remove from original sin and in a state of grace. His state of constant contemplation causes his blood to keep back too many soul spirits in the brain, so that at the moment of conception not enough of them are available to ferry his "spermatic bodies" from this usual holding place to the appropriate point of delivery. When "the rational soul is concentrating to the utmost on giving birth to its intellectual offspring ... the corporeal soul becomes weaker and less fertile," so his physical offspring turn out correspondingly "slow." This politely distances him from his social inferiors' rampant sex drives. Later examples of this same mind-set appear in the Victorian era, when Herbert Spencer and others lobbied against allowing women access to higher education on the grounds that excessive study would lead them to have feeble-minded offspring. Later still, Kanner would proclaim that autistic children tend to issue from "highly intelligent parents" who are "strongly occupied with abstractions."[19] And it may well turn out that in our time the arrival and expansion of Asperger's syndrome as an intellectual disability has occurred not in spite of but because of its accompanying paradox of high IQ, with which parents may enhance their social-intellectual self-representation.

Some historians have tried to say that this second, "accidental" type of Willis's was a modernizing move, because it removed blame from parents. However, blamelessness was *a priori* in parents of the doctor's own social class. And more importantly, this type can be traced at least as far back as Alexander of Aphrodisias, whose work was being revived and popularized at the time. Alexander had originally said:

> Why do many foolish men (*moroi*) generate clever children and many clever men generate children who are stupid? Because when the stupider ones have sex, being fully overcome by pleasure their soul is immersed in the body, and so the sperm, with its greater ability both rational and physical, produces cleverer children. However, in the case of clever, educated men, they are always exercising their thoughts and when they have sex they are reasoning about something else.[20]

He was spawning a rich textual tradition. Albert followed up by saying that "wise men mostly produce defective, foolish (*fatui*) children ... because he who is good at study is bad at sex (*malus in venereo acto*)," since "sex is the most foolish act a wise man commits in all his life" – which is why "simple men" have wise offspring. Some writers used this to argue for celibacy in priests. Others describe how the man with intellectual preoccupations cannot procreate properly because the humours in him, being particularly thick, lead to melancholy. The word they use for thick (*pinguis*) can also be translated as "dull" or "doltish": the humours and their corresponding brain functions and states can thus be similar in both the father's excessively pursued wisdom and the

---

[19] Kanner, "Infantile autism and schizophrenia," *Behavioural Science*, 10 (1965).
[20] Alexander, "Problems," in *The Problems of Aristotle; with Other Philosophers and Physicians*, G7r; I.L. Ideler, *Physici et Medici Graeci Minores*, i, 12.

son's fleshly unwisdom. Both are defined by "melancholy," albeit of different types.[21] It shows just how carefully one has to read these texts.

So when in *Twelfth Night* the melancholy fool Feste sings "Journeys end in lovers meeting / Every wise man's son doth know," what he means is: "Any fool knows that." Willis knew relevant cases among his contemporaries. The wise, ingenious and childless William Harvey had a ward, his orphaned nephew, whom historians have retrospectively diagnosed as "mentally retarded." Harvey's material body was responsible *in loco parentis* for the impairment; but this also meant that his immaterial, rational soul was free to be acknowledged as the intellectual and "spiritual father" to Willis's anatomical club.[22] (Harvey seems a particularly severe case: one of those intellectual offspring of his was the theory that sexual conception consists in the spermatic fertilization of an incorporeal "idea" in the womb.)[23] Similarly the "spermatic bodies" of Sir Christopher Wren, another club member, produced a son, "poor Billy," whom biographers have decided was mentally retarded also. Like Harvey, Wren had exhausted his soul spirits on intellectual pursuits. One such was the illustrations he drew for Willis's great anatomy textbook, among which, ironically, was a drawing of "the brain of a foolish youth" – a "changeling," as Pordage's translation has it – that Willis had dissected according to Platter's suggestion.[24]

Medical guides to sex therapy taught that orgasm requires the closest simultaneous attention from both partners, so that the soul spirits can transport the psychological faculties – the "seminal" or "spermatic *logos*" – down into the semen and thereby maximize the child's reasoning abilities. This explains how the life of Laurence Sterne's *Tristram Shandy, Gentleman* gets off to such a bad start, on the very first page. The social status ascribed to him in the title is belied by his personal and intellectual flaws, which are the result of his mother's attention deficit at the moment of conception. Later in the novel, a parodic and this time successful stimulation of the same body parts occurs when a piping hot chestnut falls off the dinner table and down into a learned philosopher's open fly. "Attention, imagination, judgment, resolution, deliberation, ratiocination, memory, fancy" rush down from his brain to his testicles along with "ten battalions" of soul spirits.

Willis's distinction between two types of antecedent cause, original and accidental, explains in one fell swoop both the Adamite degeneracy of the servile classes and the wisdom and virtue of his own elite patients. It enables him to explain foolish traits in the families of his social peers which might otherwise be embarrassing, especially in view of the increasing status of wit and learning in the honour society. He describes other accidental causes within the same client group, which are likewise linked to the soul spirits and the act of conception but whose symptoms are not a cue for mutual admiration and are cautionary instead: for example, a father's ignoble lack of temperance (Shakespeare's "expense of spirit in a waste of shame"), or his effeminacy. Such characteristics damage the soul spirits, which consequently generate offspring who lack "great and liberal wit" and threaten the future ancestral line with class degeneracy and the taint of the "original foolishness" of the masses.

When Willis says that the foolishness of the ingenious gentleman's son is an "accident," he is using the old Aristotelian language; he means that foolishness does not affect the son's prior membership of the essence "rational being." It implies, further, that the foolishness of the foolish

---

[21] Albert, *Quaestiones super De Animalibus*, in Geyer (ed.), *Opera*, xii, 299; Lemnius, *Occulta Naturae Miracula*, 11, translated as *The Secret Miracles of Nature*, 18; Hieronymus Mercurialis, *Medicina Practica*, Chapter 6; Paracelsus, *De Generatione*, 79; Alessandro Tassoni, *Dieci Libri*, Book 6; Tommaso Campanella, *De Sensu Rerum et Magia*, 202; Cardano, *Opera*, iii, 558; Browne, *Religio*, 79; Burton, *The Anatomy*, i, 213.

[22] Neugebauer, "A doctor's dilemma: the case of William Harvey's mentally retarded nephew," 569.

[23] Cited in Thomas Laqueur, *Making Sex*, 144.

[24] Adrian Tinniswood, *His Invention so Fertile*, 240; Willis, *De Cerebri Anatome*, 51.

peasant's son *is* his essence. Accident goes with disease, essence with the degeneracy of the Fall, which the labouring masses embody. In accidental foolishness the soul spirits are blunt and slow. In original foolishness they are sharp, rapid and unstable, producing behaviour that is "absurd, perverse, ridiculous and inappropriate," the "laughter-provoking ... nonsense and mimicry" we already noted in the jester model. Rather than being what Cranefield calls an "early description of schizophrenia" distinct from "mental deficiency," Willis is simply readjusting, as he says himself, certain "conventional" (*vulgo*) distinctions. When he writes about rustic masses or degenerate gentry, he uses the word *stultitia*, and the symptoms are similar in both. He uses a different term (*stupiditas*) for the wise man's "accidental" son, and it is the one that elsewhere he uses exclusively for melancholia.

Although this *stupiditas* may have a dispositional tendency to permanence, the prognosis is relatively optimistic. Grades of foolishness correspond with grades of educability. The ideal is a knowledge of "literature and liberal sciences": that is, the educational curriculum of a gentleman. The members of Willis's client group are fit subjects for anatomy in general and for the anatomy of the soul in particular because of this normative excellence of their intellects. Immediately below them are people "skilful in the mechanical arts," a routine formula of the time whose social significance is obvious (for example, Mercado's congenitally deaf people were fit only "for mechanical matters and what they can make with their hands").[25] At the next level down are those unfit for mechanical skills who nevertheless "understand country matters." Further down come people "unfit for almost any calling" who can nevertheless learn basic life-skills; and finally there are people who "scarcely understand anything at all or know what they are about [*scienter agunt*]." *All* grades below the top one are read as grades of foolishness; the criterion by which they are all excluded is the ability to "recognize the common ideas."

Such people need to be schooled in the ideas by an "indefatigable trainer." We are probably meant to take it as read that Willis is concerned about backward members of his own client group. After all, the declared aim of his book is to promote the health of the soul as the route to "the communion of saints and to *societas*," in other words the elect and the honourable, whom Willis in typical Restoration and indeed modern fashion sees as one and the same entity. The only people who need to be trained to have the common ideas are those who by virtue of their ancestral line ought to have them in the first place but by some accident do not. Everyone else is a fool anyway. Even at the lowest grade where people scarcely understand anything, training can change their nature: "However coarse and dense the [soul] spirits may be, they will nevertheless forge some tracks or channels, albeit imperfect ones, in which they can expand." And even when absence of thought (*amentia*) and movement (*stoliditas*) frustrate attempts at training, there remains the possibility of providential transformation. Epileptics, whose condition is characterized by *stupiditas*, are curable by prayer, as the Bible shows. Dull-brained children can later become capable and teachable. A hot fever can suddenly cure adults previously assumed to be foolish. Willis gives specific examples, including the cure of a "fatuous" court jester and an elderly amnesiac.

Willis's terminology for the grades of foolishness above is borrowed from the *Bacchae* of the Roman satirical playwright Plautus in which there is a single line, used by many Renaissance writers for a description of slaves, that consists solely of five cognate terms for "foolish." The papal physician Paolo Zacchia had used it earlier in the century, in his account of ignorance and melancholic foolishness.[26] Willis is tapping here into the same literary sources as his friend Dryden, who was Poet Laureate while Willis was Royal Physician and in whose satires against his fellow poets "stupidity" is the core concept. Willis deploys these terms loosely in order to describe a

---

[25] Mercado, *Opera*, 172.
[26] Plautus, *Bacchae*, line 1088; Paolo Zacchia, *Quaestiones Medico-Legales*.

continuum of deficiency; there is ultimately no separate pathological niche of the type that his translator Pordage would create.

As for the brain deficiency of country labourers, this does not fall within the disease model at all; it is an "original" non-accidental structure and substance. Treatment would therefore be wasted on them. In such people, says Willis, the soul spirits consist of a gross matter rather than their normative fineness. In this precise context it is worth noting one more link between Willis and Platter; of the scores of scientific virtuosi who claimed the spiritual paternity of Harvey, Willis alone came from parents who were both non-gentle and rural.[27]

How the praeternatural becomes the abnormal

In "foolishness," then, doctors, like the rest of the honour society, saw the intellectual disabilities of a majority: everyone except males of a certain social standing. Only later was a category invented whose degree of pathology in respect of those intellectual disabilities was inversely proportional to its size. "Later" has been a drawn-out process, in the medical model as elsewhere. In the nineteenth century, when painters such as Millet began making peasants the subjects of elevated portraiture, disapproving critics wrote of them as "types of cretins."[28] In the twentieth, Dr F.G. Crookshank's theory of "homologies" – an amalgam of social stereotypes with somatic and psychological characteristics – classified "mongoloid imbeciles" under the same species heading as the inhabitants of Mongolia, orang-utans and the English working classes.[29] Anecdote and inference might well reveal residues of this attitude among today's practitioners. It would hardly be surprising, given how all the historical evidence shows that the psychological characteristics of modern intellectual disability are a distillation of former social, racial and class stereotypes.

The question arises, however: did the medical mind-set merely extract modern intellectual disability from the legal, political and theological matrix described in earlier sections, after the event? Or were there elements already within medicine itself that positively contributed to it? Answers can be found in the changing relationship between the natural, the unnatural and the praeternatural, and in the rise of new notions of personhood. In early modern faculty psychology, cognitive impairments were not objects of pathology in the same way that "intellectual disability" now is. They were just unusual, at least among the doctor's elite clients: "unnatural" in the limited Aristotelian sense, a special manifestation of the natural. As for physical monsters, they might even be thought of as perfectly formed; in the theory known as preformationism, which maintained that the sperm or the egg is the person in miniature, "the laws of nature are not different from the will of God," and so "God is obliged to produce monsters to satisfy those laws."[30] Both monstrosity and the unnatural remained within the realm of nature, and were quite distinct from things that were praeternatural and ran counter to nature. However, the fusion that eventually occurred between the unnatural and the praeternatural was to lead to new connections being made between an unusual structure of head and brain and their accompanying cognitive faculties.

Physiognomists wondered "whether the internal faculty may be known by the external physiognomy and visage," for instance in the facial deformity of "dizzards" and jesters.[31] When Galen had dismissed the possibility of a sutural layout in which "the length of the head becomes

---

[27] Robert Frank, *Harvey and the Oxford Physiologists*, 64.
[28] Millet, "Bringing Home the New-Born Calf," Art Institute of Chicago.
[29] *The Mongol in our Midst*, 329.
[30] Pierre-Sylvain Régis, *Cours entier de philosophie*, ii, 29.
[31] Walkington, *The Optick*, iii, 17.

its depth" (the extreme X-shape), it meant that *some brain material* generally might be missing, in which case the creature could not live; but later Galenists, in allocating the internal senses more precisely to specific cerebral ventricles, raised the possibility that *some particular part of the brain* might be missing. The injury might be limited to that part, and therefore would not preclude the possibility of life. Some of them claimed to have observed Galen's "impossible" type of skull in living individuals. Pietro d'Abano said it might exist "in some monstrous dwarf"; such beings were "more or less unviable," but it was not downright impossible for them to exist. Ugo Benzi subsequently claimed not only to have observed this type in an actual four-year-old but also to have measured the child's skull.[32]

The impossible became possible chiefly through Andreas Vesalius, whose school of anatomy was more or less the first to use empirical observation of the body as a way of checking out received Galenist wisdom. He claimed to have seen "a beggar going around Bologna with a square head somewhat broader than it is long, [and] in Genoa ... a boy of about three whose head sticks out on either side."[33] A child with a similarly shaped head could be observed in Venice. More significantly for us, Vesalius calls this latter child *amens*, "mindless," though the precise content of this concept can only be guessed at; one of his followers, paraphrasing this passage, lists its symptoms only in physiological terms ("catarrh and apoplexy").[34] Vesalius himself denied that the cognitive faculties were linked to specific cerebral ventricles; and since he must have consequently thought that damage to a part caused damage to the whole, there has to be some other reason why he thought such a child might live. As someone open to the ideas of the Reformation, he may simply have been trying to indicate that a *variety* of types and individuals exists, reflecting the individuality of their relationship to God.

Several authors repeated the story. The symptoms were usually anatomical, but a couple of them reiterate Vesalius's psychological embellishment. Gabriele Falloppio (of the eponymous tubes) replaced *amens* with *stolidus*, "foolish."[35] Johannes Schenk extracted the story from its anatomical context and placed it instead in the already existing genre of monstrosity literature. Here it sits alongside the standard list of physical monsters derived from Pliny, familiar to the readers of his time.[36] To the usual accounts of two-headed monsters, conjoined twins and tribes with their faces in their chests he adds "skulls without sutures or with the sutures obliterated," including the "completely mindless" Venetian child who was "without sutures" entirely. (Vesalius had described him as the extreme X-type, not as lacking sutures. Schenk's was a frequent over-egging of the source; another author, for example, noted seeing "at a public dissection a solid, seamless cranium: such heads are known a dog's heads ... and are said to be very hard and pain-resistant.")[37] None of the other creatures on Schenk's list of monstrosities has any psychological attributes, nor did those mentioned in the monstrosity literature in general; and they all belong in the category of unnatural, rather than diabolically praeternatural.

Renaissance authors rephrased Galen's "suitable," H-shaped sutural arrangement as the "natural" one. The corresponding idea of an "unnatural" shape still carried no overtones of determinism or permanence – Vesalius noted that everyone's sutures disappear as they get older – but it did allow monstrosity to enter the discussion. The boundary between unnatural and praeternatural, previously so clear, was becoming blurred. When Vesalian anatomists announced that even the

---

[32] D'Abano, *Conciliator Controversiarum*, 120; Benzi, *Expositio*, 20r.
[33] Vesalius, *De Humani*, 16.
[34] Hofmann, *Commentarii in Galeni de Usu Partium*, unpaginated.
[35] Gabriele Falloppio, *Observationes Anatomicae*, 4.
[36] Johannes Schenk, *Observationes Medicae de Capite Humano*, 25.
[37] Benedetti, *Historia*, 244.

"unviable" X-shape occurred in the real world, it was not (and this is the important point) as a one-off, but with a degree of regularity. How then should it be categorized in relation to nature? Schenk, as we have seen, still placed it in the realm of the merely unnatural. Another writer, though, calls it "as if [*tamquam*] praeternatural," bringing in the ever-flexible pointy-headed Thersites to illustrate its "uncertain" status.[38] Vesalius himself had wavered between the two:

> Unnatural head shapes can sometimes be seen even among perfectly respectable citizens, though one rarely finds them in cemeteries. However, they would be seen to occur often if we could open up the cemeteries of people in the Styrian Alps, since these people's heads are deformed not only in this way but also in further ways that are more outlandish.[39]

"Unnatural" here means the T and X shapes. But his train of thought seems to carry him uninterruptedly along a continuum from these shapes, observed in some of his respectable peers, to something more extreme, exemplified by the oafish monstrosity of Alpine peasants.

Once again, it seems to drive home a Lutheran point about the variety among human individuals and their relationships with God. It also returns us to the point made above (see Chapter 12) about causes, and the collapse of the conventional tripartite division between natural, unnatural and praeternatural ones. For the time being it was accepted that providence and "the almighty power of God may overcome ... violent and praeternatural" defects of the "few" who are "so monstrously dull and sottish."[40] Nevertheless, a polarization had begun. The fusion between unnatural and praeternatural is so complete in modern medicine as to be unrecognizable as such; they form a single category, the "abnormal." This coincides with the rise of modern biology, which sprang partly from a drive for tighter definitions of species. The praeternatural, with its intimation of origins beyond nature, was imported into natural history, with the result that certain human-looking creatures became increasingly seen as classifiable in some non-human or interstitial category.

Growing anxiety about the borderline between humans and the other animals marks the general passage from Renaissance to Enlightenment accounts of the scale of nature. It was no antiquarian whim that led the great Enlightenment (and Calvinist) medical authority Herman Boerhaave to republish the anatomical works of the school of Vesalius from two centuries earlier. One of Vesalius's disciples, Bartolomeus Eustachius, began his textbook on cerebral anatomy with an attack on previous writers who had maliciously confused the cranial sutures of humans with those of apes.[41] What else but an atheistic ill will could explain their blurring of the line between humans and other animals? Although the Vesalian anatomists still defended Galenist theory in broad principle, they chose the evidence of their own eyes whenever their dissections contradicted it. Eustachius could therefore cast his opponents as anti-Galenists who perversely followed the ancient master without empirical justification, precisely where the poor man had been wrong. It was well known, said Eustachius, that Galen only ever dissected non-human animals, so his description of the sutures must have been inaccurate. In humans, the sutures "as drawn on the page most elegantly imitate the multiform lines of the geographer," whereas in apes "they are obscure, so that for the most part they deserve the name of sutures scarcely or not at all." Galen's description fitted the simplicity of the simian skull. In the human skull, by contrast, the sutures vary from one individual to the next; and the two arms of the lambdoid suture will often be of unequal length. Eustachius's urge to keep humans separate from apes, on the grounds of their anatomical diversity,

---

[38] Ingrassia, *In Galeni Librum de Ossibus*, 64.
[39] *De Humani*, 16.
[40] Samuel Parker, *A Demonstration*, 10.
[41] *Opuscula Anatomica*, 151; 148.

led him to insist on the viability of Galen's "impossible" type: "I publicly dissected fifteen [human] skulls in one day where the coronal suture was absent," he says. Monkeys were emblematic of the devil, and the deceptive similarity of their sutural layout to the human skull was in fact merely a crude and ridiculous *imitation*. In short, Eustachius was expressing moral difference in anatomical terms.

Locke, another medical man, expressed this moral difference in terms of a natural history of the mind. When Da Monte in the Renaissance had observed Little Johnny, he was not trying to answer the question "What does an intellectual disability look like?" Rather, he was asking, "What does it mean for an apparently human creature not to have a rational soul?" When Locke at the start of the Enlightenment observed a permanent, birth-to-death absence of reason in his "changelings," he was still asking the same question, as in some sense is today's psychologist. However, he was doing so now in a context where the soul or mind was a separate, autonomous realm of nature. Thus it is not *models of a transhistorical cognitive impairment* that follow a diagnostic continuity to modern from pre-modern; it is doctors' *attitudes to monstrosity* and, more generally, our social phobia about contamination, that do so. The continuity is an anthropological one.

It is true that some of the old diagnostic criteria did carry on. Physiognomists were still around in the nineteenth century, conducting blindfold tests on skulls to see whether they belonged to peasants or geniuses (such was the antithesis), and contributing to phrenology and eventually to intelligence testing.[42] Locke's account of the changeling, however, had been a refutation of physiognomics. A deformed body was precisely *not* a sign of deformed personality or intellect; the mind was quite capable of being deformed by itself. Nevertheless, Locke's new model of permanent disability of a strictly intellectual kind emerged partly with the aid of the old physiognomics, which succeeded in adapting to mind-body dualism and became a commonplace of eighteenth- and nineteenth-century explanations of behaviour. The transfer across to the realm of the mind was just one stage in the unceasing medical construction and reconstruction of monsters. The "darkness" and "blind ignorance" brought about by deprivation of a faculty could now be detected by what Locke called "the physiognomy of the mind."[43]

Some reflection of these changes in the wider culture can be seen in the iconography of dwarfism. Typically employed as court fools, Renaissance dwarfs like those sitting underneath Veronese's banqueting tables display no facial signs of an inferior intellectual status. But by the 1630s, when Velázquez depicted the Crown Prince of Spain alongside his dwarf, he was clearly setting off the moral and intellectual (as well as physical) perfections of the one against their assumed absence in the other. In another portrait, the short person's expression is a vacant stupor, drawn from physiognomic convention.[44] Medically, stupor was temporary or at most dispositional, but by attaching it to a permanently monstrous body Velázquez is making the expression itself, and the inner state it denotes, monstrous too. It is a foretaste of those nineteenth-century photographs depicting the gaze of the feeble-minded, the Jew, the Negro, etc. Like the supposed "vacant look" attributed to the intellectually disabled today, or the "lack of eye contact" in autism, what this stupor actually tells us about is a vacancy in the social relationship that does not (but, given other circumstances, might) come into play between them and us, as we gaze back at them.

Another vanguard text to infiltrate traditional accounts of physical monstrosity into burgeoning ones of cognitive impairment is Nicholas Culpeper's English translation, with commentary, of

---

[42] See G. Shuttleworth, *Some of the Cranial Characteristics of Idiocy*, 241; Michael Hagner, "Prolegomena to a history of radical brains," *Physis*, 36/2 (1999); G. Lanteri-Laura, *Histoire de la phrénologie*; Robert Young, *Mind, Brain and Adaptation in the Nineteenth Century*.

[43] *Some Thoughts*, 6.94.

[44] Velázquez, "Prince Baltasar Carlos with a Dwarf," Museum of Fine Arts, Boston; "Portrait of Francisco Lezcano," The Prado, Madrid.

Galen's *Art of Medicine*. Its year of publication, 1652, coincides with the English translation of Luther's seminal story about demonic changeling children (see Chapter 16), and the banning of "idiots" of the juridical type from communion (see Chapter 11). Culpeper several times interpolates "fools" into Galen's text. To take one example, Galen had simply said:

> A small head is the proper indication of a poor brain condition. A large head, however, does not necessarily indicate a good condition. But if it has become strong because the power residing in it has created matter that is useful as well as abundant, that is a good sign; if however because of abundance alone, that is not a good sign.

Culpeper's translation runs:

> A very small head is a proper indication of a vicious brain, and yet a great head doth not necessarily declare a strong brain; if there be not capacity enough in the skull to hold the brain, or a sufficient quantity of brain, the man must needs be a fool.[45]

Slack adjectives yield to the firm smack of nouns. Likewise, in their translation of Platter, Culpeper (or more probably an associate) replaces Platter's "the ignorant beget the torpid" with "drones beget drones."[46] We cannot tell whether the symptoms which Culpeper saw in his fools had much in common with those we identify in today's disabled. The novelty was rather the emergence within medicine of a substantive medical type, involving *natural* causes that are also, like reprobation, *necessary* (they "must needs be").

In the mind-set of the doctor where the image of disability is moulded and remoulded, a longer-term pattern can be seen. The Hippocratics had merely talked about four kinds of arrangement of the sutures. Galen added a hierarchy of values; one kind is "suitable" or ideal, three are progressively defective and he criticizes his predecessors for not describing a further type that would be monstrous. Even so, he said, this type can only exist in the imagination. Renaissance Galenists amplified the picture with an example of this further type which they claimed to have actually seen, even if it did not live for long: the type can exist in reality. Someone who says "It doesn't exist" is followed by someone else who feels bound to say, "Yes it does." So too with the historiography: Benzi cited his predecessor D'Abano as saying that he had seen one when in fact D'Abano had only said that it *might* exist. This ever-recurring exhaustion of doctors' state of wonder at the separateness of monsters from the rest of nature has its own dialectic, always creating a new space in which to seek out ever more outlandish discoveries. The absence of sutures is inconceivable (Hippocrates); the inconceivable becomes conceivable but unviable (Galen); the conceivable but unviable becomes the viable but wondrous (Benzi). And once late nineteenth-century physicians claimed to see sutural anomalies in the skulls of people with Down's syndrome, the viable but wondrous becomes the abnormal but mundane; an 1881 medical photograph depicts the skull of "an idiot of the mongoloid type," probably intended to show that it had only one suture.[47] In this passage from inconceivable to pathological, the wonder of nature is constantly lost and then rediscovered in precisely the form that was the previous limiting case. The limiting case would be a wonder if it could exist: then, hey presto, it does.

As an apothecary, that is, a professional medic serving the lower and middling sort, Culpeper was as great an influence on the everyday practice of medicine for the next hundred years as

---

[45] Culpeper, *Galens Art of Physick*, 11.
[46] *Platerus Golden Practice*, 1.
[47] Historical Images Collection, Wellcome Institute for the History of Medicine, London.

Sydenham and Locke were on its diagnostic method.[48] The very act of translating a major teaching tool such as Galen's *Ars Medica* into English was an act of political radicalism. In his preface Culpeper castigates the elite College of Physicians then in control of the profession, complains about their insistence on Latin to preserve their social and professional positions, and scoffs at their calculated esotericism. He applies the metaphor of monstrosity and species exclusion precisely to this professional elite and their reactionary defence of "that monster tradition, who seldom begets any children but they prove either fools or knaves, and this makes them so brutish." One of their obscurantist tricks was the custom of putting a deformed skeleton on show in their surgeries to impress new patients, "a monster in the first room."[49] But Culpeper himself, when he inserted his "fool" into Galen's text, was doing something similar. He helped to bring about a monstrosity which belonged in a separate and strictly intellectual sphere, and which had a much more rigorously determinate and excluded identity than previous kinds of monstrosity such as that in the doctor's waiting room. Far from being, as the deformed skeleton had been, a demonstration of God's power to create a rich tapestry of natural wonders (*monstrare* means to show or reveal), monsters permanently disabled from the newly prized forms of human reasoning demonstrated now, in the 1650s, the praeternatural power of the devil. In this lies the modernity of intellectual disability.

---

[48] F.N.L. Poynter, "Nicholas Culpeper and his books," *Journal of the History of Medicine*, 152.
[49] Culpeper, *A Key to Galens Method*, 139.

PART 7
Psychology, Biology and the Ethics of Exceptionalism

Chapter 15
Philosophy, the Devil and "Special People"

The conceptual basis of our natural classifications of intellectual disability spans a whole complex of biology, psychology and ethics. The modern medical model and its concept of abnormality arose within this broader context of the life sciences, their approaches to the classification and subclassification of human nature and concomitant criteria of acceptance and rejection. In this first section we deal with issues which in earlier times were seen as metaphysical, lying further back than nature – cause, identity, permanence – but which today are seen as belonging to nature, and form the starting point of scientific knowledge about our topic. We then progress to the question of how, in this natural realm, intellectually abnormal creatures appear. How are they generated: God's work? The Devil's? The parents'? These questions were being asked throughout the early modern period, and have been formative of the representation of intellectual disability prevalent today. Finally, we look at biological nature as a hierarchical scale. Where, objectively, does the possession of intellectual abilities situate human beings on this scale, and what subjective intellectual abilities of our own do we employ in assigning them there? Is there a link between these two questions? It may be a long time since any respectable biologist positioned human beings at the summit of all forms of life like a fairy on a Christmas tree, but human *intelligence* is another matter. Self-regarding illusions about it are rife, and it certainly remains the case that those deemed to be exceptionally unintelligent have remained on the lowest branches.

The ethics of indifference versus the ethics of exceptionalism

Accounts of intelligence and disability as aspects of a specifically "human nature" involve a complex of psychological, biological and ethical expertises with a religious mind-set at its root. The three appear to exist separately, impinging on each other of course, but only externally, as independent disciplines. In the long historical perspective, however, they remain a single complex. They belong together as much now as they did when they were all part of a single, divinely authored "Book of Nature," which medieval thinkers saw as complementing scripture and revealing the order of the universe.

The primary role of ethics is to obscure the fact that the complex is sustained by values rather than science. While in philosophy "ethics" (Greek) and "morals" (Latin) are the same thing, modern medicine treats them not just as different but as mutually repellent. Morals is private, individual reasoning; it is heterodox and can thus itself be idiotic. Indeed Robert Edwards, 2010 Nobel Prizewinner in Medicine, has said that morals in the sense of knowingly bringing to term a disabled child may – thanks to biotechnology – be considered a "sin."[1] Ethics by contrast is objective public reasoning, or at least public relations; it provides routine endorsements for the biologist's and psychologist's treatment of certain people as problems. The scientific description of those problems is in fact no less value-based and historically contingent than that of the private moralist. Bioethics, with its partner biotechnology, is part of the tightening of the codes designed to preserve the dominance of intelligence as the self-referential mode of bidding for status. Modern scientists have tended to see morals and ethics alike as separate from the natural world.

---

[1] Lois Rogers, *Sunday Times*, London 4 July 1999.

Ethics in our field, apart from the special case of evolutionary ethics, appears to shine a beacon from outside on a natural phenomenon. Nevertheless, scientific enquiry into people described as intellectually disabled and our ethical view of them are in fact indissoluble. How do we know the difference between them and us? How do we value them? These two questions are not just *related*, they are *one and the same* question.

Behind them lies a further, unasked question: Why classify them in the first place? At philosophy's more rarefied altitudes a non-classificatory inclusiveness has tended to prevail. Since inclusion is a binary notion dependent on that of exclusion, inclusiveness might better be called indifference: indifference, that is, to any supposed problem of social or species membership.[2] Devising criteria that classify certain individuals as proper species members and others as not begs the question: what are the problems which classification exists to solve? Philosophers have tended not to see any. Once Hobbes, for example, began writing about laws of human nature, the idea might have occurred to him of exceptions to such laws. Yet he set minimal requirements for what it means to be human or to differ from other animals, and this led him to be accommodating to "fools." Montaigne similarly cited deaf people: "Our deaf-mutes have discussions and arguments, telling each other stories by means of signs," indicating that they can access the common ideas – but also that "We are neither above nor below the animals," since animals make signs too. In this sceptical view, the distance in intellect "is more between some men and others, than it seems to be between some men and beasts ... which is but a bad business, and not much for our honour."[3] Nevertheless, they are all men. Descartes, starting from the opposite premise of a stark difference between cogitating humans and machine-like animals, arrived at the same conclusion about borderline cases. Everyone – the deaf, "those deprived of their senses (*mente capti*) ... all men, however foolish (*stupidi*)" – is at least capable of a few signs and consequently of typically human behaviour. Marginal cases belong on the human side of the line; they are the border lights revealing the adjacent darkness of beast machinery.[4] Gassendi reached the same conclusion by a different route again, a celebratory one. In intellectual difference, he said, one discovers exciting new opportunities to enrich that definition: "Our idea of man since the discovery of America is richer and more perfect than that of the ancients," and despite the variability of "sharpness" among human souls, one has to acknowledge that "no one is created with absolute mindlessness or stupidity." As one Gassendist put it, we would otherwise have to "classify foolish and mindless people (*stupidi ac amentes*) with the brute beasts" as lacking souls – an obviously absurd notion.[5]

Inclusive indifference thus encompasses positions whose premises are in most other respects antagonistic. Modern philosophy's prime example is Ludwig Wittgenstein. First, he said, the customary notion of the human mind – that it is a place where thoughts are stored as ideas about the real world, prior to being expressed in language – is an occult one. Rather, there is language itself, its meanings belonging to their particular contexts; its stability, its rules, exist only as a set of varying language games which resemble each other as family members do, rather than as revealing a systematic, certain knowledge. Secondly, he asked, if language, allegedly characteristic of our species, cannot be said to express certain knowledge, how can it indicate any difference between humans and other animals? From this came the famous aphorism, "If a lion could talk, we could not understand him." In other words, it is true that human knowledge and abilities are anthropologically diverse, relative rather than based around "common ideas"; however, this does

---

[2] Jayne Clapton, *A Transformatory Ethic of Inclusion*.
[3] Montaigne, *An Apology*, 18; 24; Charron, *Of Wisdom*, i, 381.
[4] Descartes, *Discours de la méthode*, 96.
[5] Pierre Gassendi, *Institutio Logica*, i, 95a; *Opera*, 465b; Johannes Harderus, *Exercitationes Anatomicae*, 128.

not stop them from being characteristic of the human species as a whole. Rather, our language games constitute a specifically human "form of life," with which the leonine form of life is mutually incommunicable.

Wittgenstein's notion of diversity is not that of the social constructionist or postmodernist; he leaves room for a deeper common denominator which I have elsewhere called "deep culture," a cultural difference between human and other forms of life which renders differences among humans secondary.[6] To support his argument, he uses the example of "mental defectives." He may have got this idea from his close friendship with David Pinsent, dedicatee of his *Tractatus Logico-Philosophicus*. Pinsent's mother Ellen, who corresponded with Wittgenstein, was a eugenicist and an architect of segregated "special" schools, set up to prevent the interbreeding of mental defectives with the rest of the population as part of the Edwardian social hygiene movement. She had in her kinship group several famous physicians, including the second generation of the Langdon Down dynasty, which had by now strayed from the founder's original aim of demonstrating the fully human moral worth of his patients and was supporting the eugenics movement. For Wittgenstein, however, the defective utterances of such people, incomplete though they were, belonged recognizably to the set of human language games and therefore indicated a human form of life. The existence of exactly *these* people, their participation in the deep culture of being human, was what made it possible to verify the unity of the human species, the possibility of a general human understanding and a certain knowledge that might prevail over mere relativism.[7]

For behaviourists, by contrast, absence is all. Gilbert Ryle wrote: "A lion not only cannot be good at reasoning, he cannot even be bad, and an infant or an idiot not only cannot argue logically, he cannot even argue illogically. He cannot argue at all, and so gets neither good nor bad marks for his arguments, since these do not exist."[8] But this case aside, inclusive indifference tends to prevail at elevated altitudes, and breaks down only when philosophy descends to the political and ethical arena. What we find there is something quite different: an *ethics of exceptionalism*. The idea that certain people are "special" expresses some value, whether negative or (less often) positive, and it does indeed involve ethical concerns about classification. Bioethicists, for example, view the question of who is intellectually disabled as urgently as any seventeenth-century pastor viewed that of who was reprobate. For the pastor, certain creatures existed which had a human shape but an animal's complete absence of conscience; and as we have seen, rational conscience – the defining component of the human essence for the orthodox Calvinist – was not so far from Locke's defining component, which was logical reasoning. Conscience, the accounting to oneself for one's own thoughts and behaviour, operated *by* reason. People deficient in this sense were corpses: to be dead in Christ was to be dead in one's reason. And to be in this state but also to be breathing and walking around might even mean you were the Devil who, though incorporeal, could certainly take on a human form. One might want to have eliminated such creatures from the outset.

Similar fears about an invasion of the bodysnatchers underlie the medical model of intellectual disability. From these fears has sprung the appropriate biotechnology, which today makes realizable the pastor's and the eugenicist's dream of elimination without infanticide. Of course not all bioethics is eugenicist. Even when it is not, though, one assumes that a problem exists, *a priori*: that "difficult" decisions about life and death have to be made, even where the criteria are solely intellectual and hence a historically and socially moveable feast. The diagnostic technique which launched second-wave liberal eugenics, amniocentesis, was for just such intellectual criteria.

---

[6] C.F. Goodey, "Learning difficulties and the guardians of the gene," in A. Clarke and E. Parsons (eds), *Culture, Kinship and Genes*.
[7] Ludwig Wittgenstein, *Remarks on the Philosophy of Psychology*.
[8] Gilbert Ryle, *A Rational Animal*, 4.

The justification for termination and even euthanasia on these grounds offered by utilitarian bioethicists such as Peter Singer in his *Rethinking Life and Death* reprises the ethical stance Locke reached three centuries earlier. If we could know an infant would grow up to be a non-reasoner, said Locke, infanticide might be excusable.[9] In excluding non-reasoning "changelings" from membership of the human species, he was defending man's intellectual uniqueness against those faith-based sceptics like Montaigne, who doubted the difference between humans and animals. Changelings lack the membership criterion of logical reasoning, so they have to be classified among the brutes for ethical purposes even though their physical appearance is human. Singer, as Licia Carlson points out in *The Faces of Intellectual Disability*, ignores the history, heterogeneity and instability of the concept, and can therefore add little to this picture. He is merely more optimistic about imputing intelligence to monkeys ("a rational soul to a drill," to use Locke's formula). If monkeys are capable of Sign, might they not be classified in the same species as humans despite their physical difference, and be treated as human for ethical purposes? Conversely, if a human is unable to reason logically, then is not eugenics or infanticide justifiable?

Our long-term historical perspective shows us that the simple act of posing such questions in the first place is the sign of a deeply religious mind-set. Locke and Singer both invoke the underlying principle of nominalism in order to deny species membership to the disabled. As we saw in Chapter 8, this says that only particulars (individual creatures) are real; universal categories (species) are not themselves real; they are merely names we agree on to describe sets of particulars which appear to have shared characteristics, and which are therefore potentially changeable, by consensus. In naming certain individuals as members of a category (e.g., the "human species"), we are merely following some subjective inclination that prevents our knowledge of the world from being chaotic. And if it is characteristic of the human species to be rational, a permanently non-rational human is a contradiction in terms. However, also inherent in Locke-Singer's affected humility about our ability to know real essences of species is the possibility that there is some higher authority who truly does know. As Singer himself says in the opening sentence of his *Animal Liberation*, "to end tyranny we must first understand it." Some Catholic thinkers espoused nominalism in order to justify papal control over the imposition of universal categories. Luther and Calvin were nominalists too, on the grounds that only God can know universals. Either way, the possibility that there is some superior authority somewhere who *really* knows which individuals belong to which species survives in the nominalist approach adopted by modern bioethics. If it were genuinely the case that species boundaries have no real existence in nature, there would be no absolute basis in truth for proposing members or excluding non-members. One would have to admit that one was choosing subjective criteria for membership of the species and then eliminating the exceptions, and that this was no more than an arbitrary exercise of power over the powerless. This would be impossible, unless one were a psychopath. Species boundaries must therefore be real in *some* sense, even for the nominalist.

Locke was forced as a result to come up with the novel and contradictory phrase "nominal essence"; he retained the noun and simply attached a new, oxymoronic qualifier to it. Before Locke, essences had been nothing other than "real" categories, created as such by God; sorting things into categories "nominally" suggested that categories were mere names, created by human beings, and therefore in the last resort not essences at all. Yet Locke nowhere says that real essences do not exist, only that the most we can do is approximate to them (previous nominalists had maintained that we cannot even do that). Without a similar sense of quasi-reality, and without the implicit presence of some superior authority to uphold it, today's bioethicists could scarcely support the measures of which biotechnology is now capable. If the classification of human beings were arbitrary, there

---

[9] Locke, *An Essay*, 453.

would be no difference between compassion and hatred as motives for eradicating disability. What then is that superior ethical authority? It seems in fact to be the authors' own. Locke's nominalist scepticism about the fixity of species boundaries was the stepping-stone to a new positivity about defining membership of the human species in accordance with the individual's rationality rather than his morphology. Singer in all these respects is Locke's heir. It is true that both men claim their approach is probabilistic, based on a willingness to accept a balance of evidence rather than from what they would like to be true. But where is the guarantee that they have exorcized their own teleological tendencies? Having sceptically dismantled the existing realist view of the membership criterion for being human (bodily nature), Singer has no further inclination to any scepticism: his own revised choice of criterion (rationality and intelligence) just is the right one. He himself, with that presupposition, is the higher authority. He can then oppose religion's dogmatic sanctity-of-life arguments with his own, equally dogmatic reordering of species boundaries by rationality and intelligence. Meanwhile, from the religious substructure of bioethics comes the smoke of metaphor from a really existing fire: the "Book of Life" (the human genome); "virgin birth" (parthenogenesis, embryos bred without male genetic material); and "remaking Eden" (germ-line engineering).

The modern biologist takes a purportedly nominalist approach to definitions of species: they are only ever an approximation. Nevertheless, when it comes to determining the boundaries of our own species, bioethics reverts with remarkable alacrity to straightforward realism. It just knows where the boundaries lie, and they are psychological ones. The most frequently cited ethical argument for the use of biotechnology in eliminating potential lives is not hatred but compassion: relief of suffering. But medicine's official role of preventing harm is inseparable from its shamanistic claim, based on psychology, to know what is present and absent in the mind. To attack bioethics and preventive biotechnology on the grounds that this knowledge is not value neutral, as many critics do, is only half the story. Bioethics is not just a particular view *about* this knowledge, as if it were (say) a camera giving a different take on the same event according to the values of the person operating it. It *constitutes* that knowledge: it presupposes what is and is not in the mind, and the consequent suffering of certain singled-out individuals. This presupposition is inscribed in a liberal culture whose notions of suffering can be quite trivial and, as Hans Reinders puts it, "send the message that life is more worth living the less trouble it takes."[10] Moreover, one might think that only sufferers can make judgements about their own suffering. It is hard to see how "disabled" individuals, whose disability is said to consist in a lack of understanding, can understand that they suffer from lack of understanding. On the contrary, an "autistic" person who likes dancing naked in the street when it rains clearly enjoys being autistic, whatever the problems raised in other people's minds. Intellectual suffering is no fit topic for scientific critique or empirical knowledge; and the problem is all the more acute when the supposed sufferer is a foetus rather than a living creature whom one might get to know.

The negative stereotype conceals within itself a deeper, more fundamental thought: that there may be certain lives that ought not to happen. This is not yet a thought about suffering or about intellectual disability: it is prior to any specificity as to who is being discussed. The core thought is that a potential life *of whatever kind* should not take place. This "to be or not to be," irrespective as yet of what human characteristic it is that ought not to be, already contains its own ethical premise: certain creatures exist that ought not to. The question of who exactly these creatures are takes historically shifting and contingent forms, within the longer-term utilitarian ethic of exceptionalism. In its modern form, the suffering attached to "intellectual" disability is a projected anxiety of the large in-group whose status is expressed through the mode of intelligence. From a broader historical perspective, the utilitarianism is of a deeper, more explicitly religious kind, in

---

[10] *The Future of the Disabled in Liberal Society*, xi.

which the desire to end suffering goes with a fear of the disabled person's pollution of the sacred rite of intelligence – that same rite which confirms, for the intelligent, their species membership. Jeremy Bentham may have replaced "Is this person rational?" with "Does he suffer?" as the crucial ethical concern, but there is a difference between wanting to end the imagined suffering of others and wanting to keep the imagined suffering of others away from oneself.

It is important to recognize that the ethics of exceptionalism can point in an optimistic as well as a negative direction. In the words of one Renaissance medical writer on faculty psychology, "the innocent souls of children and the foolish" do not suffer because "they do not commit sins of the flesh and therefore do not know what it is to endure deprivation of sinful bodily pleasures." One might therefore want more foolish people around rather than less.[11] What psychologists and doctors have stereotyped in Down's syndrome as an infantile affectionateness, a pathology of the developmental plateau, both Down himself and Jérôme Lejeune (discoverer with Marthe Gautier of the 21 trisomy) stereotyped instead as a gift of intense fellow feeling. The isolation of a biochemical element in Down's syndrome has led to the possibility of eliminating this characteristic, but if one did indeed see it as superior, as both those key historical figures did, one might want to engineer it into the human germ-line of the human species. Eugenic technology – Lejeune himself was a biotechnician – may go with any values it chooses. However, in both sets of values, negative and optimistic, the core component is one and the same: it is the singularity of the suffering/gift, which isolates certain people as exceptions to a classificatory rule. The alternative to both is inclusive indifference, and the distinction between indifference and exceptionalism is more fundamental than the distinction within the latter between suffering and gift.

Disability and the Devil

In order to understand how social anxieties about intelligence are transposed into natural criteria for membership of the human species, we need to know how it is generated and enters the world in the first place. The majority theory, laid down by Avicenna, was that the rational soul is generated by God, who "infuses" it into the foetus a certain (disputed) number of days after the vegetative soul, responsible for motion, and subsequently the animal soul, responsible for the external senses. His infusion of the rational soul was generic to all humans; individual differences in earthly wit were secondary and tied to the body. The existence of the rational soul was deductively proven from God's existence and was thus demonstrably present in everyone, however problematic their intellects or behaviours. By the end of the sixteenth century, inroads into this theory had come from the theory of "traducianism." "Who hath put the wisdom in the inward parts?" asks the Book of Job. Traducianists answered that it was parents who generated the rational soul and were therefore the natural cause of personality differences in offspring. Here we find a source for later, biological theories of hereditary intelligence. And if the offspring were deficient, co-participants in the act of generation were suggested: animals, or purely spiritual beings such as the Devil's *incubi* and *succubi*, who have sex with witches and then insert the semen they have gathered into women with lustful imaginations. Devil and parents alike, or together, could be sources of pollution.

Traducianism in general was an ancient theory, but its prominence in debate, like that of the Devil, was new. Both were on the increase during the seventeenth century, in tandem with the glimmerings of modern science. Although presentist historians of science like to think of devil beliefs as an archaism that gradually receded over a long historical period, in fact they were gathering

---

[11] Andrea Alpago, introduction to Avicenna, *Compendium de Anima*, 94v.

strength over the sixteenth and seventeenth centuries.[12] They were partly fuelled by the confluence between theories of nature and those of election/reprobation: "Satan findeth his own seed in us by nature ... a sprouting, and child of the house of Hell .... In Satan's fools the right principle of wisdom is extinguished."[13] Later on, in the nineteenth century, when original sin was rephrased as degeneracy, demonic pollution would be rephrased as self-pollution. It became widely known that the cause of idiocy was masturbating parents: a mundane reconstitution of *incubus* theory, with the historical gap bridged by concepts of nocturnal pollution.[14] It was from the reproductive role of the Devil among deficient, socially inferior or self-abusing parents that modern biological notions of intellectual disability emerged; the language is still being used by Langdon Down when he writes how "the largest proportion of idiocy is to be found amongst the lower orders, ... where the afflicted child is not only a consuming member, but an *incubus*, paralyzing the efforts of the productive class."[15]

Devil beliefs and the modern medical model share several tacit presuppositions. First among these is *fear*. If definitions of disability are historically short term, the ethics of anxiety and the social phobia about pollution in general are long term. We understand people from another era best, wrote the historian Raymond Aron, if we know what they feared. In a broad sense we are still afraid of the same thing. Early modern people were scared of reprobate imitators and hypocrites: that you are not who you seem to be, or you are not who you say you are, or you are not the same person you were yesterday or will be tomorrow. This fear is focused on the creature who looks human but is not, because he seems not to exhibit the defining feature of your own species essence – whether this be the reasoning conscience of 1600 or the cognitive ability of 2000. The works of the Devil re-emerge as the works of genetic abnormality.

Secondly there is *shamanism*, religion's characteristic activity of administering control over presence/absence.[16] This was encouraged by the dualistic approach to mind and body. The more the mind is seen as a natural entity in its own right, rather than (as previously) form to the body's matter, the more it can be a supernatural entity too. It is easier to spirit away an invisible mind than one that is an organic facet of a visible body. Disability as imbalance has at the same time been replaced by disability as absence, and absence implies removal – prompting the thought, removal by some malevolent being.

That thought leads, thirdly, to our preoccupation with *cause*. As we have already noted, this is something modern. Asking what causes a disability and asking who is to blame are two questions with one premise. If there were no phobia and hence no responsibility to allocate, one would not be interested in causes. The notions of explanation and abnormality are mutually reinforcing. Why, when this particular person is born, is an explanation required for his or her identity when for most others no such question arises? In proposing a cause for something, one thereby presupposes and reinforces the reality of the thing caused. The ontological fragility of a status concept like intelligence demands that causes be located in the realm of hard indisputable reality, to lend it extra credence. Causes exist along a spectrum from the microcosm of the individual to macrocosmic, universal forces: from the immediate, material nature of the body (qualities of elements, humours, soul spirits, genes), to external nature (astrological influence, parental sexual behaviour, the environment), to some supernature beyond which no further explanation is possible (God, the Devil). The power of psychiatric medicine derives from these latter, from the explanations that lie furthest back along the

---

[12] See Stuart Clark, *Thinking with Demons*.
[13] Samuel Rutherford, *The Trial and Triumph of Faith*, 31.
[14] Samuel Gridley Howe, *On the Causes of Idiocy*, 32.
[15] *The Education and Training of the Feeble in Mind*, 65.
[16] Richard Fenn, *The Persistence of Purgatory*, 71.

causal spectrum: stories of saving and negative grace, of innocence and original sin and of "Christ the physician." The world is in need of healing. Incurability provokes despair and its fellows, disgust and hatred. Medical science's interest in the causal connection from bodily difference to intellectual difference is at root an interest in our salvation. Its overwhelming power in Lockean and post-Lockean accounts of intelligence and disability marks an advance on earlier periods, when medicine and philosophy were assumed only to deal with secondary causes since God and the Devil were beyond explanation. The Devil is the ultimate cause assumed in Locke's psychopathology in the same way that God is in Newton's physics: remote, unmentioned, indispensable.

Fourthly there is the interest in moral *consequences*. Although it was the atheist Bentham who coined the term "utilitarianism," the roots of the doctrine itself are, as Fenn describes them, religious ones. When the Reformation ditched belief in purgatory, with it went the comforting thought that the spirits of the dear departed could come back from the afterworld for an occasional visit. Spirits as such were not ditched, though. Instead, they became associated with the Devil alone, whose influence in this world remained an absolute presupposition. They became the agents of the disorder he creates in our everyday world. Religious utilitarianism focused on happiness in the next life but also on these unwanted consequences for life on earth. The task of tackling the Devil's pollution of our lives, in its bioethical form, consists in the cost-benefit analysis of the supposed fiscal problems created by the presence of intellectually disabled people in the intelligence society, and their pollution of our status as its members of it; the bioethicists' precursors were the early theorists of welfare such as Vives and Baxter.

Last among these shared presuppositions between devil beliefs and the medical model is the tension between *appearance and reality*. In late medieval and Renaissance thought, there was continual dispute between those who argued that the Devil could create both illusions and real works, and those who argued that he could only create illusions. The purpose of illusions was to sow chaos. In the illusionist or apparitionist view, "devils cannot create any nature or substance, but in juggling show or seeming only"; you did not need to believe the Devil has really caused this or that in order to believe in his existence.[17] Even for apparitionists, the apparitions were in their own way real; and even realists usually denied that "the Devil can make a true creature," since "to make a true creature of any sort, by producing the same [sort] out of the causes, is a work serving to continue the creation" and that is God's work alone.[18] Nevertheless, inquisitors and witch finders would have been doing themselves out of a job if spirits and changeling children were not real in some sense. The realists interpreted the idea that such children were mere apparitions as a denial, a heresy which it was their job to purge.

Some such opposition between apparitionist and the realist views has survived from these early accounts of substituted children through to psychiatric accounts of the twenty-first century. "Coping theory," which describes how parents and families come to accept as reality the scientific diagnosis of disability in a child, is a realist doctrine of a similar and historically related kind. This axiom of psychological and medical practice identifies in parents the "natural" process of a multistage psychiatric disorder which begins with denial of the diagnosis, then leads through structured, clearly identifiable phases – typically shock, rejection of the child, guilt, anger, then a specific anger against professionals – and finally to acceptance. Moreover, it *prescribes* this ritual disorder, which parents have to agree on unless they are to be labelled deniers and heretics. They must accept the child, but with the essential precondition that they undergo these purgative stages before doing so, thus confirming that they have accepted the child's intellectually monstrous character.

---

[17] Daniel Winkler, *De Vita Foetus in Utero*, 30.
[18] Perkins, *The Workes*, iii, 635.

Chapter 16
The Wrong Child:
Changelings and the Bereavement Analogy

Coping theory is the intelligence society's desanctification ritual. Parents, so runs the formula, have to "grieve for the child they have not had" as if they had undergone genuine bereavement, before they can accept the disabled one. To put this in its longer-term historical context: if parents do not grieve, it means that they have succumbed to the apparitionist heresy by not accepting the reality of evil. They must be encouraged to do so. For the psychologist, then, parental acceptance means, if not quite in these words, "I accept the expert estimate of my child as a monster." For the social anthropologist, on the other hand, it means "I accept that my child is human, not the monster the expert led us to believe"; parents simply expand their concept of normal to include the new arrival.[1] In psychiatric terms the latter amounts to denial. Parents must come to accept, and the content of their acceptance has to be that which the theory has prescribed for them. Indeed, many accounts of coping theory subdivide the "anger" stage of parental recovery into two: anger at the event, and anger at the professional who has revealed the diagnosis – thereby accounting for any resistance to the coping model. Once this multistage process of disorder and recovery is complete, the family must then embark on a second prescribed acceptance, this time of the fact that the pathological intellect in its midst makes it a pathological institution: the "disabled family." Parents, it is said, resort to clothing themselves in a spurious normality. They may allot the child a role in the family akin to that which they allot to their other children, but this inclusive indifference is supposedly a low-level prolongation of denial: making the best of a bad job.[2]

Changeling stories: the origins

Coping theory and the bereavement analogy have their origin in past accounts of creatures substituted by devils, witches and fairies, as the explanation for the arrival of a disabled child. Having long disowned the theory in that particular form, psychiatry has conserved it by imputing the concept of child substitution to parents instead; the appearance of a disabled child implies the existence of another (normal) child who has been taken away and for whom the parents mourn. This has the effect of focusing all anxiety on the disabled child. Pieter Brueghel the Elder's painting *The Blue Cloak*, known sometimes as *The World Turned Upside Down* or *The Wrong World*, stands on the threshold of this historical shift.[3] Filled with images of sin and social disorder, including one of a devil-possessed child in the grip of an equally malign carer, it depicts a world corrupted by the Fall, where the child is not some pathological specimen but represents the malignity in all of us. Changeling theory, in its modern form, has replaced this general signifier with an image of

---

[1] See R. Bogdan et al., "Be Honest but Not Cruel," in P. Ferguson (ed.), *Interpreting Disability*; Dick Sobsey, "Family transformation," in R. Friedlander and Sobsey (eds), *Through the Lifespan*; Tim Booth, "From normal baby to handicapped child," *Sociology*, 12 (1978); Tim Stainton and H. Besser, "The positive impact of children with an intellectual disability on the family," *Journal of Intellectual and Developmental Disability*, 23 (1998); H. Reinders, *The Future*, 60.
[2] Margaret Voysey, *A Constant Burden*.
[3] Staatliche Gemäldegalerie, Berlin.

the wrong child, an individual on whom the whole weight of the world's disorder is projected. The post-Reformation redrawing of the family, as an institution giving children a more distinct status and requiring from them both closer spiritual companionship and a tighter degree of obedience on everyday matters, made those less likely to conform more visible, and more problematic.[4]

Roughly from the beginnings of the Royal Society to the early nineteenth century, "changeling" came to mean not only a substituted child but something like an intellectually disabled person in the modern sense: the term has a Protean range that will emerge in the course of this section. A modern interpretation of changeling stories is that they were a projection of the parental instinct to reject the child, an explanation that appears to traverse historical and cultural boundaries. In fact the rejection, then as now, is that of an in-group which is seeking to impose watertight natural explanations on arbitrary social exclusions. The authority of today's psychiatrist and yesterday's theologian alike is based on the claim that distinguishing the real from the merely apparitional is the route to objective knowledge, and that their own discipline is uniquely capable in this respect. The grand historical narrative assumes a complete opposition between present-day scientific explanations for disability and the "folkloric" explanations of the past. But we shall see shortly how it was psychiatry's elite theological precursors who invented the so-called folk tales in the first place.

Just as today's professional elite reproduces its anxieties about the child by projecting them on to lay parents, so the story has been projected on to primitive historical others. Here is the house journal of the British paediatric profession:

> The advance of science during the eighteenth and nineteenth centuries slowly but surely eroded the popular belief that malformed and retarded children likely were not human at all, but rather the offspring of some demon ... that could be neglected, abused and put to death with no moral compunctions. As these theological explanations for retardation gave way to medical explanations, community values and personal attitudes changed to such an extent that the very word 'changeling' ... and their equivalents in other languages now have become historical curiosities, survivals of beliefs and practice that helped our northern European forebears ... face the problems of life and death when confronted with mentally or physically defective children.[5]

The notion of the substituted child "allowed [parents] to focus their aggression directly on the child since, of course, it was not their own," and the guilt which they might otherwise have internalized and seen as punishment for their sins was projected on to it. This author runs together "popular" and "theological" as if they were the same thing. It is true that theological expertise in the past was not separated from popular culture to the degree that scientific expertise is separated from lay beliefs today. Nevertheless, theological claims were the expert ones of their time. Our assumption that the substitute child story is popular in origin comes rather from the promotional efforts of knowledge elites, whether theological or psychiatric. The same went for witchcraft beliefs. Early modern professionals made a point of distancing themselves from the taint of social vulgarity; they discarded what had once been their own doctrines by pathologizing them as popular beliefs of the lower classes, who exhibit them as a "natural" form of cognitive dysfunction.[6] In actual fact the changeling theory, at least as it relates to disability, is far from a folk myth; its origins are those of psychology itself, and of expert modern systemizations of human behaviour. Although the Brothers Grimm, the seminal modern folklore compilers, insisted on the rude and peripheral

---

[4] See Lawrence Stone, *The Family, Sex and Marriage in England 1500–1800*, 101 ff.

[5] David Ashliman, cited in J. Leask, "Evidence for autism in folklore?" *Archives of Disease in Childhood*, 90/271 (2005).

[6] Shapin, *A Social History*, 77.

roots of the story in Germanic fairy literature, the ultimate textual sources come from the core of Western theology and its growing interest in the Devil.

This process begins with Augustine's commentary on Psalm 17 of the Vulgate Bible (18 in the Authorized Version):

> Children not worthy of being called mine, aliens who were rightly told "You are of your father the Devil," have lied to me.... These estranged children [*filii alieni*], to whom I brought the New Testament that they might be restored, have retained the old man within them. And they have limped away from their path. Lame in one foot because they held to the old path, they rejected the New Testament and became cripples.

The physical disability seems to be a metaphor for the Jews' deviation from the New Testament path, which Cassiodorus a century later made explicit. "This clearly happened with the Jews," he says. They had "weak minds," "spoke irrationally" and had attention deficit, "with nothing constant in their mind."[7] Labeo Notker, the tenth-century German translator of these texts, embellished them. He, or more likely a shortsighted copyist, coined for the Jews the word *Wechselkinder* (literally, "exchanged children").[8] The underlying message remained the same: God's degenerate offspring, succoured by the Devil, were the Jews as a whole. Notker was talking about their false doctrine, not about child substitution. Luther too, despite providing elsewhere one of the chief source texts for the child substitution story, glossed this particular passage as being about a whole degenerate race rather than about substitute children.[9] Notker merely coined the word itself, *Wechselkind*; he was not responsible for the actual substitution story, though historians have made him out to be so.[10]

The earliest extant text to mention child substitution comes two centuries later from William of Auvergne, Bishop of Paris:

> You should not overlook accounts of infants who conventionally [*vulgo*] are called *cambiones* [exchanged children], which are mostly old wives' tales: that they are the children of demonic *incubi*, substituted by demons ... as if swapped and substituted to female parents for their own children. These are said to be thin, always wailing, drinking so much milk that it takes four wet-nurses to feed one. They are observed to stay with their wet-nurses for many years, after which they fly away, or rather vanish.[11]

Vulgo, in theological dispute, refers not so much to the vulgar crowd as to those fellow theologians from whom one is distancing oneself: the crowd of one's peers. William may have been arguing against doctrinaires who believed that such children have a real existence – most probably the Dominicans, who were building an academic base at the University of Paris at this time. He sees the children not as generated by some real, para-sexual means but as "malign apparitions" (hence his self-correction from "fly away" to "vanish"), possibly of demonic origin but "permitted to appear for some divine purpose." They belonged in the realm of *appearances*; only the Almighty himself could create things for real (this was the long-standing patristic view).[12] When he says

---

[7] E. Dekkers and J. Fraipont, *Sancti Aurelii Augustini Enarrationes in Psalmos*.

[8] P. Tax, *Notker Latinus*, 56; P. Piper, *Die Schriften Notkers und seiner Schule*, vi; see also Goodey and Tim Stainton, "Intellectual disability and the myth of the changeling myth," *Journal of the History of the Behavioral Sciences*, 37/3 (2001).

[9] E. Roach and R. Schwartz (eds), *Martin Luthers Wolfenbütteler Psalter*, 65.

[10] Gisela Piaschewski, *Der Wechselbag*, 12; Jean-Claude Schmitt, *The Holy Greyhound*, 75.

[11] William of Auvergne, *De Universo*, in *Opera*, 1072.

[12] For example *Canon Episcopi*, in Migne, *Patrologiae*, cxxxii, 352; cxl, 831.

the realist view is "old wives' tales" and "senile delirium," he is not referring to some supposed folklore but insulting an academic opponent.

A corresponding account of the child substitution story from the other side of the dispute comes in the *Popular Sermons* of Jacques de Vitry, William's contemporary at Paris.[13] Unlike William, who wrote on philosophical topics, De Vitry, as a Dominican, participated in the first papal inquisitions and was concerned with the practicalities of purging heresy. He wrote these sermons for ordinary priests unused to preaching; it was partly a way of training them to implement the church's centralization policy by unifying the diverse religious observances that still existed at local levels. De Vitry asked the priest to push each sermon home with an *exemplum* or moral fable "for those who find it hard to understand." The *exempla* were subsequently filleted from the volume, circulated widely (the child substitution story among them) and became the founding texts for the many collections of moral fables that were an early modern literary genre. Many of them insist on the reality of demons, a common Dominican theme. By convention *exempla* came at the end of a sermon. However, in de Vitry's original manuscript the child substitution story is not actually an *exemplum* but comes under the heading of *testimonia*; these carried the authority of previous authors and were placed at the beginning. This underlines the story's importance. Child substitution was reality, not appearance.

The story was designed to lead congregations to accept the reality of the Devil in their lives and therefore of God. It is set alongside other stories which all convey the same message: empirical evidence shows that the Devil exists, therefore religion is true and philosophy inadequate. A half-eaten loaf is the work of the Devil, not mice; when you look in the mirror and see the Devil staring back, it really is him. Likewise the substitution of children by malign, demonic forces, "children called *chamium* [sc. *cambio*] who suck dry many wet nurses yet do not benefit or grow, but have a hard, distended belly." One "purges" (cures) a doubting congregation by forcing them to admit the reality of what others regard as an apparition. The British Folk-Lore Society republished De Vitry's *exempla* alongside the Grimms' "folk" tales at the start of the twentieth century, when first-wave eugenics was at its height.[14] There are close structural comparisons between De Vitry's story and motivation and the psychiatrist's normalization of disordered parents by making them accept the reality of their bereavement and the pathology of the creature they have ended up with. Both aim to eliminate all signs of non-acceptance ("denial") as if it were heresy.

After William and De Vitry, the story was reproduced by several German theologians who endorsed the latter's realist approach. Substitute children, says Nicolas of Jauer, are "themselves demons, not … apparitions generated by demons." These authors underline the immediate presence of the supernatural and of praeternatural causes in people's lives, as an incentive to piety; if the Devil is the real source for the evil of changelings, it proves that God alone, not any earthly authority, is the real source of grace.[15] These elements then coalesce in the famous *Malleus Maleficarum* ("The Hammer of Witches") of 1486, the most frequently cited text in the later blossoming of the story. Its authors, like De Vitry, were Dominican inquisitors. Their fullest reference to the story runs:

> Some women have their own sons and daughters taken away by demons and substituted with strange children [*filii alieni*]. Commonly called *campsores*, or in German *Wechselkinder*, they come in three different kinds. Some are always emaciated and howling, even though four women's

---

[13] *Sermones Vulgares*, Bibliothèque Nationale, Paris, ms. 17509, 77.

[14] T. Crane, *The Exempla or Illustrative Stories from the* Sermones Vulgares *of Jacques de Vitry*, 129.

[15] Nicolaus of Jauer, in A. Franz, *Der Magister*, 155; Dietrich of Münster, in J. Hansen, *Quellen und Untersüchungen zur Geschichte des Hexenwahns*, 86.

milk cannot satisfy a single one of them. Others are produced by the work of an *incubus*, though they are not its sons, but sons of men whose semen the *incubus* has collected as a *succubus*, or from nocturnal pollution.[16]

The authors were trying to get local clergy to face up to the Devil's dislocation of social life: changelings were like plague. They say nothing about any cognitive elements in such creatures, though an earlier German author (on whom the authors of the *Malleus* drew heavily) had said that they were "without speech."[17] The focus here and in succeeding texts is on how changelings are generated; though the Devil lacks the ability to generate new natural creatures, he is real enough, and he uses the natural magic of *incubi* and *succubi* to transfer semen.

The fact that the *Malleus* did not become a major source for writers on witchcraft until a century after its publication helps to show how interest in the Devil and natural magic was increasing rather than diminishing over this period. The other main source for the child substitution story, Luther's, also surfaced only posthumously. His *Tischreden*, published in 1566 and first translated into English as *Colloquia Mensalia, or Table Talk* in 1652, mentions the story several times.[18] The most detailed version begins with the Devil taking the shape of a man's dead wife. Luther says that their offspring were "not right human creatures, but devils ... very horrible and fearful examples, in that Satan can plague and so torment people as to beget children." He then distinguishes between this example and a second type, where the Devil simply swaps one creature for another:

> The Devil can also steal children away ... and other children called *supposititii* or changelings [*Wechselkinder*] laid in their places .... At Dessau I did see and touch such a changed child which was twelve years of age; he had his eyes and all members like another child: he did nothing but feed, and would eat as much as two clowns or threshers were able to eat. When one touched it, then it cried out. When any evil happened in the house, then it laughed, and was joyful; but when all went well, then it cried and was very sad. I told the Prince of Anhalt, if I were prince of that country, so would I venture *homicidium* thereon and would throw it into the River Moldau. I admonished the people in that place devoutly to pray to God to take away the Devil; the same was done accordingly, and the second year after the changeling died .... Such changelings live not above eighteen or nineteen years.

On the strength of this passage, Luther has acquired a reputation for advocating the elimination of disabled people, even being cited in a 1964 German court case on euthanasia.[19] Yet the attributes corresponding to lack of soul here are not intellectual in a modern sense. Moreover, it is unreliable as evidence of Luther's actual beliefs, since the volume is not his own published text but assembled from reported conversations by a disciple who seems to reflect the second-generation Reformers' increasing focus on the Devil and witchcraft.[20]

Another version of the story in the same volume suggests that the child be suffocated, on the grounds that he is simply "a mass of flesh without a soul."[21] Locke may well have had this text in mind (it was published and widely disseminated in English during his undergraduate years) when he wrote in the *Essay concerning Human Understanding* about changelings lacking souls

---

[16] Jakob Sprenger and Heinrich Kramer [Institoris], *Malleus Maleficarum*, 2.2.8.
[17] Johannes Nider, *Praeceptorum divinae legis*, 11.
[18] Luther, *Colloquia Mensalia, or, Table Talk*, 387.
[19] T. Tappert, in *Luther's Works*, vol. 54, 397.
[20] M. Miles, "Martin Luther and childhood disability," *Journal of Religion, Disability and Health*, 5/4 (2001).
[21] Tappert, *Luther's Works*, 396.

and suggested that infanticide might therefore be appropriate. Luther's "mass of flesh" echoes Augustine's notion of fallen humanity in general as "a mass of sin"; his concern was the way the Devil creates obsessions that blind all of us to the Word, and the child's odd behaviour was symbolic of this. It was Locke, the proto-modern psychologist and natural historian, who was to draw the full conclusion: that changelings, creatures seen as entirely lacking a soul or mind, were non-human.

Citations of the *Malleus* were on the increase from the 1590s onwards. A few writers, most controversially Reginald Scot in *The Discoverie of Witchcraft*, were sceptical about the abilities of witches and devils. This was picked up by poets such as Michael Drayton, whose 1627 *Nymphidia: the Court of Fairy* criticizes credulous people who

> When a child haps to be got,
> Which after proves an idiot,
> When folk perceive it thriveth not,
> The fault therein [d]o smother:
> Some silly doting brainless calf,
> That understands things by the half,
> Say, that the Fairy left this elf,
> And took away the other.

But this was not a scepticism about natural magic as such. Scot and Drayton doubted the Devil's ability to procreate or witches' ability to consort with him, but not his actual existence. When Scot ascribed the child substitution story to the masses, it was his way of pouring scorn on its realist and apparitionist interpreters alike: substitution could be done by natural magic, which did not need supernatural means to operate. Others who wrote of it as a popular story did so with the opposite intent; they claimed that it must indicate the real existence of devils and spirits because it was so widespread (hence James I's order for Scot's book to be burnt). Either way, this was the beginning of its career as a supposed folk tale, leading in a direct line to the modern psychiatric doctrine that parents grieve for the child they have not had.

Protestants encouraged moral exempla of this kind in order to complement the reading of scripture and to spread at the grassroots the religious elite's own utilitarian belief in the Devil and his works. It was Luther who had attached to the story its anecdotal style. This made it look folkloric, but embedding doctrine in anecdote was a common preaching device which Luther himself was especially fond of. It is too easy, looking through the lens of the Grimms and their presentation of the story to modern nineteenth-century audiences, to suppose that it was of specifically German and thereby rude and popular origin, and that the earlier theologians had just been attracted by its exotic subcultural flavour. Rather, it was the latter who had dreamed the story up as a way of universalizing it, and of proving the real presence of the Devil in this world. This is clear from Luther's locating it among "the boorish Saxons" of Dessau, which subsequently became a stock feature of the story. From the very beginnings of a German high culture, Saxony had symbolized the ignorance of the fleshly, sinful and unconverted masses. It may sound convincingly specific to a folk-tale collector, but the creators of the story were already primed to set it there. William of Auvergne had placed his version of it alongside a series of other stories set in entirely mythical places; next to his account of substitute children was a story explaining that if oafish Saxons looked like bears, it was because human and bear semen were compatible.

By the 1590s, writers were going out of their way to attribute the experience of child or sperm substitution to marginal cultures. In James I's *Daemonologie*, written to advertise his role as God's absolute commander of all forces fighting the Devil, his interlocutor asks, "What is the cause that this kind of abuse is thought to be most common in such wild parts of the world?" and receives the answer: "Because where the Devil finds greatest ignorance and barbarity, there assails he grossliest." The Germans "have more experience of sorcerers because there it is quite ancient and there are more of them than in other countries," and they "maintain that from such [demonic] copulation an infant sometimes springs whom they call *Wechselkind*."[22] Whereas the German-speaking but Latin-writing authors of the *Malleus* had interpolated the German word merely to help the reader grasp an unfamiliar Latin noun, later commentators such as Caspar Bauhin, an early figure in the rise of natural history classification, glossed the authors as follows: "[They] write that the Germans think children are sometimes born from this [diabolic] union whom they call *Wechselkinder*, i.e., mutated children."[23] In fact the *Malleus* authors had said nothing about the story being German. The idea that the child substitution story was once a folk myth is itself a myth; it was precisely in being mythologized and attributed to the folk that the story could be *naturalized* and (the same thing) modernized.

Changeling theory and the rise of reason

The first OED reference to the English word changeling is 1555. There were two early types of usage. The first did indeed refer to substituted creatures; these could, however, be adults as well as children, and explanations did not involve the Devil. Titania's changeling in *A Midsummer Night's Dream*, for example, is the mundane result of a kidnapping rather than being demonically conceived. The second usage signified not substitution by some external agency but a subjective condition, the internal inconstancy of people whose will and opinions were always changing. It was this usage, rather than the first, that thereby carried overtones of deviance. Even then, however, the term itself played no part in the disputes over wardship law and "born fools"; Drayton's 1627 example above, where the concept if not the word itself appears in connection with juridical idiocy, is an isolated early example. In short, the word signified at first neither cognitive impairment nor folk myth. In his mid-seventeenth-century behaviour guide, Fuller, a regular visitor to Bedlam, talks about "a changeling, which is not one child changed for another, but one child on a sudden changed from itself," and differentiates this entirely from a "natural fool." By the 1660s however, when his great admirer Samuel Pepys observes of a servant "how ill she do any serious part ... just like a fool or changeling," it is no longer clear that the "or" is disjunctive.[24] There seems to have been a sudden shift in the 1650s or 60s; in the index of his prototype scientific dictionary, Wilkins advises his readers: "Idiot – put changeling."[25]

Reprobation was absorbed in this new concept. With religious tensions peaking in this period, changeability or "inconstancy in religion" came to be interpreted as intellectual *absence*, superseding the old model of organic imbalance. If men "are not able to give an account of their faith, nor tell any sound reason why, upon what grounds, to what end they do such and such things, can it be expected but that ... they will be drawn without much ado to change their minds?" Changeability was already gendered, being typical of "silly women, who ... never came to the knowledge of the truth: they were the fittest to become a prey unto false teachers and deceivers." However, "in these times we have to blame men as well as women for this fault."[26] The disability is both praeternatural (the deceivers are the Devil and his sidekick, the papal Antichrist) and new ("in these times").

This changeling who kept changing his mind was deficient first and foremost in his will. But from deficiency of will to deficiency of reason was a smaller step than might be supposed, as

---

[22] Jean Bodin, *De la démonamie*, 182.
[23] *De Hermaphroditorum Monstrorumque*, 262.
[24] Fuller, *The Holy and the Profane*, 182; Pepys, *Diary*, 28 December 1667.
[25] Wilkins, *An Essay towards ... a Philosophical Language*.
[26] Pemble, *Workes*, 554.

demonstrated by Breton's 1613 character-type of "a wilful Will-Fool."[27] The will, as the site of faith and especially of religious zeal, in retrospect had created civil war and social chaos, in which it was the professions of church and law, along with priests and justices themselves, that were – even more than the political regime as such – the main targets for the insurrectionary religious movements of common people. This led a critical mass of the elite to promote human reason as the prerequisite of faith ("sweet reason" was an amalgam of rational and moral piety). By the 1670s, the Nonconformists and Dissenters were going further and asserting that the workings of this new reason could be detected in the subjective mechanisms of individual and heterodox minds. For them, reason was an internal condition of religious and political liberty. For the Anglican establishment, it was a set of principles received passively from God via divinely appointed bishops. Whereas the establishment thought that toleration of heterodoxy would reignite the unreasonable wilfulness of the civil wars, Dissenters spoke about "liberty of conscience" and against "the unreasonableness of [Anglican] persecutors"; their own dissenting reason, they said, represented the "interest" of religion.[28] Each side conceived of the changeling's deficiency as the polar opposite of its own particular claim to the new reason. Since the Dissenters located reason in the liberty and responsibility of all human individuals more or less regardless of their social status, the existence of an occasional creature who lacked even this species-wide reason revealed a classification problem. The ruling Anglicans, on the other hand, feared that a reason which sprang up directly in each individual plebeian mind might subvert the kind of reason they themselves were handing down by absolute authority; it threatened a return of the excessive liberty and relativism of the 1640s and 50s. In these circumstances it made sense for the Anglicans to take the changeling label, once used to describe someone with an inconstant will, and redirect it towards people with a defective reason – by which of course they also meant a wrong, dissenting *interpretation* of reason.

On both sides, then, the new reason involved a new kind of universalism, embracing all or most human beings and replacing the old quasi-universalism of the Arminians, which had been based chiefly on belief and the will. Odd fusions and recombinations of doctrine were happening across the spectrum. The now positive relationship between reason and grace became a touchstone of politico-theological allegiance. Many leading figures in the Royal Society – Glanvill and Wilkins, for example – were Anglican clergy who had been orthodox about predestination, election and reprobation before 1660; they now fell expediently silent about it, rather than directly recanting. They began to write as if every individual holds his salvation in his own hands via a reasoned faith. As so often in the history of the human sciences, "as if" then got its feet under the table and settled in for keeps. Reason-based universalism became a tenet not only of Anglicans and many Dissenters but of a whole range of anti-establishment types: from the Socinians, who maintained that religion and revelation were fully compatible with reason, to the Baptists, who, though they stuck to a belief in grace and election, felt pressed to accommodate the new reason within it.[29] All this created a basis on which reprobation and idiotism, the antitheses of spiritual and natural intelligence respectively, were to combine. The new dispensations for reasoned behaviour had tacit predestinarian residues. By the end of the century, talk about reprobates was inadvisable, as was "talk of the Devil" (a cautionary phrase that came into use only around this time). They were no longer fit topics for the secular "polite society" that was now replacing the church as arbiter of intellectual debate. They led to impolite disputatiousness; but they existed all right, and talking about them might only entice them in.

Medicine trailed behind these political adventures of ideas. Willis's talk of certain people as *stupidi*, as we have seen, hardly amounted to the labelling of a type and was largely derived from

---

[27] Breton, *The Goode and the Badde*, 23.
[28] Penn, *The Great Case*, 11.
[29] See D. Wallace, *Puritans and Predestination*, 158.

Renaissance melancholia. When Englished as "changelings" by various contemporaries, both Anglican and Dissenter, a new direction was forged. His colleague in the Restoration's Anglican elite, Bishop Samuel Parker, adapted Willis's anatomical theory in order to advance one of his own about social behaviour. Willis's innovativeness lay in the detailed physiology of brain function; when he anatomizes "the brain of a fatuous youth," he is interested in the smallness and weakness of the intercostal nerves through which the soul controls the bodily passions, rather than in fatuous behaviour as such. Parker comments on this, labels the youth a "changeling" and remarks on his inability to control his "passions and appetites"; the changeling's soul has an "impotency and irregularity [that] consists in the nature of folly."[30] In short, this changeling is the antithesis of the Restoration's own new man, the "man of judgement." Parker mentions the intercostal nerves briefly, but that is not what he is interested in.

Then there is the Dissenter, Samuel Pordage. Historians' mistaken view of Willis as a modern pioneer on our topic comes from Pordage's translation of *De Anima Brutorum*. Not only does Pordage, like Parker, replace Willis's loose Latin adjectives with the positive label "changeling," he also smuggles in the Devil. For Willis, *all* humans have a modicum of reason in their rational (incorruptible) souls, in spite of any injuries to the sensitive or corporeal soul. He merely employed an adjective, "slow" (*bardi*), to describe the foolish or possibly melancholic offspring of wise fathers.[31] Pordage, however, marks out the latter by calling them changelings. Religious sects of the 1640s and 50s, self-appointed companies of the elect, had used this word to describe people amongst them who were suddenly "possessed"; it was the Devil's way of polluting the company's sainthood and thwarting the kingdom of heaven on earth.[32] Pordage was brought up and had continued to practise in just such a community, the Behmenists (after their founder Jakob Boehme), where his father, the community's leader, held regular conversations with angels. Dissenters across the board were particularly fond of magical or diabolic explanation since it hinted that the Restoration establishment did not have everything under its control.[33] The demonic overtones of the word "changeling" are clear in Pordage's translation.

Behmenists believed that human perfection was achievable on this earth, but also that hell and the Devil are at this very moment somewhere in the real world; and they mixed nature together with grace (or absence of it). Jesus said that a good tree cannot bring forth bad fruit; nevertheless, warns Boehme, "the forces of disorder can worm their way into the reason" by generating deficient offspring, thereby proving the Devil's real presence among us. "False essences" – deviations from the species – were an example of the chaos he could create, a demonic obstacle to human perfection because they could mimic hypocritically the manifestations of grace. Where both the fruit and the tree are bad, then

> If the parents are wicked, and indeed in the kingdom of the Devil, and that they have thus begotten their fruit out of their false essences (in which [parents] there is no faith, but only a false hypocrisy, and yet will in an apish mockery be counted Christians; and as the Devil oftentimes changes himself into the likeness of an angel, so they also send their children with the like trimmed false angels before the covenant of Christ); such doing is very dangerous .... There must be earnestness in avoiding of the Devil.[34]

---

[30] Parker, *An Account of the Nature and Extent of the Divine Dominion*, 67; see also Rina Knoeff, "The reins of the soul: the centrality of the intercostal nerves to the neurology of Thomas Willis and to Samuel Parker's theology," *Journal of the History of Medicine and Allied Sciences*, 59/3 (2004).

[31] Willis, *De Anima*, 360; Willis (trans. Pordage), "Two discourses," 311.

[32] Eugene Hynes, *Knock: the Virgin's Apparition in Nineteenth-Century Ireland*.

[33] Keith Thomas, *Religion and the Decline of Magic*, 240.

[34] Jakob Boehme, Ψυχολογια, 202; *The Works*, i, 252.

The flavour of this reoccurs in Pordage's own *Mundorum Explicatio*, a long epic poem about the creation roughly contemporary with *Paradise Lost*, where he writes about *incubi* who "shed their seed into old hags."

He also uses "changeling" to translate from Willis's text a conventional classical epithet ("more sluggish than Bacchus") which at that time signified drunkenness or melancholy. Willis did in fact contribute to Royal Society members' attempts at a scientific cataloguing of the spirit world, but in terms of medicine he had deliberately kept his distance, as his caption to the illustration in his book on brain anatomy shows; he writes that the youth is "*fatuus*, though he might vulgarly be called a spirit [*Lemur*]."[35] Pordage translates the adjective *fatuus* here again as the noun "changeling," the connotations of which are much closer to (evil) "spirit." In this sense Willis is the medical conservative, Pordage the psychological proto-modern. The distinct identity of the unreasoning changeling matches Pordage's radical Whig political beliefs. (In the year he translated the Tory physician's textbook he was also participating in the Monmouth rebellion.)

The Restoration's redefinition of reason, accompanied by a redefinition of the changeling as the creature in whom reason is absent, was not incompatible with a belief in the abilities of the Devil and perhaps encouraged it. The Devil, far from being scared off by Hobbesian materialism, had been honing his profile for a century or so. He was an absolute presupposition behind natural causes, and there was no getting round the back of him. The unitary cosmos of the Middle Ages, in which God was able to keep an eye on him, was replaced by one where he had some independence and an effective presence. By contrast with the sixteenth century – there is a mere handful of mentions of him in the 1,500 pages of Calvin's *Institutes* – the Devil met with great success in the scientific speculations of the seventeenth.

Consider this story, published in the same year as Locke's *Essay*:

> A virgin got pregnant and said that she was visited every night by a handsome youth. Her parents lay in wait for this lover and the following night found a frightful monster in their daughter's embrace. A priest was called and drove the devil out by reciting St John's Gospel. Thereupon the devil set all the bedding on fire, let off a terrible fart, and made away. The following day the daughter gave birth to a monster or fantastic abortion.[36]

This is not the folkloric relic of a bygone age; such stories were far more frequent than they had been a century earlier. It was common for a woman to dream about having been visited by a devil who leaves her pregnant, and for her husband (were she unwise enough to tell him) to take the dream literally and demand to know where the child is now. The converse case, of an actually existing child found to have the Devil as his father, was likewise written about as an everyday experience. It is true that a writer like Nathaniel Wanley, a member of both Baxter's and Boyle's circles, could call "carnal copulation with devils, either as an *incubus* or *succubus* ... a horrible absurdity," yet such a remark needs to be taken in context. "All learned physicians who do know the way that nature breeds human seed," he says, "will deride this tenet and condemn it as false and abominable .... Devils, whether conceived to be corporeal or incorporeal, ... were not created of God to generate, neither have they, nor can have any seed, or members fit for generation."[37] What Wanley is saying is that the Devil has only natural means, not supernatural ones; it is just that in the case of human reproduction, he does not have either. This did not mean that the Devil or his agents could not *transmit* semen by natural magic, merely that they could not themselves generate offspring directly.

---

[35] Willis, *De Cerebri*, 51.
[36] E. Franciscus, *Der Höllische Proteus*, cited in Carl Haffter, "The changeling."
[37] Wanley, *The Wonders*, 80 ff.

The mid-century reconceptualization of the changeling took place amidst such debates. To deny the existence of spirits would be to deny a necessary slot in the cosmological frame. One questioned how the Devil did things, not whether he existed. "Of all the delusions wherewith [the Devil] deceives mortality," says Browne, "there is not any that puzzleth me more than the legerdemain of changelings. I do not credit those transformations of reasonable creatures into beasts, or that the Devil hath a power to transpeciate a man into a horse," the archetype of unreason. But, this famous physician continues, "I could believe that spirits use with man the act of carnality, and that in both sexes ... yet ... without a possibility of generation."[38] Changelings were a key example of the Devil's methods. Even if he could not copulate with humans, he could create a whole "inner" nature in some of them, as Boyle pointed out.[39] Scot's denial of the Devil's abilities even reinforced the realist view of him against the apparitionist one. The realist view demanded hard evidence, and this was consistent with the burgeoning sense of objective scientific critique in the Royal Society; it eschewed immoderate claims but, by the same token, trusted that some claims would thereby emerge that were indeed verifiable. Hard evidence, it was supposed, would turn up, if only occasionally.

This was also the gestation period of Locke's *Essay*, which saw a revival of debate about Scot's century-old scepticism about witchcraft. His denial of it, and that of his new editor John Webster, were taken to be atheistic. Sceptical scientific experimentalists of Locke's generation such as Glanvill and More, who were among the loudest champions of the new reason, went on the attack, claiming by a typical reversal that if someone has "lost all belief that there are such things as spirits in this world," it is a sign of their own "stupor," "besottedness" and "dull sense."[40] The grand modern narrative of reason might prompt us to think that once it was espoused on both sides of the main politico-theological divide, devil beliefs faded away; but far from the existence of the Devil contradicting the new reason, they rubbed along perfectly well together. One might say they needed each other. The wise and ingenious, whether outside or within the new scientific circles, were generally more likely to cite his presence than lay people were. Doctors were particularly susceptible, since their specialism seemed to hold fewer remedies for people's problems than even the lawyer or the priest.[41] The new reason supported the idea that the Devil operated in the real world and produced dire social consequences there. According to Glanvill and More, a "disbeliever" in the existence of the Devil, spirits or witches was a disbeliever in that of God, a threat to "the greatest interests of religion" which consists in the individual employment of reason.[42] The idea of demonically conceived changelings was absolutely necessary both to the scientific method of the Royal Society and to a reasonable Christianity based on the notion of autonomous and active human subjects who follow their own developmental paths.

In fact Scot and Webster – the latter a Behmenist like Pordage – are examples of how a number of writers were reducing demonic activity to "mental operations internal to the 'hell' that was the state of mind of evil persons," among whom changelings might be counted.[43] Webster notes the stories about children "such as are real changelings or lunatics, who have been brought by such spirits and hobgoblins, the true child being taken away by them in the place whereof such are left, being commonly half out of their wits, and given to many antic practices and extravagant

---

[38] Browne, *Religio*, 34.
[39] Cited in Wanley, 214.
[40] Glanvill, *Saducismus Triumphatus*, A8r.
[41] Thomas, *Religion and the Decline*, 304; 638 ff.
[42] Glanvill, "Against Modern Sadducism," 58, in *Essays*.
[43] Clark, *Thinking with Demons*, 545.

fancies." One might see their extraordinary "passions" as instead "proceeding from the powerful influence of the planet in their nativity."[44] The notion that they are physically exchanged through the intervention of the Devil is "foolish conjecture"; by reversal, the conjecturers are themselves "natural fools." Nevertheless, "real changelings" exist. And they are still "the Devil's instruments," inasmuch as they create social havoc. In this restricted sense, Scot and Webster are realists. The Devil is not denied; he is merely not necessary to the operations of natural magic, which are seen as self-standing.

The demonic elements behind Locke's changeling had in any case already been predicted in Perkins's suggestions about the Devil's natural powers a century earlier:

> If any man in reason think it not likely that a creature should be able to work extraordinarily by natural means, he must remember that though God hath reserved to himself alone the power of abolishing and changing nature, the order whereof he set and established in the creation, yet the alteration of the ordinary course of nature he hath put in the power of his strongest creatures, angels and devils .... And this power is rather increased and made more forcible by [the] irreconcilable malice [the Devil] beareth to mankind, specially the seed of the woman.[45]

This reference to the Devil's intervention in human reproduction helps us to understand the reference which Locke's *Essay* makes to the physiological causes of the changeling's deficiency, its bodily "wheels and springs." This can be seen as *both* scientific *and* demonic at the same time: they are not mutually exclusive explanations. The Royal Society's hard-line empiricists insisted on keeping an open mind about any causes that remained occult. So internal bodily mechanisms and the Devil may well have been equal in causal status, or even colleagues. As Jonathan Edwards was to point out, the Devil could "come at" humans by bodily intervention or "some motion" of the soul spirits. He could induce the disability of the melancholic or despairing type, for example, though his sphere of intervention was limited to "the outward senses"; the "inward motions" of the psychological faculties, especially "abstraction," were inaccessible to him. Locke himself mentions the changeling's "wheels and springs" only in order to say that he does not want to account for them, or for any of the natural or physiological causes of intellectual shortcomings or absence. He simply thought it useless, in medical terms, to try and find "the hidden causes of distempers," the natural magic or "secret workmanship of nature and the several imperceptible tools wherewith she wrought."[46] That does not necessarily mean he did not believe that the Devil existed or had a hand in those shortcomings.

From the Brothers Grimm to Dr Mengele

Over the course of the nineteenth century, changeling stories entered the burgeoning literary genre of compilations of world folklore.[47] It is hard to distinguish expert theological tradition from popular folklore in the historical construction of intellectually disabled changelings, if only because nothing in the folklore tradition can be shown to predate its representation in printed texts. If it is absence

---

[44] Webster, *The Displaying*, 37; Scot, *A Discourse concerning the Nature and Substance of Devils and Spirits*, 50.

[45] Perkins, *A Discourse of the Damned Art of Witchcraft*, 18.

[46] Cited in R. Yost, "Locke's rejection of hypotheses about sub-microscopic events," in J. Yolton (ed.), *Philosophy, Religion and Science in the Seventeenth and Eighteenth Centuries*.

[47] T. Dyer, *English Folklore*; E. Hartland, *The Science of Fairy Tales*; S. Thompson, *Motif-Index of Folk Literature*.

from print that defines the folkloric, one is scarcely in a position to verify evidence of any kind; one could just make everything up. And this seems to be what actually happened. The vital source for modern histories of the changeling is the Grimms. Scholars in the field now see all of folklore as at best an interaction between the oral and the literary, and it is no longer disputed that the Grimms' stories all came from existing literary sources and nowhere else. They merely reshaped these sources into "educational manual[s] for children with good bourgeois upbringing" – moral *exempla* for the middle classes.[48] This belies the Grimms' reputation as itinerant chroniclers of tales told to them by sagacious yokels. Number 83 of their *Deutsche Sagen* is a straight paraphrase of the early German theological texts about *Wechselkinder* referred to above, merely embroidering them with a few folksy artefacts. Jakob Grimm's *Deutsche Mythologie*, which has an entry on changelings, was by contrast a scientific dictionary of mythology, with a scholarly apparatus.[49] In his footnotes to the entry Jakob gives as his sources both the theological writer Nicolaus of Jauer and the fake folk-tale he and his brother had themselves cobbled together earlier from that same writer; the two sources are cited alongside each other as discrete types of evidence, when in fact one had been manufactured out of the other by the very person doing the citing.

It is true that anthropological and historical evidence for the existence of rituals and stories about the acceptance of new-borns is widespread. In the Greek ceremony of amphidromia, to take just one example, the father carried the baby round the hearth after a ritual washing to guarantee its purity and to mark the acceptance of a new arrival in the family. But a very general phenomenon cannot be used to credit the transhistorical claims of one highly specific legend. Our particular story as it appears in the nineteenth-century folklore compilations is clustered within predominantly Lutheran areas of Germany and Scandinavia. Reified into an explanation for disability, it was then imposed on the psychiatry of the next century.

We can track the course of this reification very precisely. A generation after the Grimms, Kühn and Schwarz incorporated the changeling in a volume of stories, *Norddeutsche Sagen*, which resemble the Grimms' literary artefacts very closely but which in addition are spuriously authenticated with a folk-collector's subheadings ("Orally," "From an old workman," "From a peasant-woman" and so forth, or the name of a specific village). Johann Wolf, following up with a similar volume, was probably the first to add an intellectual element, writing about the infant's failure "to develop mentally [*geistig*]"; he also added Luther's phrase, "an unformed mass of flesh," evoking the complementary sense of *geistig*, "spiritual." This ambiguity, poised between theology and psychiatry, coincides with the latter's coming of age as a discipline.[50] Wolf also replaced the four wet nurses of the original story with seven, a magic number, thus consolidating its mythic tone.

Adolf Wuttke, in an 1860 work on German superstition, retained all these embellishments. He also turned the spiritual/mental deficiency into a more concrete diagnosis, namely the inability to develop reason or speech; and he created a formal link with medical science by suggesting that the story was a popular explanation for cretinism. A theologian, Wuttke was a leading opponent of naturalistic ethics, well-known and translated in Britain and North America. He sought instead a systematized, Christian evangelical "scientific ethics," in which the child substitution story had a role. By demoting the story to the level of mere superstition, Wuttke displaced the *natural reality of the Devil* to the *natural reality of popular belief in the natural reality of the Devil*. Like the Grimms, whose works were intended to support German cultural and political unification, his purpose thereby was to demonstrate the "deeper unity and agreement" of superstitious beliefs among "our German people." The beliefs may have been false, but precisely as such they belonged

---

[48] See Jack Zipes, *The Brothers Grimm*, 114.
[49] W. and J. Grimm, *Deutsche Sagen*, number 83; J. Grimm, *Deutsche Mythologie*, 263.
[50] *Beiträge zur Deutschen Mythologie*, ii, 303.

to the "natural man," and were a "common source" for the Germans' national unity.[51] The scientific status of the story lay precisely in this, in its being positioned at a deeper, more permanent level of the Germans' national psyche than their superficial political fragmentation might suggest. Wuttke's transposition of the story to the realm of natural superstition and belief, through a systematic anthropology and a corresponding scientific ethics, was thus part of a broader political movement to prescribe and patrol human behaviour.

The genre of fairy-tale compilations reached a climax in Britain with Edwin Hartland's 1895 volume for the British Folklore Society, which contains a whole chapter on changelings. This book is no more than a collation of the Grimms' stories, but it bears the title *A Science of Fairy Tales*, and the author was advised on it by Havelock Ellis, a man with medical training and an officer of the Eugenics Society who campaigned against the menace of the feeble-minded. The reification was now complete. In Germany, it would prove to be the trail that led from the Grimms to the Nazi euthanasia programme. Ellis's introduction to the volume says that the stories show how "man's imagination works by fixed laws," with "features absolutely identical ... between the cultured Europeans and the debased Hottentots." The changeling story thus became part of a modern, unified systematization of scientific knowledge precisely by being displaced to a universal superstitious past that allegedly persists today in the lay population, through the bereavement analogy. This is an expression of elite contempt: the story is natural to ordinary people because it is false. Evidence of this displacement can also be seen in the everyday language of insult. Etymologically, words such as idiot, imbecile, dunce, mong, moron and retard all began life as expert terms; even "fool" is probably from *follis*, a bellows or "windbag" (used of a debating opponent). They come not from the streets but from a self-styled intellectual subculture of professionals seeking to monopolize "intellect." The source of out-group labels and insults is the seminary, the study and the clinic, and only secondarily the so-called popular culture. Psychology and psychiatry share with theology a zealous divisiveness in their view of human nature, which they project upon the popular past as well as today's lay public.

We can now see the paediatric journal cited above in a fresh light. As the geneticists' religious metaphors demonstrate, it can hardly be claimed that a religious account of disability has "given way" to a scientific one. Nor is it a bygone popular culture but the modern expert one of biotechnology that has "no moral compunctions" about eliminating certain kinds of people.[52] As for the idea that one purges parents' disorder by forcing them to accept as reality that they have been bereaved, we should ask which version of this – thirteenth-century Dominican, or twenty-first-century psychiatric – is the "historical curiosity," and which the scientific axiom. And Kanner's claim, on the strength of Luther's remarks, that "mental defectives were at their worst" in the sixteenth century, and that if we now take an ethical approach to disabled people it is thanks to modern science, comes from someone who was himself a major inventor of mental defectiveness categories.[53]

Meanwhile liberal feminists have used the hints of infanticide in the changeling stories to project a kind of gender equality on the past. Women even then, it is said, were as brutally neo-Darwinian as men; they exercised their right to choose, even on a live human being.[54] In earlier times the more reliable option must have been not to terminate a foetus but to kill a living infant. Today (outside the anti-abortion movement), a clear ethical distinction is maintained between foetus and child. However, liberal feminist accounts of the changeling story, as of modern disability, obscure the additional and quite separate ethical issue around intellectual (dis)ability, which hinges

---

[51] *Der Deutsche Volksaberglaube*, 195, 1.
[52] Leask, "Evidence."
[53] *A History*, 6.
[54] Sarah Blaffer Hrdy, *Mother Nature*, 467.

on its historically and socially contingent distinction and is therefore not clear at all. Both the demonization and the justification of practices of the distant past displace the guilt from a present whose ethics is not up for examination because it cannot be disentangled from psychological and biological knowledge itself.

Whose fault is it? Parents as authors of the child's intellect

The rise of the changeling story coincided with the rise of anxiety that the passage of gentle blood from father to son could not be taken for granted, or that election might not simply be handed down to children just because the parents, as "visible church members," appeared to be elect. The Devil crept into spaces created by the dissolution of these old certainties. But he was not the only one. A causal role in generating deficient minds began to be attributed to parents as well. In the old Aristotelian tradition, the biological criterion for species membership had been the (physical) resemblance between offspring and parents. However, changelings loaded the emphasis on to intellectual resemblance, challenging the so-called Aristotelian principle that man is a rational animal. They are born of rational parents but are not rational themselves. Might not parental agency, especially when seen as compatible with diabolic agency, play a part in this otherwise inexplicable phenomenon of intellectual monstrosity?

This notion was assisted by the increasing popularity of the idea that the parents rather than God supply the human foetus with its rational soul. Such a notion was controversial. The mainstream view had always been that its creator is God, by a process known as "infusion" (though opinion differed as to how and when the rational part of the soul got into the semen). The opposing "traducianist" doctrine of parental agency remained esoteric; nevertheless, it had long been used by some – including someone as important as Augustine – to explain how original sin could be "traduced" (led across) from one generation to the next. Moreover it was compatible with the periodic revivals of interest in Averroes's theory that individual souls vary as a result of the "informative power" transmitted to them by parents. Some medieval scholars took this to mean that an individual's disposition was linked to the act of his conception. The twelfth-century medical school of Salerno, followed by philosophers such as Michael Scotus and Jean of Jandun, found room for embryology in the new physiognomic science. Michael discusses "the problem of generation" and the influence of the parental body on the embryo, though he does not mention any accompanying cognitive or moral elements.[55]

None of the above amounts to a theory of natural inheritance. While Averroes held that parental influence makes *individual souls* "subject to generation and corruption like other natural forms," he had also insisted on the existence of a divine, immortal *collective intellect* wherein every individual intellect is a chip off the divine block.[56] The presence of an informative power in the parental body explained how lower, bestial forms of existence might corrupt the soul. For example, if one of the parents had the excessively large head that signifies "a defect (*depressio*) of the rational soul" it could cause dwarfism.[57] Yet it was precisely the notion of a continuity from foetus to living creature, suggesting for us a biologically determined personhood, that for contemporaries suggested instead the creature's plasticity, and the responsiveness of its moral and intellectual state to providence.

---

[55] Cited in Danielle Jacquart, "La physiognomie à l'époque de Frédéric II," *Micrologus*, 2 (1994).
[56] Paulus Nicolettus [Venetus], *Summa Naturalium*, 5.2.37.
[57] S. Wielgus (ed.), "Quaestiones Nicolai Peripatetici," in *Mediaevalia Philosophica Polonorum*, 17 (1973).

No impairment, even one existing from before birth, could alter the creature's prior status as a rational being linked to all other rational beings through the collective intellect.

By the eve of the Reformation, traducianism had spread widely enough to require anathema from the church, on the grounds that if the rational soul were generated by parents it would be a material entity and therefore not immortal. Traducianism's appeal was that it avoided the absurdity of having God, in infusing the soul, become the author of individual imperfections and therefore of sin. Writers sticking to divine infusion pointed out that anatomists were unable to find any "organ or instrument for the rational soul" in the brain. This "inorganity" of the soul came under challenge once Descartes located it in the pineal gland, a material entity.[58] However, subsequent anatomists would note that the relative viscosity of a dissected pineal gland or the presence of stones bore no relation to the wit of the person to whom it had belonged.[59] Infusionists also clung to the idea that God creates the soul directly out of nothing. The fact that miscarried embryos tend to be deformed was proof that at this stage God had not yet infused the rational soul; if it had been there, then as form to the body's matter it would have remedied the physical deformity before birth. Traducianists claimed as supporting evidence that "wise people are born of wise parents, and conversely stupid ones (*stolidi*) from stupid parents."[60] The infusionists argued that this was not empirically adequate. Many authorities, as we have seen, testified to the opposite: "Why hath a wise man, to his son a sot? / But that he cannot make his son, God wot."[61] Traducianism was particularly popular with Anabaptists, Socinians and Levellers, among whom it had a socially subversive potential: the non-gentle ranks had no earthly honour to pass on to their children, and so might find a substitute in wit.

The theory came in various guises. One of these was "mortalism." Mortalists claimed that although parents generate the rational soul, this need not mean the soul is material or mortal. Its immortality is beyond doubt; but rather than being divinely infused in the foetus, it is bestowed only at the resurrection. This preserved a role for God, while absolving him from authorship of the soul's defects or its original sin. Milton was a mortalist for just this reason. Hobbes was a mortalist because it helped him explain how earthly human behaviour could follow mechanical laws analogous with those of the material realm. The arrival of an "anatomy of the mind," by analogy with that of the body, and the increasing separation between the two, had led by the end of the sixteenth century to theories in which parental authorship could be used to explain intellectual defect *per se*.[62] Overton, also a mortalist, went on to remark: "by [the infusionists'] grounds there can be no born fools."[63] But there are, and it could not have been an all-loving God who created people in this state.

Another version of traducianism involved reincarnation. This too freed God from any responsibility for defects. Writers of this persuasion denied that parents of fools transmitted original sin to their offspring; it did not make sense in terms of *natural* generation, since deficiencies in natural intellectual capacity are peculiar to the individual, whereas original sin was universal. According to Locke's friend Franciscus van Helmont, "Many are born blind, deaf, dumb, and some natural fools [*fatui*] and mad, possessed with unclean spirits. Now is it not a great reproach to the providence of God ... to say that God originally made those creatures so?"[64] The infusionists

---

[58] Browne, *Religio*, 41.
[59] Anton Nuck, *Opera*, 151.
[60] Johann Köhler, *De Origine Animarum Rationalium*, Argument 25, in Göckel, *Psychologia*.
[61] John Davies of Hereford, *Mirum in Modum*.
[62] For example Thomas Rogers, *The Anatomie of the Minde*.
[63] *Mans Mortallitie*, 49.
[64] *Two Hundred Queries ... concerning the Doctrine of the Revolution of Humane Souls*, 131.

claimed that God creates the soul's defects as a punishment for original sin. Not only does this seem unjust, says Van Helmont, but also "this misery fall[s] very unequally, some being born fools (*stulti*) and madmen (*fatui* [note here the precariousness of the translated terms]), others with a large capacity of natural understanding (*ingenium*); now how can this be only for *Adam*'s sin, ... seeing ... that all are equally guilty of it?" The reincarnationist idea of former earthly existences was therefore brought in to explain the *individuality* of intellectual defects.

In face of the traducianist advance, infusionists tried to finesse their position by conceding a minor role to parents. One might say that "the soul is infused into the body by God the creator, without any virtue of the generative seed" and is therefore "incorruptible," then simply add that it became corrupted at some subsequent stage through the parents' "hereditary and natural filthiness."[65] Or one could point out, as Henry Woolnor did, that bastards "have no less wisdom, wit, prudence, judgement and gifts of soul and body than other people," so allowing that the soul is not created by God alone (for whom bastardy was sinful) but also by "natural means." But even these minor concessions to the theory of parental generation were to prove fatal, opening the floodgates to ideas about the natural history and natural origins of the mind. The infusionists' own attempts at refutation or accommodation forced them to rephrase the scholastic formula about rationality as human essence ("man is a rational animal") in terms of rationality as human *nature*. They began saying, for example, that "the human *species*" (emphasis added) – that is, a natural phenomenon – "is constituted not through the body but through the rational soul."[66] The very title of the text from which this comes, a defence of the immortality and immateriality of the soul, centres on a phrase – "the nature of things" – clearly designed to recuperate for religion the terms of Lucretius's *De Rerum Natura*, the period's standard example of a materialist text.

A Pandora's box had been opened. Overton, for example, took the existence of intellectually disabled monsters to show that parental sodomy and bestial sex might be the cause.[67] For the infusionists, the fact that "buggery births" lead to lack of a rational soul means they have been "propagated out of kind"; they are not full species members, so God cannot be responsible for that lack. But, asks Overton, where in that case would the infusionists place such creatures on the scale of nature? Being generated by buggery, he says, does not just mean being out of kind (non-human). Such creatures are more than just another species: they are in addition "unnatural and cursed." God "raises and delivers" men from death at the resurrection, and he even resurrects (Overton is unusual in this respect) all the other species of animals. But he does not raise "unnatural" ones. They are done away with, as "filth which breedeth on corruption."

In pursuit of this argument, Overton draws a distinction between "mere" fools and "born" fools which prefigures the distinction made by Truman (see Chapter 11), the nineteenth century's between imbeciles and idiots, and the twentieth's between moderate and severe. We are not, says Overton, talking here about the usual course of events where there may be some "organical deficiency more or less, that is the cause that some men are less rational than others; for some have abundance of wisdom and some are mere fools." "Mere fools" are still truly human creatures, on a spectrum with the wise. A "born fool" – no ordinary fool – "would have been a better instance" of the infusionists' notion of buggery births. A born fool lacks a "rational soul." This would better support, says Overton, the infusionists' own view that nature without divinity "beget[s] mere irrational, brutish inhuman bodies," by contrast with "rationality or humanity," which for them is "a supernatural work," divinely infused.

---

[65] Primaudaye, *Académie*, 6.
[66] Lascovius, *De Homine, Magnum Illo in Rerum Natura Miraculo*, 185.
[67] *Mortallitie*, 51 ff.

Overton's whole argument hangs on this distinction between "mere" and "born" fools. The latter's "imperfections ... argue the mediate generation thereof, because no imperfection of any kind can come immediately from the hand of God; imperfections are accidental, or from the curse, therefore not of creation but of procreation" – that is to say, not of God but of the parents. Born fools must therefore be products of buggery, and as filth and corruption they are an *un*natural kind, to be disposed of. Here too the praeternatural (demonic) and unnatural (parental) forms of generation are becoming compatible. Overton's proposition that certain fools are non-species members brings a modern, pathological concept of disability into view, reducing the dangers of ambiguity and strengthening conformity to current definitions of what it is to be human. In Mary Douglas's words, "a rule of avoiding anomalous things affirms and strengthens the definitions to which they do not conform." Parental agency ("buggery," or natural causation) and diabolic agency ("the curse," or praeternatural causation) coalesce where there is fear of pollution and filth. Together they lie at the heart of modern cognitive science, making it an appropriate additional specimen for William Ian Miller's proposed "anatomy of disgust."[68]

It is worth noting, finally, the political manifestations of this. Cromwell's old tutor, Thomas Beard, had warned in a text still widely circulating in the 1640s against "the monstrous fruits of ... profane marriages" between members of the "house of God" and "worshipper[s] of images and idols," between the putatively elect and the definitely reprobate. Charles I's marriage to a Catholic might be read into this, not to mention the product of their union, the prospective Charles II. "Unlawful issue" had previously done "much wrong and violence in the world," and God had drowned them in the flood – just as Luther had recommended the drowning of changelings.[69] Above all, as today, one had to prevent them from reproducing. It is no accident that the ousting of born fools from species membership on intellectual grounds should have come from radical egalitarians such as Overton and Locke. The Leveller Overton is to the political status of idiots what Humfrey, his exact contemporary, is to their ecclesiastical status (see Chapter 11). In both men, it is the dialectic of dispute that brings them to their position. Humfrey creates the excluded category of permanent, born idiots to support his argument for open admission to the eucharist for everyone else, regardless of whether or not they belong to the company of the elect; Overton creates the excluded category of permanent, born fools to support his argument for natural political rights for everyone else, regardless of whether or not they are members of the honour society.

Planetary influences

Natural forms of external cause were also being invoked in the early modern period, if in a less important role. Climate, for example, leads to people in different regions to have different humoral dispositions. And then there are "the stars and planets, with their several positions ... under which men are born," which "incline them several ways to one thing more than to another, and in some are more predominant and vigorous than in other." These "special constellations" point to nature's inefficiency: "not being able to bring forth that which she intended, she bringeth forth that which she can."[70] One physiognomist, for instance, gives astrological significance to the rounded ears, excessively narrow nasal passages and tapering shoulders that signify "a man

---

[68] *Purity and Danger*, 48.
[69] *The Theatre of God's Judgements*, 325.
[70] Thomas Bradley, *Nosce Teipsum*, 43; Alexander, "Doth nature make any monsters?" in *The Problems of Aristotle*.

disposed to no cunning."⁷¹ Retrospective diagnosticians may see in these the physical features of Down's syndrome, but the crucial word here is "disposed." Planetary influence, being natural, is dispositional rather than determinate, unlike election or reprobation which were predestined before the Fall – and, indeed, unlike chromosomes.

Galenist accounts of external influence do not dwell at length on astrology, while Paracelsus explicitly rejects it in favour of something deeper, at least in *On the Generating of Fools*. The causes of foolishness, he says, are a matter of speculation ("philosophizing," as he calls it); they exist in a realm beyond human reasoning.⁷² It only *seems* to us that "hard zodiacal signs" are a cause; such a belief is itself stupid, coming from understandings that have been dulled by the Fall. He contrasts foolishness with madness and epilepsy in this respect. The latter have genuinely astrological causes. Significantly, the text of his that deals with them is entitled *On Lunatics*, not "On the generating of lunatics." Foolishness is the upshot of a universal Adamite corruption; mental illness, by contrast, is a specific medical condition. Foolishness and madness do not form a diagnostic dyad, and modern historians accustomed to just such a dyad are mistaken in presenting these two texts as companion pieces. They differ from each other profoundly and probably date from different periods. Fools are "simple … intelligent animals"; lunatics are "various" in their pathologies, "irrational animals."⁷³

So when a historian calls Paracelsus an early seeker for the causes of phenylketonuria, the error lies not just in the anachronism but in the assumption that in his work on foolishness he was trying to explain the causes of some particular disability, or even that he thought any natural explanation possible.⁷⁴ The causes of foolishness are "hidden," not part of any science accessible to humans such as astrology. In place of planets, Paracelsus supposes the existence of certain quasi-natural forces which he personifies as "Vulcans," a kind of super-alchemists who forge each individual human being. All we can infer, he says, is that some Vulcans are more skilled than others. Their varying degrees of inexperience lead to varying degrees of foolishness in the individuals they produce; but the production *process* is not for mere humans to discover. This occult explanation lies further back along the causal spectrum than the natural science of astrology, though not as far back as predestination and necessity. The medical innovator Jean-Baptiste van Helmont, father of Franciscus, would resuscitate Paracelsus's Vulcans a century later in the form of a single great artificer whom he calls "Archeus." However, he bundles under one heading all of Paracelsus's intellectual deficit concepts (foolishness, madness, epilepsy) regardless of their fundamentally separate classifications in the earlier man's work. The effect of this is once more to start to blur the line between necessity and nature: a move which modern psychiatry completes.⁷⁵

---

[71] John Metham, *The Works*, 118.
[72] Paracelsus, *De Generatione*, 74.
[73] Paracelsus, *Krankheiten die der Vernunft Berauben*, in Sudhoff (ed.), *Sämtliche Werke*, ii, 391.
[74] See for example Cranefield, "The begetting," 169; Kilian Blümlein, *Naturerfahrung und Welterkenntnis*, 201.
[75] Jean-Baptiste van Helmont, *Opera*, 340.

Chapter 17
Testing the Rule of Human Nature: Classification and Abnormality

If the bereavement analogy is about not having the child one expected but having a different one, supplied perhaps by the Devil, it is tacitly also about having a child who perhaps belongs not to the human species but to a different one. Having dealt with explanations provided by everyday medicine as well as those lying further back in the praeternatural or occult, we therefore turn our attention now to the story of *classification*. This can be posed in two ways. One of them has to do with natural history: where, objectively, do human beings lie on the scale of nature? The second is normative: what, subjectively, are the criteria by which we define ourselves as human? Answers cluster around one and the same item: intellectual ability. It is only from 1200 onwards that the objective framework becomes fused, and confused, with the subjective ability, in a single procedure. I examine here a few items from a vast hinterland of late medieval and early modern texts on the specific operations said to make up this ability, in particular logical reasoning and abstraction.

Logic and abstraction are among the main instruments in creating the classificatory framework for an understanding of nature (even if, on the long historical and anthropological view, this framework is only one among many possible ones).[1] Certain concepts are universals: that is, they are predicated of more than one particular. Without grouping together the individual entities which the world presents to us, we could not make sense of it. Nor could the method of objective critique characteristic of the exact sciences such as physics and chemistry have arisen without this allocation of particular items to broader conceptual categories: "sorts" or "kinds," in the vernacular language of the period. The universals which biology deals with are "species." Psychology deals with just one species or universal, "man." But its way of doing so, on the basis of certain abilities, is circular. The ability to make abstractions and to reason with logic is that subjectively existing element in the species man which leads him to his knowledge of universals, one of which says that the ability to make abstractions and to reason with logic is an objectively existing, universal characteristic of the species man.

The circularity thus described is actually a social one, and therefore ought to be able to be detected by the person who lies outside it. However, the outsider is also the person who by definition *cannot* detect it, because he lacks the ability to make abstractions or to reason logically; in other words, he is "intellectually disabled." In this respect, intelligence is – at least for the period it dominates – stronger than other self-referential status concepts such as honour or grace. Being born reprobate and beyond the reach of grace was a status one could rationalize and loudly make a virtue of, like the Marquis de Sade; the same was true of being born outside the honour society and having dragged oneself up from the gutter, like Mr Gradgrind. One cannot, however, rationalize or make a virtue of belonging to an out-group that consists of people defined by an incapacity for rationality or virtue. Yet it remains true that operative psychological concepts such as logical reasoning and abstraction present the "natural" face of what are really only insignia of social status.

---

[1] See George Lakoff, *Women, Fire, and Dangerous Things*.

Logical reasoning, abstraction and the history of psychology

In order to grasp how abstraction and logical reasoning became naturalized in this sense, we need first to consider briefly the relationship between the history of the scientific revolution and that of psychology. Periodization in the history of psychology routinely assumes that medieval accounts of intellect and the soul were broadly the same as Aristotle's; the whole conglomeration is then called primitive and separated off from the truly scientific disciplines that began to emerge at the end of the seventeenth century. The trouble with this picture, in addition to its false assumption of a continuity from Aristotle to medieval thought, is its inclusion of psychology with the rest of science. The history of psychology contains no decisive moment akin to Boyle's law or Newton's. The theologization of writings about the mind and the causes of its various states was increasing rather than decreasing through the late sixteenth and early seventeenth centuries, and it is hard to tell when thereafter this process actually ceased, if it ever has. When Rudolf Göckel (Goclenius) and his school, at the end of the sixteenth century, coined the term "psychology," it was to defend the soul's immortality. Their theory is no antique curiosity, as we shall see, and has been absorbed within modern psychology. Pastors may have been replaced by biotechnicians, but the goal of cognitive and behavioural geneticists is still the increasing perfection of an immaterial intellect.

The one seventeenth-century candidate for a Boyle in psychology might be Locke, whose empirical and modern-looking approaches to both medicine and philosophy, and his nominalist approach to the definition of species, arose partly from his familiarity with Boyle's experimental work. But whereas Boyle launched the historical process by which chemistry became disentangled from alchemy, Locke – many of whose scientific contemporaries sought an "alchemy of the soul" through the study of spirits and natural magic – never got to separate psychology from what one may call alpsychology.[2] Boyle and Newton, too, were trying in their scientific work to get inside the mind of God, but at least they had to discover something outside themselves in order to do so. No such experimental controls have accompanied hypotheses about the mind, which in Locke's case were suffused with pre-1650s Calvinism. In attributing psychological operations such as abstraction and logical reasoning to all humans on a quasi-egalitarian basis (all, that is, except the disabled "changelings" and "idiots" who test the rule), Locke had in mind a creaturely equality before God rather than an everyday meritocratic one.

Nineteenth-century psychology then started to mimic the exact sciences in earnest. Its newfound interest in measurement suited the bureaucratization of social order in Europe, helping psychology to become an academic discipline in its own right. So if not the seventeenth century, was it the nineteenth that saw a scientific revolution in the study of the soul and the mind? The gulf between late medieval accounts of intellectual operations and the nineteenth-century discipline is wide, of course, but there are bridges across it; and there is probably a sharper divide between ancient Galen and the Renaissance Galenists than between the Galenists and Galton. It was from around 1200 that a body of intellectuals armed with learned texts on abstraction and logical reasoning began to speak a shared language with social administrators. It is this medium-term historical development, unencumbered by revolution or indeed by science, that underpins the history of the discipline to which abstraction and logical reasoning are central. Theodor Adorno wrote that the abstraction of universals from particulars can be seen in market terms, as a currency of the intellect that strips individual thoughts of their singularity and makes everything in nature repeatable and commodity like.[3] Commodification of thought met with commodification of time and labour, as sophisticated

---

[2] See Somerville, *The Secularization of Early Modern England*, 153 ff.
[3] *Dialectic of the Enlightenment*, section 13.

money economies expanded from the thirteenth century. Thus the abstracting intelligence has become one of the currencies in which we exchange values about each other.

However, the interconnections between cultural and economic capital cannot be traced in any detail. Bureaucracies are a more fertile source. The medical curriculum and the expansion of philosophy and law in the first universities coincided with the thirteenth-century extension of papal power and the unification of church government and doctrine down to the local level. The distribution of the new mendicant orders such as the Dominicans who headed up this ecclesiastical expansion was planned statistically, per head of population. Meanwhile the secular authority, too, sought more control over outlying populations. The growth in trade and division of labour, the material progress and expansion of towns, the cultivation of rural wastelands and the luxurious use of surplus all made social stratification more complex and increased the mobility of landholding. Corresponding new forms of social organization called not for sapient monks but for trained administrators, in whom the ability to sort, file and abstract was a prerequisite. The growth of bureaucracy created a clerical expertise to match the increasing complexity of social organization.

If abstraction of universals from particulars is a mental filing system, it remained at this early stage fairly simple, while the social character of the out-group defined by their deficiencies in this respect was a far larger one than now. Neither women, servants nor landless peasants could or needed to do mental filing. As the out-group has since been pathologized into something much smaller, the profile of abstraction itself has become correspondingly much more complex. Take the Griffiths Test. This is a psychological assessment routinely used by paediatricians and psychologists on young children whom they already know or suspect cannot do things, and is designed to prove beyond reasonable doubt that indeed they cannot. A child, for example, may be asked to associate two objects normally unrelated, e.g., "put the rattle on the helicopter," as a way of establishing that he does not understand the concept "on." This relational task is a kind of meta-abstraction; it is unlike and goes far beyond any example a medieval philosopher would have used. Here, abstraction itself is abstracted: what it tests is whether the subject will grow up to have an intelligence equivalent to that of the psychologist doing the testing, whose own professional intellect is normative. Yet this modern meta-abstraction remains organically tied to the medieval doctrine from which it springs. If, as Karl Popper complained, the human sciences have failed to emerge from scholasticism, this has less to do with their inadequacies of method than with the fact that modern psychology is an outgrowth of notions of status, shifting class relations and new forms of social administration which all have roots in late medieval economy and society.

The theology of abstraction and logical reasoning has been absorbed directly into material and cultural production. Rather than developing scientific clarity out of religious obscurity, modern psychology has driven theology in a particular ideological direction, towards the accelerating perfection and productivity of intellectual labour. It may be historicist to say that there are thirteenth-century beginnings, however small, which point concretely towards modern psychology. But it certainly throws into relief the relative robustness of the exact sciences in the face of constructionist scepticism. In the long-term history of physics, one account of why a dropped stone falls to earth at least gives way to another account of the same phenomenon. In the long-term history of psychology, one account of a phenomenon ("intelligence," for example), while seeming to give way to another account of it, is always surreptitiously giving way to that of a different phenomenon entirely. Culture is *itself the root* of intelligence; it is not simply a lens through which we are seeing refracted some otherwise stable component of human nature.

The professionalization of logical reasoning and the place of logic in psychology

We can now look in more detail at the historical spread of logical reasoning and abstraction in turn, and at where they have positioned the human species in nature. Logic is above all a system of categorization. One might expect Aristotle to have put the capacity for logical reasoning at the centre of his categorization of the human species, but as we saw in detail in Chapter 2 the phrase "Man is a rational animal" is not only falsely attributed to him but is something he would have been incapable of saying, in the light of his general metaphysics. The phrase was in fact of Stoic origin, and got into European thought through a third-century AD introduction to Aristotle by the neo-Platonist philosopher Porphyry, who wrote (claiming to paraphrase Aristotle), "Man is a rational, mortal animal." The Stoics had also employed the adjective *logikos* in this phrase. This notion that man is "a logical animal" prefigures the way medieval philosophers would fuse logic as objective procedure with logic as subjective ability.

Porphyry's text, translated into Latin by Boethius and in this form known across medieval Europe as the "Tree of Porphyry," had a huge impact on early logic and the whole philosophical tradition: to it, early modern thought owes its ubiquitous classificatory schemata of genus, species, difference, property and accident. Another input came from Alexander, an early systematizer of Aristotle and an influence on both the Arab and the scholastic philosophers. Entrusted by the Roman state with its educational policies, he reshaped Aristotle with Stoic content. He makes Aristotle out to have said that man is "an ensouled, biped and rational creature."[4] Alexander already saw this formula in psychological terms, unlike Aristotle. According to Alexander, the essential property of man is "to *have* understanding" (emphasis added); the statement "man is receptive of understanding" (Aristotle's original and misinterpreted formula) was, he said, merely a "consequent" of this firmer, naturalistic proposition. And where Aristotle had written only about man *qua* man, Alexander derives from this a truth about individuals: "Socrates is receptive of intuited wisdom and understanding" because "man" is. A hypothetical niche was thereby established for some individual who is not receptive of wisdom or understanding, and who thus lacks the essential property of what it is to be human.

However, it was only in the late Middle Ages that writers began to embed a theory of universals in their study of the human mind and its faculties. When the Arab philosophers, commenting on Aristotle's texts, employed the formula "Man is a rational animal," they took this to be a truth inscribed in the objective structure of the cosmos. In doing so, they were also rethinking the bonds between that macrocosmic structure and the natural species "man" who was a microcosm of it. "Man is ..." in their formula was no longer (as formulae of this type had been for Aristotle) employed merely to illustrate or adjudicate disputes *about* universals, with man just one example among many. At the same time, they did not yet display the value-laden anxiety about exceptional individuals that was to accompany the new forms of psychological classification in the early modern period. In Averroes's words, "Differentia and species ... are predicated of their subjects equally, not in degrees of less and more: no man is more man than another man." If he were, then man's ranking in the cosmos in relation to other animals would no longer have its distinctive superiority and therefore he would have no special relationship with God. Any idea of intra-species difference would have threatened inter-species difference and man's special place in nature. Nevertheless, the Arabs unwittingly created the basis on which a concept of natural intra-species difference might arise.[5]

They completely reframed the relationship of "man" to logic. The general problem of what is a statement in logic and what is an empirical statement, and of their relationship to each other,

---

[4] *In Aristotelis Topicorum*, 173.

[5] Averroes, *Three Short Commentaries*, 54 ff.; *Middle Commentaries on Aristotle's* Categories *and* De Interpretatione, 39; *Middle Commentary on Porphyry's* Isagoge, 23.

has been a constant preoccupation in Western philosophy and need not concern us here. But we do need to note that a special problem arises when the so-called empirical statements are about man. When we illustrate the formal procedures of logic with an illustration using, say, "table," there is no question of our own human self-regard becoming entangled in those procedures. Their objectivity is not compromised: the distinction between the structural framework of the logic and the empirical content of the illustration remains clear. And this had been true for "man" even when Aristotle used the word in a logical context. For example, in his *Prior Analytics* it appears alongside other items – table, house, ice, triangle, cloak, etc. – which have equal status with it, as illustrations of how a syllogism may be constructed. The word "man" is as extrinsic to the syllogism as the word "table." He does assume man to have a special importance, particularly in relation to other animals (man is "cultured and literate"), but this sense of being special merely reflects certain Greek conventions that predate the rise of logic, and does not intrude into the logic itself. In the rules of logical engagement, man is no more important than a table. It is true that in *Posterior Analytics* he interpolates a psychological note when he says that the first principles of syllogizing come from man's "intuited intellect" (*nous*). However, this is unconnected to his account of how the syllogisms actually work. None of the illustrations Aristotle uses to explain their operation refers to man being an intuitively intellectual animal, or to any other psychological attribute.[6] The Arabs and scholastics, on the other hand, allowed the internal nature of man to become entangled in the structure of the syllogism. They fixed man at the centre of nature, and welded an account of his unique place in the objective, logical order of the cosmos (midway between purely rational angels and purely material animals) with what was previously an entirely separate account of the subjective processes of reasoning within him. They made the former the "necessary consequence" of the latter: "If this thing is a rational animal, it is a man."[7]

Man's logically inscribed place in the cosmic order would eventually be used to enhance the expert status of the nascent professions. Historians of logic make the case that it was only in the nineteenth century that the discipline finally shook off its origins in Aristotelianism; the logic of Ramus in the sixteenth century and Locke in the seventeenth were momentary diversions. However, these diversions were crucial to what non-philosophers of the time thought logic was, and how they made use of it. It was via the intrusion of these quasi-logical notions into everyday thought that one man did indeed become, in intellectual terms, more than another. The conceptual frameworks of the human sciences and of psychology in particular are descended from these degraded forms of logic, which early modern professionals borrowed to resolve issues of status – of man to God, of man to the rest of nature, but especially between man and man. The real thing having been left behind on its esoteric philosophical perch, this ersatz logic became a vernacular tool in the practice of humanist law, religion and later (as usual) medicine. It was their application of the vocabulary of logic to prescriptive accounts of mind and behaviour and the maintenance of social order that both demanded and produced "man" – and of course a normative definition of him – as the primary illustration of how logical systems work.

The point of logic in such texts was not, as it had been for Aristotle, to test the objectivity of thought (though that was always the claim), but to justify the categorization of abilities and personalities. Logic objectivizes status, lending the human sciences their air of authenticity and their authority. In Aristotle, the actual truth content of propositions beginning "Man is …" had been, if not irrelevant, then subordinate to the main task, which was to test out the relationship of one proposition to another and thus the validity of certain formal procedures either of analysis or simply of debate. But in Arab and scholastic philosophy, reason and man

---

[6] *Prior Analytics*, 52a; *Posterior Analytics*, 99b.
[7] Avicenna, *Psychology*, 40; *The Propositional Logic*, 73.

are embroiled with each other: these writers *begin* with the presupposition that man is a rational or logically reasoning animal, as itself a universal truth that tacitly underwrites the validity of logical propositions.

Exacerbated by the rise of humanistic systems of thinking which were less about the cosmos as such than man's place in it, this then reaches down to the professions and to the vernacular logic books that began to appear. The foremost example in England was Thomas Wilson's 1551 textbook, which went through many printings and for the next century was the first item educated people reached for when they wanted to know about logic (what they called "Aristotelian" logic, that is, the Tree of Porphyry). Wilson's very first illustration of a universal or species difference, the paradigm of such differences throughout the cosmos, is the standard "Man is a rational animal" formula. Tables and triangles are notable by their absence. In the book's opening address to Edward VI, the content of man's rationality is identified precisely with the humanist wit of the obedient professional classes, whom he presents as the elect caste of an elect nation:

> I have assayed ... to make logic as familiar to the Englishman as by diverse men's industries the most part of the other liberal sciences are, ... considering the forwardness of this age, wherein the very multitude are prompt and ripe in all sciences ... weighing also that the capacity of my countrymen the English nation is so pregnant and quick to achieve any kind or art of knowledge, whereunto wit may attain, that they are not inferior to any other.[8]

Wilson has in mind the man who has the wit to adapt and bend logic to his own career while respecting social and religious norms. Most of the book's illustrations of logic are drawn from human behaviour. This is presented in both political and religious terms, between which it seeks a balance. On the one hand, it promotes the "goodly [logical] reasoner" as the ideal citizen of a centrally and logically ordered state, and on the other it seeks in good Calvinist faith to prevent logical reasoning from overreaching itself: "Some heads are very bold to enter farther than wit can reach, or else have a mind vainly to question of ... things that should not be brought in question," such as the existence of God.

Wilson's application of this chop logic in the social realm coincides with Ramus's revolt against so-called Aristotelian logic. Ramus disliked its complexity, in which man could variously be this by essential property, that by definition, the other by difference and so on. He sought a simpler system, consisting only of universal kinds. He saw universals as a mirror, reflecting for the reader "the universal images and the generals of all things, making it much easier by means of these images to recognize each species and therefore to establish contact with that which he is seeking."[9] Ramus's most frequently worked example of a universal kind, central to his very idea of logic, was "man," to whom also he wanted to restore a biblical simplicity. His highly influential analytic technique consisted in the simple division and subdivision of such kinds. Dichotomy was popular with double predestinarians because it reinforced the simplicity of the elect-reprobate division, but it was also popular with those who, like Amyraut and Baxter, were trying to flee the starkness of predestination, and (as we saw in Chapter 11) it is what eventually produced their concept of a natural disability of the intellect.

This was not some esoteric dispute between schools of logic but part of a whole cultural transformation. In the late sixteenth century the professions, notably law and religion, were drawing on both "Aristotelian" and Ramist schools. Lawyers used them in their own handbooks on how to improve professional practice. Commenting on the charge that Ramism was plebeian ("hereby is

---

[8] Thomas Wilson, *The Rule of Reason*, A3r.
[9] Cited in Wilbur Howell, *Logic and Rhetoric in England 1500–1700*, 157.

logic ... robbed of her honour ... It comes to pass that every cobbler can cog a syllogism ... hereby is logic profaned"), Abraham Fraunce asks, "Cobblers be men, why therefore not logicians?"[10] And of course if cobblers can be logicians, so too can lawyers. Logic should not be "locke[d] up in secret corners." Human reason, public policy and the legal profession as practised by Fraunce's readers, are all identified with each other, and logic is the cement that binds them:

> If laws by reason framed were, and grounded on the same;
> If logic also reason be, and thereof had this name;
> I see no reason, why that law and logic should not be
> The nearest and the dearest friends, and therefore best agree.

Fraunce is looking for ways to police the microcosm of the individual as well as the social macrocosm. The threat represented by heterodox private reason could be cured by an injection of logic. After all, as Aristotle had said, "every common person or silly soul useth logic in some part, and practiseth of himself by natural instinct that which artificially logic doth prescribe in her several rules and constitutions; artificial logic then is the polishing of natural wit, as discovering the validity of every reason, be it necessary, whereof cometh science." Of course Aristotle had said nothing of the sort; Fraunce is trying here to bind knowledge to power, by injecting with the scientific credentials of logic a mundane and secular wit whose status needed a lift. To some degree even people outside the honour society could reason logically; the point was to harness their reasoning to the public (state) good.

But what if they could not? The new legal definition of the idiot, given a place within the simple divisions and subdivisions of Ramist logic in which "nothing is exorbitant or without the verge of that division," helped to sharpen the idea of exclusion from the human species.[11] The infiltration of legal vocabulary into discussions of human nature confirmed that the absolute category boundary involved in possession and privation was taking over from the former, fuzzier notion of the unnatural as merely an exotic expression of the natural. This had its influence on definitions of man. Wilkins, for example, in his attempt to create a universal nomenclature for simple kinds or species (aimed at stabilizing the Royal Society's investigations of the natural world), gave as his chief example of "natural power" or ability the man of "understanding, intellect, mind" and its privative, the "natural fool," "idiot," or "changeling."[12] The logic was deductive as well as dichotomous. Wilkins's category of "idioticalness," *qua* category, had to exist. Therefore, one could go out and look for people to fit it (and exactly the same is true of "intellectual disability").

As for religion, logic had already been brought into its service by Calvin, and even more by leading second-generation Protestants such as Beza and Philip Melanchthon. But what historians have seen as a humanist *application* of logic *to* religion could equally be seen as the *infiltration* of logic *by* religion, as a way of finding a language in which the prescription of doctrine and the control of behaviour might be justified. Take the doctrine of election. I cannot offer good behaviour as collateral for my election or state of grace because that would amount to thinking that I can bargain with God. So I can only detect it from my feelings of certainty. Calvin's logical-type formula for this ran: The elect are certain of their salvation; this man is not certain; therefore he is not elect. Now this might seem as if he were adapting for religious purposes the format of some already existing proposition from secular logic, say: Man is a rational animal; this man is not rational; therefore he is not a man. But in fact no one before the later seventeenth century had come

---

[10] *The Lawiers Logike*, 3.5.
[11] Cited in Howell, *Logic*, 201.
[12] Wilkins, *An Essay*, 195.

up with such a proposition. Nor could they have done, because species exclusion on the grounds of rationality demands a modern mind-set. Defects of rationality in individuals, as we have seen, had never challenged their essence or species membership; such defects were mere "accidents." Neither Locke nor anyone else could say that a man without logical reasoning was not a man until Calvin had said that a man without certainty was not elect. We have intellectually disabled people only because we once had reprobates.

The earlier part of the seventeenth century reveals the beginnings of this transition. "Man," and his division into elect and reprobate, was the primary textbook example of the Ramist subdivision of universal kinds. The first guide to Ramist logic published in English, in 1584, is full of illustrations of dichotomy running along the lines of "Faithful men must either be saved or condemned: but they shall be saved: therefore not condemned."[13] This religious doctrine about elect status, historically contingent, was crucial in the very formation of a supposedly logical, objective structure of scientific expertise about the human mind. The seepage between illustrations involving man and election and those involving man and reason occurs in several ways. First, there was the dispute among faculty psychologists as to whether damage to one of the soul's faculties remains limited to that part or whether it affects the rational soul itself. Various orthodox Calvinists took up this theme. Beza cast it in terms of grace and election. Each faculty, he said, is partly regenerate, partly unregenerate, and "that is why intelligence is not perfect."[14] Perkins drew a logic-based analogy between the individual's membership of the species ("man is a rational animal") and his membership of the company of the elect:

> [God] doth as well conclude in the heart of everyone one that believeth, that he is elected: as any man shall be able to conclude unto particular men, that every one of them is a living creature endowed with reason by this general proposition: *Every man is a reasonable creature endowed with reason*: the assumption being suppressed .... Furthermore, he publisheth it to all the elect by the Apostles in this general proposition, that *all the faithful are elect to eternal life*: the assumption (that whereby a man applies the general promise to himself) is concealed in the word of God [emphases in original].[15]

In this analogy the two concepts, one about reason, the other about election, sit together in the same pseudo-logical framework. Of course they differ from each other in certain respects; it was not the case that every particular man is elect, whereas it was the case (according to the formula as then understood) that every particular man is a reasonable creature. But analogy can of course lead to osmosis.

That was exactly what happened with Baxter's friend William Bridge, who goes beyond analogy and asks himself: if the "essential property" of man is defined on the scale of nature as "rational animal," then what exactly is the content of that rationality? Bridge answers: "To understand, to know, and to reflect upon a man's own actions .... A beast does many actions, but a beast hath not power to reflect upon his own action."[16] This was a humanist convention; as Elyot had remarked, a horse "knoweth not that he is a horse ... that ignorance that we call beastly, is in that, that beasts do not know what they themselves be, nor between them and men what is the diversity," namely possession of an immortal soul.[17] The ability to reflect on one's own actions, and the understanding

---

[13] Dudley Fenner, *The Arte of Logike*, C1r.
[14] Cited in Jeffrey Mallinson, *Faith, Reason and Revelation in Theodore Beza*, 208.
[15] *A Briefe Discourse*, 23.
[16] *Works*, iii, 7.
[17] *Of the Knowledge whiche Maketh a Wise Man*, 25v.

that this ability accounts for one's place in the hierarchy of species, were the defining components of human reason. And it is on these grounds that Bridge excludes the reprobate from the human species: "A reprobate ... does not reflect upon his own action" – i.e., he is without a conscience – "and so does not have the essential property of rational animal." By contrast, "every godly, gracious man hath this power." Rationality here is fully identified with election. The out-group consists of people lacking both simultaneously. Moreover, reasoning conscience also involves a knowledge of the necessary, divinely determined mechanism that has *caused* one's elect status, the "watches and springs" as Bridge puts it (reminiscent of Locke's "wheels and springs") that determine one's human essence. Reprobates lack the ability to detect either their own human status or its causes.

To summarize: Aristotle used the formula "Man is ..." as one illustration among many in a psychology-less logic. By the thirteenth century, the individual human mind was being seen as possessed of its own subjective logical component, a logically reasoning *ability*; by the end of the sixteenth, the mind itself, as a whole, was starting to be called the "logical faculty."[18] The union between logic as object and as subject can be seen from the title of Watts's seminal 1741 guide to education and behaviour *The Improvement of the Mind: or, a Supplement to the Art of Logic*. While logic as objective critique was contributing to the development of the exact sciences, its emergence in the human sciences came via salvation theology and preparation for the afterlife, and with modernity has ended up in what one might call a logic-less psychology.

Abstraction: its medieval roots

Locke's doctrine of abstraction as the supreme intellectual activity led Edmund Burke, scourge of "the swinish multitude," to describe "this disposition to abstractions, to generalizing and classification" as "the great glory of the human mind" (though it also led William Blake to scribble in his copy here: "To generalize is to be an idiot ... General knowledges are those knowledges that idiots possess").[19] How did abstraction reach this elevated position? In medieval faculty, psychology abstraction was just one important operation, alongside contemplation and others. The operations were in any case secondary to the faculties, and even the faculties themselves were mere "qualities" of the soul, the latter being the really "substantial" entity. Later, abstraction would take over as the distinguishing feature of the human species, with the key role of enabling the mind to know itself. We shall come across it in two guises. In medieval philosophy, abstraction meant the separation of concepts from their corresponding sense objects in the material world, or of universal concepts from particular concepts. Gradually, however, it took on a second role, as the understanding of the understanding. (I use the word "understanding" here rather than "intellect" because it helps us to grasp fully the tautology involved, as in the ubiquitous phrase "the understanding understands the understanding," *intellectus intelligit intellectum*.) Once the thinking individual had abstracted himself fully from the objects of his senses, there was only himself and his relationship with other fully abstracted entities left to think about; his likeness to God or (after the Reformation) his status with Him.

Everyone writing on the topic claimed Aristotle's *On the Soul* as his source. In fact Aristotle had not given abstraction any systematic treatment or even a dedicated vocabulary; even less did he see it as defining the human species. He uses at least five everyday terms – "to separate," "take away," "lift off," etc., – for what the Arabs, or at least their Latin translators (to be followed in English by modern translators of Aristotle himself) describe by the one technical term, "to abstract."

---

[18] Casmann, *Psychologia*, 89.
[19] Burke, *The Works of Sir Joshua Reynolds*, i, lxxxiv; Blake, *Poetry and Prose*, 777.

Aristotle does, it is true, draw a contrast between "feelings associated with the senses" and "that which is said to be at one 'remove' from them," though only with the purpose of instructing us that sensible forms are at the root of both. He also draws a contrast between "sense-perception which in practice deals with each thing" and "understanding (*episteme*) which deals with the whole" ("with universals," say modern translators, anticipating what was in fact a later philosophical development).[20] These were passing remarks, but the Arabs and scholastics turned them into an overarching theory. Aquinas, for example, wrote about abstraction as a precise operation applied to objects in the external world: "What is received from the senses becomes actively intelligible through a process of abstraction."[21] There is also the abstraction of universals from particular *concepts*: "The function of the theoretical faculty is to receive the impressions of the universal forms abstracted from matter .... If these forms are already abstract in themselves, it simply receives them; if not, it makes them immaterial by abstraction, so that no trace whatever of material attachments remains in them."[22] Hence, abstraction is an operational component of the faculty of *intellectus* or understanding: "The uncorrupted understanding is that understanding in us which is abstracted."

According to Avicenna, abstraction is one of the highest ranking of the active operations. He looks for a concrete example of how it works, and the best illustration of a completed abstraction he can find is the concept "man": "The faculty takes the unitary nature of the many [individual men], divests it of all material quantity, quality, place, and position, and abstracts from all these in such a way that it can be attributed to all men." What is abstraction? It is that which the species man does. What is the species man? We know by abstraction. Abstraction is the process by which man knows himself as an abstractor, the boundaries of this circle marking his difference from (and mastery over) the brute beasts.

Abstraction in this sense implies that the essence of "man" lies in and is defined by the ability of the human *intellectus* to know itself. But this raises the question, how can it do so if subject and object consist of the same substance? An "understanding that understands the understanding" is also needed, to understand the workings of that very idea – and so on, regressively. Aristotle had explicitly warned against going round in circles like this (the same critique is routinely made of psychology today).[23] There are limits, he urged, to what thinking can do; all there is, is a patchwork succession of thinking states – each of which will always exist only in relation to some specific thing. The Arabs tried to co-opt Aristotle, quoting him as saying that the understanding can be identical with its object. (In fact the passage they cited makes a rather different point.)[24] Moreover, they owed much also to the Platonist theory of intelligences, in which the perfect movement of the psyche is a circle. Circularity was not problematic for them, but rather a positive principle.

The Arab philosophers' Islamist critics were sceptical of the idea that the understanding could understand the understanding – not because it was regressive or circular but because they doubted whether any merely *human* being could attain any such understanding. This faith-based scepticism survived into early modern Christianity, albeit as a minority doctrine. How can the soul know itself? As one writer put it, "Properly to know that by which it knows is impossible for any creature: because to know that, is to be above it self: and to have that which it hath not. This therefore is proper to God alone, whose essence and knowledge is both one."[25] Among the Arabs, Averroes

---

[20] *On the Soul*, 417b; 432a.
[21] *Summa Theologica*, 1.1.84.
[22] Avicenna, *Psychology*, 33.
[23] For example Ilham Dilman, "Science and psychology," in A. O'Hear (ed.), *Verstehen and Humane Understanding*.
[24] *On the Soul*, 407a; 431a.
[25] Woolnor, *The True Originall*, 17.

had been particularly optimistic. He thought that philosophers might sometimes succeed in having such knowledge: that "in contemplating the understanding as the understanding, they will think its abstracted substance." This optimistic tone would come to dominate the early modern period and to presuppose the abilities of increasing numbers of people. For Averroes, the goal of philosophy was that ultimate point where "the thing which the understanding abstracts *is* the understanding as it abstracts and understands that thing."[26] In a human and partly material being, however, "the power of understanding, if it understands via its bodily instrument, does not understand itself, nor its own instrument, nor understands whether it understands." Whatever operates through a bodily organ is not capable of knowing itself. Self-understanding can only occur if "between the understanding and its own essence there is no instrument"; only then does it "understand itself and that instrument which is ascribed to it, and understand whether it understands, so that it understands through itself, not through the instrument."[27]

It was because some at least of the Arabs thought that humans were at the occasional sublime philosophical moment capable of understanding the understanding that later commentators dubbed them "intellectualists." This suggests a departure from their Greek predecessors, whose injunction "Know thyself" had strong ethical components. However, Greek philosophy was interested in the passions because they were a bar to understanding, and if the Arabs' focus seems instead to have been on the sense objects in themselves, rather than on the fleshly passions they incite, they themselves did not overlook the passions. In either case, "disability" seems to have consisted in having a body – a fairly broad catchment. This ethical core to intellectual disability remains in the later vernacular literature dealing with knowledge of the self and the mind. In Book 2 of *The Faerie Queene* for example, Spenser describes how the knight Sir Guyon, on his allegorical journey through the inner man, comes to know his true self through his resistance to the female figure of Acrasia ("Intemperance"), who symbolizes "filth and foul incontinence" in "the mind of beastly man …. That now he chooseth, with vile difference,// To be a beast, and lack intelligence."

Abstraction in the natural history of the mind

Whereas the Arabs had represented the abstraction of the understanding from sense objects and its understanding of itself chiefly as a vague transcendence, the seventeenth century brought the project down to earth by naturalizing it. Locke gave notice of the task in the opening lines of the *Essay*, when he wrote: "The understanding, like the eye, whilst it makes us see, and perceive all other things, takes no notice of itself: and it requires art and pains to set it at a distance, and make it its own object." Locke considered himself to possess the requisite art. One had to move beyond vagueness and focus on the specific detail of psychological operations and skills, of which abstraction was supreme. However fraught with problems this enquiry, however analytically difficult an animal man might be, the prospect of triumph was no longer in doubt.

In humanism's scientific project, the path to God had been through investigation of his works of nature. However, the classical sources from which this project started out (Lucretius, Pliny) were tainted with materialism. In treating the investigating entity itself, the rational soul or mind, as a work of nature too, humanism was trying to wrest its scientific project back on to sounder theological terrain. As Edward Reynolds, Dean of Christchurch during Locke's time as an undergraduate there, put it: "Hereon is grounded another reason … to prove the soul immaterial, because it depends not on the body in its operations but educeth them immediately from within itself, as is more manifest

---

[26] *Commentarium Magnum in Aristotelis de Anima Librum Tertium*, 494; 480.
[27] Avicenna, *Liber de Anima seu Sextus de Naturalibus*, 93.

in the reflexion of the soul upon its own nature."[28] The reconceptualization of the fully abstracted "rational soul" as a part of nature led to its simplification. Even in expert circles, the phrase began to be used casually, as if writers could no longer be bothered making a distinction (because everyone knew it to exist) between this immaterial entity and the sensitive or corporeal soul with its link to the corrupt material world. A requisite social stereotyping facilitated this shift in usage: "The most vulgar and illiterate," said Glanvill, "have not souls for much knowledge" – clearly, we would now read this as "minds."[29]

As we saw in Chapter 4, an erosion also occurred of the old distinction between the operations (such as abstraction) and the soul's substance and faculties. The immortality and divinity of the soul began to rub off on its operations, formerly seen as the secondary entities. Huarte, for example, argued that the operation of wit (*ingenium*) is actually a form of the infused soul itself coming directly from God, "whatsoever difference of ability" is owed to the bodily disposition.[30] For Locke, though he retained the idea of the soul having innate faculties, the real work of acquiring knowledge was done empirically, via the operations and above all via abstraction; and his successors such as Condillac then got rid of the faculties altogether.[31]

Another conceptual rearrangement facilitating the rise of abstraction was that between "passive" and "active" intellect (*nous*). We might assume that these phrases of Aristotle's stood for what we know today as ability and performance, which for us are closely linked (and for the psychometrician are indistinguishable). However, the Greeks had a strong category boundary separating ability from performance, potentiality from actuality, possession from use. Aristotle saw them as belonging to entirely distinct orders of reality; understanding for example (*episteme*, associated with actuality/activity and use) lies in a strictly separate genus from ability (associated with possession).[32] Categorically distinct, passive and active intellect are nevertheless aspects of a single thought event, relating to each other as matter does to form. In medieval philosophy "active" intellect became a divine force, activating what would otherwise remain passive in the sense of inert; hence passive intellect came to be known as "potential" intellect. The latter concept made it possible to stick to the Christian teaching that all individual rational souls are equal while allowing the more important actual/active intellect to differentiate among individuals: "If by 'rational' we mean 'actual,' it is not predicated equally."[33]

Renaissance writers began to say that "active and passive should be resolved into one," and in the post-Cartesian world, passive and potential intellect lost their significance entirely, and active intellect became identified with the now all-important operative realm of abstraction.[34] According to the anonymous author of a 1655 anatomical treatise (with "Know thyself" once more the header quotation),

> An *intellectus agens* [active intellect] is necessary for this reason, that it may make all things actually [sc. actively] intelligible …. For since every object or phantasm is material and so under the opposite condition of the power intelligent, which is abstracted and immaterial, it cannot be comprehended by the intellect until it become abstracted, immaterial, and proportionate to the

---

[28] *A Treatise*, 400.
[29] *An Essay concerning Preaching*, 54.
[30] *The Examination*, 102.
[31] Tim Stainton, *Reason's Other*.
[32] *Topics*, 119b.
[33] Levi ben Gershon, cited in H. Davidson, *Averroes*, 23; see also Zdzisław Kuksewicz, "The potential and the agent intellect," in *The Cambridge History of Later Medieval Philosophy*.
[34] Porzio, *De Humana Mente*, 26.

intellect; and this can never be done but by a power abstracted, and an essence intelligent. From this we may derive information that the office of the understanding is *agere* [to act].[35]

The distinction between the soul, as the underlying substance, and its operations had never been clearcut; but not only are the operations increasingly important here, the soul itself is reinvented as an abstracted "intelligence" – man's rather than God's – and the operations *become* this soul, so to speak, having absorbed its fundamental divinity. The "active" intellect was to be the only kind worth mentioning in the emergent discipline of empirical psychology. The category boundary between ability/potential and actuality/performance has finally disappeared, its one last refuge being in the philosophy of mind.[36] This erosion is a precondition for the very existence of psychology as an applied discipline. Failure to perform is not merely evidence of intellectual disability but completely identifiable with lack of potential. If we are asked to use our intellect but fail, then we do not have it, either actually or potentially.

Active abstraction is the centrepiece of Locke's account of human intellectual abilities in the *Essay*: the ultimate criterion for human species membership. It is no longer a divine attribute to which humans occasionally have privileged access but something specifically and commonly human, derived indirectly from Perkins's reasoning conscience. The importance of abstraction for Locke's contemporaries, and for Locke himself, cannot be grasped in isolation from its role as main bulwark in defence of the soul's immortality. A German theological text exactly contemporary with Locke's *Essay* underlines the point. This author sees abstraction as the weapon to defeat atheism, because it proves the existence of the rational soul from the study of nature itself.[37] Abstraction reveals how the understanding "in operation as well as in being" – the distinction hardly seems to matter any more – "is independent from the body ... [and] the operations of the rational soul are immaterial." It is the one operation that separates humans from animals, says the author; a sleeping dog does not see images while its body is asleep, because animals cannot abstract ("Brutes abstract not," asserts Locke). The supreme natural example of an abstractor, and equally of the abstract knowledge of his species, is man himself – and not, as for earlier philosophy, man in a temporarily shared space with God. Man knows "how to conceive the species man, the common idea of it, by discovering it in every individual man." He knows this "by abstraction, known as physics," that is, the study of nature. He knows that God exists "by abstraction, known as metaphysics," that is, the study of divinity. And finally he knows triangles and number "by abstraction, known as mathematics." But it is the first of these, knowledge of the mind, which is paramount. We can know the immortality of this human rational soul "by light of nature alone," and without it we could not then know God or mathematical truths. Abstraction here is the operator-in-chief by which the human intellect "universally comes to know universals." We know abstraction *by* abstraction, and first of all by focusing on our individual selves. And it is from this that we get an inkling of the privileged position we occupy in nature as perfectible and immortal beings, who may become (to use the transhumanists' phrase) "as radically different from our human past as we humans are from the lower animals."[38] In Paul Mengal's words – it is the seventeenth century he has in mind, but of course they apply to the present day as well – "psychology thus reconstructs the relationship of mind to body by inscribing it within a new vision of the direction of history."[39]

---

[35] Anon., *Anthropologie Abstracted: or, the Idea of Human Nature*, 19.
[36] See Anthony Kenny, *The Metaphysics of Mind*, 66.
[37] Joachim Hildebrand, *Immortalitas Animae Rationalis ex Solo Lumine Naturae*, 431; 459; 515; 423.
[38] Vernor Vinge, "The Coming Technological Singularity," *Whole Earth Review*, Winter 1993.
[39] *La naissance de la psychologie*, 17.

The immortality of the soul and the origins of the word "psychology"

At the core of logical reasoning and abstraction then, which defined the human essence and would at some point differentiate among individual humans, lay self-knowledge: of the individual and of the species. When the word psychology was first coined, towards the end of the sixteenth century, it was partly to describe this generic human understanding of the human mind, and partly to defend the existence of the immaterial and immortal soul. It arose at the height of a Europe-wide moral panic about atheism, from the theologians around Göckel at the leading Protestant university of Marburg. For these writers, "know thyself" meant: know that you have a rational soul; know that the foetus becomes human when God, not the parents, infuses its rational soul; know that this rational soul in man makes him entirely different from the other animals because it is the image of God.[40] "Psychology" at its debut, in the various recensions of Göckel and his associates, is a rephrasing of man's special relationship to the rest of nature.

Doubts about the soul's immortality and immateriality had always been around, but only as late as 1513 did the church anathematize such views: evidence that a full theoretical justification had become a political necessity.[41] There immediately followed the momentous theological scandal of Pomponazzi's assertion that philosophy alone could not prove the soul's immortality. He and his disciples pressed home the question: if the soul's component parts are subject to defect (lethargy, melancholy, etc.), can the substance of the rational soul itself be immaterial?[42] The very word "psychology" was a response to this sceptical attack, even if the scepticism rested on a religious conviction that faith was more reliable than reason. One of the Protestant psychology men, Otho Casmann, warned against taking at face value the sceptics' protestations that they were putting faith first. They claimed to be objecting to the idea that the human mind can understand itself through itself, on the grounds that this would mean we were trying to compete with God, who is in fact the "first intelligence" and the only being that can truly know his own essence. Casmann feared this scepticism might have a domino effect and discourage belief in the soul's immortality altogether. The Jesuits had answered the sceptics by saying that the human soul can at least know itself "through its appearance" (*per speciem*), if not "through its essence" (*per essentiam*). Casmann complained that this response is inadequate, and typical of the Catholic obsession with externals. The mind knows itself not "directly by its appearance" but "indirectly, by reflection."[43] The psychology men's purpose was thus to shore up – by rewriting – the principle that the mind is immaterial and immortal: it could only be true *if the human mind can actually be known, reflectively and analytically*. This reflective ability to study the soul or mind became indispensable to the principle of immateriality and immortality itself. The turn from pessimism to optimism over the prospect of doing so, and the resulting notion that disability is lack of psychologically reflective knowledge, would be neatly captured later in Glanvill's remark: "The disease of our intellectuals is too great, not to be its own diagnostic. And they that feel it not, are not less sick, but stupidly so."[44]

The main stimulus for inserting self-reflection within the study of the mind was the writers' anxiety about predestination and salvation. Göckel would later participate at the Synod of Dort, arbitrating on the doctrine of election. The search in oneself for signs of election led to the new epistemological concerns of philosophy foregrounded by Locke. As one preacher wrote,

---

[40] Göckel, *Psychologia*, "To the Reader."
[41] Jill Kraye, "The immortality of the soul in the Renaissance," *Signatures*, 1 (ISSN 1472–2178).
[42] Porzio, *De Humana Mente*, 36.
[43] Casmann, *Psychologia*, 21; Collegium Conimbricense, *De Anima Aristotelis*, 504; Casmann, *Psychologia*, 111.
[44] *The Vanity of Dogmatizing*, 62.

"How should we comfortably know that we are enriched with saving graces but by a reflexed act of the understanding, whereby we know that we have them?"[45] This meeting between philosophical tradition and worries about election and reprobation, between "man the rational animal" and "man the difficult animal," reinforced the study of the generic "self" as a burgeoning discipline that aspired to be at once a means for salvation and the starting point for knowledge of the rest of the natural world. At first "psychology" was only one among several names offered for this study. Here is another that did not catch on but might well have: "The way to God is by ourselves: it is a blind and dirty way; it hath many windings, and is easy to be lost .... He that would learn theology must first study autology."[46]

Sometimes the psychology men's very choice of title points to the doctrinal thrust of the term: for example *General Psychology: a Disputation on the Status of Souls after Death*, a work whose opening sentence is again "Know thyself."[47] In the 1575 *Quaestiones Physicae* of Ramus's friend and translator Johannes Freigius, which contains the earliest verifiable printed use of the term, *psychologia* (study of the soul) is used synonymously with *anima* (soul). There is no distinction between the thing itself and its study; this aggrandizes and reifies the soul (rather as "methodology" in social science today aggrandizes "method"). The book's contents page consists in a list of Ramist-style divisions and subdivisions. The first, unitary heading is "Perfected Entity" (*corpus perfectum*). This then divides into inanimate and animate entities. The animate branch subdivides into "Soul" (*anima/psychologia*) and "Ensouled Body" (*corpus animatum*). The *anima/psychologia* chapter turns out to be a routine description of the soul's faculties that could have been written at any time over the previous two centuries. The novelty is the word itself, psychology: a battle-cry signalling that the theory of the divinity and immortality of the soul and its *alter ego* the mind are under threat.

Whatever the due caution of historians who have insisted on the "lexical fluidity" of the word psychology in this period, it seems that all the early usages share this same doctrinal stance.[48] Only two works with the word in their titles were published outside the Goclenian circle at this time. Noël de Taillepied's 1588 *Psichologie, ou traité de l'apparition des esprits* attacks people who deny the existence of spirits, a proxy for denying the existence of the soul; and in a new edition of Boehme's *Forty Questions on the Origin of the Soul*, the word "psychology" was added to the title, perhaps in order to cleanse the original work of its traducianist views (denounced by its new editor as "heresy"). Whatever their differences, these authors share with the Goclenians a belief in the realist doctrine about spirits and the Devil, as well as a defence of the soul's immortality. "Psychology" at the moment of its invention thus seems to have been an imperialist attempt, from an initially defensive redoubt, to turn the immaterial human soul or mind into *the* overarching study. From its beginning, it was dealing with biology too, since the question of ensoulment, of *how* the rational soul arrives in the body, opens up an arena of discussion for the physical causes of defect. The titles again give a flavour: for example, Fortunius Licetus's *Human Psychology, or: On the Source of the Human Soul*, which attacks the doctrine of parental generation.[49] A work by another of Göckel's colleagues, Clemens Timpler (probably his *Twelve Theses on the Essence of the Rational Soul*), went under the nickname of "the Ensoulment Theory" (*Empsychologia*).[50]

---

[45] Estwick, Πνευματολογια: Or, a Treatise of the Holy Ghost, 88.
[46] Daniel Featley, cited in Schoenfeldt, *Bodies*, 15.
[47] Wolfgang Tüntzel, Ψυχολογια Generalis.
[48] Fernando Vidal, *Les sciences de l'âme*, 69.
[49] Ψυχολογια ανθρωπινε sive de Ortu Animae Humanae.
[50] Cited in Georg Nagel, Ψυχολογια, seu Disputatio Physica de Anima eiusque Causis.

Once again, one of the techniques employed by the psychology men was to try and recuperate the terms of their opponents. The traducianists, charged with implying that parental generation gives the soul material origins, had defended themselves by adopting Averroes's theory that there is a single immortal and incorruptible abstract intellect, held in common by all mankind over and above individual corruptible souls. The psychology men took this notion of their opponents and used it to describe instead the incorruptible element of the human essence held individually, in each human soul. It is this that Licetus, for example, then labels "the abstracted intelligence" (*intelligentia abstracta*), as it emerges from the to and fro of theological debate.[51]

From these debates there also arose, at the start of the seventeenth century and some time before Descartes, a routine subdivision of the study of man, "anthropology," into "somatology" and "psychology," body and soul.[52] Further into the century, a second wave of Marburg physician-theologians took Descartes's *cogito* and identified it with the "soul" of their Goclenian predecessors; disability was identified, accordingly, as "lack of clear and distinct ideas," of the Cartesian type.[53] There is then a connection from this second generation through to Christian Wolff, the German Enlightenment philosopher who during his stay in Marburg in the 1720s became the self-styled founder of empirical psychology. Wolff's ties to the modern discipline are well established. Prompted by Leibniz's proposal of an arithmetical calculus for the study of the soul and by Christian Thomasius's 1690 "calculus of the passions" which scored individual personalities on a numerical scale, it was Wolff who first coined the term psychometrics (*psychometriae*).[54]

Intellectual differences and human nature: difference by degree

What kind of classifiable difference between one human being and another is created by this prominence of abstraction and logical reasoning? Answers can be found in the grand, long-lived theory of natural hierarchy known as the "scale of nature." In our search for knowledge about ourselves and each other, when the going gets tough we reach for the principle, deeply embedded in our history, that order gives meaning to nature and creates a natural human hierarchy. In respect of intellectual disability, this differentiation follows three models: as part of a spectrum of degrees within a broadly human category, as an interstice between higher and lower forms of natural intellectual life and as a monstrous anomaly.

The first of these models, difference by degree, is not entirely separable from the ethical principle of inclusive indifference, since it does not challenge the actual species membership of those of the lowest degree. The very existence of humans with disabled understandings, as long as they are classed within the species, might be taken as proof of "the principle of plenitude" in the "great chain of being," showing that God has filled all the available spaces of creation.[55] In Aristotle's *On the Soul* there are just two passing references to intellectual difference: the one already noted about the sense of touch, the other about the intellectual states of old people. All Aristotle wants to say is that such differences do not challenge the fundamental rule by which the soul is "form" to the body's "matter"; only animated bodies can be thus graded, not souls by themselves. Pedagogical experts of the Roman Empire expanded on this text. Themistius, for example, in his commentary

---

[51] For example Licetus, Ψυχολογια, 253 ff.

[52] Mengal, "La constitution de la psychologie comme domaine du savoir aux XVIème et XVIIème siècles," *Revue d'histoire des sciences humaines*, 2 (2001/2).

[53] Claud Wegner, *Tentamen Primum Metaphysico-Psychologicum*, unpaginated.

[54] Cited in Roger Smith, *The Fontana History of the Human Sciences*, 202.

[55] Johann Lambert, *Cosmologische Briefe*, 106.

on Aristotle, adds blind people. It is not the sensory impairment in itself that is at issue but the *intellectual* impairment it creates. Because geometry is the paradigm of objective knowledge about the abstraction of form from matter, blind people's inability to visualize geometric shapes leads to absence of this knowledge; correspondingly, their blindness means that their own souls are not and cannot be in a state of full abstraction from their bodies, and this prevents them from knowing, subjectively, that the abstraction of form from matter (of soul from body) is denied to them. Hence, in circular fashion, they are disabled from understanding their own lack of understanding.[56]

Alexander, for whom the normative human group was "all those who are not impaired" in their understanding of universals, also noted that people are "more or less naturally endowed" with wisdom. All of us "have," in a passive or potential sense, practical wisdom (mathematics, logic) and theory (physics, metaphysics). Whether we actually use them is another matter. By "all those who are not impaired," therefore, he means people who do use them; they are those whose positions in Roman society afford them the leisure to "study" (contemplate). Alexander's psychology is suffused with concepts of honour and social class, echoing the importance Aristotle gives to fineness of touch. Horny-handed peasants are impaired, but only because they have (and ought to have) no opportunity to practise any intellectual skills. Correspondingly, when he says that the unimpaired "are guided by nature itself to the apprehension of universals," nature amounts here to training. If any determinism is involved, it is social rather than natural.[57]

Following Alexander, Avicenna doubted whether abstraction could produce in us an understanding of the sensible images obtainable from the material world; it could only ever prepare us for the revelation, by some divine being, of their corresponding "intelligible forms."[58] Averroes thought Avicenna overly pessimistic; he was conceding too much to Islamist religious sceptics, who argued that philosophy overestimated human intellectual abilities and was therefore "incoherent." Averroes's response to this scepticism, his famous *Incoherence of the Incoherence*, presents abstraction as the positive basis on which mortals themselves can occasionally achieve divine knowledge. It is the operation by which the "theoretical" faculty perceives "the real natures of intelligible things, in abstraction from matter, place and position," concepts which "the philosophers call abstract universals."[59] Whereas Avicenna saw abstraction in ideal terms, only ambiguously accessible to human beings and suspended far above the material world, Averroes saw it as a genuinely human operation – perhaps a specifically human one, since angels and divine beings did not need abstraction to access theoretical truths.

In what sort of people did this abstraction occur? Averroes's normative human type is the speculative or theoretical philosopher. In the Platonist picture of a hierarchy of immaterial or angelic intelligences, which greatly influenced Arab philosophy, only the last and lowest of these had any point of contact with the material world. And the very prospect, however unlikely, of a divine intelligence *within* mere mortals created the thin end of a wedge for hierarchical difference *among* them. Some people are further abstracted from their own materially corrupting senses than others. At the opposite pole from the philosopher's abstraction is carnal pollution. Between these two extremes are various grades of people who correspond with (rather than "are capable of") the existence of various grades of intelligible forms. "Vulgar" people are on a level with intelligibles corrupted by the material world.[60] On the next level up are novitiates undergoing an intellectual apprenticeship; they correspond with "speculative intelligibles," i.e., concepts that approximate

---

[56] Themistius, *On Aristotle on the Soul*, 432a.
[57] Alexander, *De Anima*, 81.
[58] *Avicenna Latinus*, 3.
[59] Averroes, *Incoherence of the Incoherence*, 333; 346.
[60] Averroes, *Commentarium Magnum*, 159.

better to what material things actually are and form part of the "knowledge of nature." Since this level too remains entangled with particulars, it still pertains to mere appearances; it is a "practical" level, tied to the material world as the vulgar are. Higher up are philosophers, who correspond with theory itself, i.e., with those intelligibles which are detached from the material world and which therefore constitute incorruptible, true objects of knowledge. And the summit of this grade is knowledge of the human soul: know your own essence, and you will know your creator. We know God through knowing in ourselves the image of God that we are, and this in turn is the basis of all knowledge of nature too. Most philosophers never get to this point, and even when they do, some of them know the image less well than others. Only in their optimum condition do they become, as pure intellect, the image of God. Averroes calls this transhumanist vision "a marvel of nature." Although it displays man at his best, it is not a condition that is proper to man as man, inhabiting as he does the material realm. Five hundred years later the ballast had shifted; Locke would be claiming something like the abstracting abilities of the Arabs' speculative philosophers for all – or most – humans.

Status, then, is differential intellect. Our ability to abstract denotes honour to the extent that it removes us, as intellectual beings, from the corruptions of the flesh. Averroes and Albert, however, whose commentaries on *On the Soul* launched a copious Renaissance tradition, had presented these intra-species differentials in very general terms, though Albert did suggest they had corresponding physical brain states involving a greater or lesser subtlety of the soul spirits.[61] Renaissance experts on the mind made the differentials socially specific. They rewrote Aristotle to say that the most honourable occupation of the understanding as subject is to contemplate the honourability of the understanding as object. (Actually, he had said it was mathematics.)[62] Other occupations – especially those which did not involve thinking at all, or were not professional ones – were inferior.

This social normativity of intellectual virtue was accompanied by the new emphasis on reasoning as a sign of grace; and a discussion about how the understanding and its operations represent the spectrum of individual abilities – once a largely philosophical discussion – was thereby theologized. It leads Andrea Alpago, an Arabic-reading doctor and Aristotle commentator of the sixteenth century, to expand the role of abstraction further by blurring the boundary between its subjective and objective roles; "abstractions," in his formula, simply *are* "universals," *and* the subjective process through which one arrives at them. This model for the philosopher in his optimum condition is the soul after death in beatitude:

> The soul itself, separated from the body, understands ... far nobler and more abstract things ... than it previously understood .... There are men whose lives are not immersed in worldly delectation of the senses but abstain from them ... and are only occupied in contemplation and knowledge, behaving thus because they are distanced and abstracted from the senses .... The more the soul is occupied with sense-objects, the further away it is from cognition of God, and of abstract forms.[63]

In this Dantesque condition, which some of us occasionally attain here on earth and which remains an aspiration for everyone else, the soul shares in "divine substance and other abstract substances." One is graded intellectually by one's nearness to God. The normativity of abstraction for the general population, and its differentiation by degree between some men and others, have their

---

[61] Nicholas Steneck, "Albert the Great on the classification and localization of the internal senses," *Isis*, 65 (1974).

[62] Paulus Nicolettus [Venetus], *Scriptum super Librum De Anima Aristotelis*, 197v; Ruvius, *Commentarii*, 15; 18.

[63] Alpago, *Compendium de Anima*, 38v.

historical beginnings here, at the point where honour and grace enter the frame. While "only he is a philosopher who abstracts well," abstraction is also that which *all* humans in general ought to be good at, even if only a few achieve it. Consequently it became possible that the rational soul, as such, might *itself* be "an abstraction from sensibles ... acting like the angels."[64] And so one individual human being, and one rational soul or mind, might be more perfected and rank higher with God than another.

The problem with this fusion between abstracting operations and the more fundamental substance of the rational soul was that it challenged the principle that this soul is divinely infused. Evidence had never been required to demonstrate the existence of "substances," of which the rational soul was one; substance is that which just *is*. Evidence was appropriate to abstraction however, because as an operation rather than a substance, it was observable. If the rational soul just *is* abstraction, then perhaps not all rational souls on this earth are in an equally sound condition and the differences between them are observable; traducianist beliefs about the parental origins of the soul, and thus the possibility of a variety of material influences on it, might then be right. One infusionist author confronted this problem of the soul's purity by means of a hard science analogy with alchemy and the activities of the soul:

> As for human understandings, we find by experience that the meaner and grosser they are the less they can abstract, and indeed abstraction in the understanding is a subtle act and like to extraction in chemistry, which takes the purer parts from the feculent, and resolves bodies into their several native parts, which before did lie confused in one heap and mingled together.[65]

Another consequence of this shift towards abstraction concerned predestination and grace. The elect had always been considered a smallish minority, which conflicted with an increasingly optimistic tone about the intellectual performance levels attributable to larger numbers of people and was provoked by the increasing division of labour. Edward Reynolds, writing in 1640, called for "the reflexion of the soul, upon its own nature," and continued:

> Another reason may be drawn from the condition of the understanding's objects, which have so much the greater conformity to the soul by how much the more they are divine and abstracted .... And the ground of this reason is, that axiom in philosophy that all reception is *ad modum recipientis*, according to the proportion and capacity of the receiver. And that the objects which are spiritual and divine have greatest proportion to the soul of man is evident in his understanding and his will, both which are in regard of truth or good unsatisfiable by any material or worldly objects, the one never resting in enquiry till it attain the perfect knowledge.[66]

Reynolds was a stickler for election and reprobation, but was also famed for his ability to negotiate a way through doctrinal minefields. Here he opens up the exciting prospect of *perfect* human knowledge – no longer a hubristic dream but a real possibility. Without obscuring the difference between elect and reprobate, he obscures that between rational and elect. What is it man "receives" in the above: the abstracted objects of the understanding, or grace? The more likely answer is both, indiscriminately, and moreover on a sliding scale of "capacity."

In these and suchlike texts abstraction and the rational soul stand in for each other and merge to form one side of a dualistic scheme: a single "mind," which is fully separated from the body and whose detailed operations are now the main business. George Hughes, exiled with Locke in

---

[64] Andreas Schubart, *De Abstractione*, A2; Ruvius, *Commentarii*, 3.
[65] Anon., *The Prerogative of Man: or his Soules Immortality*, 29.
[66] *A Treatise*, 400.

Holland in the late 1680s, complained that in this doctrine all the old contradictions that mind/body dualism claimed to have solved had in fact resurfaced. The doctrine presupposes "a good mind or right reason, that is to say, an uncorrupted ability (*potentia*) to judge and to distinguish true from false that is by nature equal and innate in all of us" – whereas faculty psychology reveals "so many differences in wit (*ingenium*) [and in] the speed of cogitation, the distinct facility of imagining, the capacity for and use of memory!"[67] Before Descartes, most writers had maintained a category boundary between the equality of the rational soul which exists both in "the least knowing man [and] in him who in sharpness of wit approacheth nearest to angelical and noetical spirits," and an active or "actual ability" of which "nature admits a great variety in the use and exercise."[68] All Descartes has done, says Hughes, is relocate the latter, the element of "natural" differentiation, to the soul itself. Hence intellectual difference is not due only to the fleshly corruption of the sensitive or corporeal soul, but is an attribute of the rational soul too. The abilities of the "uncorrupted intelligence" can be seen as varying from one individual to another, *qua* uncorrupted (since even in its differentiated state the Cartesian mind is fully separate from the corrupting body). The mind is a permanent and, like the body, a natural aspect of the individual's personhood. The consequence of dualism – that differences in ability exist in a purely intellectual medium which is bodiless, "arises out of itself" as Hughes puts it, and creates personal identity – are as clear to this run-of-the-mill theologian as they are to Locke, even if the latter was far less sceptical about this idea.

Who and what lay at the bottom of this human spectrum? If the supreme theoretical knowledge was understanding of the understanding, what about "ignorance of this knowledge"?[69] Returning once more to the Arab sources, we find Averroes mentioning three possible forms of it: simple ignorance (never having heard of the propositions that might lead us to knowledge), lack of opportunity to acquire knowledge by use and "deficiency (*diminutio*) in nature." This last led to a conclusion that would one day become profoundly influential: that if there are natural differences among the souls of individuals, then "we and all those who are born to acquire this knowledge are called men equivocally." This doctrine we shall discuss in more detail shortly. Pointing to more than a spectrum differential (an "equivocal" term is one that has more than one meaning), by Locke's time it would call in question the species membership of the deficient. In Averroes's time, however, "nature" was still dispositional; thus the differences the word implies were for him merely ones of degree, and until the mid-seventeenth century commentators still took them this way. Alpago, for example, took Averroes to be referring to "children and foolish people" (*stolidi*); and foolishness – even "foolishness from birth," it turns out – consists in a dispositional melancholy. They are fully human, says Alpago, with an ethical status in which the bad (lack of reasoning abilities) is balanced with the good (corresponding lack of incontinence).[70]

Just as, at the top end of the human sector of the scale of nature, the intellectual elite is also the social honour elite, so the intellectually deficient group at the bottom end is also a social one. Reynolds writes about a "double disproportion" in precisely this sense. Combining Aristotle's socio-political discussion of natural slavery with a psychological one about "abstraction ... in the objects of understanding," he continues:

> Neither is it possible for a man to be sociable, or a member of any public body, any further than he hath a proportion and measure of knowledge, since human society standeth in the communicating of mutual notions [sc. the common ideas] unto one another. Two men that are deaf and dumb and

---

[67] *Disputatio Philosophica*, unpaginated.
[68] John Maxwell, *Sacro-Sancta Regum*, 137.
[69] Averroes, *Commentarium Magnum*, 495.
[70] Alpago, *Compendium*, 94v.

blind, destitute of all the faculties of gaining or deriving knowledge, may be together, but they cannot be said to have society one with another.[71]

Given that labourers are assumed to lack the common ideas, a wide social stratum is implicated in this deficiency. Labourers and disabled alike are defined simultaneously by their exclusion from and their incapability for "human society," that is, the honour society. Lack of intellect and lack of social status are cognate characteristics, rather than the second being an outcome of the first.

Intellectual difference and human nature: interstitial difference

If the spectrum model envisages a single, broadly human class of creatures, the intellectual operations of logical reasoning, abstraction and understanding of the understanding at the same time form *boundaries* to that class. In short, intellectual *differentiation* always implies the possibility of *exclusion*. But where are we to situate the excluded on the scale of nature? Two answers come up: as monstrous anomalies (which we shall deal with shortly) or as interstices between species.

The scale of nature was sorted into sectors of ascending value: mineral, vegetable, animal, divine. Odd, interstitial creatures were said to lie between these sectors: lithodendra between minerals and plants, oysters between plants and animals. Man too was somewhat odd, overlapping the sectors both above and below him in his unique condition of being animal as well as in some sense divine (that is, by his share in reason). Rather than just filling an awkward gap like the oyster, man was therefore the very fulcrum of the whole scale, the "amphibious piece between a corporal and spiritual essence ... that links those two together, and makes good the method of God and nature."[72] According to Albert, the rational soul distinguishing man from the other animals had to indicate something more than just a species difference, since other animal species did not differ from each other by anything so significant.[73] With his aspiration to ascend the dizzying path of the *intellectus* and join the immaterial beings above him, man's greatest anxiety was the interstitial abyss between himself and the mere animals below: whatever you do, don't look down.

But what was in the interstice above? In thinking hard about nature and the cosmos, Albert must always at some point have come back to thinking about his own thinking. How did he know that what he thought about everything outside him was true? He would have pursued this question relentlessly, if only because unlike his pupil Aquinas he was something of a scientist in the modern sense; his study of nature was not entirely subsumed under his theology. So he would surely have gone on to the next question and asked himself where this intellectual ability to think about thinking was situated in the external scheme of things. And he would have recalled immediately that thinking-about-thinking already exists as an objective component of the scale, positioned on a hierarchy of relative perfection where it took the disembodied form of the angelic host. Angels have *intelligentia*. Albert, citing Avicenna, calls them the "sanctified intellect."[74] They not only have it, they *are* it. They are the perfect, completed understanding that understands the understanding, free of bodily encumbrance.

In Albert's example we can already see elements of the underlying metaphysic of modern cognitive disciplines. We begin by surmising about who might be immediately above us in the scale of perfection, and how far we may become like them. The notion that the self-reflecting

---

[71] *A Treatise*, 459; 465.
[72] Browne, *Religio*, 38.
[73] *Liber de Animalibus*, 20.6.
[74] *Summa de Creaturis*, 516 ff.

understanding has levels differentiating some human individuals from others, now as then, stems from this prior aspiration to perfectibility, and could not exist without it. Yet, unlike our transhumanists, Albert was grounded enough to know that there was a big difference between the perfected understanding and the specifically human wit of the everyday world. In fact the precise starting point for his discussion of angels was the question that forms his chapter title here: "What is the difference between man's wit (*ingenium*) and his rational soul?" Albert's answer was: a lot.

Aquinas replaced Albert's picture with a more elaborate one. Every single angel (and there was an infinite number of them) constituted a separate species on its own. Therefore the apocryphal question "How many angels can dance on the head of a pin?" implied another: "In what order of precedence?"

> Intellectual substances [sc. angels] are superior to other substances in the scale of perfection. These substances must also differ from one another in degree. They cannot differ from one another materially, since they lack matter; if any plurality is found among them, it must be by that formal distinction which establishes diversity of species .... Their degree and order must be taken into consideration. That is because, just as addition or subtraction of a unit causes variation in numbers, so natural entities are found to vary in species by the addition or subtraction of differences. For example what is merely alive differs from what is both alive and endowed with sense perception; and the latter differs from what is alive, endowed with sense, and rational .... The higher an intellectual substance is in perfection, the more universal are the intelligible forms it possesses. Of all intellectual substances, therefore, the human intellect ... has forms of the least universality, because it receives its intelligible forms from sensible things.[75]

Oscillation of this kind between optimism about man as an "intellectual substance" or subaltern angel (the bottle is half full of reason) and doubts about whether his reason can redeem him from original sin (half empty) is characteristic of all the Renaissance commentaries. The knowledge angels have represents the ideal of self-reflection; it is that of their own species essence ("they are intellectual species of a sort and are nothing else, and their existence is nothing other than their understanding that they are essences").[76] In man, the understanding cannot understand itself in its essence, only in a mediated form. There are nevertheless certain human minds which can occasionally leave the corrupted world entirely behind and so are close to angelic; hence those horizontally layered group adorations of the Godhead in paintings commissioned by bishops and princes, where saints like Aquinas and of course the commissioners themselves have their heads sticking up into the same row as the angels, above the masses. Likewise, when angels turn up in Locke's *Essay*, they are no mere nod to some obsolete convention. It is true he only mentions them in passing. But for many of his Royal Society colleagues, the position of the human mind in cosmology rested on the premise that angels existed. In the search for a new metaphysics, angels remained key agents; Francis Glisson, for example, the inspiration for some of Locke's early medical speculations, gave them pride of place in his grand attempt at a replacement of the Aristotelian classificatory system.[77] If Locke says little about them, it is because their intelligence and abstracting abilities represent what he hopes (nearly) every human will be capable of in the not-so-distant future – not because they do not exist.

What, then, about the interstice at the bottom end of the scale? Albert suggests children might be a good example. They are "quasi-intermediary" between animal and man because "like brutes they spend all day eating and drinking." The child is a mere "mass of flesh" (recalling the

---

[75] Aquinas, *Compendium Theologiae*, 69; 74.
[76] Dante, *De Monarchia*, 15.
[77] Locke, *An Essay*, 666; Glisson, *Tractatus*, 33.

changeling story). Albert extends the example to "drunks and the intemperate," since "their defects are childlike."[78] They are not brutes though, "because they possess a rational soul." Childhood and drunkenness, like melancholy, are temporary. Where the brutish behaviours are permanent, the rational soul itself has to be missing, along with its abstracting operations. Or does it? Permanent interstitial types were certainly said to exist in nature. Half-men/half-beasts – notably "pygmies" – were much discussed by scholastic philosophers. Their primary classical source, Pliny, did not give pygmies any intellectual characteristics, but Albert adds some. He defines them by their failure to be fully human at the final hurdle, which is the inability to abstract:

> Although pygmies speak, they do not argue or speak about the universals of things .... Reason has two principles. One comes from sense and memory, where the perception of experience lies; the other is that which it possesses when elevated to a unitary intellect, i.e. that which is capable of eliciting universals .... The pygmy, however, has only the first of these.[79]

There are humans, too, who lack this ability to abstract. For these, Albert uses Augustine's term *moriones*. There is no problem about classifying them as human. They are "foolish [*stulti*] by nature because they are incapable of apprehending reason, and their speech utterances resemble the pygmy's. But the pygmy lacks reason by nature, whereas *moriones* do not lack possession of reason but rather the use of it, as a result of melancholy or some other accident." "Accident," even though this might include some innate disposition, implies that the essential property of the human species remains unaffected in *moriones*; and the distinction between possession and use calls to mind Aristotle's natural slaves, who likewise are fully human.

Pygmies, by contrast, are a higher sort of monkey, separate from man as well as from the rest of the simian order: "The pygmy, inasmuch as it is an irrational animal, is the most perfect after man ... it seems to have something that imitates reason, but is deficient in this respect, and thus does not possess reason except as a shadow." Pygmies will learn something by imitation but are also capable of going away and thinking about it; "they do not immediately imitate what they see," whereas monkeys can only be taught to mimic, "without discerning what or whom they imitate." This puts pygmies above monkeys, "in whom there is no practical syllogism." They are capable of the practical part of the syllogism, but "do not progress as far as to receive the universal." Albert at least speculates about their having a soul. Just as the human soul is created "in the shadow of" the divine or Absolute Intelligence, he says, the pygmy's soul is created in the shadow of human intelligence, whereas the monkey's is merely the "imitation of a shadow." Later commentators on these passages bowdlerized them, assimilating pygmies with monkeys: "Pygmies have a human shape, they have motion and perception, but they do not have a human soul ... they are situated in a specific position immediately below the human species."[80] This move away from subtlety at the margins of definition of the human is characteristic of the early modern period.

The interstitial slot in nature can be filled with whatever our real-world surroundings suggest to us. Some historians have claimed that Albert's pygmies were orang-utans, which contemporaries believed capable of some human intellectual operations. Other historians, on the basis of racialization theory, have speculated that they were some African population whom Albert had encountered in real life.[81] Yet they might simply have been creatures of Albert's own imagination.

---

[78] *Quaestiones super De Animalibus*, 171.
[79] *Liber de Animalibus*, 21.1.1.
[80] Guglielmus de Mirica, cited in Agrimi, *Ingeniosa*, 88.
[81] See John Block Friedman, *The Monstrous Races in Medieval Art and Thought*.

The two thought processes are not necessarily incompatible. After all, institutional segregation has made "intellectually disabled" people imaginary creatures to most of us today.

Intellectual differences and human nature: difference as anomaly

Towards the end of the medieval tradition more rigid species boundaries were being sought, on the hypothesis that a human shape might disguise a non-reasoning and perhaps non-human being. Here is how the Jesuits coped with such arguments in the 1590s:

> Some people think the monster differs from the non-monster by its substantial or essential form.... The truer opinion is that the monster differs from the non-monster by its accidental form. This opinion is proved 1. It is not possible for two natures of distinct species to coalesce naturally in one species. 2. It occurs because monsters of this kind are often born solely out of human seed, and not out of a mixture of seeds. Therefore we can say about *semihomines* and *semibestiae* that they differ not in their substantial form, but in their accidental form, and the more noble partial cause is believed to prevail over the less noble, and to draw the outcome into its own species.[82]

Two traditional arguments are used here to haul monsters back on board: the impossibility of contradiction in nature, and the fixity of species. In man, the "more noble" substance that "prevails" is reason; monstrosity marks only an accidental difference. However, these authors are clearly on the defensive. By now, the very same arguments could be used to throw monsters, and particularly intellectual monsters, over the side.

The modern biology-psychology-ethics complex emerges partly from this urge for sharper demarcations of the scale of nature. Intellectual deficiency may put a question mark over membership of the human species: not less human but non-human. Complex medieval forms of classification, with their "accidents" and varying modes of differentiation, gave way to simpler taxonomies, and this in turn encouraged theories about the praeternatural origin of spuriously human-looking individuals. The path would lead to the first clinical descriptions of idiocy as a form of monstrosity in the early nineteenth century, and thence to neo-Darwinian and eugenicist theories of mental degeneracy.[83] It might be thought that the spectrum model has come to prevail more recently, given the minuteness of gradation in biochemically determined difference and the gradations of the IQ scale. Nevertheless, the law of uneven distribution at the extremes of the spectrum and especially the biological distinctiveness of single-gene or chromosomal pathologies carry within them a covert notion of species exclusion. The spectrum and its hierarchical scale of differentiation could not exist without this other, more radical division lurking somewhere in the background.

A note is required here about that word "species" and its simplification. Aristotle's biological system bears not the slightest resemblance to early modern notions of species. Medieval philosophers, largely unaware of the relevant texts, used instead the complex ramifications of the Tree of Porphyry. In the classificatory simplification of early modern life-sciences, these ramifications were replaced by "species" ("kinds," "sorts," etc.) which, whether they described real essences or merely nominal ones, were certainly seen as *resembling* logical classes: if their boundaries were not watertight, they were good enough approximations. Moreover, the early modern word "species" had a second meaning. As well as being used in this familiar classificatory sense, it was also still used to signify the form things take when they appear to our senses

---

[82] Collegium Conimbricense, *Commentariorum Physicorum Aristotelis*, 433.
[83] E.J. Georget, *De la folie*; E.S. Talbot, *Degeneracy, its Causes, Signs and Results*.

and imaginations. Ramist logicians merged the two meanings. Since the Ramist's aim was to know universals by abolishing all "Aristotelian" encumbrances, they believed it was possible for external images (species in the second sense) to mirror faithfully our internal knowledge of essences (species in the first sense). Classification simply consisted in "burnishing and polishing the mirror before it can shine and render up those images."[84] And so there was no longer a need for two separate meanings: category and appearance were one.

This tidiness about classification was also a rigidity, throwing a more intense light on those "equivocal" exceptions to the human rule that had been touched on by the Arab philosophers. The theory of equivocalism applied to differences both in number and in meaning. Number had always been important in species classification. Aristotle's biological works rank a creature in the hierarchy of nature by the number of physiological "parts" it has; Albert echoes this when he compares the souls of humans, pygmies and monkeys according to the number of parts they contain. Aquinas describes species difference in terms of items "added" or "subtracted," reason being the added item that differentiates man from the other animals. Number was therefore already a terrain on which one might plot human difference at the margins. In terms of number, equivocalism was presented as an inductive argument, since the advantages or deficits involved could be counted; but in fact it was deduced from an underlying metaphysic that attributed value to a superior number of parts.

In terms of meaning rather than of number, just as today's post-structuralist contrasts the univocal with the multivocal, so the medieval philosophers contrasted the univocal with the "equivocal" (though without making any clear distinction between a plurality of signifiers and a plurality of things signified). The supreme example of a distinction between the equivocal and the univocal was man's relationship to knowledge and the divine intellect. If the knowledge which God has and the knowledge which man has were identical, says Averroes (citing his forerunner Avempace), that knowledge would be "univocal."[85] But most of the time they are different; and this discussion about intellectual difference between man and God leads inevitably to one about intellectual difference *among men*. The question once again is whether the human understanding can access "intelligible forms" fully "abstracted" from matter, and above all whether it can know the intelligible form of the understanding itself. When a philosopher's understanding understands his understanding, his essential abilities are univocal with those of God; and "if there be those who are such as know all things through themselves, they are equivocally men, and should rather be called angels, on account of the godlike intellect they possess."[86] But what if such ability were entirely lacking? Should such "men" not rather be called something else too?

For every angelic intellectual there is, at the opposite end of the scale, a "defect in nature" turning out creatures who likewise "are men only equivocally," in Avempace's terms. To take a modern example of the genre: "Rationality is not possessed by all the beings we should describe as human, but the exceptions are not of a kind calculated to undermine the principle.... They are defective human beings who look and are physically constructed like men, but are only marginally or by a sort of prudent and humane courtesy fully human beings."[87] The idea underlying modern pathology, that on intellectual grounds some apparently human creatures differ from genuinely human ones in kind rather than by degree, has distant roots in Avempace's remarks about ignorance noted above. The understanding that understands the understanding is a form of knowledge with a basis in human nature; "the understanding *is born* to abstract it," it is something "we are born *as men* to know" (emphasis added). But because these early philosophers still maintained a strict category

---

[84] Pierre de la Ramée, *Dialectique*, 65.
[85] *Commentarium Magnum*, 490; 493.
[86] Al-Farabi, cited by Albert in *Summa de Creaturis*, 516.
[87] Anthony Quinton, "Has man an essence?" in R.S. Peters (ed.), *Nature and Conduct*.

boundary between nature and essence, they did not think of "natural" defects as challenging an individual's essence, or as we might say his species membership. The human understanding could be dispositionally impaired by corrupt intelligibles, but it was not corrupt in itself, in its underlying substantial core (*secundum substantiam*).

Despite Averroes, however, and despite the scholastics' continuing insistence on the equality of rational souls, the exclusion of some individuals from the category "man" was early on at least hypothetically conceivable. Anxiety emerged in spite of doctrine. The solution to such tensions lay as usual in a proliferation of terms. Differences between people could exist in the rational soul as *substance*, said Aquinas, without their having to be of the soul's *essence*. This influenced later doctrine, trapped as it was between notions of creaturely equality and the evident individual differences in the everyday vocations and abilities required by increasingly complex social organization. Manual labourers, with their apparent lack of wit, were said to be *substantially* on a par with animals, but their rational soul was *essentially* not in question: it was imputed to them as species members, even if they did not in fact as individuals possess it, let alone use or perform it. Moreover, it continued to be maintained that ethical qualities were no less important than intellectual ones, and that "man" was in no way an equivocal term anywhere outside of philosophy, including those areas (physiognomics, for example) where assessments of people were made and judgements passed.[88]

Renaissance commentators on *On the Soul* revived the issue of "equivocal" creatures. The idea that natural intellectual defects might pose problems of species membership coincided with the increasing tendency to emphasize the operations, concrete and observable, over the vague and static faculties. The Goclenian psychology school resisted this tendency, attacking the mistaken belief that "man is not truly man unless he exhibits human actions."[89] However, even the Goclenians were by now conceding that in principle the rational soul was corruptible. Some of them restricted their examples of this to conventional ones (old age, drunkenness, melancholy), which posed no challenge to such people's essential humanity because they did not describe a permanent identity.[90] The question of whether the rational soul was corruptible could be sidestepped by talking about such defects merely as secondary symptoms of original sin.[91] However, some members of the school went further with their concessions, turning defects of the mind from dismissible "accidents" into troubling "essences" of their own that existed from birth to death.

Georg Nagel, for example, writes about deficiency as originating in the bodiless "intellectual nature" of the foetus. Not only is the phrase a novel one in this sense (previously "intellectual nature" had been no more than a synonym for "angel"), intellectual *nature* here is identified with man's species *essence*. Göckel's argument for the immortality of the soul was that it possesses perfectible intellectual operations leading through "the steps of the operations of the understanding" to abstraction at the top, where the understanding's "reflection upon itself" finally comes to lie "above the matter of nature."[92] In Nagel, however, essence and nature coalesce. This arose from the need to make an accommodation, to think about the possibility that God and the parents are joint authors of the rational soul. While God was responsible for the child's essence, says Nagel, father and mother were responsible for its nature.[93] In extreme cases, deficiency might be the result of "some equivocal act of generation" – bestial sex, for example – "in which cause and effect relate

---

[88] Agrimi, *Ingeniosa*, 77.
[89] Licetus, *Ψυχολογια*, 216.
[90] Johann Gryn, *Utrum Anima Hominis Sit ex Traduce*, 57; 104, in Göckel, *Psychologia*.
[91] Highmore, *The History*, 12.
[92] Göckel, *Psychologia*.
[93] Nagel, *Ψυχολογια*, C3v.

to different species," a natural event in which "the name 'man' has become disjoined from the essence" it is supposed to denote. Nagel knew that regurgitating old dogma about God being sole author of the rational soul would no longer do. And with this concession came a rephrasing of what it meant to be human.

Another commentator on *On the Soul*, Antonius Ruvius, argued against the equality of rational souls on the grounds that otherwise you could not say Christ's soul was more perfect than a Jew's.[94] Even Albert, says Ruvius, at least posed it as a question whether "all souls are equal from creation, or some more excellent than others," since "some are said to excel others in natural gifts, or are more subtle than others in essence, and at understanding and remembering more easily, with a sharper wit (*ingenium*) and more perceptive understanding (*intellectus*)." What Albert had in fact said was that man is an "equivocal" term because of the variation in "theoretical abilities."[95] However, he regarded all these variations as "accidental"; they were part of the "disposition and organization of [bodily] material" and therefore of the secondary "operations," rather than of the faculty as such. Ruvius claims to agree with Albert, saying that such differences are always "in degree, not in species." But there is an ambiguity in the casual way he identifies "natural gifts" with "essence," in the above. This overturns the scholastic principle by which essence is so definitive a category that it takes more than the superficiality of an accident or even a contradiction in nature to alter it. Referring to the numerical expression of equivocal difference, Ruvius continues:

> I would say that an individual difference is not distinguished by its possessing a separate essence in a real sense, nor does it arise from the nature of the thing, but simply has some foundation in that singular thing. On the other hand this foundation is itself a real nature, a substance which is produced out of the ordinary course of events and in which certain essential elements are exhibited that constitute a specific essence; and from this real entity numerical or individual difference may be assumed, in the sense that one individual item (*individuum*) differs from another by virtue of this real entity, which exists as substance and which it possesses as distinct from the real entity of another, and indeed from this entity the essential elements of one thing are numerically distinct from those of another .... Hence the items can easily be distinguished from each other as inequal degrees of a substantial, individual perfection. So why can there not be inequalities in the specific essence or distinct species, by which the different souls of that species may be rated?

In short, Ruvius wants it both ways. There is a nod here to the old Aristotelian convention that intellectual variation among humans is accidental, but he undermines it by equating accident with "difference" (*differentia*, a stricter demarcation than "accident" in the old system). Inequalities of the rational soul or mind are turned here into quasi-real essences, a species-type difference which Ruvius knows from the basic doctrine ("Man is a rational animal") he ought not to be able to get away with.

Since an "equivocal" term implied uncertainty about the species membership of some individuals, it became entangled with the debate about nominalism. The possible kinship between equivocalism and nominalism was recognized by late medieval writers of a scientific bent such as Duns Scotus and William of Ockham,[96] and regarded as dangerous. Then with the emergence of early modern biological notions of species, it no longer mattered whether our definitions of species essences were real or nominal because they could be handled *as if* they were real, but with a get-out clause in the case of anomalies. Real essences might exist, but they were simply unknowable as

---

[94] *Commentarii*, 92; 98.
[95] Albert, *De Anima*, 12.
[96] See Amos Funkenstein, *Theology and the Scientific Imagination*.

such to mortal minds; Locke's "nominal essences," which might not or indeed *might* correspond to real ones, worked well enough as a way of classifying nature, or of approximating to it. As we noted earlier, the modesty of modern biologists about the nominalist basis of their species classifications is false. They do not say, as their medieval forebears did, that they do not know universals or species essences but God does. The possibility of someone who really knows remains open. If not God, then who? The implication is that scientists do, however much they protest that science can only ever approximate to such knowledge. Modern nominalism is partly an appeal for obedience to the human authority of the expert, just as fourteenth-century nominalism was often an appeal for obedience to the expert authority of the Pope: an appeal to certainty of a socially enforceable kind, in lieu of any other. In natural history's central case study, man, "nominal essences" formed the basis on which human authority could say what man is, thereby smuggling back a realist or essentialist agenda and enabling experts on the mind to establish surer boundaries to categories of difference.

In debates about human nature, equivocalism and nominalism alike provided the flexibility needed for tackling the contradiction between the species-wide equality of rational souls before God and increasingly important social differences in "intellectual" (vocational and professional) ability among individual species members. Some writers sought to refute both -isms as a "sophistic" response to a problem unnecessarily posed.[97] Others found them useful. Baxter, for example, posed an antithesis between "real" and "equivocal" ways of classifying the elect and of distinguishing them from the reprobate; lacking divine omniscience, we make judgements about people that are "equivocal only" (he might as easily have said "nominal only").[98] For equivocalism or nominalism here, read humility; we cannot ultimately know who is reprobate. It may well be via this theological tradition, as much as any philosophical one, that the rather less humble Locke reached his own definition of man, from whose "nominal essence" he excludes those creatures he classifies as intellectually disabled changelings. His definition of "man" in the relevant passage of the *Essay* is almost verbatim that of Baxter, as we shall see in the next chapter.

If the doctrine whereby exceptions are mere accidents and do not contradict man's species essence was by now collapsing, this was partly because it had seemed a philosophy of low expectations. If it is true that defects do not matter, how can man aspire to something better – to an angelic intellectual perfection, if not membership of Mensa? In its developed form, equivocalism turned what had formerly been accidental into something essentially different, and transformed certain individuals into a pathological type. The question as to whether one rational soul might be less perfect than another had hardly arisen earlier because "soul" and "intellect" were notionally separate entities; there were "intellectual" variations, but these could be put down as facets of the sensitive soul, with its links to the body. Mind/body dualism subsequently enabled the soul in Locke's changeling to be not *differentiated* but entirely *absent*: a numerical subtraction from what makes us human.

By the mid-seventeenth century, this equivocalist model of intellectual difference was being used to mediate the dispute between traducianists and infusionists over the origins of the rational soul. In the 1640s Browne, seeking a compromise, wrote about "equivocal and monstrous productions in the conjunction of man with beast."[99] The existence of such creatures, he says, favours the traducianist argument, since the small amount of reason these monsters do possess must have come from the human parent; they are not "merely beasts, but have also an impression and tincture of reason in as high a measure as it can evidence itself in those improper organs."

---

[97] Da Thiene, *Super Libros de Anima Aristotelis*, 6v.
[98] Letter to John Humfrey, 7 December 1654.
[99] Browne, *Religio*, 41.

Woolnor, Browne's contemporary, likewise sought "to prove ... that the production of man's soul is neither by [divine] creation nor [human] propagation but a certain mean way between both."[100] His premise ran:

> Propagation ... is that most excellent and natural faculty whereby a living creature, by seed of generation, begets his like for the continuation of the kind ..., univocal which is most properly so called when as a creature brings forth the like to itself ... and equivocal [when there is] generation of unlike, as when a plant or living creature is bred of putrefaction, as mice, flies, serpents and the like, for the continuation of the kind.

Then, narrowing the discussion down to equivocal humans:

> Not nature alone, but the efficient power of God is joined with the propagation of souls, because it is wholly denied to such copulations as are out of kind. For nature alone [i.e., by itself] would make a mixture, whereas notwithstanding we see that some kind of creatures ... which ... were at first begotten by such unkindly conjunctions, are not endowed with reasonable souls. Or if not they, yet it is possible that human seed should be mingled with other creatures (for which cause buggery is forbidden in the law), and yet such issue is altogether soulless and void of reason.

He then concludes, insulting his opponents with the customary transferred epithet, that writers "make a monstrous and profane mingle-mangle that would have man propagate his like by the power of nature merely, as other creatures do." If parents were sole authors of the rational soul, the whole world would consist of such mixed-up creatures, thereby defying the fixity of species. But if God were sole author, then he would be responsible for producing intellectual monsters and would thus (impossibly) be the cause of something profane. It was the negotiated avoidance of these two ideological extremes, dogmatic traducianism and dogmatic infusionism, that gave rise to the concept of reasonless offspring of reasoning human parents: Locke's changeling, later our "intellectually disabled" person. The theory of parental causation gained a new degree of respectability on its arrival at the negotiating table. As well as preparing the way for a recognizably modern biological explanation of inherited intelligence, it brought with it a revised doctrine of pollution by introducing buggery and/or the Devil into the discussion, and with them parental dishonour and guilt: an entirely novel chimera that would penetrate deeply the mind-set of later centuries.

---

[100] *The True Originall*, 181; 316.

PART 8
John Locke and His Successors

Chapter 18
John Locke and His Successors: the Historical Contingency of Disability

Locke's *Essay concerning Human Understanding* has been a recurring reference because it is the junction between early modern and modern, and because of his reputation as a founding father. The sixteenth and seventeenth centuries were an age of apocalyptic obsession; Locke marks not so much its demise as its secularization into a modern vision of progress and ultimate intellectual Revelation. We look now at the immediate influences on Locke, from English Puritans to French Cartesians and Jansenists, and then at the subsequent influence of his own psychology and logic on eighteenth- and nineteenth-century educational and behavioural prescriptions. We shall see in particular how his work demonstrates the historical contingency of the modern concept; his "idiots," "changelings" and "natural fools" are discrete entities arising from disparate political and theological contexts, despite the temptation to see them as interchangeable. Moreover, other phases of his career are devoid of the anxiety that surrounds these terms in the *Essay*.

Idiots and abstraction

Locke's account of idiots in Book 2 of the *Essay* is bound up with contemporary debates about the status of animals. He tackles human species difference in terms of abstraction. "Brutes abstract not" was his final word on the place of humans in the scale of nature. He was responding in part to sceptics such as Montaigne and Charron, who had refused to rank human behaviour above that of other animals. Following the widely publicized heresy trial of Daniel Sennert, who claimed that the souls of humans and beasts were alike, France had seen a great debate about animal psychology, which Locke encountered during his stay there in the late 1670s. The sceptics never seriously suggested that there should be *no* demarcation line. They merely said that brutes, while not completely lacking human-type operations, perform them more imperfectly. In any case, this was not some early form of modern comparative psychology but a faith-based doctrine about the vanity of supposing that human beings can have certain knowledge – the certainty that Descartes had been seeking to re-establish with his doctrine that animals are mere automata.

Locke's phrase thus also calls for the emphasis, "Brutes *abstract* not." We know there must be something they do not do, but what is it? The Platonists said that animals have souls but no divine illumination. The Gassendists said they have a corporeal soul but not a rational one. Descartes said they do not have *cogitatio* or souls at all. The author at the centre of the French debate, the Jesuit scientist Ignace-Gaston Pardies, rejected animal automatism, saying that animals have some aptitude for reason, but that humans alone possess the higher operations of the mind.[1] Locke refers to Pardies in his notebooks (drafts of the *Essay* dating from before his stay in France had not mentioned animal psychology). But where Pardies identified these higher operations with the innate "common ideas," Locke takes an empirical approach, building from the bottom up. Although he

---

[1] Ignace-Gaston Pardies, *Discours de la conoissance des bestes*.

retains the faculties as an underlying structure, his main focus is on the active operations "*exercised about* our ideas" (emphasis added). On the bottom rung of these operations stands perception. It is this, "in the lowest degree of it, which puts the boundaries between animals and the inferior ranks of creatures." On the next rung up is retention (divided into contemplation and memory), which is simply "secondary perception"; by this reckoning "intellectual creatures" still include songbirds. Next comes comparing: "How far brutes partake in this faculty, is not easy to determine; I imagine they have it not in any great *degree*" (emphasis added), leaving the door still ajar for the sceptics' denial of a difference in kind. Likewise, in composition and enlarging, "brutes come far short of men." Only in arriving at abstraction does Locke finally bang the door shut: "This I think I may be positive in, that the power of abstracting is not *at all* in [brutes]; and that the having of general ideas is that which puts a perfect distinction betwixt man and brute" (emphasis added).[2] Jonathan Edwards glossed Locke's account of abstraction by referring to it as "the peculiar, inimitable and unparalleled exercise of the glorious power of God" which grace produces in man. Edwards's view of what Locke meant was not far from the truth. It expresses the theological core of Locke's natural history of a specifically human mind, which he transmitted to modern psychology.[3]

Locke asserts that brutes do not abstract on implicitly nominalist grounds: *any* creature that has "no use of words, or any other general signs" must be a "brute." Not all nominalists placed such value on abstraction. Bacon, for example, saw it as implying a realist theory of universal kinds; it was a purely speculative Idol of the Tribe, blocking out "the light of experiment" and fixing that which should fluctuate – whereas for Locke it is what lets the light in, shining on what would otherwise be a chaos of "endless names." Gassendi too viewed abstraction more favourably. Like Locke, he saw it as the drawing of common or universal ideas from particular ones received empirically through the senses; unlike Locke, however, he also saw it as a matching of the imagination to the understanding, with image and concept becoming as one. This necessitated a further operation, responsible for making adjustments between the two faculties: namely ratiocination, which he ranks *above* abstraction.[4] Locke realized that if nothing is universal except names, then this separate ratiocinative stage is redundant. If words are "signs," so too are ideas themselves. That is why for Locke deaf people, whose full humanity many previous writers had considered doubtful because they could not discern words, are intellectually complete. We know "real existences" only and precisely by sorting their corresponding *ideas* from each other and giving them names. Abstraction is this denominating process. In this doctrine, abstraction (something the human mind does) takes over the role which scholasticism had allocated to universals (which are said to inhere in real objects outside the mind).[5]

It is only Locke's idiots that are capable of showing how important abstraction in the above sense is. If brutes do not have it, it is not relevant to them and no problem arises. What happens, though, if some of the creatures who ought to be able to abstract do not do so? Nominalism throws up the same problems as social administration. Difference comes alive where there are borderline cases. Decisions have to be made. If to be human is to abstract, where do we put the non-abstractor in human shape? According to the *Essay*, the idiot "scarcely reasons or puts ideas together at all .... [He] cannot distinguish, compare and abstract." Locke hovers short of making idiots non-human (here at least, though a different tone will be used for changelings). Nevertheless, it is his final remarks on the specific difference between humans and brutes that trigger his account of idiots, showing a train of thought from one to the other:

---

[2] *An Essay*, 143 ff.
[3] Edwards, *A Treatise*, 241.
[4] Gassendi, "Syntagma philosophicum," in *Opera Omnia*, 325b.
[5] Ayers, *Locke*, i, 246.

> [Brutes] are the best of them tied up within those narrow bounds, and have not (as I think) the faculty to enlarge them by any kind of abstraction. How far idiots are concerned in the want or weakness of any, or all of the foregoing faculties, an exact observation of their several ways of faltering, would no doubt discover. For those who either perceive but dully, or retain the ideas that come into their minds but ill, who cannot readily excite or compound them, will have little matter to think on. Those who cannot distinguish, compare, and abstract, would hardly be able to understand, and make use of language, or judge, or reason to any tolerable degree but only a little, and imperfectly, about things present, and very familiar to their senses.[6]

Abstraction is not a feature of "man the rational animal" but of individual rational men. One can therefore learn something about how it works in the majority by studying those individuals who are more or less disabled from doing it. And indeed, the exactness of observation of the "several," i.e., specifically different ways of faltering in the disabled subject would form the core of modern psychology's approach to intelligence.

The passage above seems to point to a difference of degree rather than kind. Locke's definition of the idiot here is poised here between the old sense of uneducated or uncultured and the "naturals" or born fools whom he mentions in the very next paragraph; idiots and naturals are not synonymous, but there is leakage from one type into the other, their common bond still underwritten by original sin. To seek coherence in Locke's treatment of idiocy, as if to him it were a psychological object, is misplaced. It is instrumental to his main aim, which is to refute the theory of innate ideas and show that knowledge is acquired in the first instance from sense data. In order to do so, he takes Aristotle's standard example of senility and expands it into one of birth-to-death personhood:

> Take one, in whom decrepit old age has blotted out the memory of his past knowledge, and clearly wiped out the ideas his mind was formerly stored with .... How far such an one (notwithstanding all that is boasted of innate principles) is in his knowledge, and intellectual faculties, above the condition of a cockle, or an oyster, I leave to be considered. And if a man had passed sixty years in such a state, as 'tis possible he might, as well as three days, I wonder what difference there would have been, in any intellectual perfections, between him, and the lowest degree of animals.[7]

As so often, the invention of idiots seems to be a device for answering some other problem; here they are mere cannon fodder in Locke's anti-innatist attack. Nevertheless the "man" in his last sentence, positioned so low as to be in the interstice between animal and vegetable, is for Locke more than a philosophical hypothesis; he is an empirically observed creature, posing social and ethical problems in the real world.

In Book 1, he has lumped idiots with a broader group that encompasses children, savages, the illiterate, Indians, "wild men of the woods" (something like Albert's pygmies), along with "at least one half of mankind" in whom innate principles and common ideas are scarcely evident: that is, the unlearned masses. But he also identifies the term with that more restricted group of congenital natural fools ("naturals"), who of all the subgroups carry the ultimate burden of the anti-innatist proof:

> It might be very well expected, that innate principles should be perfectly known to naturals; which being stamped immediately on the soul (as these men suppose) can have no dependence on the constitutions, or organs of the body, the only confessed difference between them and others .... But alas, amongst children, idiots, savages, and the grossly [sc. generally] illiterate, what general maxims are to be found? What universal principles of knowledge?[8]

---

[6] *An Essay*, 155.
[7] Ibid., 148.
[8] *An Essay*, 63.

This list closely corresponds to an almost identical one in the much earlier *Essays on the Law of Nature*, where in the place later occupied by "idiots" the word is *indocti*, "uneducated"; in the same work he also uses "deprived of their senses" (*mente capti*) – an old legal term that covered madness in general. Thus one and the same anti-innatist point can be conveyed by a multiplicity of partly overlapping usages.

In the section on retention and memory there is also a discussion of what we would now call information processing. His account of impressions and of defects in the reception and retrieval of information displays the influence of earlier writers. Descartes had used a similar vocabulary to Locke's when he described how the pineal gland links mind to body; it radiates the soul spirits around the brain until they find the track that represents the relevant impressions that have previously been "stamped" there. Willis, Locke's former physiology lecturer, wrote about brain function in the same way, as we have seen. Locke himself avoids any detailed discussion of physiology or of "how much the constitution of our bodies, and the make of our animal spirits, are concerned in this." All we know is that the tracking varies in efficiency from one person to the next. Deficits are therefore explained by a spectrum model: they differ by degree. In this context the idiot is merely the "dull man," prone to "stupidity," who is none the less human ("one man [as] compared with another").[9] Locke's tone here is quite different from the one he uses for changelings, who clearly differ from the rest of us, not by degree but in kind. We should note, however, that the "natural fools" who in Books 1 and 2 stand in for idiots, in Books 3 and 4 also stand in for changelings. All this should be a warning that Locke has no unified theory of disability, and that a writer whom this book has so far set up to be the villain of the piece may indeed be a more complex character.

Changelings and logical reasoning

Locke uses the term "changeling" to denote a creature in human physical form, born of human parents, which does not have the mind or soul that defines someone as human. By the mid-eighteenth century, the changeling had become a routine usage for someone with a so-called intellectual disability in a sense partly recognizable to the modern reader. Locke uses "changeling" rather than "idiot" when he is discussing natural history rather than faculty psychology (to put it another way, when the context is theological rather than philosophical). By the end of the seventeenth century, natural history was not only a project for clearer definitions of species but, encouraged by contemporary geographical exploration, for the discovery of *more* species.[10] One ought to consider, says Locke, whether the "drivelling, unintelligent, intractable changeling" might not be an additional, interstitial species between humans and other animals, perhaps on a par with "drills" (baboons) or even lower.[11]

Locke's changeling challenged two old Aristotelian conventions. The first of these was that the criterion for human species membership is to have human parents. Locke rejects the idea that the species membership of offspring is ultimately determined by the "originals … to which, by their descent, they seem to belong." Children often differed from their parents in terms of their wit and behaviour. His friend Penn instanced "wild" offspring born of "sober" parents and "religious" of "debauched" ones: evidence that over and above behavioural differences there was in every or nearly every individual an equal and rational soul, of which God, not the parents,

---

[9] Ibid., 153.
[10] For example Glanvill, "Of the modern improvements of useful knowledge," 29, in *Essays*.
[11] *An Essay*, 569.

was ultimate author.[12] Locke's view of the soul, so far, is compatible with the theory of divine infusion, though also (in the case of changelings) with the occasional involvement of the Devil, that other praeternatural originator, with his skills in natural magic and his employment of *incubi* and *succubi* as assistants. The changeling in this sense suits the Royal Society's aim of using mechanical philosophy to authenticate spiritual phenomena.[13] Locke's reticence about angels and the Devil in the *Essay* may well have been due as much to his determination to couch it in ordinary language as to actual disbelief; as we noted in an earlier chapter, scepticism about both was more characteristic of the seventeenth-century layman than of the great intellects.

The second convention which Locke challenged was the generic "man is a rational animal." Changelings resemble the human animal physically but lack the mind of one; they are born of rational parents – "covenanted" parents, to use Owen's theological expression of a similar thought – but are not rational themselves.[14] Locke's criterion for excluding them from the human species is their inability to reason, in the terms of the new logic as Locke himself conceives it. The term "changeling" is the right one, he says, because it is an example of plain and "civil" (public) language, by contrast with the existing abstruse Aristotelian classifications of the natural world. From this we might infer that he chose it because it was already an everyday word for someone with an "intellectual" disability. However, as we saw in Chapter 16, it was neither ordinary nor everyday, nor had it till then referred to anything intellectual or cognitive in terms recognizable to ourselves. Behind its entry into Locke's vocabulary lay a whole new role for reason. The sudden intrusion of this term may even have come from an expert consensus of some kind, perhaps as part of the Royal Society's project for a new terminological system in natural history. Bishop Jeremy Taylor, who was close to its founders, wrote a "prayer to be used in behalf of fools or changelings" in which their synonymity is clearly indicated, by contrast with Fuller's behavioural guide of a few years earlier which had insisted on quite separate meanings. The church, too, had previously had a standard "changeling" prayer, a warning to church members to remain unchanging in their faith and quite distinct from prayers such as "Upon the sight of a natural [fool]" which had a quite different moral ("O God, why am I not thus?").[15] Susceptible to the new focus on reason in religion, Taylor now defined fool and changeling alike, as creatures with "life, and no understanding."

The pathology of Locke's changeling bears similarities to that of the reprobate. When he criticizes the classification of children by the species membership of their parents and says that they do not necessarily inherit their parents' "rational" status, he employs exactly the same terms as Baxter when the latter criticizes the classification of children as elect just because their parents are hypothetically elect "church members." Furthermore, Baxter had asked who was so "dead in Christ" that they might not have even the hope of regeneration, and concluded that it was "idiots." Locke makes exactly the same point, in the same format, about changelings:

> It may as rationally be concluded, that the dead body of a man, wherein there is to be found no more appearance or action of life, than there is in a statue, has yet … a living soul in it, because of its shape; as that there is a rational soul in a changeling, because he has the outside of a rational creature, when his actions carry far less marks of reason with them, in the whole course of his life, than what are to be found in many a beast. But 'tis the issue of rational parents, and must therefore be concluded to have a rational soul. I know not by what logic you must so conclude.[16]

---

[12] Ibid., 448; Penn, *The New Witnesses*, ii, 158.
[13] See Shapin, *The Scientific Revolution*, 155.
[14] Owen, *Of Infant Baptism and Dipping*.
[15] Taylor, *The Whole Works*, xv, 355; Joseph Hall, *Works*, x, 141.
[16] *An Essay*, 571.

A human being's external shape could not be more important than the "internal perfections of the soul." Locke purified religion of the excess baggage which Baxter's work contained, but the core remains intact.

Implicit in this discussion about parents and children is an opposition between two ways of classifying the universal, "man." Locke's view was that universals, being nominal, originate in the internal processes of abstraction (in the human mind); the opposite view was that, being real and knowable, they exist in the external world (in human morphology). Through the operations of abstraction and logical reasoning, the human subject arrives at the truth about his objective place in the scale of nature; and he does so, necessarily, via the denial of rationality to some other creature with a *prima facie* claim to it that turns out to be false. The person who thinks that mere physiological externals are definitive of the human is himself deficient, in both senses of "rationality" here: both in his psychological operations and in the common ideas to which those operations should lead. To deny the necessity of changelings is to have changeling-like characteristics oneself. Changelings are unable to do the new logical reasoning, but the new logical reasoning also requires all (rational) men to nominate Locke's changelings as the creatures unable to do it. The changeling's difference is one of essence rather than mere accident, thereby excluding it from the species "man." Does it then, like that other spuriously human creature the reprobate, have a soul? Luther's recently translated *Table Talk* had implied the answer No. Locke agrees. Neither his logic nor his theory of nominal essences, nor above all his claim that the defining element of the human lies in certain precise intellectual operations, could exist without such a creature.

To grasp this fully, one needs to know that Locke thought of the *Essay* as a guide to logic ("another sort of logic," in his own phrase) and that it was regarded as such by contemporaries and for the next hundred years. This was part of a broader trend. The French Cartesian Pierre-Sylvain Régis, born in the same year as Locke, published in the same year as the *Essay* his own *Cours entier de philosophie*, which he likewise describes as a "logic" book and which gives pride of place to abstraction. The same is true of Joachim Hildebrand's 1680 text (cited earlier), which claimed that logic and abstraction could prove the immortality of the soul "by the light of nature alone."

The core doctrine of logic in the *Essay* comes in the chapter entitled "Reason," with which logic is more or less synonymous.[17] Locke, complaining that the old notion of the syllogism was a jumble, promotes instead his own account of the way logical reasoning unfolds. It does so as a "train of ideas," which in spirit if not to the letter resembles Baxter's temporally ordered contemplation. Locke's primary illustration of a correct train of ideas is drawn from debates over predestination: "Let this be the proposition laid down, 'men shall be punished in another world,' and from thence be inferred this other: 'then men can determine themselves'." What is at issue, so far, seems to be the mechanics of the logic rather than its truth content, which the anti-predestinarian Locke already takes for granted. He continues: "The question now is to know, whether the mind has made this inference right or no; if it has made it by finding out the intermediate ideas, and taking a view of the connexion of them, placed in a due order, it has proceeded rationally, and made a right inference." In this illustration, he says, it has. But in fact the presupposed truth content of the propositions leaks into the inferential mechanism of the logic. If it is true that (as the inference runs) men can determine themselves, they can do so only and precisely by means of this subjective ability of theirs to find out the intermediate ideas and put them in the right logical order in the train, since man is presupposed to be precisely the kind of creature who can do that.

This short circuit created a basis not only for the modern classification of the human species by an intelligence defined in terms of logical trains of ideas, but also for modern systems of

---

[17] *An Essay*, 668 ff.

logic-based species classification right across nature, inasmuch as the latter have always begun from the difference between human and other animals (that is, from the superior abilities of one species above the rest). In fact such systems are in turn the projection on to nature of a social and religious judgement about the status of some men in relation to others. Without the changeling, who "reasons scarcely or not at all" and is therefore not a man, the modern-looking concept of intelligence as logical reasoning, apparently definitive of the human species but actually definitive of the group defining itself as the intelligence society, could not exist. Nor, and this is crucial, could the species or the society develop. It is here that Locke cites Hooker's regret that human beings in general lack adequate reasoning skills, and that if only we had them, our descendants might thereafter progress in their religion to be as far ahead of us as we are now of fools or innocents. It is the right ambition, says Locke, but too pessimistically expressed. And that is because Elizabethans like Hooker still saw logic as consisting of innate syllogisms, bound to a divine reason. Trains of ideas will do the trick instead. People who develop trains of ideas on an empirical basis do so autonomously; they are not determined by others as changelings are, and can therefore develop personally, each as individual species members.

Locke's concept of logical trains of ideas was influenced by his own medical practice. In the four years up to 1671, when he began the first draft of the *Essay*, he and Thomas Sydenham were pioneering an approach (novel for the time) of empirical, observation-based case studies of the body, in which the physician examines how one symptom leads to the next: a train of symptoms, as it were. One might similarly trace how one idea leads to the next; for "ideas" in psychology, read "symptoms" in physical medicine.[18] In Locke's well-known theory about wrong association of ideas, expounded in the logic sections of the *Essay*, a correct *association* is also a correct *train*. One idea leads to the next; a wrong association is not a train at all, it is a sideways jump. Again, Locke refers in his introductory remarks to the parallel "trains of [bodily] motion" in the soul spirits. Descartes, Willis and Malebranche all described how soul spirits "by their continual course open out pathways [in the brain], so that with time they no longer encounter resistance," as evidence that intellectual operations vary among individuals according to their personal physiological history.[19] In some people, the pathways have run askew. For Descartes the parallel was between physiological defect and bad moral habits rather than bad logical moves; for Locke, however, the moral just *is* the logical.

Locke's fusion of the moral and the logical is clear in the way he merges the type of changeling so far discussed with a second type, where the same term is used to describe atheist libertines. Here he defends himself against the established church's charge that his concept of liberty, as freedom from episcopal and monarchical coercion, is an Antinomian-type freedom to do whatever one pleases. He relies for his answer here on Samuel Bolton's widely read text of 1645, *The True Bounds of Christian Freedom*. Libertine changelings fall short of species membership by exactly the same criterion as non-reasoning ones; they too are "determined," in this case by their pleasures and perverse wills. Locke's advocacy of religious and political toleration invited the accusation that he was stopping people from being determined by the wisdom of their ecclesiastical and political betters. His response was that one does not have to think of being free as the opposite of being determined. Libertine-type changelings illustrated the point: as the stock Puritan saying went, "libertinism is true bondage." Otherwise "nature should in vain have given us the use of reason, to discourse or to consult, or the ability to will or choose any thing." Locke compares this libertine changeling with his new, idiotic one, incapable not only of rational choice but of choice of

---

[18] Locke, *Of the Conduct of the Understanding*, 40.
[19] Malebranche, *De la recherche de la vérité*, i, 157; see also Willis (above, Chapter 14) and Descartes, *Passions of the Soul*, 1.7.

any kind. No autonomous individual reasoner, he says, would actively seek to be "less determined" by wise thoughts just so that he could consider himself free. Libertine changelings only *seem* to have freedom of will; in fact their "liberty" means that they too are totally determined by the flesh, and just like the idiotic kind have "no thought, no volition" of their own.[20]

Hence the changeling void of conscience and the changeling void of logical reasoning are overlapping types, the necessary residue of original sin in Locke's otherwise progressivist argument: more Luther's corrupt mass of flesh than Descartes's automative body or beast-machine. God does not excuse either type. Locke's logical proposition about "punishment in another world" is a religious one, but an intellectual type of disability too is implied there, since inability to abstract meant an inability to choose between good and evil; that is how contemporaries would have understood the concept. The difference between the libertine type and the intellectual type is that punishment of the latter is displaced from the afterlife to here and now. Just as Locke's "intellectual perfections" offer the fruits of election already in this life, so the intellectual disability of the idiot, and particularly the changeling, becomes a form of earthly suffering. Others close to the early Royal Society, such as Jeremy Taylor and Kenelm Digby, took the opposite tack. The Catholic Digby, invoking the notion of the holy innocent, suggests that changelings' souls are purer than others'; the Anglican Taylor, in his prayer, likewise suspects that changelings "do not deserve hell so much as we have done."[21] They are the optimistic corollary to Locke, within an overall ethics of exceptionalism.

Alongside this use of a new logic in the burgeoning human sciences came a new rhetoric, which contributed equally to Locke's changeling. Rhetoric and logic were always closely associated, "the open hand and the closed fist." Royal Society members reacted early on against the humanist style of rhetoric derived from Cicero. Wilkins's first published work *Ecclesiastes* had been a polemic against the Ciceronians' over-elaborate language, and recommended a single basic style for both preaching and science. Boyle in particular, in a work written in the 1650s that went through several subsequent editions, asserted that the plainness of scriptural prose was a better model for disseminating Christian and scientific values. A biblical, "plain" style might demonstrate God's great work of nature as clearly as it already revealed the Word. Plain language was as intrinsic to the new, simplified logic as Ciceronian floweriness had been to the over-elaborate categories of the old Aristotelian logic. Plain language also helped to create a new out-group, as Boyle reveals when he extends his experimentalist approach to psychology and the faculties. The "style of the scripture" and "the [human] understanding," he says, are interpenetrative, and this style operates upon "the generality of its readers, if they be not faultily disposed to receive impressions from it."[22] In the socio-political context of the 1650s, plain style was the ideal method for weaning the great unwashed, caught up in political processes previously closed to them, away from their dangerous sectarian enthusiasms. The Bible has a transforming effect on readers and so, muses Boyle, its plainness of style may help the common reader – literate commoners – to understand nature. The Royal Society set great store by exposing their scientific practice to a wider public than the alchemists and other occultists did. The greater part of mankind may "have not that quickness which is wont to make men pass for wits, though they may have other abilities more solid, and desirable …. And yet the Bible has a great influence upon this latter sort of intelligent readers," a group which Boyle says might extend downwards socially even as far as the self-educated ploughman. The redrawing of social categories implied in the above passage creates a new

---

[20] *An Essay*, 265.
[21] Digby, *Of Bodies*, ii, 10.
[22] Robert Boyle, *Some Considerations Touching the Style of the Holy Scriptures*, cited in Wilbur Howell, *Eighteenth Century British Logic*, 470.

exclusion, the "faultily indisposed." These are no longer everyone beyond the honour society but that much smaller group whom the Honourable Robert Boyle, second Earl of Cork, distinguishes here from the "generality" of the commons. Crediting the latter with some higher understanding was a wise move for his own honour and the intellectual and scientific trustworthiness it entailed, since the first Earl, his father, had himself been plebeian, a convicted fraudster who had notoriously used the proceeds to buy his title.

The smaller group of "faultily indisposed" will reappear in starker form in 1690 as Locke's changelings. He discusses the plain style, cultivated throughout the *Essay* itself, in the chapter entitled "The Abuse of Words," where he stresses the importance of fixing the right names for ideas.[23] Rhetoric as much as logic helps to explain the difference between a "man," a "drill" and "a monstrous foetus." Plain style demands the most appropriate words for "things as they really are." A flowery style encourages evasiveness: why not just call a spade a spade? "Changeling" describes the thing as it really is, in all its monstrosity. Moreover, it is no exaggeration to say that in Locke's overall scheme, the changeling is the *paradigm* of things as they really are. As his opening paragraphs announce, he will be proceeding by a "historical," that is, an investigative and empirically based "method" (the latter term being the signal that he is no Aristotelian). In the paragraph itself entitled "Method" he remarks: "It shall suffice to … consider the discerning faculties of a man, as they are employed about the objects, which they have to do with." And what object, he asks here, could one have to do with more important than man himself and that which defines him as man, his "understanding"? Like Boyle he targets the understanding of a putative general or common reader, whom he identifies with "native rustic reason": a calculated contradiction in terms, inasmuch as "native rustic" had previously always signified "born stupid," like a peasant or labourer.[24] Everyone, or nearly everyone, can do it. The psychological subject is about to be democratized – at the expense of changelings.

Changelings and their natural classification

Changelings are the supreme illustration of our uncertainty about real essences and about how individuals can be sorted into natural kinds. Boyle thought species should be sorted "as they deserve," that is, with as much precision as we can muster. Locke seems to go further and to mean "as we prefer."[25] His nominalist attack on the reality of species begins in Book 3 under the heading of "general terms" and "simple ideas." He is trying to pull off a difficult trick. He doubts whether the simple idea of something can refer to a "real essence" or species with secure boundaries; but at the same time he needs to maintain for species, and particularly for the human species, its proper place in a hierarchical scale of nature. Commentators treat Locke's nominalism as a lofty philosophical discussion about the status of universals in general, as if the idea of man were merely one among any number of possible illustrations in that debate.[26] But for Locke, what it is to be human was a unique problem. The only other extended illustration he uses is gold, another item of particular anxiety to him. It is true that his scholastic predecessors had also placed the human illustration at the centre of their logic and its related disciplines; realists in particular argued that if you could

---

[23] *An Essay*, 490 ff.

[24] Ibid., 679.

[25] Boyle, "The origins of forms and qualities according to the corpuscular philosophy," in M.A. Stewart (ed.), *Selected Philosophical Papers*, 49.

[26] Ruth Mattern, "Moral science and the concept of persons in Locke," *Philosophical Review*, 89/1 (1982); Evan Fales, "Natural kinds and freaks of nature," *Philosophy of Science*, 49 (1982).

not grasp that all individual, particular men are one in the species man, then you could not grasp that the several elements of the trinity are united in one God. What gives the human illustration in Locke an extra urgency is the intervening Calvinist anxiety about election and grace.

He starts out by establishing that "the common names of substances ... stand for sorts" and that the "boundary of each sort, or species whereby it is ... distinguished from others, is that we call its essence, which is nothing but that abstract idea to which the name is annexed: so that every thing contained in that idea, is essential to that sort."[27] The species "man" is not some metaphysical "mould" into which God somehow pours reason. In brief, a species is a "nominal essence." It is quite possible that real, "natural species, established by the author of nature," exist, but the material differences between them are unknowable to mere humans. There is nothing to prevent us from ranking these nominal essences hierarchically according to the scale of nature, just as if they were real ones. One can still identify and rank "perfections," it is just that one does not have to rank them according to their supposed underlying substances; the scale is simply one of valued attributes.[28] Nominal essences, perhaps because their correct definition depends on hard-won human consensus, make the hierarchy more rather than less rigid. Individual cases which seem to constitute exceptions to the human rule are no longer mere Aristotelian accidents, but sharply distinguishable from the species essence.

It is the quasi-human non-reasoners that lie at the heart of this system. They are the best possible illustration of the experimental utility of nominal essences. We "try the truth" of names by analyzing the complex ideas corresponding to them, and this will always throw up borderline cases:

> To say, that a rational animal is capable of conversation [*conversatio*, an operation of the reasoning faculty] is all one, as to say, a man. But no one will say, that rationality is capable of conversation, because it makes not the whole essence, to which we give the name man. There are creatures in the world, that have shapes like ours, but are hairy, and want language, and reason. There are naturals [sc. changelings] amongst us, that have perfectly our shape, but want reason, and some of them language too.[29]

There are also, it is reported, creatures *with* reason and language, physically unlike us because they have tails; "there are some brutes, that seem to have as much knowledge and reason, as some that are called men." However, it is the "naturals" who bear the main illustrative burden here. Locke rephrases the hierarchy of nature to fit his new account of essences:

> If it be asked, whether these be all men, or no, all of human species; 'tis plain, the question refers only to the nominal essence.... Shall the difference of hair only on the skin, be a mark of a different internal specific constitution between a changeling and a drill, when they agree in shape, and want of reason, and speech? And shall not the want of reason and speech, be a sign to us of different real constitutions and species, between a changeling, and a reasonable man? And so of the rest ....

Locke's library was full of travel literature featuring boundary crossers. He took notes from Gassendi's book on honour and nobility, which describes people who look human but when cut open have the guts and entrails of a sheep, and "in the greater Java, certain livewights of a middle nature between men and apes .... In Guinea, apes with long, grey, combed beards, almost venerable,

---

[27] *An Essay*, 438 ff.

[28] Ayers, "Mechanism, superaddition and the proof of God's existence in Locke's *Essay*", *Philosophical Review*, 50/2 (1981).

[29] *An Essay*, 450.

who stalk an alderman's pace and take themselves to be very wise."[30] This was not some sceptical Montaignian doctrine about a lack of discernible difference between human and animal behaviour. Locke is pursuing seriously his proposition that nominal essences are better boundary markers for sorting nature into a hierarchy of species than the futile ontological claims of the Aristotelians. Nominal essences lead to real knowledge as such, including real knowledge about humans, because they are "as capable of certainty, as mathematics." In fact they are even better than mathematical knowledge, which is merely the putting together of "such ideas as have no inconsistence." They are the approximation of ideas to "real existences of things" in nature.[31] The changeling and the drill (baboon) "agree in ... want of reason" not just for the sake of argument but because, as Locke says in his very next paragraph, "if history lie not, women have conceived by drills." Thus one cause of "absence of reason" in human-looking creatures was possibly bestial sex. (This was certainly Sterne's prurient reading of Locke, in *Tristram Shandy*.)[32]

To sum up, we "must ... renounce [our] sacred definition of *animal rationale*." We should, instead, "substitute some other essence of the human species." But how do nominal essences yield knowledge, if not of a realist kind? Locke replies that it is a process of making ever less inexact copies. Abstract ideas are first separated from their given names, then the names readjusted to the extent that one considers appropriate. This, and not Cartesian clarity, is how the ideas attached to real existences become "distinct" from each other. Moreover, it is just this activity that constitutes the most rarefied work the human intellect can do. On the one hand, there was justifiable anxiety about the chaos that might ensue from causing names to proliferate by this activity; as Montaigne had complained, "We change one word for another word, often more unknown. I know better what is man than I know what is animal, or mortal, or rational. To satisfy one doubt, they give me three."[33] On the other hand, says Locke, "If we rightly consider, and confine not our thoughts and abstract ideas to names, as if there were ... no other sorts of things, than what known names had already determined, ... we should think of things with greater freedom and less confusion, than perhaps we do." He seeks the middle ground. "Where men in society have already established a language amongst them, the signification of words are very warily and sparingly to be altered." Ambiguity can be tolerated most of the time. Nominal essences are thus a compromise between the moribund conservatism of real essences and a sectarian anarchy of excessive locutions. Language and classification should be renewed only where necessary, only for the sake of order.

Having established this general principle, Locke goes on to give his example of something that *does* currently require a readjusted naming scheme. And it just so happens to be that dubious creature who is defined as non-human by his inability to do readjustable naming:

> 'Twould possibly be thought a bold paradox, if not a very dangerous falsehood, if I should say, that some changelings, who have lived forty years together, without any appearance of reason, are something between a man and a beast. Which prejudice is founded upon nothing else but a false supposition, that these two names, man and beast, stand for distinct species so set out by real essences, that there can come no other species between them: whereas if we will abstract from those names, and the supposition of such specific essences made by nature, wherein all things of the same denominations did exactly and equally partake; if we would not fancy, that there were a certain number of these essences, wherein all things, as in moulds, were cast and formed, we should find that the idea of the shape, motion, and life of a man without reason, is as much a

---

[30] Gassendi, *The Mirrour of True Nobility*, 214.
[31] *An Essay*, 568.
[32] Lila Graves, "Locke's changeling and the Shandy bull," in *Philological Quarterly*, 60 (1981); *An Essay*, 451 ff.
[33] *Essais*, iii, 366.

> distinct idea, and makes as much a distinct sort of things from man and beast, as the idea of the shape of an ass with reason, would be different from either that of man or beast, and be a species of an animal between, or distinct from both. Here everybody will be ready to ask, if changelings may be supposed something between man and beast, "Pray what are they?" I answer, changelings, which is as good a word to signify something different from the signification of man or beast, as the names man and beast are to have significations different one from the other.[34]

Changelings are not susceptible to cure; he continually emphasizes their birth-to-death continuity (here "forty years together," elsewhere "sixty," "the whole course of his life" and so on). Readjustment of the name to the idea that reflects the species is crucial because in this case the creature it names is, despite treacherous physical appearances, incapable of matching or readjusting names to ideas – an intellectual operation that is constitutive of being a member of the human species, and particularly of an extended civil society. It is vital that the creature's pathological separateness from the rest of us be exposed.

Once again, Locke leaves his reader to infer how in this sense Locke's conservative opponents too are changelings, just as Eugen Bleuler, having only just coined the word "autistic" in 1911 for the excessively inward phases of mental illness, and encountering opposition to his theory from fellow clinicians, immediately explained their arguments away by calling them autistic. We can summarize Locke's position thus. The optimum human ability is abstraction; abstraction is the sorting of clear and distinct ideas into nominal essences ("a sort, or general abstract idea …"), and the clear and distinct idea that sorts human beings from other animals is our ability to abstract in this way.[35] And so the definition and place in nature of the human species or "sort" (he prefers plain language to jargon), amounts to the following: We sort ourselves as the sort that sorts. Commentators have noted that much of Book 1 of the *Essay* is a dismantling of the "self-validating circularity" of the political establishment's assumption that abilities are acquired through membership of authoritative institutions, and that the abilities of those critical of them or outside them – the forty-shilling freeholder perhaps – are therefore by definition impaired.[36] If so, then Locke has simply broadened the circumference of the circularity rather than removed it.

The intellectually disabled, in terms of their natural classification, are whatever *still* lies beyond the circumference. To reach this point I have not just pasted together two different Lockes from separate phases of his theoretical trajectory. Of course the *Essay* had an 18-year gestation period. But the timing of the relevant entries in his notebooks shows the two usages rattling around in his head at the same time: of the changeling as *non-reasoning subject*, and as the paradigm of a *correctly reasoned name for the distinct idea of a species*. On 11 November 1677 he notes:

> In the discursive [sc. reasoning] faculty of the mind I do not find that men are so apt to err, but it avails little that their syllogisms are right if their terms be insignificant and obscure or confused and indetermined, or that their internal discourse and deductions be regular if their notions be wrong …. Where a man argues right upon wrong notions or terms he does like a madman, where he makes wrong consequences he does like a fool, madness seeming to me to lie more in the imagination, and folly in the discursive.

A mere eight days later, this mention of foolishness in the human subject expands to encompass a discussion about how to name and place the foolish subject within the objective scheme of nature:

---

[34] *An Essay*, 569; 471; 569 ff.
[35] Ibid., 442.
[36] Tully, *An Approach*, 322.

> Species ... are but things ranked into orders because of their agreement in some ideas which we have made essential in order to our naming them. Though what it is to be essentially belong[ing] to any species in reference to nature be hard to determine. For if a woman should bring forth a creature perfectly of the shape of a man, that never shed any more appearance of reason than a horse nor had no articulate language, and another woman should produce an other with nothing of the shape but the language and reason of a man I ask which of these you would call by the name man? Or both or neither?[37]

Locke argues against Aristotelian conservatives who "see religion threatened, whenever any one ventures to quit their forms of speaking" and to invent new terms. They would evidently dismiss the lack of reason in a changeling as "no more but an accidental difference," a non-essential feature; they would judge the essential humanity of a new birth at baptism merely by "the outward shape and appearance of a man," and the fact that they are "of human birth." He responds:

> I am sure this is a conclusion, that men nowhere allow of. For if they did, they would not make bold, as everywhere they do, to destroy ill-formed and mis-shaped productions. Ay, but these are monsters. Let them be so; what will your drivelling, unintelligent, intractable changeling be? Shall a defect in the body make a monster; a defect in the mind (the far more noble, and, in the common phrase, the far more essential part), not?[38]

That common phrase is of course "man is a rational animal" – the conservatives' own. And so, Locke suggests, they are hoist with their own petard. This conservative who denies that the mind is the "more noble" part is, however, a straw man. The "nobler part" had been long been a standard epithet for the mind as distinguished from the body, well before Descartes. Elizabeth I's minister Nicholas Bacon, in a 1561 policy document to design a state curriculum for royal wards, had complained: "Hitherto, the chief care of governance hath been had to the land, being the meanest; and to the body, being the better, very small; but to the mind, being the best, none at all, which ... is plainly to set the cart before the horse." The most that could be said for the body was that although the "virtue" of the rational soul "could appear in deformity, yet it is more honourable in a comely personage."[39]

There is again a religious back story to Locke's ethical discussion, one that involves infanticide. He cites a "monstrous," physically impaired child who due to his outward shape might have been destroyed at birth or at least barred from the church, but was instead "declared a man 'provisionally' till time should show what he would prove," and grew up to become the Abbot of St Martin. (Locke's source here is his contemporary Gilles Ménage, who was simply illustrating the same point as Locke himself; though presented as a historical case, it is more likely the skewed residue of medieval legends about St Martin of Tours's charity towards the physically disabled.) It is deformity of mind, by contrast, that really ought to be "exclude[d] out of the species of man" and "determin[e] life and death." The only thing that stops him short of recommending infanticide for changelings is that at birth "the faculty of reason [is something] which no body could know would be wanting in its due season," a problem which modern pre-natal technology seems to have reduced. Locke may have had Luther's story in mind here which says that changelings are only baptized "in view of the fact that they cannot be known the first year." We should list as impediments to baptism only those things we can observe, and cognition and behaviour are not observable in early infancy. The doctrine of reprobation is implicit in this. Locke adds here that "the wheels, or springs ...

---

[37] R. Aaron and J. Gibb, *An Early Draft of Locke's Essay*, 98 ff.
[38] *An Essay*, 571.
[39] Nicholas Bacon, cited in Simon, *Education*, 341; Pemble, *Workes*, 6.

within, are different in a rational man, and a changeling," who is man only "in a physical sense."[40] Today we may be inclined to interpret the clock metaphor of wheels and springs as physical – that is, deterministic – in a biological sense; and as we saw above, Locke like his contemporaries may have seen the changeling as a product of bestial sex. But it must also be remembered that at the time "physical" also meant divinely determined, as reprobates were. When Locke claims that such differences are unknowable at birth, he has in mind not of course (anachronistically) the lack of a diagnostic technology such as amniocentesis but the unknowableness of God's purposes.

Infanticide had already been raised in this context by the Sidney circle's Lodowick Bryskett, who in his behavioural guide of the 1590s notes that because "children newly born ... are not able ... to give any sign or token ... that they will prove either good or evil .... So is it much more to be discommended ... that an infant newly born should be killed, though by defect of nature, want of seed, or any strain or mischance of the mother, or through abundance of ill humours or any other strange accident, it be born imperfect."[41] His fear is rather of that other spuriously human creature, the reprobate hypocrite: "Goodly personages who carry one thing in their tongue and another in their heart, be they that deserve to be hunted out of all civil society .... These be they that in very truth are crooked, misshapen and monstrous, and might well be condemned to be buried quick [sc. alive]: not simple innocent babes who, having no election, can yield no tokens either of good or evil." (This is very similar to Locke's point about the changeling.) Why then should we "esteem a person in body misshapen or deformed less worthy to be nourished, or to be admitted to magistracy?" (And this is exactly Locke's point about the Abbot of St Martin.) Bryskett goes on to rule that the distinction between elect and reprobate must override that between rational man and fool; his examples of the latter are the conventional ones of his time ("lethargies, frenzies, melancholy, drunkenness and such other passions") rather than Locke's birth-to-death absence of reason. Locke replaces an organic, behavioural and provisional model of foolishness with one that is disembodied, intellectual and permanent. Furthermore, not only is old-fashioned foolishness clearly not the precursor for this latter model, reprobation is. The real underlying and unifying threat is the deceptive morphological appearance of someone whose humanity is dubious, where "human" means susceptible to being ruled or amended.

Even physical monstrosity by itself contradicts the tired realist hypothesis of real essences as "a certain number of forms or moulds" into which God pours the relevant characteristics. Physically deformed people do not match the mould. Then how much less so does the intellectual monster:

> The frequent productions of monsters, in all the species of animals, and of changelings ... carry with them difficulties, not possible to consist with this hypothesis: since it is as impossible, that two things, partaking exactly of the same real essence, should have different properties as that two figures partaking in the same real essence of a circle, should have different properties.[42]

Descartes's immediate successors (despite his own inclusiveness) had already gone down this route of disjoining name from idea in the case of intellectual monstrosity. Louis de Cordemoy, for example, in another book in Locke's collection, extends Descartes's sceptical method to the definition of man itself. He decides he must ask himself the preliminary question, whether "all bodies which I recognize as similar to mine are necessarily joined to souls like mine; I tell myself not to believe it until I have signs so clear that I can no longer doubt it." Likewise, it is to the accompaniment of the changeling example that Locke announces his well-known general principle:

---

[40] *An Essay*, 453; 464.
[41] *A Discourse*, 34.
[42] *An Essay*, 418; see also 448.

"We cannot be too cautious, that words and species, in the ordinary notions which we have been used to of them, impose not on us."[43]

Why not? The answer seems to be chiefly an epistemological one: "from thence has rose a great part of the difficulties about truth and certainty." But there is also a social "inconvenience" behind this, namely that allowing ourselves to be imposed upon "would disturb our discourse with others." Our awareness of a lack of fit between existing names and the abstracted ideas of the species they purport to refer to shows that there *can* or *should* be matching of some kind: that there is a ground on which the human and the divinely ordained aspects of reason meet, so that consensus on some important public issues may be both possible and certain, and dangerous disputes among opinionated and competing real-essence systems avoided. It is therefore also the rationale for toleration. Toleration was incompatible with the doctrine of innate ideas, for if people were not allowed to reason out the common ideas for themselves, from their own empirical starting points, then their rulers would be encouraged to pose as the personally infallible mediators of those ideas.

The seemingly Protean concept of the changeling, the prototype of the modern intellectually disabled person, can be summarized therefore as: (1) a creature who is completely determined, the type we would all resemble if we allowed ourselves to be imposed upon – but also (2) a creature who actually *does* have to be imposed upon, for its own good and ours; (3) an illustration of the lack of fit between the names of species and the ideas which correspond to them – but also (4) an illustration of the concrete threat which this lack of fit poses, so long as it is not rectified, to a liberal politics of rational consent. In each of these respects, changelings are the paradigmatic case. And (4), it will be noted, returns us to (1).

The legal and ethical standing of idiots and changelings

As proponents of the Argument from Design were fond of pointing out, the very complexity of the world is an indicator of its perfection, and of the existence and perfection of its divine author. Therefore no one can be "so brutish" as to fail to recognize "the surprising variety" that is in nature. The archetype of the brutish and spuriously human, then, has to be he who does not understand the variety of species; he must himself be another item among that variety, different in nature from all those who do have this understanding of the idea of their own natural species, "man." Difference in nature required a corresponding revision of previous ideas about whether all (seemingly) human beings are "intelligent agents capable of a law."[44] A conventional list already existed of those whom for the purposes of law one need not treat as legally or ethically kin to oneself: prisoners of war, libertines, children, mad people. We will look briefly at how Locke views each of these groups in turn, at how they relate to the more fundamental category of idiots and changelings, and at how the conventional grounds for disqualification became distilled in the treatment of the latter.

To begin with, some background. Today we consider it self-evident that competence, in legal terms, is largely a matter of reason. To have a right (the right to consent for example), you must have cognitive competence or ability. Appeal is then made to an expert, objective assessment of this competence, whose source is assumed to lie quite outside the sphere of law itself, in the subjective nature of the individual. So on the one hand, some specific relation is implied between competence (defined as intellectual) and rights; on the other hand, though, competence and rights are radically different entities, their only relationship being a causal one. With the intellectually disabled, the causal link is from "no intellectual competence" to "no rights": the first appears to lead to the second.

---

[43] Louis de Cordemoy, *Le discernement du corps et de l'âme*, 128; Locke, *An Essay*, 573.

[44] Glanvill, "The usefulness of real philosophy to religion," 5, in *Essays*; Locke, *An Essay*, 346.

Historically it was the other way round. One had in the first instance a right (or to be more precise one had power), and therefore one had competence. The parenthesis is necessary because in fact "right," *jus*, was not then used in the way we are familiar with. Before the seventeenth century, right was a legal relationship between two parties, not the possession of either. The sole one-sided right was the power which "man" in general had over the brute beasts below him. It did not imply a right over other men (even if the word "man" was socially ambiguous: hence the frequency and seriousness with which the labouring classes were described as brute beasts).[45] It is true that the form of legal incompetence to plead known as *mente captus*, "deprived of one's senses" (from the Roman law of the Twelve Tables), existed in medieval times, but there was no notion of *individuals* having rights. Only in the early modern period did people like Francisco Suárez, Hugo Grotius, Samuel Pufendorf and, under the influence of all three, Locke, shift the word "right" so far into the subjective sphere that it became a claim on one party's side. And only once this had happened could a right come to be seen as something that exists in nature as it is in modern political constitutions, and hence as something individuals can assert, usually on the basis of their intellectual ability.

The idea of competence-based rights in its fully modern sense has its roots in the idea of individual property rights, and can be discerned in the political theories of self-ownership promoted by Locke and before him by absolutists (Hobbes) and egalitarians (the Levellers) alike. For Hobbes, the importance of self-ownership reflected that of self-preservation, in a world of competing egoisms that required an all-powerful state to control them. For the Levellers, it went with extension of the franchise and the right of resistance to the ruler's suppression of individual freedoms; a free man was free in being possessor of his own person and hence of his own abilities. For Locke, self-ownership signified an intellectual and hence moral autonomy of the individual, corresponding with the ownership of material property. Ownership of the self was a form of trusteeship; the reason I cannot belong to someone else, an absolute monarch for example, is because ultimately my self, like everyone else's, belongs to God. But this egalitarianism contains certain intrinsic exceptions. Leveller proposals for the franchise did not for the most part extend as far down as servants, who had willingly alienated their self-ownership, i.e., their ability to labour. Locke's notion of intellectual autonomy presented its own specific alienation in the form of idiots and changelings.

Thus rights and ability form a vicious circle. When we say that this person with a disability has no right because they are not able to exercise it, we have already defined "right" in advance as whatever it is that the person is unable to exercise. Many writers before Locke had explicitly refused to make exceptions on the grounds of absence of intellect alone, or to attach it to some other difference. Hobbes, for example, attributed to "fools ... a common human nature," expressly attacking the tautology by which the existence of fools offends the law of nature because they are excluded from it in the first place. Suárez refused to allow it to be attached to race, attacking fellow Spaniards who attributed a permanent "mindlessness" to indigenous Americans in order to justify their enslavement. (His criticism matched a 1537 papal bull stipulating that Americans were "rational creatures.") Pufendorf, like Suárez, criticized the theory of natural slavery, though he noted, albeit merely as an aside, that it stood up in the exceptional case of people who really were "natural" or "born fools."[46] Locke was to fasten on Pufendorf's passing surmise.

The paradigmatic case of an ethical exception to natural law in earlier times was that of the aggressor taken prisoner in a just war. He could be treated like an animal because he had ceased

---

[45] See Joan Lockwood O'Donovan, "Rights in Christian discourse," in M. Cromartie (ed.), *A Preserving Grace*.

[46] Samuel Pufendorf, *De Jure Naturae*, 3.6.3.

to be capable of a law. This did not necessarily indicate an absence of intelligence, only of agency. However, lack of reason was characteristic in most other cases. Libertine-type changelings, for example, follow their appetites alone and therefore make irrational choices. But because they are born teachable, they are the illustration that humans *can* reason and that natural law *obliges* them to do so, even if they resist. Idiot-type changelings, by contrast, are born unteachable, and this lack of potential distances them as much from the libertine type as from the captive aggressor. In Locke's *Essay*, the naturalistic framework applies to mind alone, taken separately. As a species distinct from all other animals, we are determined by the mind's operations; it is therefore the existence of idiot-type changelings above all that confuses this overridingly important natural distinction, and the onus on their mindlessness is therefore that much greater. They are denied a soul and an afterlife on grounds of their natural lack of a mind, not merely on grounds of their willful failure to exercise it.

Then there are children. In his early *Essays on the Law of Nature*, Locke, like his predecessors, still thought of natural law as binding on "all those who are endowed with a rational nature, i.e., all men in the world," by some generic essential property. But he already feels a need to add here: "There is no reason that we should deal with the case of children and fools [*fatui*]. For although the law is binding on all those to whom it is given, it does not, however, bind those to whom it is not given, and it is not given to those who are unable to understand it." Only when natural law comes to signify that which binds human beings as a species in nature, with reason no longer directly locked into divine law, does it become contradictory to say that fools are members of a rational species. Only then, therefore, does it become necessary to hedge natural law round with exceptions. The humanity of children – little monsters – is diminished in an exactly similar way, despite Locke's reputation for having an enlightened view of them. But at least children, like libertines, are hypothetically teachable, which is ruled out for idiot-type changelings. The authorially approved Latin translation of the *Essay concerning Human Understanding* renders "changeling" as *puerulus aut fatuus homo* ("childlike or foolish man"); the second adjective is old-fashioned terminology, but the first is novel and has developmental implications, reinforcing Locke's view of the understanding as a gradual, empirically based acquisition.

This view of childhood as temporary idiocy also comes up in his treatment of natural rights theory in the second of the *Two Treatises of Civil Government*, which is partly based on the theory of Grotius and Pufendorf. Here, law is not a "limitation" so much as "the direction of a free and intelligent agent to his proper interest .... Is a man under the law of England? What made him free of that law ...? A capacity of knowing that law .... Thus we are born free as we are born rational." There is no deep difference here between natural law and that of the courts, or between the history of society and that of the individual. As a result, Locke's critique of Filmer is not quite complete. He admits as much. Filmer had modelled the absolute ruler's right to authority over his subjects on the father's right to authority over his children, and Locke concedes that we are born to a freedom that is only ever *eventual*: "age and reason" are inseparable companions, and children will cross the threshold of humanity only when they reach the age of "discretion," that is, when the faculty of reasoning starts to develop its operations. Pagans in the process of conversion ("intelligent Americans" and "Indians") arrive at autonomy in the same way. Idiots are those who, by this definition of autonomy, do not and cannot. Relying on Hooker yet again, Locke asks what if "through defects that may happen out of the ordinary course of nature, anyone comes not to such a degree of reason wherein he might be supposed capable of knowing the law?" The answer is that he is "never set free from the government of his parents."

This is more than just a minor concession to Filmer's paternalist absolutism. Rather than an exception to the rule, it is a genuine and necessary survival of the original absolutist principle. Freedom is not a discrete *consequence* of adult rationality, freedom and rationality are the same thing. So are their absences, therefore. The result is that the idiot has a claim to protection which the feckless libertine, having failed to fulfill his obligation to develop his given faculties, does not. Despite the dissolution of the honour society, it remains the case in this instance that *noblesse oblige*, and our own *noblesse* today is the intelligence society as a whole (that is why, for example, we donate to disability charities).

Finally, there are mad people. In Book 2 of the *Essay* the abstract common ideas, once acquired, take on a meme-like quality, a quasi-material existence, "such as [man] has no power over, either to make or destroy." Of the potential destroyers, idiots and mad people alike illustrate the negative limits of competent abstraction, and of logical trains of ideas. How then do the two groups differ? They do not sit alongside each other in a level taxonomy but on hierarchically different rungs in the intellectual scale of nature. Idiots are to be lumped with beasts, whereas the mad belong without demur in the world of humans,

> For they do not appear to me to have lost the faculty of reasoning: but having joined together some ideas very wrongly, they mistake them for truths; and they err as men do, that argue right from wrong principles. By the violence of their imaginations, having taken their fancies for realities, they make right deductions from them. Thus you shall find a distract man fancying himself a king .... In short, herein seems to lie the difference between idiots and madmen. That madmen put wrong ideas together, and so make wrong propositions, but argue and reason right from them: but idiots make very few or no propositions, and reason scarce at all.[47]

Madness lies along a spectrum with ordinary intellect, while foolishness occupies a separate niche in nature. In a species defined, for Locke, by the operation and association of ideas, the mad are full members: "A man, who is very sober, and of a right understanding in all other things, may in one particular be as frantic, as any in Bedlam." It is the *absence* of (Lockean) ideas, not their misassociation, that bars one from membership of the species.

In medical theory, mania had usually been located in the "discursive" or inference-drawing operations of the reasoning faculty. Mania, said Willis, was an "alienation of the mind," whereas (melancholic) stupidity was an alienation of the imagination; he linked mania to excessive speed, which meant that people "very badly infer one thing from another."[48] Locke switched templates. He put madness in the imagination, and allocated idiotic stupidity to the "discursive" or reasoning faculty. In this new template it is the slow type in whom the problem is a discursive one; the mad infer correctly, albeit from wrong ideas (i.e., from an over-hasty mismatch of idea to image). We can see how this gradually emerges into the public version of the *Essay* from the entries in his private notebooks. On 15 July 1676 he asks how madness can be a fault in the reasoning faculty, if "mania be ... putting together wrong ideas and so making wrong propositions from them, notwithstanding the reason be right?" A week later, he has madness as "the wrong application of mad ideas to things that exist, as for example [those] made in fantasy [such as] him to be either king or castle." Later entries, on 5 and 11 November 1677, develop the dyad into the form later found in the *Essay*: "Madness seems to be nothing but a disorder in the imagination, and not in the discursive faculty." The mad are just like "sober" humans who get lost in a town they know a little but not well: they think they know where they are and act accordingly, but discover that they were under an illusion, whereas fools draw wrong consequences.[49]

---

[47] *An Essay*, 161.
[48] Hieronymus Mercurialis, *Medicina*, Chapter 16; Willis, *De Anima*, 350.
[49] "Medical journals," in Kenneth Dewhurst, *John Locke, Physician and Philosopher*, 70; 89.

While madness is Locke's main concern in the notebooks, the *Essay*'s greater concern with changelings, natural fools and idiots seems to belong with that work's more public aims. The published edition intensifies the fusion between a jurisprudential dyad (congenital idiots versus periodically lucid mad people) and a medical one (slothful versus furious soul spirits), and transforms it into something almost recognizable to modern psychiatry. The old mean between slow and fast is still there ("the deficit in naturals seems to proceed from want of quickness, activity, and motion, in the intellectual faculties, whereby they are deprived of reason: whereas madmen, on the other side, seem to suffer by the other extreme"); but the "activity and motion" previously attributed to material, physiological entities such as the soul spirits has here been transferred to the entity of pure mind.[50]

Policing the borders of Moral Man

Permanent absence of ideas lies beyond what is human or has a soul. A question then arises: if Locke thought definitions of species were purely nominal, how is he so certain about excluding the changeling from the human species?

In Locke, for man to be *moral* meant precisely to belong in a *natural* realm. In its surface terms this reflects the orthodox Calvinist view discussed in Part 5. An old scholastic distinction held that while "natural" qualities can vary by degree (e.g., between hot and cold), "moral" ones do not (e.g., good or evil, elect or reprobate). When Amyraut and Baxter proposed that there was a disability of the intellect that might be natural, their more orthodox opponents thought they were threatening that strictness of a *moral* divide, that between elect and reprobate. Baxter did in fact regard this divide as fixed and important above all others. As for "idiots," although he claimed only God knew whether they were saved, he tended to presume in favour of their exclusion: hence his allocation to them of their corpse-like role of being "dead in Christ," like reprobates. Again Locke is repeating Baxter (see p. 197 above) almost to the letter:

> It will be asked, if changelings are something between man and beast, what will become of them in the other world? To which I answer, 1. It concerns me not to know or enquire. To their own master they stand or fall .... But, secondly, I answer ... it may as rationally be concluded, that the dead body of a man ... has yet nevertheless a living soul in it, because of its shape; as that there is a rational soul in a changeling, because he has the outside of a rational creature, when his actions carry far less marks of reason with them, in the whole course of his life, than what are to be found in many a beast."[51]

Hence there is more than a resonance of Calvinism in Locke's application of the theory of nominal essences to human beings. There is an actual line of descent. When Baxter and others said that classification into elect and reprobate was "equivocal" (nominal) rather than "real," they meant that the pastor, in his examination of each individual, could only guess at people's inner state but also that guesswork can be empirically supported. Our sinful ways tend to be observable, as are certainly our wrong answers to catechical assessments. Even if human beings are "only equivocally called," says Baxter, we often have a shrewd idea who is who. Moreover, the nominal or equivocal is not some epistemologically lower level of knowledge: "As there is an outward effectual vocation," says Baxter, "yet that outward is real ... and not equivocal only."[52] Locke's and Baxter's aim was

---

[50] *An Essay*, 160.
[51] Ibid., 570.
[52] Baxter, *Certain Disputations*, 38; Letter to Humfrey, 7 December 1654.

the same: to screen out a category of questionably human creatures who are unprepared for the afterlife because they are incapable of rational choice. The two men differ over the secondary matter of how such creatures arrive in the world: through creation directly (Baxter), or via occult bodily mechanisms (Locke). Creation in both cases is "physical," in the sense of determined.

Locke's own early views on election and reprobation are unknown. Of the people he was in touch with on theological matters, Ferguson stuck to it while Penn, a former student of Amyraut's, rejected it. All three were conferring together regularly during the 1670s with each other and with Owen, the erstwhile high priest of election who had by now transformed himself into a defender of toleration and of "reason in faith." We can surmise that at some (probably early) point Locke must have rejected predestination. But how deep was this rejection? It was certainly not as vehement as that of the Levellers. John Howe's letters to Boyle on predestination (Howe was in exile with Locke in Holland) confirm that the new psychology arose from epistemological concerns about knowing whether one was elect. One wonders, says Howe, imputing the thought to Boyle himself, whether the anxiety about second-guessing God's plan for us "be not wholly in our own minds."[53] Why? Because "labouring under the natural defect" of an "incomprehensive narrowness ... it is very incident to our minds, to grasp at more than they can compass." The suggestion *seems* to be: let's stop trying to guess about our own inner states. But he continues: "Though the comprehension of our minds be not infinite, it might be extended much further than usually it is, if we would allow ourselves ... *gradually* [emphasis in original] to stretch and enlarge our own understandings." And by this he means the understanding of our status with God. Hence the novel idea of development – the development of a reflexive psychological knowledge – absorbs, rather than contradicts, the "old" one of election and predestination.

The notion of a developmental growth in our knowledge about our own minds and those of others was a counter to the zealous notions of sectarians, dangerous says Howe because they "disdain to be thought not able to see through everything, by the first and slightest glance of a haughty eye." The issue of whether one was elect or not became secondary to this new concern with the steady pace and sequentiality that went with "making yourself part of your own study." Nevertheless, difference was as much the ontological premise of this approach to human nature as it had been of the orthodox Calvinist's. Locke drew his own dividing line between moral man and the changeling as zealously as they had drawn theirs between elect and reprobate. Changelings may be defined by an inability to reason logically or form abstract ideas rather than by hypocrisy, but ultimately their pathology is like the reprobate's: they are fundamentally incapable of faith, to which abstract ideas are (in Ferguson's phrase) "the previous exercise." The psychology of Locke's "moral man" reconstitutes, in a new format, the status of the elect in the orthodox theology of men such as Du Moulin and Spanheim. To be moral means precisely to belong in a natural realm; Locke differs from his orthodox Calvinist forebears simply inasmuch as now the foundation of one's relationship with God lies in developing one's intellectual operations. He exhibits none of Amyraut's subtleties, which had arisen in the interim, about a part discontinuity between the moral and the natural. Despite Locke's rejection of predestination theology, then, the *Essay* is partly the product of those earlier doctrines about how one can know the signs of election in oneself: a reading of perfectibility and personal destiny.

Moreover, he is far less agnostic about people's religious status than many. Baxter was wary of claiming to know who is elect. He complains about those who have lived for a long time in doubt, albeit "very conscionable and blamelessly," who suddenly go astray when they hear Anabaptist or Familist doctrines: that is, once they hear "the doctrine of perfection in this life and suddenly been

---

[53] Howe, *The Reconcileableness*, 7.

past their fears, as if hearing of perfection had made them perfect."[54] Locke is more confident. He just knows who is the moral man and who is the changeling. He asserts it as self-evident that "man" cannot signify both a rational being and its opposite, such as a changeling, at one and the same time; to say that it can encompass both is contradictory. But this is trickery on Locke's part, since intellectually disabled changelings are not a different species in a positive sense; a changeling is something that can only be defined by reference to its failing to be a man.

Like election, faith too remains embedded in Locke's account. Although the focus was now on the operational exercise of reasoning abilities, faith was no discarded husk. Reason did not muscle faith aside but came to its rescue, reinforcing its substructure and transforming it into eighteenth-century "belief." When Locke described his "skills" in writing the *Essay* as those of "an under-labourer," the foundations he was building were reasoning ones but the edifice itself was faith, and the aim was to ensure that one might be in grace. This was certainly understood by the religious educators for whom Locke was a major resource. When Wesley said, "He that believeth shall be saved; he that believeth not shall be damned," he meant a belief not categorically distinct from reason but underpinned by it.[55] Amyraut had started the whole process by suggesting the existence of a discretely "natural" realm in respect of the intellect. However, this realm was occupied only by those with "natural disability"; ability itself was still a matter of grace. Locke and others then wrote about everyone (or nearly everyone) as having abilities in this realm of intellectual nature, as a gradual preparation for the afterlife. Locke's moral man, suggested by a new-found optimism about the developmental character of intellectual abilities, is so often seen as the prototype of Enlightenment universal man. However, he could equally be seen as the elect *homo morale* of Calvinism, supplemented with Baxter's "labouring intellect." Calvinists had long complained that the old formula *homo = animal rationale* was inadequate. Its replacement, *homo = animal morale*, seemed to breathe new life into the idea of what it is to be human. Our species is that which owes a moral duty to God on the basis of certain natural intellectual abilities which we should work at developing.

Locke wrote the *Essay*, as he said on its first page, in order to specify what those abilities were and how they worked in detail, as a preparation for higher (theological) things. What the abilities in fact comprise is not "the *moral man*, as I may call him" (the emphasis in the text), but "the moral man, as *I* may call him" – not a new coining but a readjustment of the existing Calvinist epithet described above (see Chapter 10). He will use the criterion of intellectual "skills" and "abilities" to reconstruct the definition of man, as a seamlessly natural-moral creature. But Locke could not have done so without that intervening stage of Amyraut and Baxter, in which "natural intellectual (dis)ability" had been *separated* from moral (dis)ability. It was the disability of the "changeling ... man in a physical sense" that allowed Locke to establish as a truth "capable of demonstration ... the moral man ... that ha[s] the use of reason."[56] Moral man does not construct changelings as his other; he appears as it were by their prior permission. Pathology etches in the normal. Sceptics used the existence of fools to prove that a unitary, fixed reason does not exist in man. The answer to this claim had so far been that anyone who says something like that must be a fool himself. Locke realized this was an inadequate response. His strategy was to take the sceptical challenge about fools and use it to prove that reason *does* exist naturally in man. The existence of born fools or changelings, as natural creatures lacking intellectual ability, proves that we – the rest of us, the definitively human individuals – each have within us the specific operations that characterize that ability. The name he attaches to us, "moral man," signifies our ability for

---

[54] *The Cure*, 170.
[55] Cited in C. Pinnock (ed.), *The Grace of God and the Will of Man*, 262.
[56] *An Essay*, 7; 515.

abstract ideas; our abstract ideas refer to nominal essences; the nominal essence referred to by our ability for abstract ideas is "moral man." And so the circle excludes the changeling.

But does "man," this closed natural-moral community, really embrace everyone apart from changelings? That is another matter. Locke's changelings, to judge from the way he describes them, were a tiny group, corresponding with the "severely" disabled person of today quantitatively as well as qualitatively. Yet unlike today's psychologist, Locke still maintained a distinction between lack of the ability to abstract and its non-performance. In many people non-performance was typical because of the external constraints of poverty and social rank, and the *Essay* in this sense still belongs to an old textual tradition, already noted.[57] Locke's remark here about labourers being too taken up with their croaking bellies to aspire to abstract ideas follows closely a text published in 1652 by the Restoration bishop and mathematician Seth Ward, a founding member of the Royal Society.[58] Again it was a book that Locke is likely to have known, having been published in Oxford during his attendance at the university and reprinted often over the next 20 years. Ward writes of the common ideas as "undeniable" evidence "of the *spiritual* and *incorporeal nature* of our mind, from whence will necessarily follow the *natural incorruptibility* of it, which is all that we pretend to, when we say, that it is immortal" (emphasis added). Out of the common ideas or "first and most common principles of intelligence," says Ward, the most clearly demonstrable is the immortality of the soul, so that "it must be the fool alone, as the Psalmist speaks, which can be an atheist." As for the individual subject, he continues:

> Considering the darkness of our minds, and that inability towards a strict and vigorous reflection which even in those who are most practised in the contemplation of themselves, and in the scrutiny of the ways of their own internal operations, is over frequent; and considering how little reason there is to expect it of those who by their way of living are more deeply engaged among ... the affections and circumstances of bodies and bodily motions, and perhaps may think themselves unconcerned to be busy in the knowledge of themselves, it will be requisite that we insist more particularly, that so the matter may be cleared even to the most vulgar apprehensions.

On the optimistic side, knowledge of the self is that which, even more than knowledge of mathematics, will lead to "mastery over the works of nature, and so imitate God and nature in great and marvellous conclusions." However, there are clear doubts about the possibility of instilling this self-reflecting and self-policing "ability" in ever broader social groups. The dubious status of Ward's fool is at once religious (fool as atheist) and social (fool as vulgar). Writers such as Locke, Ferguson and Truman too envisage a spiritual element ensconced within the "natural mind working in a natural way," but that word "natural" had stubbornly pejorative resonances; only with an imported nugget of divine grace is the natural mind ready to be reborn and validated as a secular psychology. There remains the question: do the labouring poor – the archetype of the old "natural man" – really belong to "moral man"? In terms of performance, if not ability, there is no category difference between Ward's fool or Locke's idiot and this broader group. At best the unimprovable condition of idiots is an object lesson to manual labourers about how they should occupy the few non-working hours they have. When Truman writes about "natural disability of the intellect," for him it still encompasses both the lack of "a sufficient estate to give" and the lack of an intellectual faculty, in a single overarching concept.[59]

In the event, the reinvention of idiots as unnatural creatures by virtue of their permanent lack of human reason or of capacity for intellectual labour is the ploy by which the rest of us are

---

[57] Ibid., 707.
[58] *A Philosophicall Essay*, 34; 72.
[59] Ferguson, *The Interest*, 144; Truman, *A Discourse*, 4.

able to present ourselves as intelligent, autonomous citizens capable of consent and democratic government. And the more Locke tends towards a universalist concept of man – not just forty-shilling freeholders but landless labourers, women, perhaps even the slaves of the colonial trading companies he invested in – the more sharply are the residual exclusions drawn, the non-elect detritus of civil society. Modern commentators routinely take the line that "Locke [maintained] that *all* men are proprietors of their reason" (emphasis in original). This only holds true if we have previously deemed any exceptions not to be men. Yet even the division by natural intellect and its absence does not overlap neatly with Locke's perceptions of the society around him. For example, he wants to point out that "*Gentlemen* should not be ignorant" (emphasis added).[60] He is anxious about the intellectual deficiencies of the social ranks for whom the book was written. At the genesis of modern psychological criteria of disability, deficiencies of intellect still operate at different degrees of strictness according to one's place in the social order. Exclusion on the grounds of some natural condition could only matter in people who had prior social grounds for inclusion.

Scientific psychology: a historical contingency

What scientific basis did Locke offer for exclusion from the species? The thinkers most influential in subverting the old "Aristotelian" certainty about man (Montaigne, Descartes, Hobbes, Gassendi) had all nevertheless retained its inclusive indifference. Gassendi is an especially good example. Although he refurbishes the *essence* of man as a "common human *nature*" (emphasis added), any natural variations or defects in the operation of the individual understanding remain as before dispositional and organic to the "corporeal" soul, leaving the rational essence and the rational soul perfectly intact in everyone: a psychology in which Gassendi, in order to preserve the principle of immortality, eschews his more usual quasi-materialist stance and demonstrates a residual Aristotelianism. He expressly denies that differences among human intellects amount to "unequal orders of perfection," because this would infer (impossibly) that they resembled the orders of angels, who are unequal in precisely this respect.[61] Locke alone does not recoil from the logical possibility of species differences among so-called men. However, he turns it into scientific fact only at a certain point during the gestation of the *Essay concerning Human Understanding*. His certainty about excluding changelings from the species of "moral man" is tied to his assertion there that "morality is capable of demonstration, as well as mathematics," and "moral knowledge is as capable of real certainty as mathematics."[62]

How did he arrive at this point? Alongside the separation of objects of knowledge into physical and moral, mentioned above, philosophers of the time also discussed a quite different kind of separation, between two *ways of knowing*: demonstrative and moral. Demonstrative certainty was absolutely certain, in an *a priori* sense, and had a divine or physical source; "moral certainty" was merely practical, and could not exist without a human agent. Locke probably absorbed this doctrine from the Cartesian logicians whom he was reading during his stay in France in the late 1670s. It is the demonstrative type that prevails in the published edition of the *Essay* when he writes about the species exclusion of changelings. This pessimistic certainty about changelings was tied to his increasingly optimistic ethical certainty about everyone else. This in turn sprang either out of desperation (when would the rational political moment actually arrive when the English might be free to prepare for glory?), or out of foresight (that moment did in fact arrive, in 1689).

---

[60] I. Shapiro, *The Evolution of Rights in Liberal Theory*, 137; Locke, *An Essay*, 710.
[61] Gassendi, *Institutio Logica*, 1.16.
[62] *An Essay*, 516; 565.

His certainty about fundamental questions of human nature thus came as much from his efforts to establish a rational ethics as from an attempt to build a psychological theory.

One can see the progression of these efforts by comparing *An Essay concerning Human Understanding* with his 1663 *Essays on the Law of Nature*. In the earlier work, he had seen no contradiction between the existence of fools (*fatui*) and the principle that reason is the essential property of all humans. His certainty here was of the old Aristotelian variety. Certainty about human nature did not have to be demonstrative; it was simply implicit in the Argument from Design. Draft A of *An Essay concerning Human Understanding*, by contrast, starts to hint at problems with "man is a rational animal." If the predicate (rational animal) is contained in the definition of the subject (man), he says, then it is a verbal truth only, "it being evident that children for some time and some men all their lives are not so rational as a horse or a dog, at which time I cannot see how the idea rational doth belong to them or can be affirmed of them." Even so, Locke has still not shaken off the old doctrine. The terms of the argument remain Aristotelian; he is merely using this example to illustrate the principle that "it is impossible for the same thing to be and not to be."[63] A child who has never seen a "negro" makes white skin a part of the definition of man and will tell you that black people are not human. Absurd maybe, says Locke, but someone else "that hath gone further" than the outward shape and has started to consider "coherent language or reasoning" would find it difficult to include deaf mutes as human. Moreover, "he may demonstrate, that infants, changelings and maniacs are no men, and I have discoursed with very rational men who have actually denied it." The more rational such men are, of course, the more likely they are to regard this exclusion as demonstrative and scientific. Nevertheless at this stage all he is doing is being open about the need for new approaches. Besides, he writes, "it is no very material question to our present purpose," though between this draft and the published version of the *Essay* idiocy will have become a very material question indeed.

With the typical caution of the early drafts we are said to have knowledge of all ideas "only in particulars (unless we will think mathematical demonstrations to be universal, of which I will not here dispute but all the rest are certainly particulars)" – and that includes ideas about the mind.[64] In order to have really certain knowledge, you would need to know "the precise bounds and extent of the species its terms stand for." Draft B then complains about the "time and sedulity" required for this. The chief illustration as usual is ourselves: "I think none of the definitions of the word man, nor descriptions of that sort of animal has done so perfectly and exactly as to satisfy a considerate inquisitive person." This is all very tentative by comparison with the old-fashioned certainties of the *Essays on the Law of Nature* or the novel ones of the eventual published version of the *Essay concerning Human Understanding*. In the latter the problems of time and sedulity seem to have been overcome. He claims that his definition of the human, the readjusted idea of moral man, is equally accessible to *a priori* demonstration as the properties of a triangle. In that case, there is no difference between the moral and the demonstrative certainty about either "man" or "triangle." One may as well say it is a *moral* certainty that the precise essence of a triangle is such-and-such, since that is just the consensual way in which human reason conceives of triangular bodies and no divine intellect needs to come from outside to say so; likewise one may as well say it is a *demonstrative* certainty that the things "moral names" stand for are "moral man" and "changeling." They are identical types of statement, he says. Hence it would appear that the certainty of the laws of human nature is the same as the certainty of, say, the law of gravity.

---

[63] Peter H. Nidditch and G.A.J. Rogers, *Drafts for the* Essay concerning Human Understanding; Nidditch, *Draft A of Locke's* Essay concerning Human Understanding, 106.

[64] Ibid., 121.

Locke's new stance is that not only do we have the same kind of certainty about human nature as about mathematics, we have it from a specifically human source, that of our own intellectual "abilities." This provoked the question as to whether all ideas about human nature are not tainted by their imperfectly human origins. Locke responded by saying that in the phrase "man is subject to law," man itself can only mean a "corporeal rational creature," and "whether a child or changeling be a man in a physical sense, may amongst the naturalists be as disputable as it will, it concerns not at all the moral man, as I may call him, which is this immoveable unchangeable idea, a corporeal rational being."[65] Sceptics who said that "rational being" was a merely verbal and therefore shifting definition would be right, were it not for the fact that a firmed-up account of it has emerged in the "moral man" as demonstrated by Locke himself. His confidence is misplaced, however. His demonstrative certainty about the underlying reality of the moral man is glued imperceptibly in place by his exclusion of the changeling. Uncertainty therefore remains unresolved. If the precise essence of a triangle is the way in which human reason conceives of triangular bodies, then the precise essence of human reason is the way in which human reason conceives of human reason. And so the definition of man remains changeable and open for power bids as to what that reason consists of.

Of course this scientization of psychology did not have to lead to pessimistic ethical conclusions about the intellectually deficient. It led certain other writers in the opposite direction, giving the ethics of exceptionalism an optimistic spin. Digby, for example, had used the notion of demonstrative certainty to claim that when one compares "the ranks of intelligence" from "the most contemptible idiot" to "the greatest clerk that ever lived," one finds that "the lowest knows as much as the highest," since "indifferent knowledge in this world, shall be replenished with all knowledge in the next … This amplitude of knowledge is common to all human souls (of whatever pitch soever they seem to be here), when they are separated from their bodies."[66] The idiot's soul "climbs up by degrees" to this knowledge of itself, says Digby, by exactly the same method that mathematicians compose their demonstrations. Digby can be optimistic because he is talking about the afterlife; the afterlife was important for Locke too, but he thought the hard intellectual graft had to be done here on earth, and everyone had to be prepared for it.

Can changelings be persons after all?

More fluctuations in Locke's outlook can be seen from the famous chapter on personal identity which he added to the *Essay*'s second edition. Here the correlation between his pessimism about the changeling and his optimism about everyone else recedes once more.

Locke's concept of personhood owes much to Puritan and Jansenist notions of the moral responsibility of the person over a whole lifetime and thus on his intellectual unity; indeed, there could be no modern intellectually disabled identity without the historical arrival of the person in this more fundamental sense. The ancient Greek medical texts contain pre-natal explanations for physical disability, but none for intellectual states; the core concept of a birth-to-death self is absent from ancient thought in general.[67] Autobiography, as a self-conscious genre, is largely modern. When Augustine wrote his *Confessions* it was a religious therapy, marking the cataclysmic

---

[65] *An Essay*, 516.
[66] Digby, *Of Bodies*, ii, 95.
[67] Hippocrates, *On Joints*, in *Hippocrates III*; see also Giuseppe Roccatagliata, *A History of Ancient Psychiatry*; Richard Sorabji, "Soul and self in ancient philosophy," in M. James and C. Crabbe (eds), *From Soul to Self*.

moment of a total spiritual transformation rather than reflecting on a life considered as a whole. Correspondingly, intellectual impairment did not describe a permanent personality; even senile dementia was curable by divine intervention before death. And in medical accounts of idiocy, it was as late as the end of the nineteenth century that the vital ingredient of incurability took hold definitively.

Pre-Lockean thinkers had conceived personhood not in terms of time but of space; the *persona* was that aspect of the human being which is "one in itself," like the trinity – not an individual member of the species but a hypothetically abstracted unit of rational nature as a whole. Theology explicitly rejected any notion of a permanent intellectual identity because this would have implied a denial of providential intervention. One's character, like one's body, was transient because temporal, by contrast with one's immaterial rational soul which was God's creation and thereby transcendent, not bounded by notions of time (or thus even of permanence) at all. Even if the instruments and operations of the faculties failed to operate throughout someone's life, this did not affect the transcendent permanence of their rational soul. The modern disabled person, in the sense of someone whose absence of intellect determines the personality over a lifetime, is not only absent from medieval thought but inconceivable, moreover *morally* inconceivable, since before the seventeenth century any talk of incurability is only ever a reference to original sin and so to humanity as a whole.

Locke on the other hand wrote in the first published edition of the *Essay* about the "intractable" changeling: his unteachable condition lasts inevitably for the whole of his life. In denying a role for providence, Locke had his forebears. In 1646 Overton, from his prison cell, had challenged the state by extending the notion of equality from the religious sphere of souls equal before God to an earthly political sphere of "self propriety," based on "natural rights" to which "all men are equally and alike born."[68] This was a psychological as well as a juridical usage of the word "propriety" (property), evoking both legal ownership and the philosophical sense of a defining characteristic (in this case, the essential property of "rational animal"). In yoking the words "self" and "property" together, Overton was shifting the grounds for defining humanity. Where previously it had been taken as a whole, here it is coming to be an aggregate of individual selves. The result is that "accidents" in the old sense become pathologies. Locke's changeling, and the modern "intellectually disabled" person, came about once individuation began to be seen in terms not of mere seedlings planted out from a universal humanity, but of individual *selves* who each *represent* that humanity on a one-by-one basis. Overton excludes certain accidents from the species, along lines that foreshadow Locke. He cites Montaigne's proposition that the difference between man and beast is one of degree only; to see a difference in kind would be to overlook the fact that "some [men] … have no more souls than beasts, and some less." Montaigne was of course just trying to shock everyone into behaving properly, but for Overton it is serious scientific stuff. Overlooking Montaigne's irony, he takes lack of a soul to indicate a difference in kind. "Fools" are the exception that really tests the rule, since they "are born, live and die without souls" and do not even have a soul to be given them on the day of judgement. In Overton's pessimistic ethics of exceptionalism, permanent foolishness is the positive opposite of the uncorrupted innocence it represents for the optimists.

Franciscus van Helmont asks similarly, "How is Christ said to 'enlighten every man that cometh into the world' (John I.9) that they may believe and be saved, seeing there are many born fools or idiots, and possessed with a deaf and dumb spirit; and yet are very unclean and wicked, and so die?" In short, they surely die in the same unregenerate condition in which they were born:

---

[68] *An Arrow against All Tyrants*, A2.

> Doth not all divine illumination presuppose and pre-require a capacity of understanding in some measure, in order to the improvement thereof? ... Does it not hence appear then, that all such as from the womb have *never* had the use of their understandings [emphasis added], have lived in former times, and enlightened by Christ, but are now, for some extraordinary abuse of their understandings then signally punished, suitable to their crimes? And shall not all such, if this be not their last hour, or that the day of their visitation be not over, yet come to live again in the word, and have the use of their understandings, and a divine illumination as well as other men?[69]

Van Helmont's belief in the transmigration and the possible restoration of souls only serves to highlight the "misery" of "being born fools," and the finality of foolishness over any one individual lifetime.

The religious element of confessional was not so much replaced by birth-to-death personhood as absorbed within it. The new ways of conceiving personhood that Locke typifies were new ways of assessing moral responsibility: the submission to divine authority of an audited account of actions undertaken over one's entire life, thereby co-operating rationally with God's grace. Where Locke writes of personal identity as "owning one's own actions," we should be aware that in the English of that time "owning" meant not just possessing but confessing or "owning up to." Locke replaces Descartes's spatial notion of a thinking substance with the temporal one of consistency and unity over time, the whole lifetime of an individual. What makes the "person" is his consciousness, which is etymologically related to "conscience" or the rendering of accounts with God. Conversely, in today's pathological identity, where biological conception is linked to the impossibility of cure, absence of moral worth amounts to absence of personhood.

Locke, however, does not reprise the changeling theme in this context. Precisely here, he seems to relax once more the qualifications for species membership. His focus on the lifetime leads him to minimize the difference between humans and other animals; they all participate "in the same continued life, by constantly fleeting particles of matter, in succession vitally united to the same organized body."[70] This principle of continuity "makes an embryo, one of years, mad, and sober, the same man." The threshold for being a "person" may look at first as steep as it did for being moral man, inasmuch as it "stands for ... a thinking intelligent being, that has reason and reflection, and can consider itself as itself, the same thinking thing in different times and places; which it does only by ... consciousness." But consciousness, while "inseparable from thinking, and ... essential to it," is not here some high-flying ability of its own but a mere accompaniment to all the mind's operations, including even the most basic ones such as perception, "it being impossible for any one to perceive, without perceiving that he does perceive." Hence it is an inclusive concept. In his attempt to extricate himself from the problem of dualism – that it reproduces within the realm of mind alone all the old Aristotelian contradictions which dualism sought to simplify – Locke finds himself retreating from a scientific to a commonsense, non-demonstrative definition of the human for support:

> For I presume 'tis not the idea of a thinking or rational being alone, that makes the idea of a man in most people's sense; but of a body so and so shaped joined to it; and if that be the idea of a man, the same successive body not shifted all at once, must as well as the same immaterial spirit go to the making of the same man.

Although he has not actually relaxed the qualifications for species membership, the emphasis is different. Exceptions to the rational rule are dealt with leniently:

---

[69] *Two Hundred Queries*, 75.
[70] *An Essay*, 331 ff.

> I think I may be confident, that whoever should see a creature of his own shape and make, though it had no more reason all its life, than a cat or a parrot, would call him still a man; or whoever should hear a cat or a parrot discourse, reason, and philosophise, would call or think it nothing but a cat or a parrot; and say, the one was a dull irrational man, and the other a very intelligent rational parrot.

The tone of voice, if nothing else, has changed. Unadjusted names (a "man" who none the less has "had no reason all his life") may not be accurate, but they will do. The chapter on personal identity is about the individual self as such, not about its relationship to the species; correspondingly, the treatment of supposedly inadequate individuals swings towards inclusive indifference and an everyday account of what it is to be human.

We should note finally that even within the first edition, Locke's exceptionalism is dependent upon context. For example, differential psychology is brought up yet again under the heading of "Probability," but in this context it suits him to depict differences of ability as gradual. It is true, he says, that "if we will compare the understanding and abilities of some men, and some brutes, we shall find so little difference, that 'twill be hard to say, that that of the man is either clearer or larger"; nevertheless, the point of saying this here is to show that the scale of nature has "gradual and gentle descents," rather than the precise interstitial categories he mentions elsewhere such as lithodendra, oysters and changelings.

From theology to psychology – and vice versa

In a final twist, Locke's *On the Conduct of the Understanding*, unfinished at his death, manages to be more pessimistic even than the first edition of the *Essay*. The logic of the earlier work was not an end in itself but a ground-clearing exercise for the directly theological themes of the *Conduct*, which he had always had in mind as being the final destination of the trajectory he had mapped out in 1671. The express purpose of this last work was to identify the "great many *natural* defects in the understanding capable of *amendment*" (emphasis added), in preparation for the afterlife.[71] As our own nature-versus-nurture reflex might lead us to expect, he distinguishes such natural defects from "differences which arise from acquired habits." But equally clearly he demarcates a further, internal distinction within the realm of nature itself: between "want of a due improvement" of natural defects, and "want of parts" or "lack of natural faculties." We might think that by natural defects, therefore, he means some pathological condition with the prospect of some improvement within strict limits. However, that is not what he means: he is referring to the majority of human beings. Amendment of their natural defects is a plausible aim, and it thereby throws into much sharper relief the actual *absence* of faculties in a small minority. "Want of parts" is not natural at all but *un*natural, because unamendable. Locke, expert in the operations by which one arrives at the common ideas, is lead climber on the ascent to intellectual perfection: not yet at the summit but with an idea of the best, if not the sole route. The rest of us will follow in our own ways. His changeling is the person who, by contrast, does not have any equipment to start with.

The *Conduct* is pessimistic even about those large numbers of people whose faculties are amendable. If we compare it with the *Essay*'s positive account of those people who are restricted only by social circumstance, such as malnourished labourers or gospel-less Americans, we find in the later work that although "Americans [are] not all born with worse understandings than the Europeans ... we see none of them have such reaches in the arts and sciences." In general, "We are born to be if we please rational creatures but 'tis use and exercise only that makes us so, and we are

---

[71] *Of the Conduct*, 158.

indeed so no farther than industry and application has carried us."[72] That "industry" is intellectual and professional. He writes about the man "of low and mean education who ha[s] never elevated [his] thoughts above the spade and the plough nor looked beyond the ordinary drudgery of a day-labourer ... used for many years to one tract, out of that narrow compass he has been all his life confined to; you will find him no more capable of reasoning than almost a perfect natural," that is, a born fool. "Tract" recalls the term used by Descartes and Willis to denote the physical pathways carved out in the brain by the soul spirits, with the addition of a further, social resonance: the one-track mind is also the track or furrow ploughed by the country labourer.

This time, it is not only changelings that challenge the principle "man is a rational animal," but natural defects of this far more widespread type. "Wherever a man's rational faculty fails him and will not serve him to reason there we cannot say he is rational how capable soever he may be by time and exercise to become so" – time and exercise that for so many of the working population remained entirely hypothetical. The concept of rationality presented here is even more firmly linked than it was in the *Essay* to that of development. It is also – and therefore – more firmly linked to social status: the highest "knowledge and science in general is the business only of those who are at ease and leisure." In the *Conduct* the requirement is not that everyone become a Lockean philosopher but, as his early Calvinist upbringing had taught him, that everyone has the reason appropriate to their calling. Hence his advice during the 1680s to a friend about the latter's "blockheaded" son, affected by what has been retrospectively diagnosed as encephalitis (but which Locke refers to as "melancholy"). Locke suggested finding the boy a calling he could cope with, so that he might lead his earthly existence in a social niche which, while it did not correspond with his ascribed rank in the honour society, was still as close to honourable as possible. He proposed "a handicrafts trade"; this could still fit a "gentleman's calling," he said, as long as – crucially – he did not depend on it for his living. (Basket weaving springs to mind.) In addition to the professional calling there are certain natural graces – "concern in a future life" and "thoughts in religion" – which are not related to social status at all. *No one* can be excused from "understanding the words and framing the general notions relating to religion right"; after all, as scores of earlier Protestant writers had said, there were "instances of very mean people who have raised their minds to a great sense and understanding of religion."[73] If they can do it, says Locke to his readers, so can you.

So much for those whose failure to try is not to be excused. As for those others who do not have the natural ability to try in the first place, Locke's intuition is not that they should therefore be excused but the opposite. In them, the very *grounds* for excusal are absent. Absolute absence of any such natural graces, of the basis for any calling at all, logically means "levelling them with the brutes and charging them with a stupidity below the rank of rational creatures." Those who simply do not try "might be brought to be rational creatures and Christians," whereas the second type "can hardly be thought to be so who wearing the name know not so much as the very principles of that religion" (a description which he allocates to both the idiotic and the libertine changeling).[74] He follows up immediately by asserting that knowledge of the mind is the necessary precondition for all other types of scientific knowledge: "Great advancements might be made in knowledge of all kinds especially in that of the greatest concern and largest views if men would make a right use of their faculties and study their own understandings." The seeming switch here from an understanding of religion to understanding of the mind is not a switch at all because they are the

---

[72] Ibid., 119.

[73] Letter to Edward Clarke, 6 February 1687; Marshall, *A Kind of Life Imposed on Man*, 89; *Of the Conduct*, 170.

[74] *Of the Conduct*, 171.

same thing. The notion of what constitutes intelligence, in being rescued from old conventions, is also being rescued from pagan influence or Catholic ones.

The application of logical forms to the study of one's own understanding and to the human sciences in general would become increasingly common after Locke's death. The line runs from the *Essay* and the *Conduct*, through his influence on eighteenth- and early nineteenth-century nonconformist educators and behaviour experts, and thence into modern applied psychologies. Whereas (as we saw in Chapter 17) the emphasis in logic had once been on the consistency of its procedures, Locke and his eighteenth-century followers invested a greater importance in the truth content of the propositions handled by those procedures. Verbal statements used in the exposition of logical procedures now had to correspond rigidly with their corresponding factual states. This kind of logic turned out to be the framework in which modern scientific theorems could be cast. It would certainly work for practical purposes in physics. In the human sciences, though, a problem arose. An ideological statement could become a factual statement simply by being proposed in a logical format. One could then assert as scientific truth whatever one liked. Take the example of the eighteenth-century logician and Locke disciple William Barron, who wrote: "Truth relates to the enunciation of knowledge, and is the agreement of ideas with words. If I assert that the British is a free government, and that the English are more industrious than any other nation in Europe, I maintain truth, because my words actually correspond to the accurate ideas of the facts."[75] Indeed, palpably value-laden truths of this kind were to form the content of the verbal components of early IQ tests. But Barron's proposition is no passing travesty. Locke's own model of logic used religious examples that were similarly value laden, as we have seen. Whatever he said in the *Essay* and the *Conduct* about his intellectually disabled creatures being non-human because they lacked a rational soul, he believed at the moment of writing. He was not just shuffling an array of "well-established doctrines" which he may or may not have endorsed, and was certainly not playing devil's advocate.

But if the burden in logic had come to lie as much on the truthfulness of its constituent propositions as on their consistency with each other, the very starting point for this shift, across the board, was a religious proposition – a dogma, in fact, with God as its unchallengeable guarantor – about the centrality of man's place in nature and of his logically reasoning intellect in relation to other creatures. What about the truth content of *that* proposition? Ray and Linnaeus launched modern forms of biological classification on the basis of a logic that likewise developed out of this prior theory of man's relationship to God; but while modern biology has undergone a critical process enabling it in many respects to migrate to the land of objective scientific critique, the psychology of intelligence remains in the land of its birth. Without the benefit of a scientific revolution of its own, its theological core has never dissolved. Human reason's vision of its own self remains tethered (if tacitly) to God, to stop it from simply blowing away. The kinship between psychology and religion is a familiar theme in critical histories of the discipline; but the relationship is more than one of mere analogy, or of similarity of their respective professional roles in the social order. The twenty-first-century psychologist's secularism is as flimsy as the eighteenth-century gentleman's Anglican faith was once said to be.

Logical "trains of ideas" thus emerged from the substructure of the Protestant ethic. Locke applies Baxter's notion of "intellectual labour" to the detail of the intellectual operations, in a proto-industrial concept of mind. Education means coaxing children into continuous trains of ideas; that is why Locke was against corporal punishment (it confuses and interrupts the train). Political and religious ideas should likewise be free from external compulsion, so that individual opinions can negotiate their own route more easily towards the single revealed truth. In this respect the *Conduct*

---

[75] Cited in Howell, *Eighteenth Century British Logic*, 296.

brings up another component of intelligence, attention span. Where once the relevant pathology was "instability of opinion" about the common ideas, now it is a discontinuity in the trains by which one reaches them. Locke comments in this respect, "He that will observe children will find that even when they endeavour their utmost they cannot keep their minds from straggling."[76] This found its way into the eighteenth century's everyday culture and behavioural advice. Isaac Watts emphasizes how necessary it is to "fix attention": "a student should labour, by all proper methods, to acquire a steady fixation of thought. Attention is a very necessary thing in order to improve our minds. The evidence of truth does not always appear immediately, nor strike the soul at first sight." Watts cites mathematics as the best pedagogy in this respect, because it is the most abstract form in which "a perpetual chain of connected reasonings" occurs. Mathematical trains are the model for moral and religious ones; scientific and exact, they are the best exercise for learning one's catechism and the ideal "young gentleman and lady's monitor," a social control mechanism.[77]

The need to labour at knowing one's own internal psychological operations and making them more efficient, says Watts, is a constituent of faith itself, thus endorsing Locke's assertion in the *Conduct*: "God has made the intellectual world harmonious and beautiful without us but it will never come into our heads all at once; we must bring it home piecemeal and there set it up by our own industry or else we shall have nothing but darkness and a chaos within, whatever order and light there be in things without us."[78] Watts's 1724 *Logic* was published in countless editions well into the nineteenth century; it transmitted the logic of Locke's *Conduct* to the burgeoning public education system, in the form of a theology of the inner person that corresponded with the public functions and prescriptions of reason and emotion in everyday human life. Once again the work's full title demonstrates the point: *Logick: or the Right Use of Reason in the Enquiry after Truth with A Variety of Rules to guard against Error, in the Affairs of Religion and Human Life, as well as in the Sciences*. It is true that Watts is not Locke's star pupil. Often he seems to be trying to shoehorn the latter's logic back into some older Aristotelian framework. And when he paraphrases Locke's theory of nominal essences, he unwittingly gives the master's well-guarded secret away: nominal essences are real enough, he says; they only need to be flexible when species boundaries are threatened as in "monstrous births." In short, they are a way of having your cake and eating it. Watts's examples of a logical proposition are nearly all drawn from religious knowledge. Logical trains of (religious) ideas thus become a textbook method for inculcating appropriate behaviour, more open to monitoring and assessment. Students' abilities, as he says elsewhere, can be differentiated by their capacity to "take in propositions," from those who "can take in a long train of propositions" to those who can only take in two at a time, for whom "it is hard for them to discern the difference between right and wrong in matters of reason on any abstracted subjects; these ought never to set up for scholars."[79]

The other writer of mass influence to inherit Locke's logic and embed it in behavioural and educational prescriptions was John Wesley. He too tries at first to wiggle it into a conventional Aristotelian framework. However, he also reports faithfully Locke's description of logic as a set of rules for "the proper use of words."[80] Wesley starts off with simple terms, the "common word or noun." The very first of these, as we might expect, is "man." The first subsequent division is then: "a man or a brute." From here he proceeds to "Definition." In the case of man, "Homo is defined

---

[76] *Of the Conduct*, 210.
[77] Watts, *The Improvement of the Mind; or, a Supplement to the Art of Logic*, 150; John Hamilton Moore, *The Young Gentleman and Lady's Monitor*, 2.
[78] *Of the Conduct*, 224.
[79] Watts, *The Improvement*, 168.
[80] Wesley, *A Compendium of Logic*, 1.1.1.

nominally, which ... is: accidentally, a two-legged unfeathered animal; logically, a rational animal; physically, a being consisting of an organized body and a reasonable soul." For Wesley, logic is a therapy. Its job is to clarify the intellectual operations; and clarified intellectual operations are those which can understand intellectual operations in all their clarity. Their condition correlates with the individual's state of grace and status with God. Wesley's examples are exclusively of the type "Every wicked man is miserable; Every tyrant is a wicked man; therefore Every tyrant is miserable," or "All the faithful are dear to God; Some, that are afflicted, are faithful; therefore Some, that are afflicted, are dear to God." And so on. It would be easy to think that he was just using a rhetorical device familiar among preachers, imparting to dogmatic assertions about faith a scientific logical structure to which the statement is obviously not suited; but in fact the logic and the faith were integral to each other, from the beginning.

Watts, Wesley and Jonathan Edwards, all of whom minimized reprobation out of good taste as much as doctrine (thus leaving room for it to spring up in some other guise), probably had a greater influence on the general culture, and hence on the school curricula from which the everyday practices of psychology would later emerge, than did any writers on higher-level matters, and certainly more than any medical men. David Hume elevates the discussion of changelings on to the plane of a liberal argument about the social limits of justice. He posits "a species of creatures intermingled with men which, though rational" may be of such "weakness of mind" that we "should not, properly speaking, lie under any restraint of justice with regard to them"; the qualification "though rational" appears to suggest that, however arbitrarily we may act towards them in ethical terms, we should at least not classify them out of the species. Adam Smith identifies idiocy in pre-Lockean terms as the lack of formal education and lack of a personal sense of honour. Thomas Reid's discussion of Locke on abstraction and nominal essences steers clear of intellectual monstrosity entirely, even though he acknowledges elsewhere the existence of people who lack reason, that "gift of heaven" (and does not see them as problems).[81] As for the medical men, they did not open their doors to Locke's natural history of the mind immediately and indeed spent most of the eighteenth century attacking it, for the same old reason that their predecessors had attacked Epicureanism: he was threatening the equality and immortality of the soul. Sometimes they take the positive step of insisting that the "changelings" are fully human and have souls.[82] The same insistence featured in eighteenth-century London's obsession with Peter the Wild Boy, and in his feral successor Victor of Aveyron (since retrospectively diagnosed with "mental retardation" or "autism," according to taste).

Only later in the century did doctors develop proto-psychiatric classifications of intellectual pathology, which nervously begin to ape those of bodily disease. The framework for this was the Lockean logical paradigm: the moment for his proposed "observation of [the] several ways of faltering" had arrived. François Boissier de Sauvages, acknowledging Locke's principle that "names are the signs for ideas," followed by William Cullen, Philippe Pinel and others, provided the classificatory basis for those nineteenth-century categories of idiocy and imbecility with which historians have already familiarized us.[83] Typically, John Mason Good's *The Study of Medicine* finds a spot for our topic at "Class 4 (Neurotica), Order 1 (Phrenica), Genus 6 (Moria or Fatuity), Species 2 (Moria demens), Variety 3 (Anoea or Idiotism)." However the question, as always, is: what was

---

[81] Hume, *Enquiry concerning the Principles of Morals*, 190; Smith, *The Theory of Moral Sentiments*, 260; Reid, *Essays on the Intellectual Powers of Man*, 190 ff., 232.

[82] Henry Lee, *Anti-Scepticism, or Notes upon Each Chapter of Mr. Lock's* Essay concerning Humane Understanding, 261.

[83] See also Suzuki, "Anti-Lockean Enlightenment? Mind and body in early eighteenth-century English medicine," in R. Porter (ed.), *Medicine in the Enlightenment*.

the symptomatic content of the patient's idiotism? In this respect the full impact of the Lockean paradigm had yet, even then, to be felt. Most of the symptoms Boissier lists under *amentia* still evoke Galenist tradition. It would take the arrival of the formal disciplines of psychology, under the influence of the everyday behavioural mind set inculcated by Watts, Wesley and Edwards, before lack of abstraction and logical reasoning became embedded in medical and psychiatric descriptions of disability.

Locke and our history

Like his fellow Royal Society members, Locke sought a language in which all terms have the precision of mathematics. Human reason, needed to maintain a perfectly ordered commonwealth, lay in the public effectiveness of ordered language. However, in the term for the species "man" – that is, the term language users apply to themselves – precision and order emerged upon forfeit of a sacrifice, namely the intellectually disabled changeling. The sacrificing of some piece or other to make the whole comprehensible is of course characteristic of science in general:

> Such stability as there is in a system of knowledge comes entirely from the collective decisions of its creators and users. It derives from the active protection of parts of the network. That is to say: from the requirement that certain laws and classifications be kept intact .... The rest of the network then becomes a field of resources to be exploited to achieve this end – a place where thresholds can be moved with relative ease; where complexity or blame can be conveniently located, or troublesome cases relegated.[84]

But as we have seen throughout this book, psychology in this sense is a very special system indeed. What is the stable network that Locke wants kept intact? The link between human beings and reason – a link that formerly went under the classification "Man is a rational animal." Why is a moving of the classificatory threshold, the readjustment to "moral man," necessary? Because reason is now the responsibility of imperfect but hopefully perfectible beings, of individuals, rather than a ready-made and uniform divine gift. What must now therefore be protected against? Not so much relativism, as absence. The special characteristic of systems of psychological knowledge, unlike our knowledge of physics or chemistry, is that the system under observation is not the conceptual handling of objects in the external world but that of the system's creators and users themselves; and correspondingly, the troublesome and blameworthy case is not only a *conceptual* one, it is troublesome and blameworthy *people*, the system's non-users. Intellectually disabled people, as people, are absent from a system of knowledge in which both object and subject are the intellectually able species "man." However, as a concept, they are key to it. The system cannot exist without their separate conceptual classification, yet their real existence as people threatens it. Or would threaten it, if ever those people might miraculously present the abstracted and logically reasoning abilities that are the entry ticket to the system, according to its own creators' and users' rules of self-representation and status – but of course, this is impossible as they cannot, by definition, abstract or reason logically. Hence modern man (that is, the intelligence society) more than "relegates" them, it turns them into objects of "ritual avoidance," both in an existential sense and in our social institutions.[85]

---

[84] David Bloor, "Durkheim and Mauss revisited: classification and the sociology of knowledge," *Studies in the History and Philosophy of Science*, 13/4 (1982).

[85] Douglas, *Purity and Danger*, 54.

An Enlightenment concept of man was subsequently generated, and could only have been generated, by excluding *a priori* from that concept certain "men." With the positive establishment of the human mind as a natural and quasi-secular realm of its own came intellectual disability as its generalized negative. Locke's theory of consent promotes liberty as key to plucking ecclesiastical and social order out of a volatile political environment; but accompanying the strange birth of liberal England were some other, anomalous offspring. Inhuman changelings, incompetent, totally determined and at the opposite end of the scale from liberty, were necessary to the theory of consent. Locke's out-group, conceived out of a particular political conjuncture, has been taken by modern psychology to be a self-evident fact of nature. Of course Locke too presented it as if it were, at the time. However, his invocation of nature was merely an ad hoc remedy, a bandage for the fissures in a doctrine of human reason that was wide open to sceptical attack. As Montaigne had remarked, "They cannot even dream up an ordinance for man, let alone find a true one, without there being some sound or cadence which they cannot quite fit in, however abnormal or monstrous they make their contrivance and however much they try and botch it up with a thousand false and fantastical patches."[86]

How does one combat debilitating scepticism? The *Essay* is partly a response to a widely debated exchange from earlier in the century. Lord Herbert of Cherbury had argued for the innateness of the common ideas on the grounds that if they are innate they must also be beyond doubt. There are, he said, ideas that are certain because all members of the human race agree about them. Back came the sceptics, such as Gassendi: a madman might not agree.[87] All right then, says Herbert, everyone *except* madmen or "idiots" (this probably still included the labourers on his estate), and for good measure the sceptics themselves: everyone who ignores or doubts the common ideas is "insane, addled, weak-brained, unreasoning, witless, and stupid." But in that case, returns the sceptic, how can we be certain who is right in the head and who not? Enter Locke with a fully scientific rejoinder, grounded in the idea that the autonomous mind has its own separate existence in nature. It is not the actual *content* of the common ideas, he says, but the *operations leading there* that are innate and can be known with certainty. It follows that these operations, in reconstituting what "ability" means, have their own specific impairments, in which madmen remain human (the operations run askew) but not changelings (the operations are absent).

In a liberal society that defines human ability in terms of autonomy, consent and rational choice, the idea of intellectual disability as natural absence gives the psychology of intelligence a place on which to stand, and to move its intellectual universe. Locke was, if momentarily, as desperate as our own bioethicists for an ethical certainty about what it is to be human; without the "intellectually disabled" changelings and idiots he describes, all his anti-sceptical efforts would have been in vain. This shows us that exclusions from the magic circle of intelligence are in fact the freakish product of a particular set of circumstances in the relatively recent past. There were and will be other ways of sizing up other people, and other ways of promoting one's own self-esteem.

---

[86] *An Apology*, 112.

[87] Herbert of Cherbury, *De Veritate*, 83; Gassendi, Letter to Elie Diodati, 29 August 1634, in *Actes du congrès du tricentenaire de Pierre Gassendi*.

Works Cited

Certain texts of very recent origin are treated in this book as objects of anthropological as well as historical investigation and are therefore listed here as primary sources.

Primary sources

D'Abano, Pietro, *Conciliator Contraversiarum, quae inter Philosophos et Medicos Versantur,* Venice 1548.
Ibn Abbas, Ali, *Liber Totius Medicinae,* Lyons 1523.
Aeschylus, *Prometheus Bound,* in *Aeschylus I,* Cambridge MA 1926.
Akakia, Martin, *Claudii Galeni Ars Medica,* Venice 1544.
Albertus Magnus, *Commentarii in Octo Libros Politicorum Aristotelis,* in *Opera Omnia* (A. Borgnet ed.), viii, Paris 1896.
———, *Summa de Creaturis,* in *Opera Omnia* (A. Borgnet ed.), xxxiv, Paris 1896.
———, *Liber de Animalibus* (R. Stadler ed.), Munich 1916.
———, *Quaestiones super De Animalibus,* in *Opera Omnia* (B. Geyer ed.), xii, Münster 1955.
———, *De Anima,* in *Opera Omnia* (B. Geyer ed.), vii, Münster 1968.
Alexander of Aphrodisias, *The Problems of Aristotle; with Other Philosophers and Physicians,* London 1647.
———, *De Anima* (I. Bruns ed.), Berlin 1887.
———, *In Aristotelis Topicorum Commentaria* (M. Wallies ed.), Berlin 1891.
———, *On Fate* (R. Sharples ed.), London 1983.
———, *Ethical Problems* (R. Sharples ed.), London 1990.
———, *Scripta Minima* (R. Sharples ed.) in W. Kullmann et al. (eds), *Gattungen wissenschaftlicher Literatur in der Antike,* Tübingen 1998.
Allestree, Richard, *The Whole Duty of Man,* London 1659.
L'Alouette, François, *Traicté des nobles et des vertus dont ils sont formés,* Paris 1577.
Alpago, Andrea, *Compendium de Anima,* Venice 1546.
Amyraut, Moise, "Eschantillon de la doctrine de Calvin, touchant la prédestination," in *Six sermons de la nature,* Saumur 1636.
———, *Fidei circa Errores Arminianorum,* Saumur 1646.
———, *Speciminis Animadversionum Specialorum in Exercitationes de Gratia Universali,* in *Specimen Animadversionum,* Saumur 1648.
———, *La vie de François, seigneur de La Noue,* Leiden 1661.
———, *De Libero Arbitrio,* Saumur 1667.
Andrewes, Lancelot, *XCVI Sermons,* London 1629.
Anon., *The Prerogative of Man: or, his Soules Immortality,* Oxford 1645.
Anon., *Anthropologie Abstracted: or, the Idea of Human Nature,* London 1655.
Anon., *A Modest Plea for an Equal Commonwealth, against Monarchy,* London 1659.
Anon., *An Antidote against Mr Baxter's Palliated Cure of Church Divisions,* London 1670.
Anon., *The Heraldry of Nature,* London 1785.
Aquinas, Thomas, *Compendium Theologiae,* St Louis 1952.
———, *Summa Theologica,* New York 1947.

Aranzi, Guilio Cesare, *Hippocratis Librum de Vulneribus Capitis*, Leiden 1579.
Argenterio, Giovanni, *In Artem Medicinalem Galeni Commentarii Tres*, Turin 1566.
Aristotle, *Nicomachean Ethics*, Cambridge MA 1926.
———, *Politics*, Cambridge MA 1932.
———, *Metaphysics*, Cambridge MA 1935.
———, *On the Soul*, Cambridge MA 1936.
———, *Categories*, Cambridge MA 1938.
———, *Prior Analytics*, Cambridge MA 1938.
———, *Posterior Analytics*, Cambridge, MA 1960.
———, *Topics*, Cambridge MA 1960.
———, *On the Parts of Animals*, Cambridge MA 1961.
Aristotle (attrib.), *Physiognomics*, Cambridge MA 1963.
Arminius, James, *Works*, London 1825.
Ascham, Roger, *The Scholemaster*, London 1570.
Ashley, Robert, *Of Honour*, San Marino CA 1947.
Monsieur D'Aubray, *Le satyre Menippée*, Paris 1594.
Averroes, *Commentarium Magnum in Aristotelis de Anima Librum Tertium* (F. Crawford ed.), Cambridge MA 1953.
———, *Incoherence of the Incoherence* (S. van den Bergh ed.), Cambridge 1954.
———, *Middle Commentary on Porphyry's* Isagoge (H. Davidson ed.), Berkeley 1969.
———, *Three Short Commentaries on Aristotle's* Topics, Rhetoric, *and* Poetics (C. Butterworth ed.), Albany 1977.
———, *Middle Commentaries on Aristotle's* Categories *and* De Interpretatione (C. Butterworth ed.), Princeton 1983.
Avicenna, *Compendium de Anima* (F. Rahman trans.), Oxford 1952.
———, *Psychology* (F. Rahman ed.), Oxford 1952.
———, *Avicenna Latinus* (S. van Riet ed.), Leiden 1968.
———, *Liber de Anima seu Sextus de Naturalibus*, Leiden 1972.
———, *The Propositional Logic* (N. Shehaby trans.), Dordrecht 1973.
Bacon, Francis, *Essays*, London 1601.
———, *Works* (B. Montagu ed.), iv, London 1826.
———, *The Life and Letters of Francis Bacon* (J. Spedding ed.), ii, London 1857.
———, *Essays Civil and Moral*, London 1909.
Banister, John, *The Historie of Man*, London 1578.
Baron-Cohen, Simon, *The Essential Difference: the Truth about the Male and Female Brain*, London 2004.
Bartolus (de Saxoferrato), *Tractatus de Insigniis et Armis*, Bonn 1883.
Bates, William, *The Whole Works*, London 1815.
Bauhin, Caspar, *De Hermaphroditorum Monstrorumque*, Oppenheim 1614.
Baxter, Richard, *Letters*, Dr Williams Library London.
———, *The Right Method for a Settled Peace of Conscience*, London 1653.
———, *Apology*, London 1654.
———, *The Reduction of a Digressor*, London 1654.
———, *Certain Disputations of Right to Sacraments*, London 1657.
———, *Directions and Perswasions to a Sound Conversion*, London 1658.
———, *Of Saving Faith*, London 1658.
———, *The Holy Commonwealth*, London 1659.
———, *The Cure of Church Divisions*, London 1670.

———, *The Duty of Heavenly Meditation*, London 1671.
———, *Gods Goodness Vindicated*, London 1671.
———, *Catholicke Theologie*, London 1675.
———, *The Poor Mans Family Book*, London 1684.
———, *The Universal Redemption of Mankind*, London 1694.
———, *Reliquiae Baxterianae*, London 1696.
———, *Compassionate Counsel to All Young Men*, in (W. Orme ed.) *The Practical Works of Richard Baxter*, xv, London 1830.
Beard, Thomas, *The Theatre of God's Judgements* (fourth edition), London 1648.
Benedetti, Alessandro, *Historia Corporis Humani*, Florence 1998.
Benzi, Ugo, *Expositio super Libros Tegni Galeni*, Venice 1498.
Berners, Juliana, *The Boke of Saint Albans*, London 1881.
Beverley, John, *Unio Reformantium*, London 1659.
Binet, Alfred "Méthodes nouvelles pour le diagnostic du niveau intellectuel des anormaux", *L'année psychologique*, 11 (1905).
———, *Les idées modernes sur les enfants*, Paris 1910.
——— and Théodore Simon, *A Method of Measuring the Development of the Intelligence of Young Children*, Chicago 1913.
Blake, Martin, *The Great Question*, London 1645.
Blake, William, *The Poetry and Prose of William Blake* (G. Keynes ed.), London 1956.
Bodin, Jean, *De la démonamie des sorciers*, Anvers 1586.
De le Boe, Franciscus [Sylvius], *The Practice of Physick*, London 1717.
Boehme, Jakob, *Ψυχολογια: Vera I.B.T. XL Quaestionibus Explicata*, Amsterdam 1632.
———, *The Works*, London 1764.
Bonours, Christophle, *Eugeniaretologie, ou discours de la vraye noblesse*, Liège 1616.
Bostrom, Nick, "How long before Superintelligence?" *International Journal of Futures Studies*, 2, 1998.
Boswell, James, *The Life of Samuel Johnson*, London 1783.
Boudon, Henri-Marie, *La science sacrée du catéchisme*, Paris 1678.
Bourne, Immanuel, *A Defence and Justification of Ministers Maintenance by Tythes and of Infant Baptism, Humane Learning, and the Sword of the Magistrate*, London 1659.
Boyle, Robert, *Some Considerations touching the Style of the Holy Scriptures*, London 1661.
———, "The origins of forms and qualities according to the corpuscular philosophy," in M.A. Stewart (ed.), *Selected Philosophical Papers*, Indianapolis 1991.
Bradley, Thomas, *Nosce Teipsum, in a Comparison between the First, and the Second Adam*, York 1668.
Braham, Humfrey, *The Institucion of a Gentleman*, London 1555.
Brant, Sebastian, *Navicula sive Speculum Fatuorum*, Strasbourg 1510.
Brathwait, Richard, *The English Gentleman* (second edition), London 1633.
Breton, Nicholas, *The Goode and the Badde*, in S. Brydges (ed.) *Archaica*, London 1815.
———, *The Court and Country*, in W. Hazlitt (ed.) *Tracts Illustrating English Manners*, London 1868.
Bright, Timothy, *A Treatise of Melancholie*, London 1586.
Brooke, Robert, *The Nature of Truth, its Union and Unity with the Soule*, London 1640.
———, *A Discourse Opening the Nature of that Episcopacie, which is Exercised in England*, London 1642.
Brooks, Thomas, *A Golden Key* (1675), Glasgow 1763.
Browne, Sir Thomas, *Religio Medici*, London 1643.

Bryskett, Lodowyck, *A Discourse of Civill Life*, London 1606.
Bull, George, *Examen Censurae*, London 1676.
Bullinger, Heinrich, *The Decades of Henry Bullinger*, Cambridge 1849.
———, *Antidotus against the Anabaptistes*, Amsterdam 1973.
Bunyan, John, *Reprobation Asserted*, London 1674.
———, *The Pilgrim's Progress*, London 1678.
———, *The Holy War*, London 1682.
Buridan, Jean, *Aristotelis de Anima*, in George Lockhart, *Quaestiones et Decisiones Physicales Insignium Virorum*, Paris 1518.
———, *Quaestio in Octo Libros Politicorum Aristotelis*, Oxford 1640.
Burke, Edmund, Supplement to E. Malone (ed.), *The Works of Sir Joshua Reynolds* (second edition), London 1798.
Burroughs, Jeremiah, *Irenicum, to the Lovers of Truth and Peace*, London 1645.
Burt, Sir Cyril, *Mental and Scholastic Tests* (fourth edition), London 1962.
Burton, Robert, *The Anatomy of Melancholy*, London 1932.
Butler, Samuel, *Characters*, Cleveland 1970.
Calvin, Jean, *Institutes*, Louisville 1960.
Cameron, John, *Opera Omnia*, Frankfurt 1642.
Campanella, Tommaso, *De Sensu Rerum et Magia*, Paris 1637.
Cardano, Girolamo, *De Subtilitate*, in *Opera Omnia*, Lyons 1663.
Casmann, Otho, *Psychologia Anthropologica; sive Animae Humanae Doctrina*, Hanover 1594.
Castiglione, Baldesar, *The Book of the Courtier*, London 1967.
Cattell, James, "Mental tests and measurement," *Mind*, 15 (1890).
De Caumont, Jehan, *De la vertu de noblesse*, Paris 1586.
Celsus, Aurelius Cornelius, *De Re Medica*, Paris 1772.
Champier, Symphorien, *Le fondement et origine des titres de noblesse*, Lyons 1547.
Charron, Pierre, *Of Wisdom*, London 1707.
Cicero, *De Officiis*, Cambridge MA 1913.
———, *Tusculan Disputations*, Cambridge MA 1927.
———, *On Oratory*, Cambridge MA 1942.
———, *Topics*, Cambridge MA 1949.
Clichtovaeus, Jodocus, *De Vera Nobilitate*, Paris 1512.
Coeffeteau, Nicolas, *A Table of Humane Passions*, London 1621.
Coke, Sir Edward, *The First Part of the Institutes of the Lawes of England*, London 1628.
Collegium Conimbricense, *In Tres Libros de Anima Aristotelis Stagiritae*, Cologne 1600.
———, *Commentariorum Physicorum Aristotelis Stagiritae*, Cologne 1625.
Collinges, John, *The Preacher (Pretendedly) Sent, Sent Back*, London 1658.
Columbus, Realdus, *De Re Anatomica*, Frankfurt 1593.
Combe, George, *Elements of Phrenology*, London 1828.
Conway Morris, Simon, *Life's Solution*, Cambridge 2003.
de Cordemoy, Louis, *Le discernement du corps et de l'âme*, Paris 1666.
Cotton, John, *The Grounds and Ends of the Baptisme of the Children of the Faithfull*, London 1646.
Cowell, John, *The Interpreter*, Cambridge 1607.
Crane, Thomas, *The Exempla or Illustrative stories from the Sermones Vulgares of Jacques de Vitry*, London 1890.
Crooke, Helkiah, *Microcosmographia: a Description of the Body of Man*, London 1615.
Crookshank, Francis, *The Mongol in our Midst*, New York 1931.
Cudworth, Ralph, *The True Intellectual System of the Universe*, London 1678.

Culpeper, Nicholas, *A Key to Galens Method of Physick*, London 1651.
———, *Galens Art of Physick*, London 1652.
Dampmartin, Pierre, *Bonheur de la cour*, Anvers 1592.
Dante, *De Monarchia*, R. Kay (trans.), Toronto 1998.
Darwin, Francis, *The Life and Letters of Charles Darwin* (second edition), London 1887.
Davenant, John, *Dissertatio de Morte Christi*, Cambridge 1650.
Davies, John (of Hereford), *Mirum in Modum*, London 1602.
———, *Witts Pilgrimage*, London 1605.
Davies, Sir John, *Nosce Teipsum: of Humane Knowledge*, London 1599.
Dawkins, Richard, *The Extended Phenotype*, Oxford 1982.
Dekkers, E. and Fraipont, J., *Sancti Aurelii Augustini Enarrationes in Psalmos*, Turnhout 1956.
Descartes, René, *Discours de la méthode*, Paris 1925.
———, *Passions of the Soul*, Indianapolis 1989.
———, *Regulae ad Directionem Ingenii*, Amsterdam 1998.
Diderot, Denis, *Letter on the Blind, for the Use of Those who can See*, in M. Jourdain (ed.) *Diderot's Early Philosophical Works*, Chicago 1916.
Digby, Sir Kenelm, *Observations upon* Religio Medici, London 1643.
———, *Of Bodies, and of Mans Soul*, London 1669.
Dio Chrysostom, *Discourses*, Cambridge MA 1939.
Diogenes Laertius, *The Lives of the Philosophers*, Cambridge MA 1925.
Donne, John, *Satires, Epigrams and Verse Letters*, Oxford 1967.
Drake, Roger, *A Boundary to the Holy Mount*, London 1653.
———, *The Bar, against Free Admission to the Lords Supper, Fixed*, London 1656.
De Dryvere, Jérémie, *In Τεχνην Galeni Commentarii*, Lyons 1547.
———, *Universae Medicinae Methodus*, Leiden 1592.
Duke, Francis, *The Fulness and Freeness of Gods Grace*, London 1654.
Dulaure, Jacques-Antoine, *Histoire critique de la noblesse*, Paris 1790.
Dyer, Thiselton, *English Folklore*, London 1878.
Earle, John, *Microcosmographie, Or a Peece of the World Discovered, in Essayes and Characters*, London 1628.
Edwards, Jonathan, *A Treatise concerning Religious Affections*, Boston 1746.
Edwards, Robert, "Test-Tube Revolution," in *The Sunday Times*, 4 July, London 1999.
Elyot, Thomas, *The Governour*, London 1531.
———, *Of the Knowledge whiche Maketh a Wise Man*, London 1533.
Erasmus, Desiderius, *Familiarum Colloquiorum Opus*, Frankfurt, 1555.
———, *The Manual of the Christian Knight*, London 1905.
Erastus, Thomas, *Disputationum de Nova Philippi Paracelsi*, Basle 1572.
Estwick, Nicholas, *Πνευματολογια: or, a Treatise of the Holy Ghost*, London 1648.
Eustachius, Bartolomeus, *Opuscula Anatomica*, Leiden 1707.
Eysenck, Hans, "The concept of intelligence: useful or useless?" *Intelligence*, 12 (1988).
Du Fail, Noël, *Baliverneries*, Paris 1548.
Falloppio, Gabriele, *Observationes Anatomicae*, Venice 1561.
Faret, Nicholas, *The Honest Man: or, the Art to Please in Court*, London 1632.
Fenner, Dudley, *The Artes of Logike*, Middelburg 1584.
Fenner, William, *Wilfull Impenitency the Grossest Selfe-Murder*, London 1656.
Ferguson, Robert, *A Sober Enquiry into the Nature, Measure and Principle of Moral Virtue*, London 1673.
———, *The Interest of Reason in Religion*, London 1675.

Ferne, John, *Blazon of Gentrie*, London 1586.
Fiera, Battista, *Commentaria Novae Doctrinae in Artem Medicinalem Galeni*, Mantua 1515.
Firmin, Gabriel, *The Real Christian, or a Treatise of Effectual Calling*, London 1670.
Flavell, John, *The Method of Grace*, London 1681.
Flint, J. and Yule, W., "Behavioural phenotypes," in M. Rutter et al. (eds), *Child and Adolescent Psychiatry*, Oxford 2002.
Franz, Adolph, *Der Magister Nikolaus Magni von Jawor*, Freiburg 1898.
Fraunce, Abraham, *The Lawiers Logike*, London 1588.
Freigius, Ioannis, *Quaestiones Physicae*, Basle 1579.
Fuller, Thomas, *The Holy and the Profane State*, London 1642.
Furetière, Antoine, *Dictionnaire universel*, Paris 1690.
Furneaux, W.D., "Intellectual abilities and problem-solving behaviour," in H. Eysenck (ed.), *Handbook of Abnormal Psychology*, London 1960.
Galen, Claudius [Galenus], *The Art of Medicine*, in C. Kühn (ed.), *Opera Omnia*, i, Hildesheim 1964.
———, *De Usu Partium*, in *Opera Omnia*, iii.
———, *Quod Animi Mores*, in *Opera Omnia*, iv.
———, *De Locis Affectis*, in *Opera Omnia*, viii.
———, *Commentary on Hippocrates* Epidemics 6, in *Opera Omnia*, xvii.
———, *De Ossibus*, in *Opera Omnia*, xvii.
Galton, Francis, *Hereditary Genius: an Inquiry into its Laws and Consequences*, London 1869.
———, *Inquiries into Human Faculty and its Development*, London 1883.
Gassendi, Pierre, *The Mirrour of True Nobility*, London 1657.
———, *Opera Omnia*, Lyons 1658.
———, *Institutio Logica, et Philosophiae Epicuri Syntagma*, London 1660.
———, Letter to Elie Diodati, *Actes du congrès du tricentenaire de Pierre Gassendi*, Paris 1957.
Gazzaniga, Michael, *The Ethical Brain*, Chicago 2005.
Georget, Etienne, *De la folie: considérations sur cette maladie*, Paris 1820.
Gibbon, Edward, *Autobiography*, London 1971.
Gillespie, George, *Aaron's Rod Blossoming*, London 1646.
Glanvill, Joseph, *Scepsis Scientifica, or The Vanity of Dogmatizing*, London 1661.
———, *Essays on Several Important Subjects in Philosophy and Religion*, London 1676.
———, *An Essay concerning Preaching*, London 1678.
———, *Saducismus Triumphatus: or, Full and Plain Evidence concerning Witches and Apparitions* (second edition), London 1682.
Glisson, Francis, *Tractatus de Natura Substantiae Energetica, seu de Vita Naturae*, London 1672.
Glover, Robert, *Nobilitas Politica vel Civilis*, London 1608.
Göckel, Rudolf [Goclenius], *Psychologia, hoc est, de Hominis Perfectione, Animo et in Primus Ortu hujus*, Marburg 1590.
Good, John Mason, *The Study of Medicine*, London 1822.
Gracián, Baltasar, *Oráculo manual y arte de prudenza*, New York 1993.
Grantham, Thomas, *The Infants Advocate*, London 1688.
Greville, Fulke, *Poems and Dramas of Fulke Greville*, Oxford 1945.
Grimm, Jakob, *Deutsche Mythologie*, Göttingen 1835.
Grimm, Wilhelm and Jakob, *Deutsche Sagen*, Berlin 1816–1818.
Gundisalvus, Dominicus, *Liber de Anima*, Toronto 1940.
Gwillim, John, *A Display of Heraldrie*, London 1610.

Haier, Richard, "Cortical glucose metabolic rate correlates of abstract reasoning and attention studied with positron emission tomography," *Intelligence*, 12 (1988).
Hall, Joseph, *Works* (P. Wynter ed.), Oxford 1863.
Hall, S. et al, "Structural and environmental characteristics of stereotyped behaviors," *American Journal of Mental Retardation*, 108 (2003).
Haller, Albrecht von, *Elementa Physiologiae*, Lausanne 1763.
Hammond, Henry, *The Miscellaneous Theological Works*, Oxford 1847.
Hansen, Joseph, *Quellen und Untersüchungen zur Geschichte des Hexenwahns*, Bonn 1901.
Harderus, Johannes, *Exercitationes Anatomicae et Medicae*, Basle 1682.
Hartland, Edwin, *The Science of Fairy Tales*, London 1895.
Hartley, David, *Observations on Man*, London 1749.
Van Helmont, Franciscus, *Two Hundred Queries Moderately Propounded concerning the Doctrine of the Revolution of Humane Souls*, London 1684.
Van Helmont, Jean Baptiste, *Opera Omnia*, Frankfurt 1707.
Herbert, Lord Edward (of Cherbury), *De Veritate*, Paris 1624.
Heron, Haly, *The Kayes of Counsaile*, Liverpool 1954.
Hetherington, W. (ed.), *Notes and Debates of Proceedings of the Assembly of Divines at Westminster*, Edinburgh 1846.
Highmore, Nathaniel, *The History of Generation*, London 1651.
Hildebrand, Joachim, *Immortalitas Animae Rationalis ex Solo Lumine Naturae*, Celle 1680.
Hippocrates, *Airs, Waters, Places* in *Hippocrates I*, Cambridge MA 1923.
———, *On Joints*, in *Hippocrates III*, Cambridge MA 1928.
———, *On Regimen*, in *Hippocrates IV*, Cambridge MA 1959.
———, *On Injuries of the Head*, in E. Littré (ed.), *Opera Omnia*, iii, Amsterdam 1982.
———, *Places of Man*, in *Opera Omnia*, vi, 1982.
Hobbes, Thomas, *Leviathan*, Cambridge 1991.
Hofmann, Caspar, *Commentarii in Galeni de Usu Partium Corporis Humani*, Frankfurt 1625.
Hooker, Richard, *The Lawes of Ecclesiastical Politie*, London 1594.
Hooker, Thomas, *The Convenant of Grace Opened*, London 1649.
Howe, John, *The Reconcileableness of God's Prescience of the Sins of Men, with the Wisdom and Sincerity of his Counsels ... in a Letter to the Honourable Robert Boyle Esq*, London 1777.
Howe, Samuel Gridley, *On the Causes of Idiocy*, Edinburgh 1858.
Huarte, Juan, *The Examination of Mens Wits*, London 1594.
Hughes, George, *Disputatio Philosophica*, bound in Wegner, *Tentamen Primum* [below].
Hume, David, *Enquiry concerning the Principles of Morals*, in H. Aiken (ed.) *Hume's Moral and Political Philosophy*, New York 1948.
Humfrey, John, *An Humble Vindication of a Free Admission unto the Lords Supper*, London 1652.
———, *A Second Vindication of a Disciplinary, Anti-Erastian, Orthodox Free Admission to the Lords Supper*, London 1656.
Humfrey, Lawrence, *The Nobles, and of Nobility*, London 1563.
I.M., *A Health to the Gentlemenly Profession of Serving-Men*, London 1598.
Ideler, Julius, *Physici et Medici Graeci Minores*, Berlin 1841.
Ingrassia, Gian Filippo, *In Galeni Librum de Ossibus Commentaria*, Palermo 1603.
Irwing, Paul, and Richard Lynn, "Is there a sex difference in IQ scores?" *Nature*, 442 (2006).
James VI of Scotland, *Daemonologie*, Edinburgh, 1597.
Jensen, Arthur, "Reaction time and psychometric g," in H. Eysenck (ed.), *A Model for Intelligence*, New York 1982.
Johannsen, Wilhelm, *Elemente der exakter Erblichkeitslehre*, Jena 1926.

Jones, John, *A Briefe, Excellent, and Profitable Discourse, of the Naturall Beginning of all Growing and Living Things*, London 1574.

———, *The Arte and Science of Preserving Bodie and Soule*, London 1579.

Jonston, John, *A History of the Wonderful Things of Nature*, London 1657.

Kanner, Leo, "Infantile autism and schizophrenia," *Behavioral Science*, 10 (1965).

Kant, Immanuel, *Critique of Teleological Judgement*, Oxford 1952.

Kelley, Truman, *Scientific Method*, New York 1932.

Kenyon, John, *The Stuart Constitution 1603–1608: Documents and Commentary*, Cambridge 1966.

Knox, John, *The First Blast of the Trumpet against the Monstrous Regiment of Women*, Edinburgh 1895.

Köhler, Johann, *De Origine Animarum Rationalium*, bound in Göckel, *Psychologia* [above].

Kühn, Adalbert and Wilhelm Schwartz, *Norddeutsche Sagen*, Leipzig 1848.

Lambert, Johann, *Cosmologische Briefe*, Augsburg 1761.

Lane, Edward, *Du Moulin's Reflections Reverberated*, London 1681.

Langdon Down, John, *The Education and Training of the Feeble in Mind*, Belfast 1867.

Langland, William, *The Vision of Piers Plowman* (B-Text), London 1995.

Lascovius, Petrus Monedulatus, *De Homine*, Wittenberg 1585.

Lavater, Johannes Caspar, *Essays on Physiognomy*, London 1789.

Lee, Henry, *Anti-Scepticism, or Notes upon Each Chapter of Mr. Lock's* Essay concerning Humane Understanding, London 1702.

Da Legnano, Giovanni, *De Bellis, de Represaliis et de Duello*, Washington DC 1917.

Leigh, Gerard, *The Accedence of Armorie*, nl 1612.

Lemnius, Levinus, *Occulta Naturae Miracula*, Antwerp 1559.

———, *De Habitu et Constitutione Corporis*, Erfurt 1582.

Lenton, Francis, *Characters: or, Wit and the World in their Proper Colours, in The Young Gallants Whirligigg*, London 1629.

Leoniceno, Niccolò, *Galeni Ars Medicinalis*, Leiden 1532.

Lewis, M., "Ultradian rhythms in stereotyped and self-injurious behavior," *American Journal of Mental Deficiency*, 85/6 (1981).

Licetus, Fortunius, Ψυχολογια Ανθρωπινε sive de Ortu Animae Humanae, Frankfurt 1606.

Lightfoot, John, *Horae Hebraicae et Talmudicae: Hebrew and Talmudical Exercitations upon the Gospels*, Cambridge 1658.

Locke, John, *Two Treatises of Civil Government*, London 1924.

———, *An Early Draft of Locke's* Essay (R. Aaron and J. Gibb eds), Oxford 1936.

———, *Essays on the Law of Nature*, Oxford 1954.

———, *Some Thoughts concerning Education*, London 1964.

———, "Medical notebooks," in K. Dewhurst, *John Locke, Physician and Philosopher*, London 1966.

———, *An Essay concerning Human Understanding*, Oxford 1975.

———, *Of the Conduct of the Understanding*, Utrecht 2000.

Long, A.A. and D.N. Sedley (eds), *The Hellenistic Philosophers*, Cambridge 1987.

de Lorraine, Monsieur le Cardinal, *Discours sur le congé impétré*, Paris 1565.

Loyseau, Charles, *Traité des ordres et simples dignités*, Paris 1610.

Lull, Ramón, *Book of the Ordre of Chyvalry*, London 1926.

Luther, Martin, *Colloquia Mensalia, or, Table Talk*, London 1652.

———, *Gesamtausgabe Werke*, Weimar 1883.

Lynn, Richard, "Skin color and intelligence in African Americans," *Population and Environment*, 23/4 (2002).

Malebranche, Nicolas, *De la recherche de la verité*, Paris 1674.

———, "Mémoire: pour expliquer la possibilité de la transsubstantiation", in *Oeuvres*, xvii, Paris 1960.

Manardi, Giovanni, *Annotationes in Artis Medicinalis Galeni*, Basle 1541.

Mancin, Dominike, *The Mirrour of Good Maners*, Manchester 1885.

Markham, Francis, *The Booke of Honour*, London 1625.

Marois, Claude, *Le gentil-homme parfaict*, Paris 1631.

Maxwell, John, *Sacro-Sancta Regum*, Oxford 1643.

Mayow, John, *Tractatus Quinque Medico-Physici*, London 1674.

Mede, Joseph, *Works* (fourth edition), London 1667.

Mercado, Luis, *Opera Omnia*, Frankfurt 1608.

Mercurialis, Hieronymus, *Medicina Practica*, Frankfurt 1602.

Metham, John, *The Works of John Metham*, London 1916.

Migne, J.-P., *Patrologiae Cursus Completus*, Paris 1841.

Mill, James, *Analysis of the Phenomena of the Human Mind*, London 1869.

Milles, Thomas, *The Catalogue of Honor*, London 1610.

———, *The Treasurie of Aunciept and Moderne Times*, London 1619.

Milton, John, *De Doctrina Christiana*, Cambridge 1825.

Mommsen, Theodor et al. (eds), *The Digest of Justinian*, Philadelphia 1985.

De Montaigne, Michel, *Essais* (F. Strowski, ed.), Paris 1906–12.

———, *An Apology for Raymond Sebond*, London 1987.

Da Monte, Giambattista, *In Artem Parvam Galeni Explanationes*, Lyons 1556.

Moore, John Hamilton, *The Young Gentleman and Lady's Monitor, and English Teacher's Assistant*, London 1802.

Morani, Moreno, *Nemesii Emeseni de Natura Hominis*, Leipzig 1987.

More, Henry, *The Life of the Learned and Pious Henry More*, London 1911.

Moreno, Bernabé (de Vargas), *Discursos de la nobleza de España*, Madrid 1659.

De Mornay, Philippe, *The True Knowledge of a Mans Owne Selfe*, London 1602.

Du Moulin, Pierre, *The Anatomy of Arminianisme*, London 1620.

———, *Esclaircissement des controverses Salmuriennes*, Leiden 1648.

Mulcaster, Richard, *Positions wherin those Primitive Circumstances be Examined, which are Necessarie for the Training up of Children*, London 1581.

Müller, Johannes, *Elements of Physiology*, London 1842.

Nagel, Georg [Nagelius], Ψυχολογια, *seu Disputatio Physica de Anima ejusque Causis*, Wittenberg 1624.

Nenna, Giambattista, *A Treatise of Nobilitie*, London 1600.

Nicole, Pierre, *Essais de morale*, Paris 1715.

———, "Honneur", in *Pensées de Pascal suivies d'un choix des pensées de Nicole*, Paris 1907.

Nidditch, Peter H., *Draft A of Locke's* Essay concerning Human Understanding, Sheffield 1980.

——— and G.A.J. Rogers, *Drafts for the* Essay concerning Human Understanding: *Drafts A and B*, Oxford 1990.

Nider, Johannes, *Praeceptorum Divinae Legis*, Frankfurt 1485.

Nivelon, Francis, *The Rudiments of Genteel Behaviour*, London 1737.

Norden, John, *The Mirror of Honour*, London 1597.

Nuck, Anton, *Opera*, Leiden 1733.

O'Brien, G. and W. Yule (eds), *Behavioural Phenotypes*, London 1995.

Degli Oddi, Oddo, *Expositio in Librum Artis Medicinalis Galeni*, Venice 1574.

De Oncieu, Guillaume, *La précédence de la noblesse*, Lyons 1593.

Overbury, Thomas, *Characters*, London 1614.
Overton, Richard, *Mans Mortallitie*, Amsterdam 1643.
———, *An Arrow against All Tyrants*, London 1646.
Owen, John, *The Death of Death in the Death of Christ*, London 1648.
———, *Pneumatologia*, London 1674.
———, *Meditations and Discourses on the Glory of Christ*, London 1684.
———, *Of Infant Baptism and Dipping*, London 1839.
———, *Works*, vii, Edinburgh 1850.
Palazzini, Pietro, *Dictionarum Morale et Canonicum*, Rome 1965.
Palmer, Anthony, *A Scripture-Rale to the Lords Table*, London 1654.
Paracelsus, *De Generatione Stultorum*, in *Sämtliche Werke* (K. Sudhoff ed.), xiv, Munich 1933.
———, *Krankheiten die der Vernunft berauben*, in *Sämtliche Werke*, ii, 1933.
Pardies, Ignace-Gaston, *Discours de la conoissance des bestes*, Paris 1672.
Parker, Samuel, *An Account of the Nature and Extent of the Divine Dominion*, Oxford 1666.
———, *A Demonstration of the Divine Authority of the Law of Nature*, London 1681.
Pascal, Blaise, *Pensées*, London 1995.
Paulus Nicolettus [Venetus], *Summa Naturalium*, Venice 1476.
———, *Scriptum super Librum de Anima Aristotelis*, Venice 1481.
Peacham, Henry, *The Art of Drawing with the Pen*, London 1606.
———, *The Gentleman's Exercise*, London 1607.
———, *The Compleat Gentleman*, London 1622.
Pelletier, Thomas, *La nourriture de la noblesse*, Paris 1604.
Pemble, William, *The Workes*, Oxford 1659.
Penn, William, *The Great Case of Liberty of Conscience Once More Debated*, London 1671.
———, *The New Witnesses Proved Old Hereticks*, London 1672.
Pepys, Samuel, *Diary*, London 1893.
Perkins, William, *A Briefe Discourse, Taken out of the Writings of Her. Zanchius*, London 1595.
———, *A Discourse of Conscience*, Cambridge 1597.
———, *A Discourse of the Damned Art of Witchcraft*, Cambridge 1610.
———, *The Workes*, Cambridge 1616.
Piper, P. (ed.), *Die Schriften Notkers und seiner Schule*, Freiburg 1882.
Plater, Felix, Abdiah Cole, Nicholas Culpeper, *Platerus Golden Practice of Physick*, London 1664.
Plato, *The Sophist*, Cambridge MA 1921.
———, *Theaetetus*, Cambridge MA 1921.
———, *Protagoras*, Cambridge MA 1924.
———, *Gorgias*, Cambridge MA 1925.
———, *Philebus*, Cambridge MA 1925.
———, *The Statesman*, Cambridge MA 1925.
———, *The Laws*, Cambridge MA 1926.
———, *Epistles*, Cambridge MA 1929.
———, *Timaeus*, Cambridge MA 1929.
———, *The Republic*, Cambridge MA 1930.
Platter, Felix, *Observationum in Hominis Affectibus*, Basle 1614.
———, *Praxeos Medicae*, Basle 1656.
Plomin, Robert, "Behavioural genetics," in P. McHugh et al., *Genes, Brains and Behavior*, New York 1992.
Poiret, Pierre, *Cogitationum Rationalium*, Amsterdam 1685.
Porzio, Simone, *De Humana Mente Disputatio*, Florence 1551.

Powell, Thomas, *The Attourney's Academy*, London 1623.
De la Primaudaye, Pierre, *Académie Françoise*, London 1586.
Prynne, William, *A Vindication of Foure Serious Questions*, London 1645.
Pufendorf, Samuel, *De Jure Naturae et Gentium*, Frankfurt 1684.
De la Ramée, Pierre, *Dialectique*, Paris 1555.
Régis, Pierre-Sylvain, *Cours entier de philosophie*, Amsterdam 1691.
Reid, Thomas, *Essays on the Intellectual Powers of Man*, Edinburgh 1785.
Reisch, Gregor, *Margarita Philosophica*, Freiburg 1517.
Reynolds, Edward, *A Treatise of the Passions and Faculties of the Soule of Man*, London 1640.
Rich, Barnabie, *Faultes, Faults, and Nothing Else but Faultes*, London 1606.
Ibn Ridwan, Ali, *Galeni Liber qui Techni Inscribuntur*, bound in Ibn Abbas, *Liber* [above].
Riolan, Jean, *In Artem Parvam Galeni Commentarius*, Paris 1631.
De Rivault, David, *Les estats, esquels il est discouru du Prince, du Noble, & du tiers Estat*, Lyons 1595.
Roach, E. and R. Schwarz (eds), *Martin Luthers Wolfenbütteler Psalter*, Leipzig 1983.
Rogers, Thomas, *The Anatomie of the Minde*, London 1586.
De la Roque, Gilles, *Traité de la noblesse, de ses differentes espèces*, Paris 1678.
Rowland, Samuel, *The Letting of Humours Blood in the Head-Vaine*, London 1600.
Rushton, J. Philippe, *Race, Evolution and Behaviour*, New Brunswick NJ 1995.
Rutherford, Samuel, *The Trial and Triumph of Faith*, London 1645.
———, *Christ Dying and Drawing Sinners to Himselfe*, London 1647.
Rutter, Michael, et al., "Genetic influences on mild mental retardation," *Journal of Biosocial Science*, 28 (1996).
Ruvius, Antonius, *Commentarii de Anima*, Cologne 1613.
Ryle, Gilbert, *A Rational Animal*, London 1962.
Salkeld, Thomas, *The Compleat Gentleman*, London 1730.
Di Santa Sofia, Galeazzo, *Libellus Familiarium Introductionum in Artem Parvam Galeni*, Hagenau 1533.
Santorio, Santorio, *Commentaria in Artem Medicinalem Galeni*, Venice 1630.
Schenk, Johannes, *Observationes Medicae de Capite Humano*, Basle 1584.
Schubart, Andreas, *De Abstractione*, Jena 1652.
Sclano, Salvo, *Commentaria Praeclarissima Artis Medicinalis Galeni*, Venice 1597.
Scohier, Jehan, *L'estat et comportement des armes*, Brussells 1597.
Scot, Reginald, *The Discoverie of Witchcraft*, London 1584.
———, *A Discourse concerning the Nature and Substance of Devils and Spirits*, London 1665.
Segar, William, *The Book of Honor and Armes*, London 1590.
———, *Honor, Military and Civil*, London 1602.
Selden, John, *Table Talk*, London 1689.
De Sepúlveda, Juan Ginés, *Tratado sobre las justas causas de la guerra contra los Indios*, Mexico 1941.
Sermoneta, Giovanni, *Quaestiones Subtilissimae*, Venice 1498.
Sextus Empiricus, *Against the Mathematicians*, London 1933.
Shuttleworth, George, *Some of the Cranial Characteristics of Idiocy*, London 1881.
Sidney, Sir Philip, *A Defense of Poesy*, Manchester 2002.
Simons, Menno, *The Complete Writings*, Scottdale PA 1956.
Skuse, D. et al., "Evidence from Turner's syndrome of an imprinted X-linked locus affecting cognitive function," *Nature*, 387 (1997).
Smith, Adam, *The Theory of Moral Sentiments*, Indianapolis 1982.

Smith, Sir Thomas, *De Republica Anglorum*, London 1583.
Song, F., et al, "Screening for fragile X syndrome: a literature review and modelling," *Health Technology Assessment Publications*, 7 (2003).
Spilsbery, John, *A Treatise concerning the Lawfull Subject of Baptism*, London 1652.
Sprenger, Jakob, and Heinrich Kramer [Institoris], *Malleus Maleficarum*, Leiden 1669.
Taine, Hippolyte, *De l'intelligence*, Paris 1870.
Talbot, Eugene, *Degeneracy, its Causes, Signs and Results*, London 1898.
Tassoni, Alessandro, *Dieci Libri di Pensieri Diversi*, Venice 1608.
Tax, P. (ed.), *Notker Latinus*, Tübingen 1972.
Taylor, Jeremy, *The Whole Works*, London 1822.
Teretius, Gregorius, *Confessio et Instructio Idiotae*, Kraków 1653.
Testard, Paul, *Synopsis Doctrinae de Natura et Gratia*, Blois 1633.
Themistius, *On Aristotle on the Soul*, London 1996.
Theophrastus, *Characters*, London 1870.
Da Thiene, Gaetano, *Super Libros de Anima Aristotelis*, Vicenza 1486.
De Thierriat, Florentin, *Trois tractez, savoir de la noblesse de race*, Paris 1606.
Thompson, Stith, *Motif-Index of Folk Literature*, Bloomington 1932.
Thorndike, Edward, *The Measurement of Intelligence*, New York 1927.
Timson, John, *The Bar to Free Admission to the Lord's Supper Removed*, London 1654.
Todd, T. and D. Lyons, "Cranial suture closure, its progress and age relationship: endocranial closure in adult males of Negro stock," *American Journal of Physical Anthropology*, 8 (1925).
Tombes, John, *Anti-Paedobaptism*, London 1654.
Tomkis, Thomas, *Lingua; or the Combat of The Tongue and the Five Senses for Superiority*, London 1607.
Torrigiano, Pietro [Turisanus], *Plusquam Commentum in Parvam Galeni Artem*, Venice 1557.
Tozzi, Luca, *In Artem Medicinalem Galeni*, in *Opera Omnia*, Venice 1711.
Truman, Joseph, *A Discourse of Natural and Moral Impotency*, London 1671.
———, *The Great Propitiation*, London 1672.
Tüntzel, Wolfgang, Ψυχολογια *Generalis*, Jena 1633.
Turquet, Théodore (de Mayerne), *La monarchie aristodémocratique*, Paris 1611.
Twisse, William, *De Praedestinatione, Gratia, & Libero Arbitrio*, Amsterdam 1649.
———, *De Vindiciis Gratiae*, Amsterdam 1652.
Tyndale, William, *The Obedience of a Christen Man*, Antwerp 1528.
———, *Doctrinal Treatises and Introductions to Different Portions of the Holy Scriptures*, Cambridge 1848.
Ussher, James, *The Power Commanded by God to the Prince*, London 1661.
Vallés, Francisco, *Galeni Ars Medicinalis Commentariis*, Alcalá de Henares 1567.
Van Foreest, Pieter, *Observationum et Curationum Medicinalium ac Chirurgicarum*, Frankfurt 1634.
Vesalius, Andreas, *De Humani Corporis Fabrica*, Leiden 1725.
Vinge, Vernor, "The coming singularity: how to survive in the post-human era," *Whole Earth Review*, Winter 1993.
De Vitry, Jacques, *Sermones Vulgares*, Bibliothèque nationale, Paris, ms.17509.
Vives, Juan Luis, *De Anima et Vita*, Basle 1538.
———, *De Subventione Pauperum*, Florence 1973.
Walkington, Thomas, *The Optick Glasse of Humors*, London 1607.
Wanley, Nathaniel, *The Wonders of the Little World*, London 1678.

Ward, Seth, *A Philosophicall Essay*, Oxford 1652.
Watts, Isaac, *Logick: or the Right Use of Reason in the Enquiry after Truth*, Edinburgh 1781.
———, *The Improvement of the Mind: or, a Supplement to the Art of Logic*, London 1811.
Webster, John, *The Displaying of Supposed Witchcraft*, London 1677.
Wegner, Claud, *Tentamen Primum Metaphysico-Psychologicum*, Copenhagen 1708.
Weigel, Valentin, Γνωθι Σεαυτον, *Nosce Teipsum, Erkenne dich selbst*, Neuenstadt 1618.
Wesley, John, *A Compendium of Logic*, London 1756.
Wielgus, S. (ed.), "Quaestiones Nicolai Peripatetici," *Mediaevalia Philosophica Polonorum* 17, 1973.
Wilkins, John, *Ecclesiastes, or, the Art of Preaching*, London 1646.
———, *An Essay towards a Real Character, and a Philosophical Language*, London 1668.
William of Auvergne, *De Universo*, in *Opera Omnia*, Orléans 1674.
Willis, Humphrey, *Englands Changeling, or the Time Servers Laid Open in their Colours*, London 1659.
Willis, Thomas, *De Cerebri Anatome*, Amsterdam 1664.
———, *De Anima Brutorum*, London 1672.
———, *De Anima Brutorum*, (trans.) Samuel Pordage as "Two discourses on the soul of brutes," London 1683.
Wilson, Thomas, *The Rule of Reason*, London 1551.
Winkler, Daniel, *De Vita Foetus in Utero*, Jena 1630.
Wittgenstein, Ludwig, *Remarks on the Philosophy of Psychology*, Oxford 1980.
W.M., *The Middle Way of Predetermination Asserted*, London 1679.
Wolf, Johann, *Beiträge zur Deutschen Mythologie*, Göttingen 1852–1857.
Womock, Laurence, *Arcana Dogmatum Anti-Remonstrantium*, London 1659.
Woolnor, Henry, *The True Originall of the Soule*, London 1641.
Wordsworth, William, Letter to John Wilson, June 1802, in E. de Selincourt (ed.), *The Early Letters*, Oxford 1935.
Wuttke, Adolf, *Der Deutsche Volksaberglaube der Gegenwart*, Hamburg 1860.
Wyrley, William, *The True Use of Armorie*, London 1592.
Zacchia, Paolo, *Quaestiones Medico-Legales*, Rome 1621.
Zanchius, Jerome, *Confession of Christian Religion*, Cambridge 1599.
Zúñiga, Francesillo, *Crónica burlesca del emperador Carlos V*, Salamanca 1989.
Zwingli, Huldrych, *The Defence of the Reformed Faith*, Allison Park 1984.

Secondary literature

Aaron, P.G., *Dyslexia and Hyperlexia: Diagnosis and Management of Developmental Reading Disabilities*, Dordrecht 1989.
Adorno, Theodor, *Dialectic of Enlightenment*, Stanford 2002.
Agrimi, Jole, *Ingeniosa Scientia Naturae: studi sulla fisiognomica medievale*, Florence 2002.
Allderidge, Patricia, "Management and mismanagement at Bedlam, 1547–1633," in C. Webster (ed.), *Health, Medicine and Mortality in the Sixteenth Century*, Cambridge 1979.
Armstrong, Brian, *Calvinism and the Amyraut Heresy*, Madison 1969.
Ashcraft, Richard, *Revolutionary Politics and John Locke's* Two Treatises of Government, Princeton 1986.
Ashworth, William, "Memory, efficiency, and symbolic analysis: Charles Babbage, John Herschel, and the industrial mind," *Isis*, 87 (1996).

Ayers, Michael, "Mechanism, superaddition and the proof of God's existence in Locke's *Essay*," *Philosophical Review*, 50/2 (1981).
——, *Locke: Epistemology and Ontology*, London 1994.
Balme, David, "Aristotle's biology was not essentialist," in A. Gotthelf and J. Lennox (eds), *Philosophical Issues in Aristotle's Biology*, Cambridge 1987.
Baroja, Julio Caro, "Religion, world views, social classes, and honour," in J. Peristiany and J. Pitt-Rivers (eds), *Honour and Grace in Anthropology*, Cambridge 1992.
Baruzzi, A., "Der Freie und der Sklave in Ethik und Politik des Aristoteles," *Philosophisches Jahrbuch*, 77 (1970).
Barzun, Jacques, *From Dawn to Decadence*, London 2000.
Battegay, Raymond, "Felix Platter und die Psychiatrie," in U. Tröhler (ed.), *Felix Platter in seiner Zeit*, Basle 1991.
Beek, Henri, *De Geestesgestoorde in de Middeleeuwen*, Harlem 1969.
Bell, H.E., *An Introduction to the History and Records of the Court of Wards and Liveries*, Cambridge 1953.
Benschop, Ruth, and Douwe Draaisma, "In pursuit of precision: the calibration of minds and machines in late nineteenth-century psychology," *Annals of Science*, 57 (2000).
Berger, Harry, *The Absence of Grace: Sprezzatura and Suspicion in Two Renaissance Courtesy Books*, Stanford 2000.
Bergvall, A., "Reason in Luther, Calvin and Sidney," *Seventeenth Century Journal*, 23/10 (1992).
Berrios, German, "Mental retardation," in Berrios and R. Porter (eds), *A History of Clinical Psychiatry*, London 1995.
—— and I. Markova, "Conceptual issues," in H. D'haenen et al. (eds), *Biological Psychiatry*, London 2002.
Berry, J., "Radical cultural relativism and the concept of intelligence," in Berry and P. Dasen (eds), *Culture and Cognition: Readings in Cross-Cultural Psychology*, London 1974.
Bickert, Vera, *Calderons El alcalde de Zalamea als soziales Drama*, Frankfurt 1977.
Billington, Sandra, *A Social History of the Fool*, London 1984.
Bitton, Davis, *The French Nobility in Crisis, 1560–1640*, Stanford 1969.
Bloor, David, "Durkheim and Mauss revisited: classification and the sociology of knowledge," *Studies in the History and Philosophy of Science*, 13/4 (1982).
Blümlein, Kilian, *Naturerfahrung und Welterkenntnis*, Frankfurt 1992.
Bogdan, R. et al., "Be Honest but Not Cruel," in P. Ferguson (ed.) *Interpreting Disability*, Williston 1991.
Booth, Tim, "From normal baby to handicapped child," *Sociology*, 12, 1978.
Boring, E., *A History of Experimental Psychology*, New York 1929.
Bourdieu, Pierre, "Epreuve scolaire et consécration sociale," *Actes de la recherche en sciences sociales*, 39 (1981).
——, *The Logic of Practice*, Cambridge 1990.
Bouvier, Michel, "Le naturel," *XVIIe siècle*, 39 (1987).
Brann, Noel, *The Debate over the Origin of Genius during the Italian Renaissance*, Leiden 2002.
Bray, John, *Theodore Beza's Doctrine of Predestination*, Nieuwkoop 1975.
Brozek, Josef and Maarten Sibinga, *Origins of Psychometry: Johan Jacob de Jaager, Student of F.C.Donders*, Nieuwkoop 1970.
Brunt, P., *Studies in Greek History and Thought*, Oxford 1993.
Bruyn, George, "The seat of the soul," in F. Rose and W. Bynum (eds), *Historical Aspects of the Neurosciences*, New York 1982.

Buess, Heinrich, "Basler Mediziner der Barockzeit," in *Beiträge zur Geschichte der Naturwissenschaften und der Technik in Basel*, Olten 1959.
Bush, Michael, *The European Nobility*, Manchester 1988.
Cantor, Geoffrey, *Quakers, Jews, and Science: Religious Responses to Modernity and the Sciences in Britain, 1650–1900*, Oxford 2005.
Carlson, Licia, *The Faces of Intellectual Disability*, Bloomington 2010.
Carson, John, *The Measure of Merit: Talents, Intelligence, and Inequality in the French and American Republics, 1750–1940*, Princeton 2007.
Caspari, Fritz, *Humanism and the Social Order in Tudor England*, Chicago 1954.
Castro, Américo, *Le drame de l'honneur dans la vie et dans la littérature espagnoles du XVIe siècle*, Paris 1965.
———, *Spanien, Vision und Wirklichkeit*, Cologne 1957.
Clapton, Jayne, *A Transformatory Ethic of Inclusion*, Rotterdam 2009.
Clark, Stuart, *Thinking with Demons*, Oxford 1997.
Claus, David, *Toward the Soul*, London 1981.
Clegg, Jennifer, and R. Lansdall-Welfare, "Death, disability, and dogma," *Philosophy, Psychiatry and Psychology*, 10/1 (2003).
Craig, W., "Middle knowledge," in C. Pinnock (ed.), *The Grace of God and the Will of Man*, Minneapolis 1989.
Cranefield, Paul, "A seventeenth-century view of mental deficiency and schizophrenia: Thomas Willis on 'stupidity or foolishness,'" *Bulletin of the History of Medicine*, 35 (1961).
———, "The discovery of cretinism," *Bulletin of the History of Medicine*, 36 (1962).
——— and Walter Federn, "Paracelsus on goiter and cretinism: a translation and discussion of *De Struma, vulgo der Kropf*," *Bulletin of the History of Medicine*, 37 (1963).
——— and Walter Federn, "The begetting of fools: an annotated translation of Paracelsus' *De Generatione Stultorum*," *Bulletin of the History of Medicine*, 41 (1967).
Cummings, Brian, *The Literary Culture of the Reformation: Grammar and Grace*, Oxford 2002.
Danziger, Kurt, *Constructing the Subject*, Cambridge 1990.
Dasen, Véronique, *Dwarfs in Ancient Egypt and Greece*, Oxford 1993.
Daston, Lorraine, "Enlightenment calculations," *Critical Inquiry*, 21 (1994).
Desmond, Adrian, and James Moore, *Darwin*, London 1991.
Devyver, André, *Le sang épuré: les préjugés de race chez les gentilshommes français de l'Ancien Régime*, Brussels 1973.
Dilman, Ilham, "Science and psychology," in A. O'Hear (ed.) *Verstehen and Humane Understanding*, Cambridge 1996.
Dols, Michael, *Majnun: the Madman in Medieval Islamic Society*, Oxford 1992.
Douglas, Mary, *Purity and Danger*, London 1966.
Draaisma, Douwe, *Metaphors of Memory*, Cambridge 2000.
Duby, Georges, *The Chivalrous Society*, London 1977.
Dunn, John, "From applied theology to social analysis: the break between John Locke and the Scottish Enlightenment," in I. Hont and M. Ignatieff (eds), *Wealth and Virtue*, Cambridge 1983.
Elias, Norbert, *The Court Society*, Oxford 1983.
Ellis, Jack D., *The Physician-Legislators of France: Medicine and Politics in the Early Third Republic*, Cambridge 1990.
Evans, G.R., *John Wyclif, Myth and Reality*, Downers Grove, 2005.
Eyal, Gil, et al., *The Autism Matrix: the Social Origins of the Autism Epidemic*, London 2010.
Fales, Evan "Natural kinds and freaks of nature," *Philosophy of Science*, 49, 1982.

Fancher, Raymond, "Francis Galton and phrenology," in *Proceedings of Tennet IV*, Montreal 1983.
———, *The Intelligence Men*, New York 1987.
Fenn, Richard, *The Persistence of Purgatory*, Cambridge 1995.
Ferguson, Philip, *Abandoned to their Fate*, Philadelphia 1995.
Fiering, Norman, *Jonathan Edwards's Moral Thought and its British Context*, Chapel Hill 1981.
Fine, Cordelia, *Delusions of Gender: the Real Science behind Sex Differences*, London 2010.
Flynn, James, *What is Intelligence?* Cambridge 2001.
Fortenbaugh, William, "Aristotle on slaves and women," in J. Barnes et al. (eds), *Articles on Aristotle*, ii, London 1977.
Frank, Robert, *Harvey and the Oxford Physiologists*, Berkeley 1980.
French, Roger, and Andrew Cunningham, *The Invention of the Friars' Natural Philosophy*, Aldershot 1996.
Friedman, John Block, *The Monstrous Races in Medieval Art and Thought*, Syracuse 2000.
Fudge, Erica, *Perceiving Animals*, London 2000.
Funkenstein, Amos, *Theology and the Scientific Imagination*, Princeton 1986.
Gardner, Howard, *Frames of Mind: the Theory of Multiple Intelligences*, New York 1983.
Garnsey, Peter, *Social Status and Legal Privilege in the Roman Empire*, Oxford 1970.
Gernsbacher, Morton Ann et al., "Three reasons not to believe in an autism epidemic," *Current Directions in Psychological Science*, 14/2 (2005).
Gerrish, B., *Grace and Reason: a Study in the Theology of Luther*, Oxford 1962.
Gigon, O., "Die Sklaverei bei Aristoteles," in Fondation Hardt (ed.), *La 'Politique' d'Aristote*, Geneva 1964.
Gill, Christopher, "The question of character development," *Classical Quarterly*, 33 (1983).
Le Goff, Jacques, *The Birth of Europe*, Oxford 2005.
Goodey, C.F., "Mental disabilities and human values in Plato's late dialogues," *Archiv für Geschichte der Philosophie*, 74/1 (1992).
———, "John Locke's idiots in the natural history of mind," *History of Psychiatry*, 5 (1994).
———, "On Aristotle's 'animal capable of reason,'" *Ancient Philosophy*, 16 (1996).
———, "Learning difficulties and the guardians of the gene," in A. Clarke and E. Parsons (eds), *Culture, Kinship and Genes: towards Cross-cultural Genetics*, London 1997.
———, "Politics, nature and necessity: were Aristotle's slaves feeble-minded?" *Political Theory*, 27/2 (1999).
———, "From natural disability to the moral man: Calvinism and the history of psychology", *History of the Human Sciences*, 14/3 (2001).
———, "Foolishness in early modern medicine and the concept of intellectual disability," *Medical History*, 48/3 (2004), Copyright The Trustee, The Wellcome Trust.
———, "Intellectual ability and speed of performance: Galen to Galton," *History of Science*, 42 (2004).
———, "Blockheads, roundheads, pointy heads: intellectual disability and the brain before modern medicine," *Journal of the History of the Behavioral Sciences,* 41/2 (2005).
———, "Behavioural phenotypes in disability research: historical perspectives," *Journal of Intellectual Disability Research*, 50/6 (2006).
——— and Tim Stainton, "Intellectual disability and the myth of the changeling myth," *Journal of the History of the Behavioral Sciences*, 37/3 (2001).
Gould, Stephen Jay, *The Mismeasure of Man*, New York 1981.
Graves, Lila V., "Locke's changeling and the Shandy bull," *Philological Quarterly*, 60 (1981).

Green, Ian, *The Christian's ABC: Catechisms and Catechizing in England c.1530–1740*, Oxford 1996.
Hacking, Ian, *The Taming of Chance*, Cambridge 1990.
———, *The Social Construction of What?* Cambridge MA 1999.
Haffter, Carl, "The changeling: history and psychodynamics of attitudes to handicapped children in European folklore," *Journal of the History of the Behavioral Sciences*, 4/1 (1968).
Hagner, Michael, "Prolegomena to a history of radical brains," *Physis*, 36/2 (1999).
Harvey, Ruth, *The Inward Wits: Psychological Theory in the Middle Ages and Renaissance*, London 1975.
Herzog, Don, *Happy Slaves: a Critique of Consent Theory*, Chicago 1989.
Hexter, J.H., "The English aristocracy, its crises, and the English Revolution, 1558–60," *Journal of British Studies*, 8/1 (1968).
Hidalgo-Serna, E., "The philosophy of 'ingenium'," *Philosophy and Rhetoric*, 13 (1980).
Higonnet, Patrice, *Goodness beyond Virtue: Jacobins during the French Revolution*, Cambridge MA 2001.
Hill, Christopher, *From Reformation to Revolution*, Harmondsworth 1969.
———, *The Intellectual Origins of the English Revolution*, Oxford 1996.
Hilton, Boyd, *A Mad, Bad, and Dangerous People? England 1783–1846*, Oxford 2006.
Hilts, V., "Obeying the laws of hereditary descent: phrenological views on inheritance and eugenics," *Journal of the History of the Behavioral Sciences*, 18/1 (2006).
Howell, Wilbur, *Logic and Rhetoric in England, 1500–1700*, Princeton 1961.
———, *Eighteenth Century British Logic and Rhetoric*, Princeton 1971.
Hrdy, Sarah Blaffer, *Mother Nature: Natural Selection and the Female of the Species*, London 1999.
Hughes, Ann, "The frustrations of the godly," in J. Morrill (ed.), *Revolution and Restoration*, London 1992.
Hynes, Eugene, *Knock: the Virgin's Apparition in Nineteenth-century Ireland*, Cork 2008.
Ingram, Martin, "From Reformation to toleration," in T. Harris (ed.), *Popular Culture in England, c.1500–1800*, London 1995.
Jackson, Mark, *The Borderland of Imbecility*, Manchester 2000.
Jacquart, Danielle, "La physiognomie à l'époque de Frédéric II," *Micrologus*, 2 (1994).
James, M.E., "English politics and the concept of honour, 1485–1642," *Past and Present*, supp. iii (1978).
Joseph, Jay, *The Gene Illusion*, Ross-on-Wye 2003.
Joutsivuo, Timo, *Scholastic Tradition and Humanist Innovation*, Helsinki 1999.
Kanner, Leo, *A History of the Care and Study of the Mentally Retarded*, Springfield IL 1964.
Keeble, N., *Richard Baxter: Puritan Man of Letters*, Oxford 1982.
Kenny, Anthony, *The Metaphysics of Mind*, Oxford 1989.
Kessler, Eckhard, "The intellective soul," in C. Schmitt and Q. Skinner (eds), *The Cambridge History of Renaissance Philosophy*, Cambridge 1988.
Kevles, Daniel, *In the Name of Eugenics*, Cambridge MA 1985.
Kilmister, Clive, "Genius in mathematics," in P. Murray (ed.), *Genius: the History of an Idea*, Oxford 1989.
Klineberg, Otto, "An experimental study of speed and other factors in 'racial' differences," *Archives of Psychology*, 93 (1928).
Knoeff, Rina, "The reins of the soul: the centrality of the intercostal nerves to the neurology of Thomas Willis and to Samuel Parker's theology," *Journal of the History of Medicine and Allied Sciences*, 59/3 (2004).

Kraye, Jill, "The immortality of the soul in the Renaissance," *Signatures*, 1, ISSN 1472–2178.
Kuksewicz, Zdzisław, "The potential and the agent intellect," in N. Kretzmann et al. (eds), *The Cambridge History of Later Medieval Philosophy*, Cambridge 1982.
Kusukawa, Sachiko, *The Transformation of Natural Philosophy*, Cambridge 1995.
Lakoff, George, *Women, Fire and Dangerous Things*, Chicago 1990.
Lamont, William, *Richard Baxter of the Millennium*, London 1979.
Lanteri-Laura, Georges, *Histoire la phrénologie*, Paris 1970.
Laplanche, François, *Orthodoxie et prédication: l'oeuvre d'Amyraut et la querelle de la grâce universelle*, Paris 1965.
Laqueur, Thomas, *Making Sex: Body and Gender from the Greeks to Freud*, Cambridge MA 1990.
Leahy, Thomas, *A History of Modern Psychology* (second edition), Englewood Cliffs 1991.
Lear, Jonathan, *Aristotle: the Desire to Understand*, Cambridge 1988.
Leask, J., "Evidence for autism in folklore?" *Archives of Disease in Childhood*, 90/271 (2005).
Lendon, J.E., *Empire of Honour: the Art of Government in the Roman World*, Oxford 1997.
Levitas, Andrew S. and Cheryl S. Reid, "An angel with Down syndrome: a sixteenth-century Flemish nativity painting," *American Journal of Medical Genetics*, 116 (2003).
Lewontin, Richard, et al., *Not in Our Genes: Biology, Ideology and Human Nature*, London 1984.
Luttmer, Frank, "Persecutors, tempters and vassals of the devil," *Journal of Ecclesiastical History*, 51/1 (2000).
McDonagh, Patrick, *Idiocy: a Cultural History*, Liverpool 2009.
Mackenzie, Donald, *Statistics in Britain*, Edinburgh 1981.
Mallinson, Jeffrey, *Faith, Reason and Revelation in Theodore Beza*, Oxford 2003.
Mans, Inge, *Zin der Zotheid*, Amsterdam 1998.
Marshall, Paul, *A Kind of Life Imposed on Man: Vocation and Social Order from Tyndale to Locke*, Toronto 1996.
Marston, Jerrilyn, "Gentry honor and royalism in early Stuart England," *Journal of British Studies*, 13/1 (1973).
Mattern, Ruth, "Moral science and the concept of persons in Locke," *Philosophical Review*, 89/1 (1982).
Mazzacurati, Giancarlo, *Il Renascimento dei moderni*, Bologna 1985.
Meininger, Herman P., "Authenticity in community: theory and practice of an inclusive anthropology," *Journal of Religion, Disability and Health*, 5 (2001).
Mengal, Paul, "La constitution de la psychologie comme domaine du savoir aux XVIème et XVIIème siècles," *Revue d'histoire des sciences humaines*, 2 (2001/2).
———, *La naissance de la psychologie*, Paris 2005.
Michell, Joel, *Measurement in Psychology: a Critical History of a Methodological Concept*, Cambridge 1999.
Midgley, Mary, *Science and Poetry*, London 2001.
Miles, M., "Martin Luther and childhood disability," *Journal of Religion, Disability and Health*, 5/4 (2001).
Miller, William Ian, *The Anatomy of Disgust*, Cambridge MA 1998.
Mitchell, Joshua, *Not by Reason Alone: Religion, History and Identity in Early Modern Political Thought*, Chicago 1993.
Moore, R.I., *The Formation of a Persecuting Society*, Oxford 1987.
Motley, Mark, *Becoming a French Aristocrat*, Princeton 1990.
Müller, R., "La logique de la liberté dans la *Politique*," in P. Aubenque (ed.) *Aristote politique*.
Murray, Alexander, *Reason and Society in the Middle Ages*, Oxford 1978.

Neugebauer, Richard, "Medieval and early modern theories of mental illness," *Archive of General Psychiatry*, 36 (1979).
———, "A doctor's dilemma: the case of William Harvey's mentally retarded nephew," *Psychological Medicine*, 19/3 (1989).
———, "Mental handicap in medieval and early modern England," in D. Wright and A. Digby (eds), *From Idiocy to Mental Deficiency: Historical Perspectives on People with Learning Disabilities*, London 1996.
Norton, Rictor, "Gay history and literature," *The Homosexual Literary Tradition*, London 1972.
Nyhan, William, "Behavioral phenotypes in organic genetic disease," *Pediatric Research*, 6 (1972).
O'Donovan, Joan Lockwood, "Rights in Christian discourse," in M. Cromartie (ed.), *A Preserving Grace: Protestants, Catholics and Natural Law*, Washington DC 1997.
Orme, Nicholas, *Medieval Schools*, New Haven 2006.
Otto, Beatrice, *Fools are Everywhere: the Court Jester around the World*, Chicago 2001.
Ottosson, Per Gunnar, *Scholastic Medicine and Philosophy*, Naples 1984.
Pagden, Anthony, *The Fall of Natural Man*, Cambridge 1982.
Park, Katharine, "Albert's influence on late medieval psychology," in J.A. Weisheipl (ed.), *Albertus Magnus and the Sciences*, Toronto 1980.
———, "The organic soul," in C. Schmitt and Q. Skinner (eds), *The Cambridge History of Renaissance Philosophy*, Cambridge 1998.
Pearl, Sharrona, *About Faces: Physiognomy in Nineteenth-Century Britain*, Cambridge MA 2010.
Piaschewski, Gisela, *Der Wechselbag: ein Beitrag zum Aberglauben der nordeuropäischen Volker*, Breslau 1935.
Pick, Daniel, *Faces of Degeneration: a European Disorder, c.1848–c.1918*, Cambridge 1989.
Pinnock, C. (ed.), *The Grace of God and the Will of Man*, Minneapolis 1989.
Pitt-Rivers, Julian, "Honor," in E. Sills (ed.), *International Encyclopedia of the Social Sciences*, New York 1968.
———, *The Fate of Schechem*, Cambridge 1977.
———, "Postscript: the place of grace in anthropology," in J. Peristiany and J. Pitt-Rivers (eds), *Honour and Grace in Anthropology*, Cambridge 1992, 215–46.
Porter, Theodore, *Trust in Numbers: the Pursuit of Objectivity in Science and Public Life*, Princeton 1995.
Poynter, F.N.L., "Nicholas Culpeper and his books," *Journal of the History of Medicine*, 17 (1962).
Privateer, Paul Michael, *Inventing Intelligence: a Social History of Smart*, Oxford 2006.
Quinn, E.V. and J.M. Prest, *Dear Miss Nightingale: a Selection of Benjamin Jowett's Letters*, Oxford 1987.
Quinton, Anthony, "Has man an essence?", in R.S. Peters (ed.), *Nature and Conduct*, London 1971.
Reinders, Hans, *The Future of the Disabled in Liberal Society*, Notre Dame 2000.
Richards, Graham, "Getting the intelligence controversy knotted," *Bulletin of the British Psychological Society*, 37 (1984).
———, *Mental Machinery*, London 1992.
———, *"Race", Racism and Psychology: towards a Reflexive History*, London 1997.
Richards, Jennifer, "'A wanton trade of living'? Rhetoric, effeminacy, and the early modern courtier," *Criticism*, Spring 2000 (BNet).
Richardson, Ken, *The Making of Intelligence*, London 1999.

Rivers, Isabel, *Reason, Grace and Sentiment: a Study of the Language of Religion and Ethics in England, 1660–1780*, Cambridge 2000.
Robinson, Daniel, *An Intellectual History of Psychology*, Madison 1986.
Rocca, Julius, "Galen and the ventricular system," *Journal of the History of the Neurosciences*, 6 (1997).
Roccatagliata, Giuseppe, *A History of Ancient Psychiatry*, Westport 1986.
Roffe, David, "'A novel and a noteworthy thing?' The guardianship of lunatics and the crown in medieval England," ms.
Rose, Lynn, "The courage of subordination: women and mental retardation in ancient Greece," ms.
Rose, Steven, et al., *Not in our Genes: Biology, Ideology and Human Nature*, London 1984.
Ross, Sarah Gwyneth, *The Birth of Feminism: Woman as Intellect in Renaissance Italy and England*, Cambridge MA 2009.
Rubinstein, Lene, "The Athenian political perception of the *idiotes*," in Paul Cartledge et al. (eds), *Kosmos: Essays in Order, Conflict and Community in Classical Athens*, Cambridge 2002.
Rummel, Erika, *The Confessionalization of Humanism in Reformation Germany*, Oxford 2000.
Russell, Conrad, *Times Higher Education*, 23 November, London 2001.
Schaffer, Simon, "Babbage's intelligence: calculating machines and the factory system," *Critical Inquiry*, 21 (1994).
Schalk, Ellery, *From Valor to Pedigree: Ideas of Nobility in France in the Sixteenth and Seventeenth Centuries*, Princeton 1986.
Scheerenberger, Richard, *A History of Mental Retardation*, Baltimore 1983.
Schlaifer, R., "Greek theories of slavery from Homer to Aristotle," *Harvard Studies in Classical Philology*, 47 (1936).
Schmitt, J., *The Holy Greyhound*, Cambridge 1983.
Schoenfeldt, Michael, *Bodies and Selves in Early Modern England*, Cambridge 1999.
Schofield, Malcolm, "Ideology and philosophy in Aristotle's theory of slavery," in Patzig, G. (ed.), *Aristoteles 'Politik,'* Göttingen 1990.
Shapin, Steven, *A Social History of Truth: Civility and Science in Seventeenth Century England*, Chicago 1994.
———, *The Scientific Revolution*, Chicago 1996.
Shapiro, I., *The Evolution of Rights in Liberal Theory*, Cambridge 1986.
Shulsky, Abraham, "The 'infrastructure' of Aristotle's *Politics*," in *Essays on the Foundations of Aristotelian Political Science*, C. Lord and D.K. O'Connor (eds), Berkeley 1991.
Simon, Joan, *Education and Society in Tudor England*, Cambridge 1966.
Simpson, Murray K., *Modernity and the Appearance of Idiocy: Intellectual Disability as a Regime of Truth*, forthcoming.
Singer, Peter, *Rethinking Life and Death: the Collapse of our Traditional Ethics*, New York 1996.
Smail, Daniel, "Predestination and the ethos of disinheritance in sixteenth-century Calvinist theatre," *Sixteenth Century Journal*, 23 (1992).
Smith, Jay, *Nobility Reimagined*, Ithaca 2005.
Smith, N., "Aristotle's theory of natural slavery," in D. Keyt and F. Miller (eds), *A Companion to Aristotle's* Politics, Oxford 1991.
Smith, Roger, *Inhibition: History and Meaning in the Sciences of Mind and Brain*, Berkeley 1992.
———, *The Fontana History of the Human Sciences*, London 1997.
Sobsey, Dick, "Family transformation: from Dale Evans to Neil Young," in R. Friedlander and Sobsey (eds), *Through the Lifespan*, Kingston Ontario 1996.

Somerville, C. John, *The Secularization of Early Modern England*, Oxford 1992.
Sorabji, Richard, "Soul and self in ancient philosophy," in M. James and C. Crabbe (eds), *From Soul to Self*, London 1999.
Squibb, George, *The High Court of Chivalry*, Oxford 1959.
Stachniewski, John, *The Persecutory Imagination: English Puritanism and the Literature of Religious Despair*, Oxford 1991.
Stainton, Tim, *Reason's Other: the Historical Construction of Intellectual Disability*, forthcoming.
—— and H. Besser, "The positive impact of children with an intellectual disability on the family," *Journal of Intellectual and Developmental Disability*, 23 (1998).
Steneck, Nicholas, "Albert the Great on the classification and localization of the internal senses," *Isis*, 65 (1974).
Stevenson, W., *Sovereign Grace: the Place and Significance of Christian Freedom in John Calvin's Political Thought*, Oxford 1999.
Stone, Lawrence, *The Family, Sex and Marriage in England 1500–1800*, Harmondsworth 1990.
Stratford, Brian, "Down's syndrome at the court of Mantua," *Maternal and Child Health*, 7 (1982).
Sutherland, Gillian, *Ability, Merit, and Measurement: Mental Testing and English Education, 1880–1940*, Oxford 1984.
Suzuki, Akihito, "Mind and its Disease in Enlightenment British Medicine," unpublished PhD thesis, University College London 1992.
——, "Anti-Lockean enlightenment? Mind and body in early eighteenth-century English medicine," in Roy Porter (ed.), *Medicine in the Enlightenment*, Amsterdam 1995.
Tappert, T., *Luther's Works*, Augsburg Fortress Edition, Philadelphia 1967.
Thomas, Keith, *Religion and the Decline of Magic*, Harmondsworth 1982.
Thomson, Mathew, *The Problem of Mental Deficiency: Eugenics, Democracy, and Social Policy in Britain c.1870–1959*, Oxford 1998.
Tinniswood, Adrian, *His Invention so Fertile: a Life of Christopher Wren*, London 2001.
Trent, James, *Inventing the Feeble Mind*, Berkeley 1994.
—— and Steven Noll (eds), *Mental Retardation in America: a Historical Reader*, New York 2004.
Tsouna, Voula, "Doubts about other minds and the science of physiognomics," *Classical Quarterly*, 48 (1998).
Tully, James, *An Approach to Political Philosophy: Locke in Contexts*, Cambridge 1993.
Velicu, Adrian, *Civic Catechisms and Reason in the French Revolution*, Farnham 2010.
Vidal, Fernando, *Les sciences de l'âme, XVIe–XVIIIe siècle*, Paris 2006.
Voak, Nigel, *Richard Hooker and Reformed Theology*, Oxford 2003.
Voysey, Margaret, *A Constant Burden: the Reconstitution of Family Life*, London 2009.
Wagner, Anthony, *Heralds and Heraldry in the Middle Ages*, Oxford 2000.
Wallace, D., *Puritans and Predestination: Grace in English Protestant Theology 1525–1695*, Chapel Hill 1982.
Warwick, Andrew, *Masters of Theory: Cambridge and the Rise of Mathematical Physics*, Chicago 2003.
Weintraub, K., *The Value of the Individual*, Chicago 1978.
Weisheipl, J.A., "Ockham and the Mertonians," in J. Catto (ed.), *The History of the University of Oxford*, Oxford 1984.
White, Stephen, *Custom, Kinship and Gifts to Saints*, Chapel Hill 1988.

Wiberg, J., "The anatomy of the brain in the works of Galen and Ali Abbas," *Islamic Medicine*, 40 (1914/1996).
Williams, Bernard, *Shame and Necessity*, Berkeley 1993.
Winship, Michael, *Making Heretics: Militant Protestantism and Free Grace in Massachusetts, 1636–1641*, Princeton 2002.
Wish, Harvey, "Aristotle, Plato, and the Mason-Dixon Line," *Journal of the History of Ideas*, 10 (1949).
Wober, M., "Towards an understanding of the Kiganda concept of intelligence," in J. Berry and P. Dasen (eds), *Culture and Cognition: Readings in Cross-Cultural Psychology*, London 1974.
Wood, James, *The Nobility of the Election of Bayeux*, Princeton 1980.
Wooldridge, Adrian, *Measuring the Mind: Education and Psychology in England*, Cambridge 1994.
Wright, David, *Mental Disability in Victorian England: the Earlswood Asylum*, Oxford 2001.
Wyatt-Brown, Bertram, *The Shaping of Southern Culture: Honour, Grace, and War*, Chapel Hill 2001.
Wyss, Heinz, *Der Narr im schweizerischen Drama des 16.Jahrhunderts*, Berne 1959.
Yost, R., "Locke's rejection of hypotheses about sub-microscopic events," in John Yolton (ed.), *Philosophy, Religion and Science in the Seventeenth and Eighteenth Centuries*, Rochester NY 1990.
Young, Michael, *The Rise of the Meritocracy*, London 1958.
Young, Robert, *Mind, Brain and Adaptation in the Nineteenth Century*, Oxford 1970.
Zihni, Lilian, "A History of the Relationship between the Concept and the Treatment of People with Down's Syndrome in Britain and America, 1867–1967," unpublished PhD thesis, University College London 1990.
Zipes, Jack, *The Brothers Grimm*, London 1989.
Zupko, Jack, "What is the science of the soul? A case study in the evolution of late medieval natural philosophy," *Synthese*, 110 (1997).

Index

General Terms

Ability (*dunamis, potentia*) 29, 35, 55–6, 66, 114, 132, 157, 161, 169, 174, 190, 196, 203, 240, 292–3, 297, 300
   "ability time" 42, 45–6
   in children 174, 182
   as landed property 77, 84, 90, 96, 104, 113, 117, 146
   moral *versus* natural ("physical") 171–2, 190–201, 331–7
   and receipt of grace 169–70
Absolutism, political 73, 86, 89, 93–5, 107, 117, 121, 127, 151, 164, 208–9, 268, 328
Abstraction
   an operation of intellect 41, 44, 97, 130, 169, 175, 187, 209, 220, 231, 242, 272, 313–45
   its place in conceptual history 10, 12, 15, 39, 43, 45, 52, 71, 124–7, 228, 281–309
Acceptance (of disability) 207, 253, 260–64, 273–4
Affections, and receipt of grace 169
Alchemy 123, 279, 282, 299, 320
Alienation, mental 238–40, 328, 330
Americans, first-nation 25, 39, 110, 193, 211, 315, 328–9, 340
American Psychiatric Association 214
American democracy 124, 177
Amniocentesis 210, 255, 326
Anabaptism 95, 151, 168, 181–2, 187, 276
Anatomy, medical 53, 132, 151, 193, 212, 221, 223, 230, 232, 241, 243–4, 246–8, 269–70, 276
Angels 11, 55, 59, 80, 110, 167, 179, 210–11, 269, 272, 285, 297, 299, 301–2, 305, 317, 335
Animals
   lacking abstraction 126, 293, 313–16
   lacking self-knowledge 167, 288
   in the scale of nature 16–18, 22, 25–6, 31, 72, 93, 95, 115, 124, 128, 133, 138–9, 164, 214, 224, 247, 254–6, 284–5, 294, 301, 305–6
Animal spirits, *see* soul spirits
Anthropology
   and historical method 2, 63–9, 103–4, 110, 219, 248, 254–5, 273, 281
   origins of the discipline 193, 296
Antinomianism 66, 99, 199, 319

Appearance and reality 1, 9, 63–4, 214–15, 260, 263–4
Arab philosophy 114, 284–6, 289–91, 297–300, 305, 329
Argument from Design 212, 327, 336
Aristocracy, *see* Gentry
Arminianism 157, 161, 163, 170–71, 184, 189–93, 195, 198–9, 268
Arrivistes, upstarts 59, 65, 80, 105–6, 111, 114, 116, 120, 127, 137–8, 140
Artisans, handicraftmen 20, 33, 60, 95, 106, 117, 127
Asperger's syndrome 75, 242
Astrology 259, 278–9
Atheism
   doctrinal dangers of 53, 154, 163, 247, 271, 293–4, 319
   fools as atheists 100, 201, 210, 227, 334
Attention
   maintenance of 10, 12, 15, 44, 71, 226
   deficit (ADHD) 214, 217, 219, 228–33, 243, 263
   and mental training 343
Autism
   arbitrariness of definition 65, 214, 217, 248
   and genes 214, 217
   historical arrival of 3, 218, 242, 324, 344
   as private thinking 73, 84, 98, 257
Autonomy, personal 4, 10, 25, 27, 29, 65–7, 84–6, 92, 94, 100, 107, 110, 113, 131–2, 136, 138–9, 155–6, 161–2, 168, 182, 271, 319–20, 328–9, 335, 346

Backwardness 4, 26, 174
Baptists 162, 268
Barbarians 16, 25, 28, 33
Bastards 65, 140, 277
Bedlam (Bethlehem Hospital) 220, 267, 330
Behavioural phenotypes 213–19
Behaviourism 214, 255
Behmenism 269, 271
Benefit of clergy 131
Bestial sex, *see* Buggery births
Bereavement analogy 261–74
Bioethics 253, 255–7
Biology
   biological classification, *see* Scale of nature

and psychology 1–3, 10, 15, 27–8, 30, 32–6, 71–2, 75, 84, 105, 111, 121, 140, 142, 145, 155, 207–8, 212, 215–17, 222–3, 253, 257–9, 275, 281, 295, 304–9, 326
Biotechnology 46, 210, 253, 255–7, 274
Black people
    and grace 183
    and honour 81, 122, 124, 130
    and intelligence 6, 74, 132, 231–2, 236, 248, 336
    and instability of opinion 230–32
    oppression and liberation 4, 30, 218
Blindness 36, 199, 236, 276
    as intellectual disability 297, 300–301
    unlike intellectual disability 192, 212
Bloodline, *see* lineage
Bodies
    corrupting the faculties 58, 99–100, 114–15, 119, 134, 199, 219–31, 238–48, 258, 260, 269, 272, 275–7, 291–3, 297–300, 307–8, 317–19
    relationship to minds/souls 15, 27, 29–33, 36, 40, 50, 53, 55–7, 69, 85, 89, 127, 132, 169, 173, 191–5, 207–18, 259, 295–6, 316, 325–6, 337–9
Bourgeoisie 15, 67, 69, 82–5, 105–6, 112, 120–23, 139–41, 170, 273
Brain, the
    functions of 40, 42, 45, 170, 238–45, 269, 298, 316, 319, 341
    health of 50–51, 58–9, 134
    structure of 53–5, 132, 220–33, 245–9
"Buggery births," and bestial sex 277–8, 306, 309, 323, 326
Bureaucracy and intellectual skills 39, 56, 107, 282–3

Calculation, calculative skills 17, 21–2, 35, 41–2, 58, 107, 160, 175, 208, 296
Calling, the (Protestant concept of) 73–4, 81, 106, 131, 146, 172, 176, 180–81, 197, 222, 244, 341
Calvinism 70, 88, 90, 153–4, 156, 159, 162, 164, 169, 173, 178, 180, 196, 200, 247, 282, 322, 333, 341
    orthodox doctrine of "limited atonement" 79, 82, 162–3, 168, 170, 172, 189, 192–3, 198, 201, 255, 286, 288, 331–2
    middle-way doctrine 161–6, 170–73, 184, 188, 189–198
Capable subjects 96, 182, 200
Capitalism, expansion of 11, 39, 51, 82, 105
Catechism 83, 91–2, 159, 166, 174–8, 189, 204, 331, 343

Causes of disability, medical doctrine of 15, 27, 32–3, 83, 120, 154, 200, 212–15, 219, 224, 238–43, 247, 249, 259–60, 270, 272, 279, 295
Changelings 9, 90, 131–2, 159, 229, 238, 243, 248–9, 256, 260, 261–75, 302–3, 308–9, 316–46
Character types, characterology 51, 99, 109, 138, 186, 268
Charisma, intelligence as 69
Charitable giving 176, 325, 330
Children
    child development 39, 46, 67, 93–4, 98, 134, 173–4, 239, 242, 244, 275–8, 283, 302–3, 329, 336
    childlike adults 26, 47, 174–5, 181–5
    corporal punishment of 176, 342
    and the Devil, 259–75, 281
    and election 71, 183–4, 202, 317
    gifted 6, 77, 143–4, 175
    and segregated education 71–2, 216
City state (*polis*) 20, 27–8, 30–32, 36
Class, social 8, 15, 28, 53, 69–71, 81, 86, 89, 93–7, 99, 103, 105, 122–3, 125–30, 133, 135, 137, 139–40, 145, 168, 175–7, 180, 187, 194, 209, 219, 229, 230–33, 239, 242–3, 245, 249, 259, 262, 283, 297
Clerks and *literati* 56, 86, 283
Climate, influence on psychology 232, 278
Communitas, the Commons 127, 134, 138, 168, 170, 185, 321
Competence 3, 15, 21, 27, 31, 94, 109, 130, 141–6, 169–70, 178, 181, 193, 201, 220, 237, 327–30
Conscience 84, 88–9, 91, 163–7, 255, 259, 289, 293, 320, 339, 346
Consciousness, self-knowledge, self-reflection 84, 91, 158, 165–7, 288–9, 294, 301–2, 306, 334, 338–9
Consensus, the source of psychological classification 1, 42, 46, 68, 75, 121, 207, 214–18, 317, 322, 327, 336
Consent, rational 1, 10, 25, 27, 88, 93–4, 124, 129, 134, 327, 335
Conservatism 8, 30, 72–4, 144, 270, 323–5
Constructionism 1–2, 5–9
Contemplation (*contemplatio*) 55–6, 87–91, 114, 166–7, 173, 175, 181, 231, 237, 242, 289, 291, 297–8, 314, 318
Contract, theory of 66, 68, 105, 152, 161, 168, 188, 190–92
Convention (*nomos*) 25–9, 33, 36, 115, 153
Coping theory 260–61
Counter-Reformation 73, 81, 156, 158, 160, 168

Court of Chivalry 105, 108
Court of Wards, *see* Wardship
Covenant theology 152, 184–5, 188–9, 192, 317
Cranial sutures 224–8, 230, 247
Credulity, a symptom of foolishness 97, 137, 146, 229, 231–2, 266
Cretinism 4, 10, 236, 239, 245, 273
Curability, *see* incurability

Deafness 184, 199, 202, 219, 228–9, 236, 239, 241, 244, 254, 276, 300, 314, 336, 338
Deformity, physical 225, 232, 236, 245, 276, 325
Degeneracy 65, 71–2, 78, 95–6, 116, 119, 124, 132–4, 138, 140, 219, 230, 243–4, 259, 263, 304
Deliberation 31–3, 40, 55, 209, 237–8
Demonstrative proof (of human identity) 50, 54, 164, 333, 335–7, 339
Determinism 11, 28–9, 33, 67–8, 112, 121–3, 140, 142, 199, 318–19, 332
   as fate 107
   genetic, physiological 212, 215, 222–3, 227–8, 230, 246, 250, 275, 279, 297, 304, 326
   religious 70, 82, 95, 152–6, 158–61, 165–72, 183, 185, 190–94, 203, 279, 289
Developmental plateau 32, 47, 174, 258
Devil, the 1, 65, 90, 97, 129, 160, 186, 202, 212–14, 238–41, 250, 253–75, 281, 295, 309, 317
Diagnostic and Statistical Manual of Mental Disorders (*DSM*) 213
Disability, "intellectual"
   ancient Greek accounts of 15–36
   and grace 179–204
   and honour 125–47
   as *impotentia* 133, 147, 169, 190–91, 198, 226
   Locke's account of 313–46 *passim*
   medical accounts of 207–52
   moral 190–96, 201
   natural intellectual disability, early concepts of 26–7, 31, 189–201
   and physical 1, 3–4, 15, 192, 213, 219, 227, 263, 337
   and speed of intelligence 39–62
   and status 93–102
Discretion (*discretio*) 55, 91, 135, 144, 188, 227, 329
Discourse (*discursus*) 55, 110, 177, 232, 324
Dishonour, *see* shame
Dispositions (definitive of "nature") 33, 84, 111, 142, 152–4, 188, 196, 219, 223–4, 228, 244, 279, 300, 306–7
Dissenters (*see also* Nonconformists) 189, 198, 200, 268–9
Dissenting Academies 177

DNA 1, 16, 30, 67, 153, 213–14, 216
Down's syndrome 10–11, 45, 146, 210–11, 217, 245, 249, 258, 279
Drapetomania 217–8
Dualism 55, 57, 71, 192, 207–8, 213–14, 231, 248, 259, 299–300, 308, 339
Dullness (*hebetudo*) 4, 128, 133, 135, 137, 185–6, 196, 199, 202, 220, 227, 238, 242, 244, 247, 271, 316
Dwarfism 225, 239, 246, 248, 275

Ease of learning (*eumathia*) 16–19, 21, 49, 51–2, 55, 57
Effeminacy, as intellectual deficiency 130–32, 181, 243
Egalitarianism 5, 74–5, 78, 86, 96, 124, 154, 176, 178, 222, 278, 282, 328
The elect (*see also* Reprobates; Epistemology)
   and social class 71, 79, 80–83, 90, 92, 95, 97, 179–81, 230, 244, 278, 286–7
   idiots elect or not 125, 184–5, 187–8, 197, 202–3, 259, 317
   pagans elect or not 160, 162, 183, 199, 235, 329
   as precursors of the intelligent 65–6, 68, 70, 77, 85, 88, 94–6, 151–78, 189–91, 195, 199, 201, 268–9, 287–9, 294, 299, 320, 326, 332–3
Embryo, see Foetus
Emotions (*see also* Affections) 2, 9, 68, 75, 152, 167, 169, 239, 343
Empathy (*see also* Autism) 98, 214, 220
Empiricism 9, 15, 42, 50, 54, 57, 67, 74, 151, 207, 211–12, 246–7, 264, 272, 282, 284–5, 292–3, 296, 313–5, 319, 321, 327, 331
English civil wars and revolution 89, 93, 96, 143, 153, 162, 229, 268
Enthusiasm, religious 40, 59, 162–3, 166, 170, 268, 320, 332
Epicureanism 210, 344
Epilepsy 131, 223, 227, 244, 279
Epistemology, and the signs of election 16, 159, 294, 327, 332
Equality of souls 79, 80–81, 92–3, 95–7, 116, 137, 179, 182, 187, 222, 231, 282, 300, 306–8
Equivocalism 300, 305–9, 331
Erastianism 202
Essence (of "man")
   real or nominal 133, 256, 304, 307–8, 318, 321–4, 327, 331, 334–7, 343–4
   distinct from essential property 34, 199
Essentialism, univocalism (and human nature) 5, 7, 9, 70, 74, 182, 243–4, 277, 305–9

Ethics
  ethics of "exceptionalism" 11, 26, 36, 41, 55, 203, 249–58, 284, 320, 337–8, 340
  and morals 253
  naturalistic/scientific 273–4
Eucharist
  communicants' understanding of 65, 145, 166–8, 171, 183, 188–9
  exclusion from 79, 97, 183–4, 186, 201–4, 249, 278
Eugenics 8, 18, 26, 30, 45, 65, 69, 82, 123–7, 213, 216, 218, 255–8, 264, 274, 304
Euthanasia 256, 265, 274
Exams, educational 41, 45, 66, 70, 72
Exchange, principle of 66, 85, 151–3, 283

Faith 70, 81, 84, 88, 187, 222, 235
  in children 181–4
  and reason 90, 151–3, 155–6, 158, 160–63, 165, 167, 170, 173, 180, 191–3, 196–200, 268, 32–3, 343–4
Families 1, 70–71, 80, 90, 104–6, 109–13, 123, 134, 143–6, 176–7, 208, 216, 218, 222, 242–3, 254, 260–63, 273
Familist sects 332
Fascism, Nazism 26, 46, 123, 274,
Fate 67, 107, 154, 193
  as predestination 153
  and Stoicism 125, 154
Feeble-mindedness 4, 26, 28, 30, 186, 242, 248, 274
Feminism 131
  liberal 274
  radical 98
Feudalism
  and education systems 98, 142
  and social structure 83, 112, 130, 177
Foetus
  ethical status of 257, 274, 321, 339
  development of 172, 174, 180, 211, 257–8, 275–7, 294, 306
Folklore, and the changeling myth 262–7, 270–74
Foolishness (*stoliditas, stultitia, stupiditas, fatuitas*) 79, 135–7, 180, 254, 258, 300, 303, 324, 326, 330, 338–9
  literary treatments of 90–92, 122, 139
  medical accounts of 219–20, 227–8, 230–32, 235–46, 269, 279
Fools
  artificial 122, 140
  born 141, 145, 239, 241, 267, 276–8, 315, 328, 333, 338–9, 341
  holy 237
  lacking inhibition 47, 237
  natural 10, 129, 145, 199–200, 203, 226, 267, 272, 276, 287, 313, 315–16, 331
  professional 3, 95, 137–40, 186–7, 219, 225, 227, 232–3, 237–8, 240, 244–5
  "fool sonnets" 146
Fragile X syndrome 214
French revolution 105, 108, 178
Frenzy, *see* phrenitis

Galenism 40, 50, 53–4, 137, 192, 212–13, 216, 221–7, 232–3, 238–9, 241, 246–9, 279, 282, 345
Genealogies 66, 84–5, 90–91, 99, 107–8, 117–21, 124, 137, 140, 156, 184, 194
Genes 33, 69, 213–19, 221, 259
Genetics, cognitive 1, 4–5, 8, 11–12, 46, 65, 71, 82, 153, 160, 179, 183, 213–19, 230, 257, 259, 274, 282
Genius 15, 41–2, 46, 50, 59–60, 66, 69–70, 75, 124, 215, 248
Genotypes 214–17
The Gentleman's Magazine or Monthly Intelligencer 70
Gentry, nobility, aristocracy 49–60, 65–7, 71, 77–90, 108, 103–21, 124, 140, 156–7, 180, 221, 225, 231, 233, 237, 240, 243–5, 275–6, 322, 330, 335, 341, 343
Godly learning 160, 162–3
Goitre, as symptom of foolishness 10, 228, 236, 239–41
Golden Age arguments 4, 16, 118
Grace, as bid for status 63–99, 151–207 *passim*, 221–3, 229, 242, 260, 268–9, 281, 287, 295, 298–9, 314, 322, 333–4, 339, 341–4
  common 155, 197
  general 96
  imitative (*sprezzatura*) 80, 99, 139
  natural 57, 59, 67, 80, 85–8, 94–5, 98, 155, 158, 160–61, 163, 168–70, 173, 187, 196, 341
  special (divine, spiritual, effective) 59, 73, 80, 83, 86–94, 96, 108, 151, 155–7, 161, 163–4, 171, 173, 175, 191, 334
  sufficient 157
Griffiths Mental Development Scale 283

Hand-flapping 216
Heraldry, coats of arms 65, 68, 78–9, 82–4, 91, 116–24, 128, 136–42, 157, 177, 197
  heraldic science 105–13, 222
Heresy 53, 56, 81, 98, 108, 161, 175, 193, 194–5, 201, 207, 209–10, 260–61, 264, 295, 313
Heterodoxy 93, 209, 230, 253, 268, 287
Honesty, bourgeois 67, 105, 112, 121, 170

Honour
- as bid for status 63–92, 103–148 *passim*
- Christianization of 115–16, 227
- the honour society, *societas* 65, 78, 80, 84–6, 91, 94–7, 103–8, 113–16, 125–30, 133–6, 119, 141, 143, 145, 156–9, 168, 179–80, 207, 230, 242–5, 278, 281, 287, 301, 321, 330, 341
- national 81, 123–4, 178

Hospitals, long-stay 2, 15, 211
Humanism 11, 52, 54–6, 59, 85, 89, 116, 131, 143, 152–3, 160, 166, 180, 191, 199, 210, 221–2, 240, 285–8, 291, 320
Human sciences 12, 16, 72, 110, 212, 268, 283, 285, 289, 320, 342
Humours 11, 40, 58, 75, 181, 193, 219, 221–2, 239, 242, 259, 326
Hypocrites (religious) 65, 67, 158, 175, 185–6, 189, 201, 203, 218, 222, 238, 259, 269, 326, 332

Iconography 10–11, 79, 84, 103, 109, 181, 200, 231, 236, 245, 248, 261, 302
Ideas
- association and misassociation of 43, 59, 215, 319, 330
- common (*communes notiones*) 26, 53, 126–7, 131, 171, 180, 187, 191, 198–9, 209, 230–31, 244, 254, 300–301, 313–15, 318, 330, 334, 346
- trains of 174–7, 319, 330, 340, 342–3

Idiocy writs 141–2, 145–6
Idiots
- country or village 90, 95, 137–8, 145, 180, 240, 242, 244–5, 341
- legal 142, 144, 197
- natural 97, 145, 184
- unlearned 41, 116, 126–7, 134, 136–7, 158, 162, 180, 202

Idolatry 11, 40, 137, 183
Imagination, faculty of 41–2, 53–8, 79–80, 88, 91, 115, 122, 135, 137, 142, 164, 180, 221, 226–7, 232, 238, 241, 305, 314, 324, 330
Imbeciles, imbecility 4, 124, 140, 180, 199, 238, 245, 274, 277
Incubi and *succubi* 258–9, 263, 265, 270, 317
Incurability, curability 100, 147, 186, 193–7, 203, 212, 220, 223, 228, 235–6, 240, 244, 260, 338
Infanticide 18, 255–6, 266, 274, 325–6
Information-processing 15–16, 45, 50
Infusionism (divine authorship of the rational soul) 276–7, 299, 308–9
Inheritance, *see* Lineage

Inhibition, lack of 47, 237
Instability of opinion 130, 228–33, 343
Insult, language of 98–100, 130–31, 137, 146, 274, 309
Intellect (*intellectus*, *see also* Understanding, the)
- civic (*phronesis, prudentia*) 17–19, 21, 25, 31, 34, 40, 88, 130, 209, 222, 226
- intuited (*nous*) 17, 22, 29, 53, 69, 166, 285, 292
- as labour 8, 45, 117, 119, 167, 198, 283, 334, 341–2
- potential and actual 55, 66, 157, 174, 292–3, 297
- professional 5–6, 9, 51–2, 58–9, 73–5, 81, 85–6, 95, 98, 105–9, 115–23, 127–8, 137, 142, 144, 146, 221, 242, 250–51, 261–2, 274, 283–9, 298, 308, 341
- differentiated from reason 160
- spatial *versus* temporal model of 123, 174, 181, 339

Intelligence
- artificial 45
- as individual possession 64–5, 80, 105, 108
- *intelligentia*, usages of 107, 191, 210–11, 296, 301
- machine intelligence 42
- natural 107, 112, 169, 182, 204, 268
- the nine intelligences, 110, 210
- social 208

IQ, cognitive ability, psychometrics 5–9, 39–46, 65, 68, 71–2, 74, 89, 106–7, 109, 111–12, 121, 125, 140–41, 175, 177, 242, 292, 296, 304, 342

Jacobinism 84, 124
Jansenism 84, 156, 178–9, 113, 337
Jews 46, 56, 79, 81, 122, 130, 193, 231, 248, 263, 307

Labourers 94, 124–6, 135, 145, 179–81, 194, 197, 200, 209, 230–33, 245, 301, 306, 321, 333–5, 340–41, 346
The Ladies' Diary 70
Law for the Prevention of Hereditarily Diseased Offspring 46
Lazarillo de Tormes 118
Learned ignorance 41
Learning difficulty (*dusmathia*) 4, 16–19, 22, 50, 227
Lepers 56, 107
Lethargy 11, 40, 100, 210, 220, 223, 227, 294, 326
Levellers, the 94, 154, 183, 187, 197, 276, 278, 328, 332
Libertines, as fools 98, 229, 319–20, 327, 329–30, 341

Lineage, bloodline, inheritance 77–124, 140, 145, 216, 225, 229, 275
Literacy 17, 41, 50, 56, 89, 95, 97, 105, 119–20, 131, 146, 158, 161–2, 166, 168, 177, 196, 202, 239, 292, 315, 320
Logic
   professionalization of, and the human sciences 284–9
   and changelings, in Locke 316–21, 342–5
   Ramist 190–91, 285–8, 295, 305
Logical reasoning
   as definitively human 15, 43, 45, 124, 175, 187, 209, 220, 255–6, 294, 296, 316, 318–20, 345
   logical structure and the human subject 50, 52, 281–9
   Piagetian "mental logic" 39, 182
Lunacy, legal distinction from idiocy 141–2, 146, 220
Lutheranism 200, 247, 273

Macrocephaly 228
Madness 1, 3, 5, 8, 19, 21, 36, 144, 180, 193, 202–3, 219, 279, 316, 324, 330–31
Magic
   general theory of 68, 112
   natural 60, 265–6, 270–73, 317
Materialism 23, 53–5, 100, 270, 277, 291, 335
Medical model, of intellectual disability 207, 213, 218–19, 230, 245, 253, 255, 259–60
Melancholy 56, 58, 116, 142, 144, 193, 202, 210, 219, 227–8, 236–9, 241–4, 269–72, 294, 300, 303, 306, 330, 341
   and social class 134, 147, 180
   religious 176, 185, 222–3, 230
   slow or fast 40, 60, 135
   in women 180–81
Memes 10, 330
Memory, faculty of 42, 53–4, 57, 88, 91, 136, 158, 167, 170, 184, 226–7, 238, 300
Mental age tests 44, 71, 178
Mental physiology 43
Mental retardation, see "disability, intellectual"
Merchants
   economic power of 51, 73, 82, 103, 105–6, 113, 120
   lack of honour in 66 , 83, 108, 118–19, 122–3, 127, 141
Merit, meritocracy 63, 66–7, 69, 72–4, 80–82, 85, 92, 95, 98, 104–8, 114, 117, 120–24, 127, 157, 159, 161, 170, 175, 189, 282
Microcosm and macrocosm 39, 85, 123, 134, 174, 183, 259, 284, 287
Middle-way (Calvinist) doctrine 161–5, 171–3, 184, 188–90, 197–8

Monkeys 247–8, 256, 303, 305, 316, 321–3
Monsters, monstrosity 17, 67, 96, 99–100, 123, 127, 134, 140, 159, 179, 186, 191, 197, 204, 210–13, 224–8, 232–3, 236, 245–50, 260–61, 270, 275, 277–8, 301, 304, 308–9, 313, 321, 325–6, 329, 343–4, 346
Moors (Spanish), psychology of 81, 122, 183, 231–2
Moral man, Calvinist concept of 159, 195, 199–200, 331–9, 345
Moriones 187, 196, 237, 249, 303
Morons, moronism 4, 218, 274
Mortalism 276
Multitude, the 77, 96–7, 123, 130, 134, 168, 179, 286, 289

Natural history 15, 58, 111, 115, 164, 169, 194, 200, 208, 247–8, 267, 277, 291, 308, 314–17, 344
Natural kinds 1–2, 4, 6, 9, 278, 321
Natural law 96, 114, 152–4, 193, 204, 208–9, 328–9
Nature, natural
   tripartite relationship with nurture and necessity 15, 33, 71, 95, 111, 115, 117, 121, 123, 153–5, 215, 228, 239, 340
   tripartite relationship with unnatural and praeternatural 127, 199, 212, 245–7, 277–8, 287, 334, 340
Necessitarianism 70, 155, 174, 188, 212
New man 80, 98, 106, 269
Nobility, *see* Gentry
Nonconformism (*see also* Dissenters) 59, 70, 97, 155, 175, 215, 268, 342
Normal/abnormal 2, 9, 15, 42, 47, 58, 72, 83, 197, 211–14, 217–18, 220, 230, 245–50

Old age, and intellectual deficiency 15, 193, 219, 238–9, 296, 306, 315, 338
Oppositional Defiant Disorder (ODD) 98, 214, 216, 218
Original sin, as cause of deficiency 65, 87, 91, 153–7, 160–61, 163, 165–6, 179, 181, 190–92, 194, 199, 201, 230, 236, 238, 240, 244, 261, 266, 279
Oxford Anatomical Club 241

Paediatrics 11, 262, 274, 283
Paganism 53, 95, 154, 160, 162, 183, 193, 199, 203, 235–6, 329, 342
Papacy, the Pope 152, 156, 158, 221, 244, 256, 264, 267, 283, 328
Parents 1, 33, 78, 104, 109, 121, 123, 126, 128–9, 131, 140, 145, 184, 214, 216–18, 222, 240–45, 306

as authors of the rational soul 258, 275–7, 295–6, 299, 308–9
and changelings 90, 261–78
parental guilt 46–7, 309
sexual performance and intelligence of offspring 132, 241–3, 259
Patriarchy, paternalism 93–4, 98, 329
Patrilinealism 104–5, 143
Peasants 19, 60, 77, 81, 90, 92, 105, 122, 127, 130, 145, 163, 180, 202, 222, 228, 236–7, 239–40, 244–5, 247–8, 283, 297, 321
Pelagianism 156–7, 161, 187, 190–93
Perfectibility, human 65, 85, 88, 114, 118, 123–4, 153, 163, 165, 172, 173, 176, 178, 182, 184, 211, 269, 282, 293, 301–2, 308, 320, 332–3, 340, 345
Periodization, in the history of psychology 282
Personhood 31, 66, 80, 160, 245, 275, 300, 315, 337–9
Phenylketonuria (PKU) 218, 279
Philosophy of science 5, 7, 45
Phlegmatic humour 11, 195, 221, 228, 233
Phrenitis, frenzy 40–41, 147, 194, 219, 223, 239, 326
Phrenology 216, 248
Physics, unlike psychology 5, 7, 12, 32, 46, 59, 164, 172, 175, 260, 283, 293, 342, 345
Physiognomics 10, 211–12, 216, 220–25, 228, 232, 237, 245, 248, 275, 278, 306
Pineal gland 132, 276, 316
Platonism 164, 171, 211, 284, 290, 297, 313
Pollution 11, 56, 65, 71, 79, 81, 83, 90, 93, 112, 122, 155, 159, 178, 186, 188–9, 198, 202–3, 207, 213, 248, 258–60, 269, 278, 309
Polygenism 231
Poor Law 197, 203
Positivism 3–4, 6–7, 111
Predestination (*see also* Necessitarianism, The Elect, Reprobates) 153–7
Preformationism 245
Prerogativa Regis 141
Presentism 3–4, 258
Primogeniture 82, 105, 111–12, 143
Printing, invention of 162
Prisoners of war
not ethical beings 327
as "slaves by convention" in Aristotle 25–6
Probability 200, 340
Prophets, intellectual ability of 41, 55, 59, 70, 166, 237
Providence, providential cure 127, 145, 152, 191, 193, 227, 235, 247, 275–6, 338
Psychology
animal 215, 313

cognitive 15, 49, 173,
developmental 151–78 *passim*
educational 7, 44–5, 58, 65, 119, 174, 190
experimental 7, 72
faculty 12, 53–8, 128, 135, 160
history of 42, 114, 122, 147, 192, 221, 226, 245, 289, 316
and speed of intellect 43, 49–58
as gossip 42
industrial 45
origins of the word 282, 294–6
and scholasticism 12, 52, 283
and the theology of grace 147–204 *passim*
as transhistorical concept 3, 6, 8, 10, 23, 26, 64, 110, 128, 213, 237, 248, 273
Psychophysics 43
Purgatory 41, 173–5
Purity of blood/in-group 65, 82, 105, 113, 122, 147, 198, 273, 299
Pygmies, *semi-homines* 115, 303–5

Qualities of elements 40, 193, 213, 219, 212–13, 225, 232, 259

Racism
and IQ testing 6, 8, 44, 46, 124
and the psychology of slaves 25–6
scientific 33, 82, 132, 211, 231–2
Racial hygiene 215, 218
Rational animals
conflated with the elect 287–9, 295
as natural species 199–200, 275, 277, 279
Locke's treatment of 315, 317, 322, 325, 336, 338, 341, 344–5
medieval origins and usage 147, 168, 182, 284–6, 303, 307
phrase misattributed to Aristotle 25, 34–6
Rational choice 10, 39, 200, 319, 329, 332, 346
Reaction times 40–44
Reason
congruous 168
differentiated from intellect and understanding 160
divine 74, 91, 95, 153, 165, 211, 237, 319
right (*recta ratio*) 160, 164, 166, 300
sweet 161, 268
Reasoning, human (faculty of, *see also* Logical reasoning) 17, 21–2, 35, 53–7, 90–91, 115, 122, 135, 201, 221, 298, 300, 329–30
its relationship to faith 151–78, 186, 188–9, 196, 198, 236, 238, 333
and the cerebral ventricles 132, 226–7, 232
Recapitulation theory 211

Reincarnation of souls 18, 276–7
Repetitive behaviours ("stereotypy") 214–16
Reprobates
    and the elect 65, 69, 82, 92, 95, 156, 159, 161, 166, 171, 175–7, 268, 286, 289, 295, 299, 308, 331–2, 344
    as precursors of "the intellectually disabled" 72, 77, 94, 151, 155, 168, 178–203, 218, 223, 227, 249, 255, 259, 267–8, 278–9, 288, 317–18, 325–6, 332
    and social class 77, 79–80, 97, 229
Rhetoric 19–20, 51, 89
    and the "changeling" 320–21
Rights 4, 82–3, 94, 143, 154, 278, 327–9, 338
Royal Commission on Heraldry 107–8, 141
Royal Earlswood Hospital 15, 211
Royal Society 58–9, 89, 96, 128–9, 160, 164, 181, 208, 262, 268, 270–72, 287, 302, 317, 320, 334, 345

Satire 8, 79, 98–9, 108, 118, 139, 144, 146–7, 185, 229, 244
Scale of nature, biological classification 16–17, 34, 72, 83, 115, 167, 200, 247, 277, 281–311, 318, 321–2, 330, 340, 342
Scepticism
    constructionist 3–6, 9, 283
    faith-based 79, 254–7, 257, 266, 271, 290, 294, 297, 313–17, 323, 333, 337, 346
    materialist 55, 147
Schizophrenia 244
Schools 2, 71, 77–8, 120, 124, 127, 143, 177–8, 203, 207, 239, 244, 255, 344
Segregation, social 2–4, 6, 8, 15, 46–7, 56, 65, 69, 71, 107, 144, 178, 186, 198, 211, 218, 255, 304
Self-examination at holy communion 88, 166–9, 203
Self-knowledge, *see* Consciousness
Self-ownership, theological significance of 328, 339
Self-reflection, *see* Consciousness
Self-representation, intelligence as 2, 63–4, 103, 120, 127, 242, 345
Senses
    external 40, 43, 49, 52–3, 85, 100, 114–15, 135, 164, 194, 225, 227, 232, 258, 272, 289–90, 297–8, 304, 314
    internal 133–4, 180, 220, 246
Servants, social and intellectual status of 80, 90, 97–9, 105, 118, 124, 145, 175, 177, 222, 229, 283, 328
Shamanism 257, 259

Shame, dishonour 78–80, 91, 105, 108–9, 115, 117, 119–20, 125, 129, 134, 136, 140, 146, 181, 187, 243
Skulls, shape and size of 30, 110, 213, 216, 218, 223–4, 228, 230, 232, 246–9
Slavery
    Greek accounts of 18, 20, 25–33
    early modern accounts of 25–7, 79, 100, 110, 124, 130, 209, 212, 218, 232, 244, 300, 303, 328, 335
Social administration (*see also* Bureaucracy) 11, 39, 42, 45–6, 51, 56, 67, 74, 86, 97, 105, 120, 138, 197–8, 203, 211, 221, 282–3, 314
Social mobility 77, 99, 103–7, 127, 129, 134, 187, 283
Socinianism 175, 268, 276
Sophists 16–21, 25–9, 33, 39, 49–51, 99, 221, 308
Soul
    psyche 17–22, 26–32, 35–6, 40, 49–50, 53–4, 126, 207, 290
    anima 54, 207, 241–2, 269, 292, 300, 313, 335
    rational 53–8, 85, 90, 130, 147, 165, 173–4, 179, 210–11, 226, 236, 241–3, 248, 256, 258, 275–7, 288, 291–5, 299–303, 306–9, 316–17, 325, 331, 335, 338, 342
    sensitive 173, 184, 210, 241, 269, 292, 300, 308
Soul spirits 40, 58, 69, 85–6, 115, 119, 133, 138, 169–73, 191, 209, 213, 216, 218–21, 225–33, 241–5, 259, 272, 298, 316, 319, 331, 341
Species, human
    anomalies and interstitial types 67, 75, 90–91, 104, 115, 127–9, 182, 193–200, 211, 259, 268–9, 275–8, 281–309, 316–46
    circular definition of 9, 165, 324
    modern definitions of 1, 5, 15, 25, 36, 58, 245, 247
    and the scale of nature 16, 33, 35, 123, 193–200, 223, 254–8
Speed of intellect 16, 21, 39–60, 84–5, 90, 92, 97, 113, 130, 158, 184, 220, 300, 330–31
Statistics 6, 42, 46, 108, 121, 158, 211–16, 283
Status
    ascribed *versus* achieved 67, 91, 95, 104, 125, 132, 133, 135, 138, 143, 145, 182, 243, 341
    self-referential bids for 63–70, 77–8, 84–93, 95, 97
Stoics 28, 32, 34, 36, 49, 125–6, 154, 193, 227, 284
Syllogisms
    and social class 134, 287
    objectivity of 50, 52, 285
    practical 166–9, 303
    replacement by "trains of ideas" 175, 318–19
Synod of Dort 156–7, 171, 183, 189–90, 195, 294

Temperament, bodily 53, 85, 128, 155, 195, 223–7, 231, 241
Theology
    and medicine 53–6
    fusion with psychology 2, 12, 51, 114–15, 126, 137, 159, 162–3, 168–9, 182, 188–9, 223, 262, 268, 271, 273–4, 282–3, 289, 291, 293, 295–6, 298, 314, 317, 340–45
Thersites, as disabled archetype 129–30, 225, 227, 232, 247
Thinking states (*dianoia, noiesis*)
    in Aristotle 17, 224, 290
    in Galen 221, 223–6
The Thirty-Nine Articles of Religion 156
Touch (sense of) and social class 25, 297
Transhumanism 45, 173, 293, 298, 302
Tree of Porphyry 284, 286, 304
Turner's syndrome, 217
Twin studies 46, 82, 186, 217

Understanding, the
    episteme 17, 34–6, 290, 292
    human 87–8, 91, 110, 118, 159, 163–5, 169, 174, 187, 208, 255, 294, 299, 305–6
    intellectus, see Intellect
    logic-related (contrasted with "quick thinking") 50, 52
    understanding of the understanding 163–5, 176, 289–90, 300–301, 305

Villeins 105, 108, 118, 120, 130, 133–4, 136–7, 169
Virtue 19, 21–2, 31–3, 79–82, 84, 86, 95, 103–24, 130–31, 133–5, 139, 141, 144, 163, 180, 195, 209, 281

Wardship 109, 141–7, 189, 196, 203, 267
Wechsler Intelligence Scales 45
Weekly Memorials for the Ingenious 70
Welfare, welfarism 198, 260
Westminster Assembly 186, 195, 201
Wet-nurses 140, 221, 263–4, 273
Will, the 2, 59, 113, 151–3, 156–7, 160–63, 166–8, 170–71, 190–91, 198, 208, 229, 232, 245, 268, 319
Witchcraft
    and changelings 258, 260–65
    scepticism about 266, 271
Wit
    "erection" of 87–90
    as *ingenium* 52–9, 85, 87, 115, 222, 227–8, 238–9, 242, 277, 292, 300, 302, 307
Women
    and grace 78, 98
    and honour 67, 70, 98, 125, 147, 197
    and infanticide 274–5
    and melancholy 179–81
    and instability of opinion 230–31, 267
    and intellectual ability 6, 18, 27, 30, 32, 74, 97–8, 129–32, 139, 156, 219, 283, 335
Working class 26, 71, 97, 126, 168, 245

Names

D'Abano, Pietro 246, 249
Ibn Abbas, Ali 228, 230
Adorno, Theodor 282
Albert the Great [Albertus Magnus] 52, 55, 57, 58, 115, 126, 127, 130, 242, 298, 301–3, 305, 307, 315
Alderotti, Taddeo 52
Alexander of Aphrodisias 114, 125–6, 154, 242, 284, 297
Allestree, Richard 170
Alpago, Andrea 298, 300
Amyraut, Moïse 189–90, 191–4, 195, 196, 198, 199, 200, 201, 204, 286, 331, 332–3
Andrewes, Lancelot 158
Anton, Robert 146
Aquinas, Thomas 12, 54, 73, 92, 115, 131, 136, 154, 155, 201, 208, 209, 230, 290, 301–2, 305–6
Argenterio, Giovanni, 55,
Aristotle, 2, 16–17, 25–36, 50, 51–2, 53, 63, 83, 86–7, 113–14, 126, 130, 151, 153, 160, 162, 182, 190, 209, 214, 223–5, 230, 282, 284–5, 287, 289–90, 292, 296–8, 300, 303–5, 315
Arminius, Jacobus 157, 160, 183
Aron, Raymond 259
Ascham, Roger 59, 86
Ashley, Robert 133
Auden, W.H. 5
Augustine, St 156, 185, 187, 211, 239, 263, 266, 275, 303, 337
Austin, J.L. 219
Avempace [Ibn Bajja] 305
Averroes [Ibn Rushd] 140, 275, 284, 290–91, 296, 297–8, 300, 305–6
Avicenna [Ibn Sina] 51, 222, 225, 226, 258, 290, 297, 301

Babbage, Charles 41–2, 45
Bacon, Francis 81, 89, 107, 147, 160, 162, 183, 212, 314
Bacon, Nicholas 325
De Balzac, Honoré 140
Baron-Cohen, Simon 98
Bartolus of Saxoferrato 87, 115, 116

Bauhin, Caspar 238, 267
Baxter, Richard 41, 95–6, 113, 153, 155, 162, 164–5, 168, 169, 171–2, 173, 174–7, 180–82, 185, 189, 195–201, 203, 204
Beard, Thomas 278
Bentham, Jeremy 258, 260
Benzi, Ugo 246, 249
Beza, Théodore 82, 156, 166, 287, 288
Billington, Sandra 3
Binet, Alfred 7, 42, 44, 70, 71–2, 178, 216
Bleuler, Eugen 324
Bloch, Marc 69
Boehme, Jakob 269, 295
Boerhaave, Herman 247
Boethius 284
Boissier de Sauvages, François 344–5
Bolton, Samuel 319
De Bono, Edward 103
Boswell, James 129
De Boulainvilliers, Henri 123, 140
Bourdieu, Pierre 65, 69, 73
Boyle, Robert 1, 60, 69–70, 89, 119, 164, 170, 172, 208, 270–71, 282, 320–21, 332
Brant, Sebastian 235–6, 239
Breton, Nicholas 146, 268
Bridge, William 288–9
Brooke, Robert 164
Browne, Thomas 113, 121, 179, 212, 271, 308–9
Brueghel the Elder, Pieter 261
Bryskett, Lodowick 173, 326
Buffon, Comte de 83, 155
Bull, George 199–200
Bullinger, Heinrich 152, 180
Bulwer, John 229
Bunyan, John 79, 174, 180, 188, 201, 229
Burke, Edmund 289
Burt, Cyril 7, 44, 46, 71
Burton, Robert 147
Butler, Samuel 99, 144

Calderón de la Barca, Pedro 81, 92
Calvin, Jean 67, 68, 82, 86, 87, 88, 97, 152, 156, 157, 160, 163, 166, 167, 170, 172, 177, 185–8, 192, 195, 196, 211, 240, 256, 270, 287–8
Cameron, John 189–92, 195
Canguilhem, Georges 8
Carlson, Licia 256
Carson, John 73
Cartwright, Samuel 217
Della Casa, Giovanni 98–9
Casmann, Otho 294
Cassiodorus 263

Castiglione, Baldesar 80–81, 85, 98–9, 103, 131, 134, 137
Cattell, James 43
Celsus, Aurelius 232
De Cervantes, Miguel 118, 122
Charles I of England 84, 142, 152, 221, 278
Charles II of England 96, 110, 143, 278
Charron, Pierre 57, 128–9, 313
Cicero 52, 86, 108, 112, 115, 154, 187, 320
Colet, John 120
Collinges, John 204
Collingwood, R.G. 207
Combes, Emile 71
De Condorcet, Nicolas 178
Connolly, John 199
Coppo di Marcovaldo 10–11
De Cordemoy, Louis 326–7
Cranach, Lucas 180
Cranefield, Paul 3, 187, 235–6, 239, 241, 244
Cranmer, Thomas 143–4
Cromwell, Oliver 68, 81, 84, 151, 153, 162, 72, 278
Cromwell, Thomas 120
Crooke, Helkiah 220
Crookshank, F.G. 245
Cullen, William 344
Culpeper, Nicholas 248–50

Dante Alighieri 136
Danziger, Kurt 6, 8–9
Darwin, Charles 70, 146, 213
Darwin, Erasmus 70
Davies, Sir John 147, 151
Davies of Hereford, John 146, 169
Defoe, Daniel 203
Descartes, René 55, 57–8, 64, 132, 160, 175, 208, 227, 241, 254, 276, 296, 300, 313, 316, 319–20, 325–6, 335, 339, 341
Dickens, Charles 15, 90
Diderot, Denis 213
Digby, Kenelm 320, 337
Donders, Franz 43
Donne, John 99, 220–21
Douglas, Mary 11, 278
Drake, Roger 202–4
Drayton, Michael 266–7
Dryden, John 8, 137, 244
De Dryvere, Jérémie 55
Dumas, Alexandre 82
Duns Scotus, John 100, 133, 307
Dürer, Albrecht 181

Edwards, Jonathan 169, 177, 208, 272, 314, 344–5
Edwards, Robert 253

Elizabeth I of England 59, 77, 86, 91, 131, 143, 147, 325
Elyot, Thomas 86–8, 113, 116, 118, 127, 233, 288
Erasmus, Desiderius 41, 109, 115–16, 120, 160, 222, 235, 239–40
Esquirol, Jean-Etienne 178
Essex, Earl 120, 131, 147
Eustachius, Bartolomeus 247–8
Eysenck, Hans 7, 44

Falloppio, Gabriele 246
Faret, Nicole 95
Fechner, Gustav 43
Fenn, Richard 172, 260
Ferguson, Robert 200–201, 332, 334
Fielding, Henry 137
Fiera, Battista 56
Filmer, Robert 93–4, 329
Fine, Cordelia 98
Firmin, Gabriel 165–6, 168–9, 175
Flavell, John 172
Flynn, James 7
Van Foreest, Pieter 228
Fortescue, John 106
Foucault, Michel 9
Foxe, John 81
Francis, St 107
Fraunce, Abraham 287
Freigius, Johannes 295
Freud, Sigmund 155
Fuller, Thomas 226, 237, 267, 317

Galen, Claudius 40, 50–53, 56–8, 114, 132, 221–32, 240, 245–50, 282
Galton, Francis 42–4, 53, 65, 70–72, 113, 124, 186, 215–16, 282
Gardner, Howard 7, 43
Gassendi, Pierre 241, 254, 314, 322, 335, 346
Gauss, Carl Friedrich 41
Gautier, Marthe 258
Gibbon, John 110–12
Glanvill, Joseph 87, 96, 171, 173, 181, 268, 271, 292, 294
Glisson, Francis 302
De Gobineau, Arthur 82
Göckel, Rudolf [Goclenius] 282, 294–5, 306
Goddard, Henry 218
Gomarus, Franciscus 156–7, 183
Good, John Mason 344
Gracián, Baltasar 64, 146
Greville, Fulke 147, 162
Grimm, The Brothers 262–6, 272–4
Grotius, Hugo 152–3, 208, 328–9

Hacking, Ian 6, 42, 217
Hammond, Henry 171
Hardy, Thomas 26
Harrington, James 197
Hartley, David 59
Harvey, William 221, 243, 245
Von Helmholtz, Hermann 42–3
Henri IV of France 121
Henry VI of England 144
Henry VII of England 90
Henry VIII of England 67, 80, 86, 98, 107, 120, 141, 143, 156
Herbert of Cherbury, Lord 346
Herbert, George 92
Hierophilos 212
Hildebrand, Joachim 318
Hippocrates 40, 58, 224–5, 227, 249
Hitler, Adolf 46
Hobbes, Thomas 17, 64, 146, 154, 175, 182, 208, 254, 276, 328, 335
Homer 50, 129, 225, 232
Hooker, Richard 88–9, 97, 144, 161, 183, 319, 329
Howe, John 332
Huarte, Juan 73, 131, 152, 292
Hughes, George 299–300
Hume, David 177, 344
Humfrey, John 202–4, 278
Hunt, James 211
Hutchinson, Anne 97, 158

James I of England 105, 117, 156, 220, 266
James, Mervyn 87, 103
Jean of Jandun 221, 275
Jensen, Arthur 44
Johannsen, Wilhelm 215
John of Salisbury 119
Johnson, Samuel 129
Jonson, Ben 89
Jowett, Benjamin 26

Kanner, Leo 3–4, 75, 218, 242, 274
Kant, Immanuel 210, 213
Kelley, Truman 7, 72
Kingsley, Charles 190
Knox, John 131
Kühn, Adalbert 273

Lamarck, Jean-Baptiste 121
Lamont, William 173
Langdon Down, John 210–11, 255, 259
Langland, William 55–6, 237
Lavater, Johann 212
Lely, Peter 84

Lemnius, Levine 222
Leoniceno, Niccolò 52, 54, 56
Licetus, Fortunius 295–6
Lilburne, John 94, 146
Linnaeus, Carl 342
Locke, John 2, 9, 12, 53–4, 59, 87, 89–90, 93–6, 110, 113, 126, 129, 131, 142, 147, 152–3, 159, 164–5, 171, 173, 175–6, 181, 183, 189, 194–5, 198, 200, 208–11, 241, 248, 250, 256–7, 260, 265–6, 270–2, 276, 278, 282, 285, 288–9, 291–4, 299–300, 302, 308–9, 313–46
Lope de Vega, Félix 63, 81
Louis XI of France 121
Louis XIV of France 82–3, 140
Lucretius 277, 291
Lull, Ramón 87, 113
Luther, Martin 73, 151–2, 162, 236, 249, 256, 263, 265–6, 273–4, 278, 318, 320, 325
Lyly, John 147

Malebranche, Nicolas 319
Mans, Inge 3
Mantegna, Andrea 10–11
Marston, John 147
Marx, Karl 42, 69
Mauss, Marcel 66, 68, 151
Mede, Joseph 202
Melanchthon, Philip 287
Ménage, Gilles 325
Mendel, Gregor 215
Mengal, Paul 293
Mercado, Luis 228, 244
Michael Scotus 221, 275
Michelangelo 208
Middleton, Thomas 134, 139, 143, 147
Mill, James 59
Milton, John 54, 175, 200, 276
Molière 120, 135, 140
De Montaigne, Michel 54, 57, 79, 254, 256, 313, 323, 335, 338, 346
Da Monte, Giambattista 56–7, 228, 232–3, 248
Moore, R.I. 56
More, Thomas 86
Moreno de Vargas, Bernabé 122
De Mornay, Philippe 88, 147, 160, 193
Mulcaster, Richard 43, 77–8, 86, 90, 144, 154
Müller, Johannes 42
Murray, Alexander 163

Nagel, Georg [Nagelius] 306–7
Nemesius 226
Neugebauer, Richard 3, 142, 144–5

Newton, Isaac 1, 41, 59, 70, 89, 111, 153, 172, 260, 282
Nicholas of Cusa 41
Nicolas of Jauer 264, 273
Nivelon, Francis 103
Notker, Labeo 263
Nyhan, William 215–16

Degli Oddi, Oddo 55
Overbury, Thomas 99
Overton, Richard 154, 276–8, 338
Owen, John 153, 171, 195, 317, 332

Paine, Thomas 124
Paracelsus 132, 137, 235–40, 279
Pardies, Ignace-Gaston 313
Parker, Samuel 269
Pascal, Blaise 58, 152
Paul, St 79, 155, 236
Peacham, Henry 103, 109, 112–13, 119, 121, 131, 135–6, 141
Pearson, Karl, 6, 44, 211
Pelagius, 156
Pemble, William, 184–5, 188
Penn, William, 94, 316, 332
Pepys, Samuel, 267
Perkins, William, 79, 109, 156, 158, 166–7, 172, 185–6, 201, 272, 288, 293
La Peyrère, Isaac 193, 231
Philip II of Spain 56
Piaget, Jean 39, 182
Pinel, Philippe 178, 344
Pinker, Steven 12
Pinsent, David 255
Pinsent, Ellen 255
Piscator, Johannes 190
Pitt-Rivers, Julian 64, 98, 112
Plato, 2, 16–23, 25–6, 28, 35, 49–51, 57, 59, 71, 128, 181
Platter, Felix 235, 238–41, 243, 245, 249
Platter, Thomas 240
Plautus 244
Pliny 111, 121, 246, 291, 303
Pomponazzi, Pietro 54, 294
Popper, Karl 283
Pordage, Samuel 241, 243, 245, 269–71
Porphyry 284, 286, 304
Priestley, Joseph 70, 174, 177
Privateer, Paul Michael 6
Proust, Marcel 114, 124
Pufendorf, Samuel 153, 208, 328–9

Quételet, Adolphe 42

De la Ramée [Ramus], Pierre 190, 285–6, 295
Ray, John 200, 342
Régis, Pierre-Sylvain 318
Reid, Thomas 177, 344
Reinders, Hans 257
Reynolds, Edward 291, 299–300
Richard II of England 77
Richards, Graham 59
Ibn Ridwan, Ali 225–6
Rivet, André 192
Rose, Lynn 32, 125
Rousseau, Jean-Jacques 47
Rowland, Samuel 135, 145
Rüdin, Ernst 46
Ruvius, Antonius 307
Ryle, Gilbert 255

Scheerenberger, Richard 3, 238
Schenk, Johannes 246–7
Schwarz, Wilhelm 273
Sclano, Salvo 55
De Scohier, Jehan 111
Scot, Reginald 266, 271–2
Séguin, Edouard 199
Selden, John 106
Sennert, Daniel 313
De Sepúlveda, Juan Ginés 25
Shakespeare, William 52, 91–2, 98, 131, 137–9, 143, 210, 221, 231–3, 243
Shapin, Steven 89, 103
Sidney, Philip 80, 87–91, 113, 162, 173, 326
Silver, Lee 160
Simpson, Murray 4
Singer, Peter 256–7
Smith, Adam 344
Smith, Roger 237
Spearman, Charles 44, 211
Spencer, Herbert 44, 242
Spenser, Edmund 65, 80, 90–91, 142, 291
Spinoza, Benedict 160
Sterne, Laurence 243, 323
Stock, Gregory 45
Suárez, Francisco 152, 328
Swift, Jonathan 139
Sydenham, Thomas 241, 250, 319

De Taillepied, Noël 295
Taine, Hyppolite 124
Taylor, Frederick 45
Taylor, Jeremy 317, 320
Testard, Paul 192
Themistius 296

Theophrastus 51, 99, 133
Thomasius, Christian 296
Thucydides 29
Tiepolo, Giambattista 119
Timpler, Clemens 295
Titian 166
Torrigiano, Pietro 51–2, 56, 230
Tozzi, Luca 58
Trent, James 6
Truman, Joseph 198–201, 277, 334
Turner, Richard 132
Twisse, William 195, 197, 199, 201
Tyndale, William 158

Vallés, Francisco 56
Velázquez, Diego 248
Vesalius, Andreas 240, 246–7
De Vitry, Jacques 264
Vives, Juan Luis 54, 57, 152, 198, 228, 260
Voltaire 109

Wanley, Nathaniel 270
Ward, Seth 334
Watts, Isaac 41, 59, 177, 187, 289, 343–5
Weber, Max 83, 174
Webster, John 271–2
Weigel, Valentin 238
Wesley, John 177, 333, 343–5
Whitman, Walt 177
Wilkins, John 129, 170, 267–8, 287, 320
William of Auvergne 263, 266
William of Ockham 158, 307
William of Wykeham 105, 116
Willis, Thomas 235, 241–5, 268–70, 316, 319, 330, 341
Wills, William Henry 15
Wilson, Thomas 286
Wittgenstein, Ludwig 254–5
Wolf, Johann 273
Wolff, Christian 296
Woolnor, Henry 277, 309
Wordsworth, William 41, 93
Wren, Christopher 243
Wundt, Wilhelm 43–4

Young, Michael 72, 127

Zacchia, Paolo 244
Zanchius, Jerome 159, 167
De Zúñiga, Francesillo 237
Zwingli, Huldrych 151–2, 168, 180, 183, 240

Printed in Great Britain
by Amazon